Test	SI Units	Conventional Units	Conversion
Gamma GT			
Male	11–51 IU/L	11–51 IU/L	–
Female	7–33 IU/L	7–33 IU/L	
Glucose, fasting	3.5–5.5 mmol/L	64–100 mg/dL	0.055
Growth hormone, adult	0–10 micrograms/L	0–10 ng/mL	1.0
Homocysteine	2.8–18.5 µmol/L	2.8–18.5 µmol/L	1.0
IGF-1	123–463 micrograms/L (age related)	123–463 ng/mL (age related)	1.0
Insulin, fasting	35–145 pmol/L	5–20 µU/mL	7.175
Iron	7.9–28.6 µmol/L	44–160 micrograms/dL	0.18
Iron-Binding Capacity	44.8–71.6 µmol/L	250–400 micrograms/dL	0.18
Lactic acid (lactate)	0.5–2.2 mmol/L	4.5–19.8 mg/mL	0.11
LDH	118–273 IU/L	118–273 IU/L	–
Luteinizing hormone			
Male	0.5–11.2 IU/L	0.5–11.2mIU/mL	1.0
Female	1–18 IU/L	1–18 mIU/mL	
Postmenopausal F	15–62 IU/L	15–62 mIU/mL	
Magnesium	0.8–1.3 mmol/L	1.8–3.0 mg/dL	0.4114
Osmolality, serum	285–295 mmol/kg	285–295 mOsm/kg	1.0
Parathyroid hormone	10–65 ng/L	10–65 pg/mL	1.0
Potassium	3.5–5.0 mmol/L	3.5–5.0 mEq/L	1.0
Phosphate	0.84–1.45 mmol/L	2.6–4.5 mg/dL	0.3229
Progesterone			
Male	0–1.2 nmol/L	0–0.4 ng/mL	3.180
Female, follicular	<4.8 nmol/L	<1.5 ng/mL	
Female, luteal	18.1–89.4 nmol/L	5.7–28.1 ng/mL	
Postmenopausal F	<0.6 nmol/L	<0.2 ng/mL	
Prolactin	4–30 micrograms/L	4–30 ng/mL	1.0
Prostate-specific antigen	<4 micrograms/L	<4 ng/mL	1.0
Protein, total	60–85 g/L	6.0–8.5 g/dL	10
Renin, normal sodium			
Supine	0.1–0.4 ng/L/sec	0.5–1.6 ng/mL/hr	0.278
Upright	0.5–1.0 ng/L/sec	1.9–3.6 ng/mL/hr	
Sodium	135–145 mmol/L	135–145 mEq/L	1.0
Testosterone, total			
Male	10.4–34.7 nmol/L	350–1000 ng/dL	0.035
Female	0.52–2.08 nmol/L	15–60 ng/dL	
Thyroid-stimulating hormone	0.49–4.67 uIU/mL	0.49–4.67 µU/mL	1.0
Thyroxine, T4			
Free	9.14–23.81 pmol/L	0.71–1.85 ng/dL	12.87
Total	64.3–167 nmol/L	5–13 micrograms/dL	
Triglycerides	< 2.26 mmol/L	< 200 mg/dL	0.0113
Troponin-T, Normal	< 0.2 micrograms/L	< 0.2 ng/mL	–
Troponin I, Normal	< 0.4 micrograms/L	< 0.4 ng/mL	–
Tri-iodotyronine, T3			
Total	1.23–3.39 nmol/L	80–220 ng/dL	0.0154
Free	2.23–5.35 pmol/L	144–347 pg/dL	0.0154
Urea	2.8–6.4 mmol/L	8–18 mg/dL	0.3570
Uric acid			
Male	<420 µmol/L	<7.1 mg/dL	59.48
Female	<340 µmol/L	<5.7 mg/dL	
Vitamin B12	147–590 pmol/L	200–800 pg/mL	0.7378
Vanillylmandelic Acid (VMA), urine	5–44 µmol/24 hr	1–8 mg/24 hr	5.05

OXFORD MEDICAL PUBLICATIONS

Oxford Handbook of
Clinical Diagnosis

Published and forthcoming Oxford Handbooks

Oxford Handbook for the
Foundation Programme 4e
Oxford Handbook of Acute
Medicine 3e
Oxford Handbook of Anaesthesia 3e
Oxford Handbook of Applied Dental
Sciences
Oxford Handbook of Cardiology 2e
Oxford Handbook of Clinical and
Laboratory Investigation 3e
Oxford Handbook of Clinical
Dentistry 6e
Oxford Handbook of Clinical
Diagnosis 3e
Oxford Handbook of Clinical
Examination and Practical Skills 2e
Oxford Handbook of Clinical
Haematology 3e
Oxford Handbook of Clinical
Immunology and Allergy 3e
Oxford Handbook of Clinical
Medicine – Mini Edition 8e
Oxford Handbook of Clinical
Medicine 9e
Oxford Handbook of Clinical
Pathology
Oxford Handbook of Clinical
Pharmacy 2e
Oxford Handbook of Clinical
Rehabilitation 2e
Oxford Handbook of Clinical
Specialties 9e
Oxford Handbook of Clinical
Surgery 4e
Oxford Handbook of
Complementary Medicine
Oxford Handbook of Critical Care 3e
Oxford Handbook of Dental
Patient Care
Oxford Handbook of Dialysis 3e
Oxford Handbook of Emergency
Medicine 4e
Oxford Handbook of Endocrinology
and Diabetes 3e
Oxford Handbook of ENT and Head
and Neck Surgery 2e
Oxford Handbook of Epidemiology
for Clinicians
Oxford Handbook of Expedition and
Wilderness Medicine
Oxford Handbook of Forensic
Medicine
Oxford Handbook of
Gastroenterology & Hepatology 2e
Oxford Handbook of General
Practice 4e

Oxford Handbook of Genetics
Oxford Handbook of Genitourinary
Medicine, HIV and AIDS 2e
Oxford Handbook of Geriatric
Medicine 2e
Oxford Handbook of Infectious
Diseases and Microbiology
Oxford Handbook of Key Clinical
Evidence
Oxford Handbook of Medical
Dermatology
Oxford Handbook of Medical Imaging
Oxford Handbook of Medical
Sciences 2e
Oxford Handbook of Medical
Statistics
Oxford Handbook of Neonatology
Oxford Handbook of Nephrology
and Hypertension 2e
Oxford Handbook of Neurology 2e
Oxford Handbook of Nutrition and
Dietetics 2e
Oxford Handbook of Obstetrics and
Gynaecology 3e
Oxford Handbook of Occupational
Health 2e
Oxford Handbook of Oncology 3e
Oxford Handbook of Ophthalmology 3e
Oxford Handbook of Oral and
Maxillofacial Surgery
Oxford Handbook of Orthopaedics
and Trauma
Oxford Handbook of Paediatrics 2e
Oxford Handbook of Pain
Management
Oxford Handbook of Palliative Care 2e
Oxford Handbook of Practical Drug
Therapy 2e
Oxford Handbook of Pre-Hospital
Care
Oxford Handbook of Psychiatry 3e
Oxford Handbook of Public Health
Practice 3e
Oxford Handbook of Reproductive
Medicine & Family Planning 2e
Oxford Handbook of Respiratory
Medicine 3e
Oxford Handbook of Rheumatology
3e
Oxford Handbook of Sport and
Exercise Medicine 2e
Handbook of Surgical Consent
Oxford Handbook of Tropical
Medicine 4e
Oxford Handbook of Urology 3e

Oxford Handbook of
Clinical
Diagnosis

Third edition

Huw Llewelyn

Formerly Consultant Physician, Kings College Hospital,
London. Honorary Departmental Fellow, Aberystwyth
University, Ceredigion, UK

Hock Aun Ang

Honorary Senior Lecturer in Medicine, Penang Medical
College, Senior Consultant Physician, Seberang Jaya
Hospital, Penang, Malaysia

Keir Lewis

Associate Professor, College of Medicine,
Swansea University. Chest Consultant Hywel Dda
University Health Board, UK

Anees Al-Abdullah

General Practitioner, Meddygfa Minafon,
Kidwelly, Carmarthenshire, UK

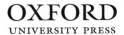

OXFORD
UNIVERSITY PRESS

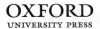

OXFORD
UNIVERSITY PRESS

Great Clarendon Street, Oxford, OX2 6DP,
United Kingdom

Oxford University Press is a department of the University of Oxford.
It furthers the University's objective of excellence in research, scholarship,
and education by publishing worldwide. Oxford is a registered trade mark of
Oxford University Press in the UK and in certain other countries

© Huw Llewelyn 2014

The moral rights of the authors have been asserted

First edition published 2006
Second edition published 2009

Impression: 1

Published in the United States of America by Oxford University Press
198 Madison Avenue, New York, NY 10016, United States of America

British Library Cataloguing in Publication Data
Data available

Library of Congress Control Number: 2014937826

ISBN 978-0-19-967986-7

Printed and bound in China by
C&C Offset Printing Co., Ltd.

Foreword to third edition

Last year, I celebrated my 30th year as a doctor and my son began his training as a (graduate entry) medical student. I have come to enjoy the intergenerational 'grand rounds' in which one of us describes a case in the time-honoured format—starting with a structured history, going on to the clinical examination and adding diagnostic tests that progress from the simple and non-invasive to all the wonders and dreads of modern technology—while the other tries to guess the diagnosis from as few clues as possible. Given that most medical knowledge now lies in the category 'forgotten by the mother and not yet encountered by the son', this book is likely to become well thumbed by both of us as we play our diagnostic game.

Much of this book reflects the fact that Huw Llewelyn is a mathematician and logician as well as a highly experienced physician. In many cases, diagnosis can and should be a process of deduction that begins with a 'diagnostic lead' (a single symptom or sign, such as 'right iliac fossa pain', that gets you started), the cause of which can be progressively narrowed and refined by incorporating factors such as age and gender; the timing and speed of onset; the pattern of associated symptoms, signs and pre-existing conditions; and the results of investigations. Frontal headache in a teenager who was well until yesterday is likely to have a different cause from frontal headache that has been present for many months in a 65-year-old with hypertension and depression. Evidence can often be collected in the history and clinical examination that is 'suggestive' or 'confirmatory' (use these terms with care—they are defined in the book) of particular diagnostic possibilities. More rarely, certain tests or combinations of tests can effectively 'rule in' or 'rule out' certain diagnostic options.

You probably knew all that already, so what will you learn from this book that goes beyond standard teaching on clinical diagnosis? For me, the added value was in the sophistication with which the principles of probability and decision science have been applied to the many and varied challenges of clinical practice. The book's (mainly implicit) message is that if you take a logical and step-wise approach, using your experience, history-taking skills, and clinical acumen to select the best diagnostic leads and add granularity to your decision tree, you will often render costly and unpleasant diagnostic tests redundant. Less commonly, you will justify the expense and inconvenience of such tests in selected patients.

The skilled diagnostician is not the one who rattles off a long list of differential diagnoses for every symptom, applies algorithms mechanically, ticks all the boxes on a blood request form or scans the head of every patient with blurred vision. Rather, the skilled diagnostician is the one who combines thoughtful history-taking, focused clinical examination, and judicious investigation so that each successive step contributes to an emerging picture of the problem and informs the selection of the next step. As the authors say (p.20), 'It is important to understand that clinical diagnosis is not a static classification system based on diagnostic criteria or their probable presence. It is a dynamic process.'

The bulk of the book is a treasure-trove of diagnostic puzzles from red throat to wasting of the small muscles of the hands, from which I predict hours of fun for students and seasoned clinicians alike. There are also sections on biochemical conundrums such as hyponatraemia, and radiological old chestnuts such as a round opacity on the chest X-ray. Reassuringly, theoretical sections such as 'Grappling with Probabilities' and 'Bayes' and other rules' are relegated to a final chapter that can be safely omitted by those whose interests are more clinical than mathematical.

Despite its emphasis on deductive logic, this book is by no means an uncritical offering to the gods of decision science. Llewelyn and his coauthors are careful to point out (as Dave Sackett and colleagues did back in the 1970s) that many diagnoses are made intuitively—for example via the pattern recognition that allows us to look at a patient and instantly think 'Down's syndrome' or 'chicken-pox'. They also remind us that mild symptoms are often both non-specific and self-limiting (hence may need no more active management than advising the patient to return if not improving), and they warn us of the dangers of over-diagnosis and that increasingly common problem in modern diagnostics, the 'incidentaloma'.

Like the birth of a third child, the publication of a third edition of a book is cause for much celebration: it tends to both reflect and build on significant success with earlier versions. Perhaps it is too early to encourage the authors of the *Oxford Handbook of Clinical Diagnosis* (3rd edition) to contemplate a companion volume to this magnum opus. But if they were open to such a suggestion, I would encourage them to team up with experts in public understanding of science and produce a version of the book aimed at patients and carers. After all, if your patients were reading the wisdom distilled in these pages, that would surely make for some interesting and productive conversations.

Trisha Greenhalgh OBE
Professor of Primary Health Care and Dean for Research Impact
Barts and the London School of Medicine and Dentistry
Queen Mary University of London
2014

Preface

This book helps doctors and students to arrive at a diagnosis, and to explain and to justify their reasoning, especially when seeing patients with new problems that lie outside their personal range of experience. This will happen very frequently to students, frequently to house officers, but will still happen regularly to very experienced senior hospital doctors and general practitioners.

The book adopts the approach used by experienced diagnosticians, by focusing on the finding with the shortest differential diagnosis (i.e. the best diagnostic lead). It describes the differential diagnoses of such findings that may be encountered by a reader in the history, examination and usual preliminary tests and how the diagnoses can be confirmed. It describes what tactics to adopt in order to find better leads, while not losing sight of the patient's original concern. The probability and set theory of this process is explained in Chapter 13.

The entries on each page of the book resemble a traditional past medical history with multiple diagnoses. The reader scans down the page to see which of the diagnoses with its findings match the patient's findings so far. The compatible findings can then be used as evidence for the diagnosis and treatment, to be shared with the patient and other members of the multidisciplinary team, such as nurses, pharmacists, physiotherapists, and other professionals allied to medicine. It can be used to create high-quality discharge or handover summaries.

Patients or their carers may wish to share in the diagnostic and decision-making process. In order to do this, they need to know what problems have been identified and the tests and treatments being proposed. They will need to know which of these diagnoses explain each problem and treatment. They may also need to know which findings are being used to confirm each diagnosis, and to choose its treatments and to mark the outcome. The book describes how this information can be provided in writing. The patient or carer will then be in a position to explain all this to another doctor, if necessary.

In this third edition, there are sections on each page that show how the diagnosis may be finalized by the outcome of management. This replaces the section in the second edition that described the 'initial management' of the condition. The purpose of this is to show how the response of treatment, etc., affects the diagnostic process. Chest X-ray images have been added to illustrate the findings in Chapter 12. The appendix of the second edition has been replaced by Chapter 13 in this third edition and explains the basis of evidence-based differential diagnosis and diagnostic confirmation.

Huw Llewelyn
2014

Dedication

For Angela.

Contents

Acknowledgements x
Advisors xi
Symbols and abbreviations xii

1 The diagnostic process 1
2 Interpreting the history and examination 25
3 General and endocrine symptoms and physical signs 61
4 Skin symptoms and physical signs 123
5 Cardiovascular symptoms and physical signs 173
6 Respiratory symptoms and physical signs 235
7 Gastrointestinal symptoms and physical signs 287
8 Urological and gynaecological symptoms and physical signs 399
9 Joint, limb, and back symptoms and physical signs 423
10 Psychiatric and neurological symptoms and physical signs 453
11 Laboratory test results 543
12 Chest X-rays 573
13 Making the diagnostic process evidence-based 615

Index 643

Acknowledgements

This book is based on ideas and teaching methods developed by Dr Huw Llewelyn at King's College Hospital London with the support of Professor Alan McGregor, the late Professor Sir James Black FRS and the late Professor John Anderson, for which he is very grateful. We thank staff and students at Singleton Hospital Swansea, Prince Philip Hospital Llanelli, West Wales General Hospital Carmarthen, Luton and Dunstable Hospital, Eastbourne District General Hospital, Newham University Hospital, the Whittington Hospital, Pinderfilelds Hospital Wakefield, the Great Western Hospital Swindon, Kettering General Hospital, Queen's Hospital Burton on Trent, Nevill Hall Hospital Abergavenny, Dorchester District Hospital, Manor Hospital Walsall, Good Hope Hospital Sutton Coldfield, and Solihull Hospital for their help. We also thank Dr Arthur Miller, formerly Head of the Department of Chemical Pathology at the University College and Middlesex Hospitals London for his helpful advice.

We are grateful to the staff at Oxford University Press for their support and patience, particularly Mr Michael Hawkes.

Advisors

Dr Rhys Llewelyn
Registrar in Radiology
Royal Cornwall Hospital
Truro

Dr Ilana Raburn
House Officer in Medicine
Queen Alexandra Hospital
Portsmouth

Symbols and abbreviations

OHCD	*Oxford Handbook of Clinical Diagnosis*
➔	cross reference
↑	increased
↓	decreased
→	leading to
+ve	positive
−ve	negative
±	with or without
>	greater than
<	less than
≥	equal to or greater than
≤	equal to or less than
α	alpha
β	beta
®	registered
1°	primary
2°	secondary
ABG	arterial blood gas
AC	acromioclavicular
ACE	angiotensin-converting enzyme
ACL	anterior cruciate ligament
ACTH	adrenocorticotropin
ADH	antidiuretic hormone
AER	albumin excretion rate
AF	atrial fibrillation
AFB	acid-fast bacilli
ALT	alanine transaminase
ANA	anti-nuclear antibody
ANCA	anti-neutrophil cytoplasmic antibody
A–P	antero-posterior
APTT	activated partial thromboplastin time
ARB	angiotensin receptor blocker
ARDS	acute respiratory distress syndrome
5-ASA	5-aminosalicylic acid
ASOT	anti-streptolysin O titre
AST	aspartate transaminase

ATLS	advanced trauma life support
AXR	abdominal X-ray
bd	twice daily
BMI	body mass index
BP	blood pressure
Ca^{2+}	calcium
CCU	coronary care unit
CIN	cervical intraepithelial neoplasia
CNS	central nervous system
CO_2	carbon dioxide
COPD	chronic obstructive pulmonary disease
CPK	creatinine phosphokinase
CRP	C-reactive protein
CSF	cerebrospinal fluid
CT	computed tomography
CVP	central venous pressure
CXR	chest X-ray
d	day
DC	direct current
dL	decilitre
DIC	disseminated intravascular coagulation
DNA	deoxyribonucleic acid
DOB	date of birth
DU	duodenal ulcer
DVT	deep vein thrombosis
ECG	electrocardiogram
ECT	electroconvulsive therapy
EEG	electroencephalogram
EMG	electromyography
ELISA	enzyme-linked immunosorbent assay
ERCP	endoscopic retrograde cholangiopancreatography
ESR	erythrocyte sedimentation rate
FBC	full blood count
FEV_1	forced expiratory volume in 1 second
FFP	fresh frozen plasma
FH	family history
FSH	follicular stimulating hormone
FT3	free T3
FT4	free T4
FVC	forced vital capacity

GALS	gait, arms, legs, spine
GCS	Glasgow Coma Score
γGT	gamma glutamyl transpeptidase
GI	gastrointestinal
G6PD	glucose-6-pyruvate dehydrogenase
GnRH	gonadotropin-releasing hormone
GTN	glyceryl trinitrate
GTT	glucose tolerance test
GU	gastric ulcer
h	hour
Hb	haemoglobin
HBsAg	hepatitis B surface antigen
hCG	human chorionic gonadotropin
HCV	hepatitis C virus
HDU	high dependency unit
5-HIAA	5-hydroxyindole acetic acid
HIV	human immunodeficiency virus
HMMA	4 hydroxy-3-methoxymadelic acid
HPC	history of presenting complaint
HOCM	hypertrophic cardiomyopathy
HRT	hormone replacement therapy
IC	intercostals
IgM	immunoglobulin M
IHD	ischaemic heart disease
IM	intramuscular
IP	interphalangeal
ITU	intensive treatment unit
IUCD	intrauterine contraceptive device
IV	intravenous
IVC	inferior vena cava
IVU	intravenous urography
JVP	jugular venous pressure
K⁺	potassium
kg	kilogram
L	litre
LFT	liver function test
LH	luteinizing hormone
LIF	left iliac fossa
LMW	low molecular weight
LP	lumbar puncture

LRLQ	localized right lower quadrant
LVF	left ventricular failure
MCP	metacarpophalangeal
mg	milligram
MI	myocardial infarction
min	minute
mL	millilitre
mmHg	millimetre of mercury
mmol	milllimole
MMSE	mini-mental state examination
mo	month
MR	magnetic resonance
MRCP	magnetic resonance cholangiopancreatography
MRI	magnetic resonance imaging
MS	multiple sclerosis
MSU	midstream urine
MTP	metatarsophalangeal
Na^+	sodium
NB	*nota bene*
NG	nasogastric
NIV	non-invasive ventilation
NNT	number needed to treat
NSAID	non-steroidal anti-inflammatory drug
NSAP	non-specific abdominal pain
NSTEMI	non-ST elevated myocardial infarction
O_2	oxygen
OBAS	observation, bracing, and surgery
od	*omni die* (once daily)
OGD	oesophagogastroduodenoscopy
P2	pulmonary component of 2nd heart sound
P–A	postero-anterior
PC	presenting complaint
PCL	posterior cruciate ligament
PCR	polymerase chain reaction
PE	pulmonary embolism
PEG	percutaneous endoscopic gastrostomy
PET	positron emission tomography
PEFR	peak expiratory flow rates
PMH	past medical history
PND	paroxysmal nocturnal dyspnoea

PO	*per os* (by mouth)
PPI	proton pump inhibitor
PR	*per rectum* (by rectum)
prn	as required
PSA	prostatic-specific antigen
PT	prothrombin time
PUVA	psoralen UVA
qds	*quater die sumendus* (four times daily)
RA	rheumatoid arthritis
RBC	red blood cell
RF	rheumatoid factor
RICE	rest, ice, compression, and elevation
RLQ	right lower quadrant
RNA	ribonucleic acid
RUQ	right upper quadrant
S2	2nd heart sound
SALT	speech and language therapy
SH	social history
SHBG	sex hormone-binding globulin
SLE	systemic lupus erythematosus
SSRI	selective serotonin reuptake inhibitor
SVC	superior vena cava
SVT	supraventricular tachycardia
T4	thyroxine
TB	tuberculosis
tds	*ter die sumendus* (three times daily)
TSH	thyroid stimulating hormone
TFT	thyroid function test
TURP	transurethral resection of prostate
U&E	urea and electrolytes
UTI	urinary tract infection
URTI	upper respiratory tract infection
US	ultrasound
UV	ultraviolet
V/Q	ventilation/perfusion
VMA	vanillylmandelic acid
WBC	white blood cell
WCC	white cell count
wk	week
y	year

Chapter 1

The diagnostic process

The purpose of this book 2
When and how to use this book 3
'Intuitive' reasoning 4
'Transparent' reasoning 5
Diagnostic leads and differentiators 6
Changing diagnostic leads 7
Confirming and finalizing a diagnosis 8
Evidence that 'suggests' a diagnosis 9
Confirmatory findings based on general evidence 10
Findings that suggest diagnoses based on general evidence 11
Explaining a diagnostic thought process 12
An evidence-based diagnosis and plan 13
Medical and surgical sieves 14
Diagnoses, hypotheses, and theories 15
Imagining an ideal clinical trial 16
Diagnostic classification, pathways, and tables 18
Dynamic diagnoses 20
Explaining diagnoses to patients 21
Informed consent 21
Minimizing diagnostic errors 22

The purpose of this book

This book explains how to interpret symptoms, physical signs and test results during the diagnostic process. There are many books that provide lists of differential diagnoses. However, this one also explains how you should use these lists. Each section describes:

- The main differential diagnoses of a single diagnostic 'lead'
- How to 'differentiate' between these differential diagnoses
- How to confirm the diagnosis and also to 'finalize' it using the outcome of treatment (see ➔ 'Transparent' reasoning, p.5, ➔ Changing diagnostic leads, p.7 and ➔ Confirming and finalizing a diagnosis, p.8).

Making diagnostic reasoning and decisions transparent

The book explains how to outline your diagnostic reasoning on paper. It does this by showing you how to write a list of differential diagnoses and established diagnoses, each with its supportive evidence so far, which includes the result of management (see ➔ An evidence-based diagnosis and plan, p.13). This can be used in a draft management plan and later in a hospital hand-over or in a discharge summary. The differential diagnoses in the sections of this book, with their evidence and initial management, are described in the same format and can be used as example entries when writing out an outline of the diagnoses and evidence, which includes the result of the management for a patient.

Understanding the reasoning of others

This book helps you to understand the diagnostic reasoning and decisions of others. In order to do so, you (and patients, carers, nurses, and other health professionals) have to ask:

- What is the current management plan (the pieces of advice, treatments, tests, and follow-up arrangements)?
- For each of these items, what are the diagnoses (provisional, probable, definitive, and final)?
- What is the evidence for each diagnosis (how it presented, how it was confirmed, and its markers of progress or outcome)?

Look up the 'problem findings' and diagnoses in this book so that you know what type of answers to expect to these questions. You can write them out in a similar format (see ➔ An evidence-based diagnosis and plan, p.13). After hearing these answers, you may wish to make your own notes in response.

Checking a clinical impression and explicit reasoning

It is important to check all diagnoses and decisions. Reasoning alone using knowledge from a book of this kind is not enough. Such reasoning should be checked by discussing it with someone who is familiar with the situation from past experience and who can recognize if the reasoning makes sense. However, it is equally important to check that diagnoses and decisions made 'intuitively' make sense when compared with transparent reasoning of the type described in this book.

When and how to use this book

This book can be used:
- When assessing a patient, e.g. after the history of presenting complaint, after completing the full history, after completing the examination, and when the test results come back
- In the same way during problem-based learning with case histories
- During private study and revision to allow you to solve clinical problems later without having to refer to the book
- When asking someone else to explain a diagnosis and decision to you.

If the presenting complaint is severe (e.g. pain or breathlessness), disabling (e.g. inability to move a limb or speak), or unusual (e.g. coughing or vomiting blood), then it will tend to be good lead with a shorter differential diagnosis. The most useful diagnostic leads are described in this book—look at the 'Contents' list of each section so that you can recognize them.

Remember that many symptoms and other findings are due to self-limiting conditions that are transient or are corrected within hours or days by the body's own restorative mechanisms. Such self-limiting conditions always have to be considered as part of any differential diagnosis. If the finding is mild and has only been present for a short time and is not accompanied by other features, then it is more probable that it will resolve spontaneously without its cause being identified. However, it is important to review such patients to ensure that there is improvement or resolution, by asking the patient to return if the problem persists. The ability to deal with such self-limiting conditions is a very important skill that has to be learnt by experience. Severe and persistent findings will often turn out to have a cause that requires medical attention.

If the presenting complaint is not a good lead but has a long differential diagnosis, then consider what systems (e.g. cardiovascular or respiratory) it came from and ask 'direct questions' directed at this system to try to find better leads. Also, focus on that system first in your examination. Note the speed of onset; this will suggest the underlying disease process. Onset within seconds suggests an 'electrical' cause, e.g. a fit or rhythm abnormality; onset over seconds to minutes suggests an embolus, a trauma, or rupture; onset over minutes to hours suggests a thrombotic process, over hours to days an acute infection, over days to weeks a chronic infection, weeks to months a tumour, and months to years a degenerative process.

Read this book during private study or revision by covering the column of diagnoses on the left side of the table and testing your ability to recognize the diagnoses when you read the nature of the diagnostic lead associated with the table, and the suggestive and confirmatory findings on the right side of the table. If you are able to do this successfully, you will soon learn to take a history and examine a patient without having to use this book. Do it first with the symptoms and physical signs that are common in your current (and next) clinical attachment so that you are prepared.

'Intuitive' reasoning

Most of the time, experienced doctors use a non-transparent reasoning process. This seems to involve recognizing combinations or patterns of findings consciously or subconsciously, which suggest or confirm a diagnosis, or indicate that some treatment should be given. This is a skill that is improved by repetition. This book will encourage you to do this sooner. However, all doctors specialize and the information in this book will be of help to experienced doctors with patients outside their specialty.

If you were told that a patient had suffered sudden onset of sharp chest pain over seconds to minutes, then this 'diagnostic lead' will make you think consciously or subconsciously of a pneumothorax, pulmonary infarction, etc. If another patient has suddenly started coughing up blood, then this lead would suggest acute bronchitis, pulmonary infarction, bronchial carcinoma, pulmonary tuberculosis, etc. However, if both happened in the same patient, your mental links would 'intersect' on pulmonary infarction and it would surface to consciousness.

If you were to come across this combination of features and had read in this book during private study that they 'suggested' pulmonary infarction, then you might think of this diagnosis directly. If you came across these findings many times and a diagnosis of pulmonary infarction was usually confirmed on CT-pulmonary angiogram, then you would soon recognize that the combination of findings as suggesting pulmonary infarction (like recognizing someone's face). The psychological process that leads to such recognition is sometimes described as 'Gestalt' (German for an overall impression). Instead of writing 'diagnosis' many doctors will write 'Impression:' to indicate this.

If the findings so far do not point to a single diagnosis with certainty, then you will have to consider a number of other possibilities. It may then be reasonably certain that the diagnosis will turn out to be one of these. A device for doing this is not to specify a list of diagnostic possibilities, but to write down a term that represents a group of diagnoses, e.g. 'pulmonary lesion' or 'autoimmune process'.

If a diagnosis or small number of differential diagnoses do not come to mind readily in one of these ways, then it is important to turn to the 'transparent' reasoning process. You will always come across unfamiliar situations, however experienced you become, so the 'transparent' approach will always be important.

'Transparent' reasoning

Diagnostic reasoning is transparent if the findings used to arrive at a diagnosis are specified clearly and if the interventions resulting from that diagnosis are also specified. The combination of findings used might have been recognized by the diagnostician at the outset. However, in many cases, the combination of findings would have been assembled by a reasoning process of elimination (see ➲ Diagnostic leads and differentiators, p.6).

A diagnosis will only be certain or 'definite' if the findings so far are 'sufficient' or 'definitive' by an agreed convention. For example, two fasting blood sugars of at least 7mmol/L on different days by convention provide a 'sufficient' criterion for confirming diabetes mellitus. There are other 'sufficient' criteria, e.g. two random sugars over 11mmol/L. All the different sufficient criteria collectively make up the 'definitive' criteria. This means that it is 'necessary' to have at least one of these various criteria. At least one fasting glucose of at least 7mmol/L is also 'necessary' (but not 'sufficient') to confirm the diagnosis, so if the first of a pair of fasting blood sugars is below 7mmol/L, the diagnosis is logically 'eliminated' because they both can no longer be over 7mmol/L.

If the first of two fasting sugars is 7.1mmol/L, then this makes diabetes mellitus more probable than not. The differential diagnosis will also include 'impaired fasting glucose' (if the next result is less than 7mmol/L). Medical conditions change and even though a diagnosis is 'eliminated', any borderline tests may be repeated quite soon. In reality, few diagnoses are defined precisely in this way and a doctor may 'confirm' a diagnosis if the probability of benefit from its advice or treatment is judged to be high and cite in a transparent way the findings on which this confirmation is based.

'Over-diagnosis' is said to occur if patients are labelled with a diagnosis when a high proportion show little prospect of benefiting from any advice or treatment directed at that diagnosis. For example, 'diabetic albuminuria' is said to be present if the urinary albumin excretion rate (AER) is between 20 and 200 micrograms/min on at least two out of three collections, provided that other findings indicate that there is no other cause of albuminuria present. However, there is no difference in those developing diabetic nephropathy within 2 years between those taking placebo or active treatment for the 1/3 of patients with an AER between 20 and 40 micrograms/min, suggesting that there is 'over-diagnosis' as this group of patients do not benefit. Diagnostic criteria need to be based closely on treatment outcomes to avoid this.

A diagnosis becomes final when all the findings that led to the diagnosis being considered can be 'explained' by that diagnosis. For example, if a patient complained of persistent fatigue and this did not respond to the treatments and advice for diabetes, then an additional diagnosis has to be considered. The diagnosis of diabetes mellitus may have been confirmed definitively, but the diagnostic process will not be finalized until other reasons for the fatigue have been confirmed or excluded. It is only then that the process stops. The 'final diagnosis' is then a 'theory' and no longer a hypothesis to be tested further, at least for the time being.

Diagnostic leads and differentiators

A combination of features that identifies a group of patients within which the frequency of those with a diagnosis is high (or even 100%) might well be recognized at the outset. If not, a combination of findings can be assembled 'logically' by using reasoning by elimination. This would be done by first considering the possible causes of a single finding, called a 'diagnostic lead' (e.g. localized right lower quadrant abdominal pain). The possible diagnostic explanations for this 'lead' are then considered, one is chosen (e.g. appendicitis) and findings looked for that occur commonly in that chosen possibility and less commonly (ideally rarely or never) in at least one other possibility.

If a finding (e.g. being male) occurs often in a diagnosis being pursued (e.g. appendicitis) but cannot happen in a differential diagnosis (e.g. ectopic pregnancy), then that diagnosis can be ruled out, being female being a 'necessary' condition for suffering an ectopic pregnancy! However, if a finding such as guarding occurs commonly in the diagnosis being chased (e.g. appendicitis) and less frequently in another diagnosis (e.g. non-specific abdominal pain—NSAP) then NSAP will become less probable, not ruled out.

The 'lead' and the new finding will form a combination within which the frequency of the diagnosis being chased (e.g. appendicitis) becomes more frequent and the diagnosis in which the finding occurs less often becomes less frequent in that combination of findings.

The frequency with which a finding occurs in a diagnosis is often described as its 'sensitivity' by epidemiologists, i.e. the frequency with which the finding 'detects' the diagnosis when screening a population. Statisticians also call the 'sensitivity' the 'likelihood' of the finding being discovered when the patient is known to have the diagnosis. If the finding is 'likely' to occur in a diagnosis being chased and is 'unlikely' to occur in one of its differential diagnoses, then the ratio of the two likelihoods represents the finding's ability to differentiate between those two diagnoses. This makes one more probable and the other less probable. This book describes such findings under the headings of 'Suggested by' and 'Confirmed by'. It is findings that cannot occur by definition in other diagnoses that 'confirm' a diagnosis—'definitely'.

Eddy and Clanton analysed the thought processes of senior doctors participating in the Clinico-Pathological Conferences at the Massachusetts General Hospital[1]. They pointed out that choosing a diagnostic lead, e.g. localized right lower quadrant abdominal pain (which they called a 'pivot') was central to these experienced doctors' explanations when solving diagnostic problems. They also noted that during diagnostic reasoning, other findings (e.g. guarding) were used to 'prune' some of the differential diagnoses (e.g. pruning away NSAP).

There has been a re-awakening of interest in all this as 'stratified' or 'personalized' medical research. The aim is to have more differential diagnostic sub-divisions so that each predicts treatment response more accurately.

Changing diagnostic leads

A patient presenting with breathlessness will have a long list of differential diagnoses. A diagnostician might suspect a 'cardiac' or 'respiratory' reason and after asking for cardiovascular and respiratory symptoms and looking for physical signs, might ask for a chest X-ray (CXR) in the hope of getting a better diagnostic lead. A circular shadow on a CXR will have a much shorter list of differential diagnoses and a CT scan showing a lesion contiguous with a bronchus an even shorter one. A biopsy might provide a diagnostic criterion for a bronchial carcinoma. However, this may only be a working diagnosis even if it is confirmed or definite. All the diagnoses applicable to that patient will not become final until the patient's symptoms have been cured, stabilized, or predicted correctly and no follow-up or other action needs to be taken.

If we come across a powerful finding or combination of findings (e.g. a dense, round shadow on a CXR), this will form a stronger lead with a shorter list of differential diagnoses. It is easier to make a fresh start with such a powerful new finding than to try to work out which of a long list of original diagnostic possibilities (e.g. breathlessness) are being made more probable or less probable by the new finding. Therefore, another measure of a powerful finding is the number of differential diagnoses required to explain, say 99% of patients with that finding. The better the lead, the fewer the differential diagnoses.

Care has to be taken to consider spurious and self-limiting causes for any lead (e.g. a CXR appearance), especially if the differential diagnoses of that lead finding cannot explain any of the patient's symptoms. The same consideration applies when a screening test is performed, e.g. a mammogram. If the patient is asymptomatic, then it is important to consider the possibility that a new finding might be due to a self-limiting condition that might resolve spontaneously without medical assistance. One option would be to repeat the test after a short interval to see if there has been regression. Asymptomatic conditions that are detected incidentally are often labelled wryly as 'incidentalomas'. In many cases they are investigated aggressively and the patient sometimes subjected to potential harm (e.g. radical surgery) with adverse consequences only to find out that the lesion was innocent after all. This is sometimes described as 'over-diagnosis' and 'over-treatment'.

Confirming and finalizing a diagnosis

A diagnosis can be confirmed in different ways. The different confirming (or 'sufficient') criteria taken together form the 'definitive criteria' of the diagnosis. The definitive criteria thus identify all those and only those with the diagnosis. Such criteria can be based on symptoms, signs, and test results (and, in some cases, on the initial result of treatment). However, few patients with a diagnosis will require all the advice or treatments suggested by that diagnosis (e.g. not all patients with diabetes mellitus will need insulin). Further findings may have to be looked for called 'treatment indications', which often form sub-diagnoses. For example, the presence of a very high blood sugar, weight loss, and persistent ketones in the urine would be one such 'indication' for giving insulin; that patient might also be diagnosed as having 'Type 1 Diabetes Mellitus or Type 2 Diabetes Mellitus with severe insulin deficiency'.

In many cases, a diagnostician will start treatment when a diagnosis is probable or suspected without waiting for formal criteria to be fulfilled (e.g. a treatment given on suspicion of meningitis). In such a situation, the diagnostician might imagine the existence of a large number of identical patients who were randomized into different treatment limbs of a randomized clinical trial. The treatment chosen would be the one 'imagined' (i.e. 'predicted', ideally with a known track record of success) to produce the best outcome, bearing in mind the benefits and adverse effects. If the patient improves on treatment, then this may also be regarded as confirmation of the diagnosis, if patients with no other diagnosis could have improved in that way. However, if the patient and diagnostician were satisfied that nothing else needed to be done, then the diagnosis would become 'final'. This could happen even if the diagnosis was only probable, e.g. if a severe headache had been suspected of being meningitis, had resolved on antibiotics but no bacteria had grown in the laboratory, then the final diagnosis would be 'probable bacterial meningitis'.

There may be no formal criteria that are suitable for use in day-to-day clinical care. One approach is to provide a trial of therapy, and if the patient improves, to regard this as a confirmatory result and no other explanation is looked for. The confirmatory findings in this book are based on all of the approaches outlined here. They reflect typical approaches used in the authors' experience. However, none of these approaches are ideal; future medical research may improve matters.

Some patients with a diagnosis have mild conditions so that treatment is not necessary; others may be so severe that it is too late to treat, while others are treatable—this subdivision is known as 'triage' in emergency settings. The group with a diagnosis may also contain subgroups with causes and complications that also require treatment. Therefore, diagnoses (probable or confirmed) may be thought as 'envelopes' that enclose subgroups of patients with other diagnoses for which different actions are indicated. The way in which evidence can be sought to form diagnostic indications and sub-diagnoses is described in Chapter 13.

Evidence that 'suggests' a diagnosis

It is important to remember what 'evidence' means. Evidence is made up of facts, which are records of observations and actions that took place at a place and time. A 'fact' becomes 'evidence' when it is used to make a prediction—in the context of this book, about the presence of a diagnosis (which leads to other predictions that include what could be done to improve matters). A diagnosis is the title to what we picture or predict is happening now, has happened in the past, and what will happen to a patient in the future. This will include causes and complications of the diagnosis. Some of this may be pictured with certainty (i.e. what has been observed already) or with different degrees of probability, depending on the available evidence.

Evidence may be based on facts such as symptoms, signs, and test results recorded in a particular patient. This is 'particular' evidence from a particular patient, which is a 'particular' proposition in logic. In contrast to this, 'general' evidence will be based on facts related to groups of patients such as the result of a clinical trial, which is a 'general' proposition in logic. In order to practice evidence-based medicine, we have to relate the 'particular' evidence from a particular patient to 'general' evidence about groups of similar patients that we have observed and documented carefully or published by others in the medical literature.

The predictions based on 'particular' evidence are diagnoses with different degrees of probability about what is wrong with a patient and what to do. If the listener is going to accept such an opinion on the basis of the evidence, there has to be agreement as to what is acceptable as evidence, which includes how the evidence was obtained. This book contains typical evidence that is used to 'suggest' probable diagnoses and to 'confirm' diagnoses according to definitive criteria that are accepted at present by most doctors in their day-to-day work. These conventions will no doubt change as more 'general' scientific evidence is published.

Each differential diagnosis in every section is followed by the evidence that 'suggests' the probable presence of the diagnosis. The diagnosis is considered to be 'definite' when the confirmatory 'sufficient' criteria are present. In each section, the confirmatory evidence for each diagnosis is provided under another subheading.

For example, localized right lower quadrant abdominal pain with guarding 'suggests' that the diagnosis will probably be appendicitis (see ➲ Localized tenderness in left or right lower quadrant p.363). The diagnosis of appendicitis is 'confirmed' by the appearances at laparotomy and by the resulting definitive histological examination. It is important to note that not all the available findings from the patient have to be used in the reasoning process to confirm a diagnosis. The findings selected may be called the 'central' evidence'. For example, a patient with a large number of findings that includes localized right lower quadrant (LRLQ) pain and guarding can be regarded as a member of a set of such patients with LRLQ and guarding within which the frequency of appendicitis is high (see ➲ Picturing probabilities, p.618).

Confirmatory findings based on general evidence

A confirmatory finding identifies a group or set of patients that 'envelopes' all those with indications for treatment 'explained' by the diagnosis. If new treatment indications are discovered that are explained by the diagnostic theory, then 'the envelope' may need to be expanded. For example, it was discovered some years ago that many patients with features of diabetic retinopathy requiring treatment had blood sugars outside the criteria for diabetes mellitus. Because of this, the World Health Organization and the American Diabetes Association suggested that the 'envelope' for diabetes should be expanded by lowering the diagnostic cut-off point of fasting blood glucose.

It is also possible that new tests may be discovered in the future that select patients more efficiently for treatment. If these new treatable patients lie outside the diagnostic group that was previously considered for treatment, then it might be appropriate to use the new test to identify patients who should be deemed to have the diagnosis. So if 'confirmatory' tests are to be chosen in an evidence-based way, then they should be shown to be superior to rival tests by including more patients who respond to the advice or treatments directed at the diagnosis and excluding more patients with no prospect of responding.

Many diagnoses are based on test results that are 'abnormal', i.e. above or below two standard deviations of the test result in the general population. This means that the 2.5% of patients above and 2.5% of those below these two standard deviations could be regarded as 'abnormal'. The use of two standard deviations is arbitrary and not 'evidence-based'. For example, patients with diabetes mellitus are 'diagnosed' as having 'diabetic microalbuminuria' if their AER are above two standard deviations of the mean (i.e. >20 micrograms/min).

However, in a clinical trial on patients with type 2 diabetes mellitus where their blood pressures had been controlled, there was no difference between those on treatment and placebo in the proportion of patients developing nephropathy within two years if they had an AER between 20 and 40 micrograms/min.[2] This suggests that the cut-off point should be 40 micrograms/min. However, before changing the definition, it would be important to ensure that the patients inside the envelope with an AER between 20 and 40 micrograms/min might not benefit in other ways, e.g. by some being prevented from developing peripheral or coronary artery disease.

Ruling diagnoses in and out

A diagnosis is 'ruled in' if at least one of its confirming (or sufficient) criteria is present. A diagnosis is 'ruled out' if it can be shown that the patient lies outside the diagnostic envelope by showing that one of its 'necessary' criteria is absent. Another way of doing this is to show that not one of the possible confirming (or sufficient) features is present. Another way is to show that a single necessary feature is absent, which must occur in those with the diagnosis, e.g. that the patient is not female and, therefore, cannot have an ectopic pregnancy. Such a constant diagnostic finding is called a 'necessary' criterion, of course.

Findings that suggest diagnoses based on general evidence

The best findings for 'suggesting' probable diagnoses are those which, when used alone or in combination with others, predict the presence of 'confirmatory' test results with the highest frequency of success. The general evidence for the ability of findings to do this during population screening is usually offered in the form of indices such as sensitivity, specificity, and likelihood ratios (the use of such indices can be misleading, however; see ➲ Things that affect 'differential' and 'overall' likelihood ratios, p.627). However, in order to assess the usefulness of tests during the differential diagnostic process, other indices have to be used. One index is the number of diagnoses required to explain most (e.g. 99%) of the differential diagnoses of a diagnostic lead—the fewer the better.

Another index is the ability of a test to differentiate between pairs of diagnoses in such a lead. If a test result occurs commonly in patients with confirmatory findings of one diagnosis and uncommonly in patients with another diagnosis, then that test will help to differentiate between them. The difference in these frequencies of occurrence can be measured by their ratio.

Statisticians describe the frequency of a finding that occurs in those known to have a diagnosis as the 'likelihood' of it occurring (the 'likelihood' is also known to epidemiologists as the 'sensitivity'). The difference between these 'likelihoods' for two different diagnoses can be represented by the ratio of the two likelihoods. As this ratio refers to a pair of differential diagnoses, we can call it a 'differential likelihood ratio'. This is different to the 'overall likelihood ratio', which is the frequency of a finding in patients with a confirmed diagnosis divided by the frequency of the same finding in *all* those confirmed *not* to have that diagnosis. This 'non-differential' or 'overall' likelihood ratio is more useful when screening populations by using one test to detect one diagnosis. The 'overall' likelihood ratio is not as helpful for differential diagnoses (see ➲ Evidence for a finding's role in reasoning by elimination, p.625 for a discussion about likelihood ratios).

Explaining a diagnostic thought process

You may well have arrived at differential diagnoses by using intuitive, non-transparent, pattern recognition and not considered in an explicit way how it was done. Alternatively, you may have recorded your team's consensus opinion. However, you may be asked by a patient, student, nurse, or doctor to explain your thinking. In fairness, the way that your own mind (let alone someone else's mind) has actually worked subconsciously may be impossible to explain.

The first step is to write a summary of the positive findings, diagnoses, evidence, and management, as shown in ➔ An evidence-based diagnosis and plan, p.13. The original evidence for established diagnoses (e.g. type 2 diabetes mellitus) may not be available. However, for new diagnoses, choose from the evidence the best lead with the shortest differential diagnosis. Use the other findings to show that the one (or some) diagnoses are more probable or confirmed, and others less probable or ruled out.

If these conclusions of the non-transparent and transparent thought processes are not the same, you may wish to revise your opinion and list of differential diagnoses. By doing this, you will be checking diagnoses by using a different mental process in the same way as you would check the answer to arithmetic addition by adding up the list of numbers in a different order.

In order to avoid overlooking diagnoses, jog your memory by using 'sieves' to use 'recognition' to and help 'recall' by listing the possible broad anatomical and physiological explanations (see ➔ Medical and surgical sieves, p.14).

An evidence-based diagnosis and plan

Positive findings summary
Central chest pain for 4h with jaw discomfort, sweating, and nausea (1/10/13). PMH of hypertension for 10y. History of mild jaundice during febrile illnesses for years. BP 146/88 on admission (1/10/13). ECG: T wave inversion S2, AvF, V4, and V5. Latest HbA1c=8.7% (5/8/13).

Assessment and plan
?Unstable angina

?Non-ST elevated myocardial infarction (NSTEMI)
Outline evidence: central chest pain for 4h with jaw discomfort, sweating and nausea (1/10/13). ECG: T wave inversion S2, AvF, V4, and V5.
Plan: for troponin I immediately and 12h after onset of pain. Aspirin 300mg stat, bisoprolol 5mg od, isosorbide mononitrate 10mg bd.

?Gilbert's disease

?Cholelithiasis
Outline evidence: jaundiced sclera, history of mild jaundice during febrile illnesses for years, none of liver disease (1/10/13).
Plan: check bilirubin, urobilinogen, AST, γGT.

Other active diagnoses

Essential hypertension
Outline evidence: history of raised BP for 10y. Current BP 146/88 on admission (1/10/13).
Plan: continue bendroflumethiazide 2.5mg od, perindopril 2mg od.

Type 2 diabetes mellitus
Outline evidence: latest HbA1c = 8.7% (5/8/13).
Plan: stop gliclazide 160mg bd. Start insulin sliding scale.

Medical and surgical sieves

Check that you have not forgotten something by using a 'medical sieve'. For example:

- Social system and environment
- Locomotor system
- Nervous system
- Cardiovascular system
- Respiratory system
- Alimentary system
- Renal and urinary tract
- Reproductive system
- Endocrine and autonomic system
- Haematological and immune system.

Consider each of these systems by using the 'surgical sieve'. Is there a problem that is congenital, infective, traumatic, neoplastic, or degenerative?

There are many such 'sieves' in use; choose the ones that appeal to you.

The information in the pages of the OHCD is also set out in the same format as the Assessment and Plan (compare diagnoses of 'unstable angina' and 'NSTEMI' with those in ➲ Chest pain—alarming and increasing over minutes to hours, p.174). The section on chest pain gives some differential diagnoses with typical suggestive and confirmatory evidence that could also be added to those in ➲ An evidence-based diagnosis and plan, p.13. You may refer to these as examples when writing your own assessments and plans.

Diagnoses, hypotheses, and theories

Although the findings used to confirm a diagnosis can be observed, all things pictured or imagined under the title of the diagnosis cannot be confirmed by observation, e.g. molecular changes in damaged tissue or what would have happened in a particular patient if a treatment had not been given. Not only does this apply to hypotheses for individual patients, it also applies to what is imagined about populations of patients in scientific hypotheses and theories. It is thus possible that something else will be imagined or pictured in future that is also compatible with findings previously explained by another theory.

This is why the philosopher of science, Karl Popper, argued that general hypotheses and theories cannot be proven or confirmed in their entirety (see also ➋ Reasoning with hypotheses, p.637). However, if a new observation is inconsistent with one aspect of the hypothesis, it will have been 'falsified'. It will thus have to be changed to some degree (perhaps completely or slightly) to take the new observation into account.

Raised ST segments on an ECG in someone with severe central chest pain were formerly part of the criteria for confirming 'myocardial infarction', which suggested that a part of the myocardium was dead. However, one aspect of this theory has been 'falsified' because it has been discovered that some (or all) of the 'infarcted' myocardium is salvageable. With our new understanding, we use the same findings to 'confirm' an 'ST elevated myocardial 'infarction'. (It would be more accurate to say 'ST elevated acute myocardial ischaemia'.) We have modified the theory and now think that the process of 'infarction' is not complete and that the 'ischaemia' can be stopped with treatment, with reversal of many changes.

However, it is important to assess the reliability of the 'falsifying' fact. This is done by estimating the probability of the 'falsifying' observation being *replicated* by other scientists (or another doctor if the hypothesis is a diagnosis about an individual patient based on particular evidence). If the probability of replication of the evidence is high about a 'general' observation, then the observation may be accepted by the scientific community (but many may go to the trouble of repeating the study to make sure). If the P value is low or the 95% confidence intervals are narrow, then the probability of non-replication due to chance observations alone will be low. However, before we can conclude that the probability of replication is high, we must also be satisfied that the probability of non-replication due to other reasons is low (e.g. non-replication because of the presence of contradictory results in other studies, poor or idiosyncratic methodology, dishonesty, etc.). This is discussed further in ➋ Estimating the probability of replication with reasoning by elimination, p.636.

Imagining an ideal clinical trial

The findings used to define a 'diagnostic envelope' should enclose the best treatment indication criteria. These criteria should be chosen ideally from a number of candidate criteria. The chosen treatment criterion should be the one that produces the clearest outcome difference between the treatment and control in a comparative trial when all patients with some prospect of benefit are included. For example, when method A for measuring micro-albumin in urine chose patients for a trial, 15.3% developed nephropathy on placebo and 7.7% developed nephropathy on treatment, the proportion benefiting being 7.6% (NNT=13.1). However, with method B, 25.9% developed nephropathy on placebo and 11.1% developed it on treatment, the proportion benefiting being 14.8% (NNT=6.9). This would suggest that method A was not identifying patients who benefited so well and would be inferior to method B. This is discussed in detail in ➔ Analysing clinical trials to 'stratify' diagnostic and treatment criteria, p.633; ➔ How to improve treatments by better selection or 'stratification' of patients, p.634; ➔ Studies to establish treatment indication and diagnostic cut-off points, p.635.

In the absence of detailed trial data, a doctor may have to guess whether a patient's findings would identify a group of patients who would benefit from the treatment more than a placebo, bearing in mind side-effects, costs, etc. If, on balance, this would be the case, the doctor could apply a diagnostic term that would summarize his theoretical explanation as to why giving that treatment to a patient with that combination of findings would be better than not doing so.

Decision analysis

Decision analysis is a discipline that models mathematically what would happen if a detailed clinical trial were performed to compare the treatment options being considered for a particular patient. A 'decision tree' is constructed first to show all the possible diagnoses. The tree is extended to show the possible interventional limbs into which the patient could be randomized, followed by all the possible outcomes of each treatment. The branches would end with the effect that each outcome would have on the overall well-being of the patient.

An estimate is then made of the proportions of patients with each diagnosis, the proportions opting for each treatment and the proportions of those experiencing various degrees of well-being. These proportions are then multiplied together to estimate the average degree of well-being experienced by patients sharing each treatment outcome. Each of these average degrees of benefit is regarded as the 'expected' degree of well-being that would be experienced by an individual patient with each outcome. This is regarded as a representation of what an experienced doctor would do when he or she estimates the effect on the patient of the different interventions available.[3, 4]

Medical science aims to provide diagnostic criteria, treatment indication criteria, and treatments that, when used together, will predict with a high-est possible degree of certainty which treatment will work best for each patient (or would not help at all). This old aim is also the aim of 'stratified' or 'personalized' medicine. Such well-designed diagnostic systems would make it easier to choose the best option and to justify it using evidence in the form of data. This will not be possible without a clear understanding of the diagnostic process and criteria for confirming diagnoses that also indicate the best treatment for that patient as discussed in Chapter 13 (see ➲ Evidence-based diagnosis and decisions, p.616).

Diagnostic classifications, pathways, and tables

A diagnostic pathway or algorithm is a way of representing diagnostic reasoning processes or a diagnostic classification (see Fig. 1.1). The same reasoning processes can be displayed using a table of the kind shown in Table 1.1. This is also how information in this book is displayed. It is flexible and also allows findings to be shown that do not form part of the diagnostic criteria. The reader can scan down such a table to find the diagnoses that are compatible with the findings so far. The entry can then be copied into a table in the patient's records as a draft entry for that diagnostic possibility.

Table 1.1 Diagnostic table for the differential diagnoses of jaundice

Carotinaemia (not 'real' jaundice)	*Suggested by:* onset over months. Skin yellow with white sclerae, normal stools, and normal urine. Diet rich in yellow vegetables/fruits).
	Confirmed by: no bilirubin, no **urobilinogen** in the urine, and normal **serum bilirubin**. Normal **liver function tests (LFT)**. Response to diet change.
'Pre-hepatic' jaundice due to haemolysis	*Suggested by:* jaundice and anaemia (the combination seen as 'lemon' or pale yellow). Normal dark stools and normal-looking urine.
	Confirmed by: ↑(unconjugated and thus insoluble) **serum bilirubin**, but normal (conjugated and soluble) bilirubin and thus no ↑bilirubin in urine. ↑**urobilinogen in urine** and ↓**serum haptoglobin**. Normal LFT. ↑**reticulocyte count**.
'Hepatic' jaundice due to congenital enzyme defect	*Suggested by:* jaundice. Normal-looking stools and normal-looking urine. Jaundice worse during febrile illnesses.
	Confirmed by: ↑**serum bilirubin** (unconjugated), but no (conjugated) bilirubin in urine. No **urobilinogen in urine** and **normal haptoglobin**. Normal **LFT**.
'Hepatocellular' jaundice ('hepatic' with some 'obstructive' jaundice)	*Suggested by:* onset of jaundice over days or weeks, pale stools but dark urine.
	Confirmed by: ↑serum (conjugated) **bilirubin** and thus ↑**urine bilirubin**. Normal **urine urobilinogen**. **LFT** all abnormal, especially ↑↑**ALT**.
'Obstructive' jaundice	*Suggested by:* onset of jaundice over days or weeks with pale stools and dark urine. Bilirubin (i.e. conjugated and thus soluble) in urine.
	Confirmed by: ↑ **serum conjugated bilirubin** and **urine bilirubin**, but no ↑**urobilinogen** in urine. Markedly (↑↑) **alkaline phosphatase**, but less abnormal (↑) **LFT** and ↑γ**GT**.

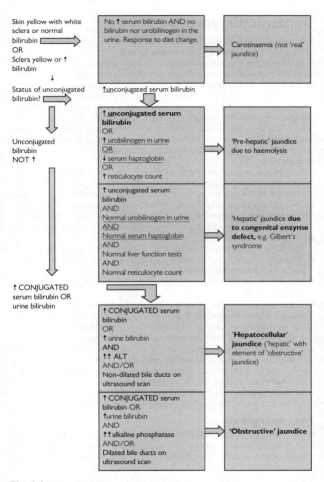

Fig. 1.1 A diagnostic pathway for jaundice.

Dynamic diagnoses

It is important to understand that clinical diagnosis is not a static classification system based on diagnostic criteria or their probable presence. It is a dynamic process. Diagnostic algorithms 'classify' patients by following a logical pathway based mainly on diagnostic criteria. Other systems predict the probable presence of diagnostic criteria. All these methods can be regarded as 'diagnosing' a snap-shot of what is happening at a particular time.

The diagnostician has to imagine the presence of a dynamic process that changes with time. There may be several processes taking place at the same time, some progressing over years (e.g. atheromatous changes), some over minutes to hours (e.g. a thrombosis in a coronary artery), some over minutes or seconds (e.g. ventricular tachycardia), and others instantaneously (e.g. a cardiac arrest).

A diagnostic process leading to treatment may have to happen in stages and for a number of diagnoses at the same time. It might be more appropriate to think of the process as one of 'feedback' control. In this way, the doctor would be acting as an external control mechanism support the patient's failing mechanisms. After the initial history and examination, the feedback information may come from electronic monitoring, nursing observations, ward rounds, hospital clinic, or primary care follow-up.

There are three types of mechanisms of interest to the diagnostician:
- Those that control the 'internal milieu' by keeping temperature, tissue perfusion, blood gases, and biochemistry constant.
- Those that control the body's structure by effecting repair in response to any damage.
- Those that control the 'external milieu' of day-to-day living.

These are all interdependent. If one mechanism fails, then it may unmask other weaknesses by causing other failures. It may not be enough to treat the main failure. It is often necessary also to treat the causes and consequences, as they may be unable to recover on their own. For example, a coronary thrombosis may be treated with stenting of the coronary artery, but any resulting rhythm abnormalities may need to be treated and also the causative risk factors (e.g. smoking) that could result in recurrence. So when we explain our diagnostic thought processes, it helps to think of each diagnosis as a subheading with its own evidence and decision.

The whole patient

A 'diagnosis' does not imply that only one solution needs to be discovered. The complete diagnosis (or diagnostic formulation) may have to include various causes, consequences, interactions, and other independent processes. As well as internal medical processes, it has to include external factors, such as circumstances at home and the effects on self-care, employment, and leisure.

There may be many diagnoses that have been confirmed previously and for which the patient is on established treatment. Therefore, the diagnostician must imagine what is happening to the 'whole patient'. This requires a broad medical education that allows a range of phenomena to be pictured, from molecular events to events in the home and outside world.

Explaining diagnoses to patients

The patient may already be imagining with some trepidation what might be happening. It is important to find out what the patient is imagining and to use this as a starting point for your own explanation. The patient's own views are usually sought and documented at the end of the history of the presenting complaint.

Patients and relatives usually ask questions spontaneously or request an appointment for time to be set aside to do this. Some may be too shy and need encouragement to do so, in which case this important aspect of care will be omitted. Others may be too ill to listen and may prefer relatives or carers to ask on their behalf. If questions are not asked spontaneously, it is best to ask patients tactfully if they or anyone else with their consent have any questions.

Although patients and relatives may understand explanations and other answers to questions at the time they are given to them, even the most intelligent may forget unfamiliar technical terms and their meaning within a short time, especially if they are ill. Therefore, it is important to provide a written reminder of such terms and how they are related. This can be done by giving the patient a printed summary similar to that in ➔ An evidence-based diagnosis and plan, p.13. This can also allow the patient to ask further questions if they wish.

Informed consent is also based on similar questions and discussion. The process is more effective if the patient is able to ask the questions (i.e. if the process is 'patient-centred'). Such a process may be facilitated if they refer to a summary such as that shown in ➔ An evidence-based diagnosis and plan, p.13.

Ideally, patients should know the presenting complaint for their latest problems, the primary diagnosis or differential diagnoses, and what actions are being taken in terms of tests and treatments. They should also be aware of their past medical history: the various diagnoses, how they presented and were confirmed, their treatments, follow-up arrangements, and markers of progress. Again, the relevant technical terms and how they are linked can be summarized for them as shown in ➔ An evidence-based diagnosis and plan, p.13.

Informed consent

In order for a patient to consent to treatment, he or she must understand what has been said and be able to retain that explanation. A basic understanding means the patient must know what actions have been agreed and the possible diagnoses in each case. In order to understand each diagnosis, it is essential to know which symptoms it explains and how these symptoms or some other markers are progressing. Few patients are able to retain all of this, especially if there are many technical terms that are unfamiliar to them. Therefore, it would be a sensible policy to provide the patient with a typed explanation setting out these basic relationships as shown in ➔ An evidence-based diagnosis and plan, p.13. This would then become the next 'past medical history' when the patient is asked to provide it by another doctor or nurse. It would thus allow patients to ask a doctor or nurse to remind them of the meanings of the various terms.

Minimizing diagnostic errors

The diagnostic and decision-making process usually takes place in busy clinics, wards, operating theatres, and emergency rooms. Therefore, most diagnoses have to take place by some rapid conscious or subconscious pattern recognition, and there is usually little time for reflection. Mistakes are kept to a minimum by good training, especially listening carefully and writing out what has been observed, thought, and done.

Another important principle to bear in mind is that even the most expert and well-founded diagnoses and decisions can only be successful in a proportion of cases. Therefore, there must be a strategy to monitor their outcome and to change diagnoses and decisions, if possible.

Diagnostic errors can be classified in terms of cognitive psychology[5] into:

- Faulty triggering
- Faulty context information
- Faulty verification
- No fault errors
- Faulty information gathering and processing.

Faulty triggering

This is a failure to consider appropriate diagnostic possibilities, often attributed to a weakness of medical education, which focuses on disease processes instead of the diagnostic processes. This type of error can be kept to a minimum by using the suggestions in the sections from ⮕ 'Transparent' reasoning, p.5 to ⮕ An evidence-based diagnosis and plan, p.13, and by referring to the differential diagnoses in the other sections. Finally, this error can be reduced by not only writing down the differential diagnoses, but also by writing down the findings from which were chosen the leads that 'triggered' them as shown in ⮕ An evidence-based diagnosis and plan, p.13. This can be given to the patient to be shown to other doctors who might also spot any omissions.

Faulty context information

This is focusing on one diagnosis and failing to consider others that may also be present. It involves jumping to conclusions. This can be avoided by using the sieves in ⮕ Medical and surgical sieves, p.14, referring to the appropriate section in this book, and writing out an overall plan as shown in ⮕ An evidence-based diagnosis and plan, p.13, so that other doctors might spot any errors. Again, this can be given to the patient (to show to other doctors who might spot any errors).

Faulty verification

This is failure to ensure that the patient's presenting symptom and other markers of poor health have been controlled or stabilized as well as possible. This is discussed in ⮕ Confirming and finalizing a diagnosis, p.8. It also helps to set out each diagnosis with its evidence as shown in ⮕ An evidence-based diagnosis and plan, p.13, which includes the markers being followed and their latest results. Again, this summary can be given to the patient to be shown to other doctors who might spot such omissions.

No fault errors

Even the most expert and well-founded diagnoses and decisions can only be successful in a proportion of cases. This is why diagnoses and decisions are qualified with probabilities. Therefore, there must be a strategy to monitor the outcome of all diagnoses and decisions and to change them, if possible. If a summary of the kind shown in ➲ An evidence-based diagnosis and plan, p.13 is given to the patient to be shown to other doctors, they will be able to understand the basis of previous decisions and take appropriate action.

Faulty information gathering and processing

This is poor use of leads and differentiators in appropriate settings. This book focuses on this process. It is important to know the differential diagnoses of leads and the frequency with which they occur in different clinical settings. It is also important to know the frequency with which findings occur in pairs of diagnoses. At present, this is gained from personal experience. Little research is done into diagnostic leads, differential likelihood ratios, optimizing treatment indication, and diagnostic criteria because the main focus of research is currently on sensitivity, specificity, and overall likelihood ratios. The way in which the situation can be improved is outlined in Chapter 13 (see ➲ Evidence-based diagnosis and decisions, p.616).

References

1. Eddy DM, Clanton CH (1982) The art of diagnosis: solving the clinico-pathological conference. *N Engl J Med* 306, 1263–8.
2. Llewelyn DEH, Garcia-Puig J (2004) How different urinary albumin excretion rates can predict progression to nephropathy and the effect of treatment in hypertensive diabetics. *J Renin Angiotensin Aldosterone Syst* 5, 141–5.
3. Llewelyn H, Hopkins A eds (1993) *Analysing how we reach clinical decisions*. Royal College of Physicians of London, London.
4. Dowie J, Elstein A eds (1988) *Professional judgement: a reader in clinical decision making*. Cambridge University Press, Cambridge.
5. Kassirer JP, Kopleman RI (1999) Cognitive errors in diagnosis: instantiation, classification and consequences. *Acad Med* 1999; 74: S138–43.

Interpreting the history and examination

Thoughtful history taking 26
Interpreting the case history 29
Sore throat 31
The systems enquiry 32
The past medical history 36
The drug history 38
Interpreting the physical examination 40
Interpreting the investigations 42
Writing the diagnosis and management 44
Case presentations 45
Clinical opinions 46
The 'open mind' approach 47
The plan of the remainder of this book 48
Plan of the general examination 49
Cardiovascular system 50
Respiratory system 51
Alimentary and genitourinary systems 52
Nervous system 54
The full neurological assessment 56
Mental state examination 58
Basic blood and urine test results 59
Abnormal chest X-ray appearances 60

Thoughtful history taking

The aim of the diagnostic process is to build up a picture of what is happening to the patient. 'Diagnosis' is derived from the Greek 'to perceive through knowledge' (i.e. to predict from experience what is beyond the history, examination, etc.).

The diagnosis (or diagnostic formulation) may have to include prediction about past, present, and future, causes, consequences, interactions, and other independent processes. As well as internal medical processes, it has to include external factors such as circumstances at home and the effects on self-care, employment, and leisure.

It is important to establish very clearly why the patient has sought help. This is known as the presenting complaint. Ask about its severity and duration. Be prepared to act immediately to give symptomatic relief (e.g. for pain) if the patient is distressed.

In some cases, the presenting complaint may not explain the decision to seek help. The patient may be too ill, shy, guilty, or embarrassed to describe what is happening accurately. In other cases, it may be someone else who is unduly worried. Be alert to the real reason.

Having established the presenting complaint(s), establish the factual details of 'place and time'. It is the ability to give a place and time that establishes the complaints as 'facts' as opposed to vague 'anecdote'.

Listen without prompting first but, if necessary, ask where they were and what they were doing when the problem was first noticed. This will help the patient's recall and help your diagnostic thought process.

Establish the speed of initial onset and subsequent change in severity with time. Onset within seconds suggests a fit or heart rhythm abnormality, over minutes a bleed or clotting process, hours to days an acute infection, days to weeks a chronic infection, weeks to months a tumour, and months to years a degenerative process.

If there are other complaints, note the same details. Ask about other associated, aggravating, and relieving factors, especially as a result of the patient's own actions and other professional care.

Ask what the patient thinks is going on and is afraid of. This will be the starting point for your own explanation and suggestions to the patient later about what is to be done.

The history also allows patients and supporters to identify the issues that they want addressed in terms of discomfort, loss of function, and difficulties with day-to-day existence. Final diagnoses are based on the initial history because they have to explain it completely. If the diagnoses arrived at cannot explain the entire history and the effects of various treatments, then the diagnoses will be incomplete—others will have to be considered.

Write out your history in a systematic way, e.g. as shown in the next section, and go over it with the patient, if possible, to check that it is right.

This is a lot to remember, especially if you are trying to put it into practice in a busy, noisy environment. However, writing out your findings according to a plan each time will help you to remember.

The plan in Box 2.1 is an example—make up your own.

Box 2.1 A plan for writing out the history

History taker's name: *Date of assessment:*

Patient's name: *DOB:*   *Age:*   *Occupation:*
Patient's address:

Admitted as an emergency/from the waiting list on (date) at (time)

Presenting complaints (PC)
1st symptom—duration
2nd symptom—duration
etc.

History of each presenting complaint (HPC)
1. Nature of complaint (e.g. pain in chest), circumstances, and speed of onset, progression (change with time—picture a graph), aggravating and relieving factors, associated symptoms (describe under 2, etc.)
2. Next associated symptom, etc. described as in (1).

Add response to direct questions from chasing up some diagnostic possibilities that come to mind as the history is taken.

Add the patient's opinion or fear about what may be happening.

Past medical history (PMH)
1st diagnosis and when—evidence—treatment—name of doctor
2nd

Drug history (DH)
Name, dose, and frequency—diagnostic indication—evidence—prescriber
Next drug etc.
Alcohol and tobacco consumption, other 'recreational' drugs
Drug sensitivities and allergies

Developmental history
(especially in paediatrics and psychiatry): pregnancy, infancy, childhood, puberty, adulthood

Family history (FH)
Age Illnesses
(Arrange around 'family tree', if preferred)
Mention especially:

Parents	*Tuberculosis?*
Siblings	*Asthma? Eczema?*
Children	*Diabetes? Epilepsy?*
Spouse	*Hypertension?*

Social history (SH)
Home and domestic activity support—job and financial security—travel and leisure. (Consider the effect of all these on the illness and the effect of the illness on these.)

History by A N Other   3.00 p.m. 19 October 2013
Miss AM (DOB: 28/2/85) Aged 29 Secretary
23, Smith Square, Old Town
Emergency admission 19 October 2013 at 2.00 p.m.

PC:

1. Severe sore throat, sweats, and malaise for 2 days

2. Sudden loss of consciousness in A&E at 2.00 p.m.

HPC: The patient was well until last Friday afternoon 18 October when she developed a **sore throat** at work. It was relieved that day by warm drinks and paracetamol, but when she woke this Saturday morning, it was very severe. She remembered that she had been told to report sore throats because she was taking carbimazole and to get a white cell count. She was worried that she might have developed a low white cell count because of this drug. She came to A&E because it was a Saturday. When she got up from her seat in the waiting room after being called, she felt dizzy, blacked out, and fell to the floor, striking her head. She recovered consciousness within a minute.

Interpreting the case history

There are two striking symptoms: (1) a severe sore throat that is getting worse and (2) the sudden loss of consciousness. Both are examples of findings with short lists of causes: good diagnostic 'leads' or 'pivots'.

Most readers will have experienced a sore throat and will be aware that it is usually due to a viral pharyngitis, bacterial tonsillitis (e.g. due to a haemolytic *streptococcus*), or glandular fever. It could also be due to bone marrow dysfunction (e.g. due to drug effect) or something else in a small proportion of cases (see ➔ Sore throat, p.31). The onset over days is compatible with all these possibilities. A white cell count might give results that would differentiate between these possible causes (see Table 2.1).

The sudden loss of consciousness with rapid recovery is known as 'syncope'. It is also a good lead with a well-defined differential diagnosis. It can be due to a vasovagal attack, cough, micturition or carotid sinus syncope, postural hypotension, transient cerebral ischaemia, a Stokes–Adams attack, aortic stenosis, hypertrophic cardiomyopathy (HOCM), hypoglycaemia, or epilepsy (see Table 2.1). The fact that it happened after the patient got up from a chair suggests postural hypotension (because this always occurs in this condition, but rarely, if ever, in the others). Postural hypotension may be due to fever and dehydration so although the two leads have common causes, postural hypotension could be a consequence of any infection. Therefore, the syncope does not differentiate between any of the causes of a sore throat. The patient has expressed a fear that the sore throat could be drug-induced because she has been warned about this.

These thoughts can be summarized in the problem-structuring note in Table 2.1. You can write this on a sheet of paper, perhaps in pencil for easy editing, on a computer, or on a black or white board when discussing a case with colleagues. Such thoughts are usually considered mentally without writing them down, which is why the diagnostic thought process can be difficult to learn from senior colleagues.

Outline findings

After outlining your thoughts in the problem-structuring note as shown in Table 2.1, turn to the appropriate page in this book by looking up 'sore throat'. Check that you have not forgotten to include something. The entry in this book for 'sore throat' is shown in ⮕ Sore throat, p.31 and in ⮕ Sore throat, p.320. You may wish to read this before moving on to the next step.

Table 2.1 Female. Aged 29. Severe sore throat for 2 days, getting worse. Taking carbimazole for 6 months. Sudden loss of consciousness after getting up from chair, recovery within a minute.

Diagnoses	Outline evidence	Management
Viral pharyngitis?	Severe sore throat for 2 days, getting worse. (19/10/13)	Paracetamol 500mg 6 hourly PRN. Examine throat. Request **WCC**: ↓neutrophils, ↑lymphocytes?
Acute bacterial (or follicular) tonsillitis (mainly streptococcal)?	Severe sore throat for 2 days, getting worse. (19/10/13)	Paracetamol 500mg 6 hourly PRN. Examine throat. Request **WCC**: ↑neutrophils?
Glandular fever (infectious mononucleosis due to Epstein–Barr virus)?	Severe sore throat for 2 days, getting worse. (19/10/13)	Paracetamol 500mg 6 hourly PRN. Examine throat. Request **WCC**: lymphocytes atypical? Paul–Bunnell or Monospot® +ve?
Drug-induced agranulocytosis? (this is what the patient fears)	Severe sore throat for 2 days, getting worse (19/10/13). Taking carbimazole.	Paracetamol 500mg 6 hourly PRN. Examine throat. Request **WCC**: ↓granulocytes (neutrophils, eosinphils, basophils)?
Postural hypotension syncope? Due to dehydration?	Sudden loss of consciousness after getting up from chair, recovery within a minute (19/10/13). Evidence of acute infection.	Look for fall in BP when standing. Request U&E. Consider fluids IV to rehydrate.
Thyrotoxicosis now controlled?	Taking carbimazole.	Examine for tremor, etc. Carbimazole 5mg od. FT4 and TSH normal?

Sore throat

Initial investigations (other tests in bold): FBC, U&E, throat swab, Paul–Bunnell test (Table 2.2).

Table 2.2 Main differential diagnoses and typical outline evidence, etc.

Viral pharyngitis	*Suggested by:* sore throat, pain on swallowing, fever, cervical lymphadenopathy, and injected fauces. WCC: ↑lymphocytes, leucocytes normal. *Confirmed by:* negative **throat swab** for bacterial culture, self-limiting: resolution within days. *Initial management:* analgesics, e.g. paracetamol.
Acute follicular tonsillitis (streptococcal)	*Suggested by:* severe sore throat, pain on swallowing, fever, enlarged tonsils with white patches (like strawberries and creamy lines). Cervical lymphadenopathy, especially in angle of jaw. Fever, WCC: ↑leucocytes. *Confirmed by:* **throat swab** for culture and sensitivities of organisms. *Initial management:* analgesics, antibiotics, e.g. benzyl-penicillin IM or Penicillin V orally; if no allergy, good fluid intake.
Infectious mononucleosis (glandular fever) due to Epstein–Barr virus	*Suggested by:* very severe throat pain with enlarged tonsils covered with grey mucoid membrane. Petechiae on palate. Profound malaise. Generalized lymphadenopathy, splenomegaly. **WCC:** ↑atypical lymphocytes. *Confirmed by:* **Paul–Bunnell or Monospot® test** +ve. **Viral titres:** ↑Epstein–Barr. *Initial management:* analgesia, no antibiotics (amoxicillin may cause skin rash).
Candidiasis of buccal or oesophageal mucosa	*Suggested by:* painful dysphagia, white plaque, history of immunosuppression/diabetes/recent antibiotics. *Confirmed by:* **oesophagoscopy** showing erythema and plaques, **brush cytology:** spores and hyphae. *Initial management:* local antifungal agents, e.g. miconazole oral gel or nystatin oral suspension. Parenteral administration if systemic involvement.
Agranulocytosis	*Suggested by:* sore throat, background history of taking a drug, or contact with noxious substance. *Confirmed by:* ↓ or absent neutrophil count. *Initial management:* stop potential causative drugs, antibiotic cover until resolved.

The systems enquiry

The systems enquiry may take place at various points in the history. The questions given here are detailed. They can also be asked as broad prompts (e.g. do you have any chest, abdominal, bladder symptoms, etc.?). Some may prefer to perform the systems enquiry immediately after the history of presenting complaint because they would not have enough knowledge to ask the questions to differentiate between the initial differential diagnoses (e.g. asking about generalized lymph node enlargement that might differentiate between glandular fever and the other causes of a sore throat). If the patient said 'yes' to a question during the systems enquiry, it could be added to the problem-structuring note and looked up later in this book.

If a direct question turns up a positive response, it has to be treated with caution. It may be a 'false-positive' response to a leading question. A positive response has to be treated as an extra presenting complaint, added to the original list and explored carefully with the history of presenting complaint. They can also be looked up in the pages of this book.

If there is a negative response to a direct question, this is more reliable (unless the patient is very forgetful or is purposely withholding information). The absence of all symptoms under a heading indicates that it is less probable that there is an abnormality in that system.

Systems enquiry

Locomotor symptoms
- No pain and stiffness in the neck, shoulder, elbow, wrist, hand, or back
- No pain and stiffness in the hip, knee, or foot
- No pain or stiffness in any joints and muscles.

Negative responses make locomotor abnormalities less probable. If any are positive, then a 'GALS' examination screen is performed under the headings of Gait, Arms, Legs, Spine. Care can be taken with painfully inflamed or damaged joints.

Skin, lymph nodes, and endocrine
No heat or cold intolerance (e.g. wanting to open or close windows when others are comfortable).
Sweats and shivering for 2 days
- No drenching night sweats
- No episodes of rigors
- No rashes and itching.
No skin lumps or lumps elsewhere

No heat or cold intolerance makes an abnormality of thyroid metabolism less probable (suggesting that the carbimazole is probably controlling the thyrotoxicosis). Positive findings (e.g. sweats and shivering for 2 days) can be looked up in this book—they will be found to be poor leads and differentiators (because they occur often in each condition), and not very helpful in differentiating between the causes of a sore throat.

No further information is gained with the following responses. However, they provide an opportunity to reflect on the function of each system.

Cardiovascular symptoms

No tiredness and breathlessness on exertion (non-specific)
Syncope after rising from chair in A&E—see HPC
No leg pain on walking

Negative responses make cardiac output and peripheral vascular disease less probable.

No ankle swelling

A negative response makes a right-sided venous return abnormality less probable.

No exertional dyspnoea
No orthopnoea
No paroxysmal nocturnal dyspnoea

Negative responses make a left-sided venous return abnormality less probable.

No palpitations
No central chest pain on exertion or at rest

Negative responses make a cardiac abnormality less likely.

Respiratory symptoms

No chronic breathlessness
No acute breathlessness

Negative responses make abnormality of overall respiratory and blood gas abnormality less probable.

No hoarseness
No cough, sputum, haemoptysis
No wheeze

Negative responses make airway disease less probable.

No pleuritic chest pain

A negative response makes pleural reactions and chest wall disease less probable.

Alimentary symptoms

No loss of appetite (non-specific)
No weight loss (non-specific)
No jaundice, dark urine, pale stools
Negative responses make metabolic gut and liver disease less probable.
No nausea or vomiting (non-specific)
No haematemesis or melaena
No dysphagia but sore throat—see HPC
No indigestion
No abdominal pain
No diarrhoea or constipation
No recent change in bowel habit
No rectal bleeding ± mucus

Negative responses make gastrointestinal disease less probable.

Genitourinary symptoms

Menstrual history—date of menarche, duration of cycle, and flow normal
Volume of flow and associated pain normal
Any pregnancy outcomes normal
No dyspareunia and vaginal bleeding
No vaginal discharge

Negative responses make gynaecological disease less probable.

No haematuria or other odd colour
No urgency or incontinence
No dysuria
No polyuria or nocturia
No loin pain or lower abdominal pain

Negative responses make urological disease less probable.

No impotence or loss of libido
No urethral discharge

Negative responses make male urological disease less probable.

Nervous system symptoms

No vision loss, blurring, or double vision
No hearing loss or tinnitus
No loss of smell and taste
No numbness, pins and needles, or other disturbance of sensation
No disturbance of speech
No weakness of limbs
No imbalance
No headache
No sudden headache and loss of consciousness

Dizziness and blackouts in A&E—see HPC
No vertigo
No 'fit'
No transient neurological deficit

Negative responses make neurological disease less probable.

Psychiatric symptoms

No fatigue, not tired all the time
No mood change
No odd voices or odd visual effects
No anxiety and sleep disturbance
No loss of self-confidence
No new strong beliefs
No phobias, no compulsions, or avoidance of actions
No use of recreational drugs

Patients may hide or forget many symptoms. There is a school of thought that regards symptom reviews as being of little value, and that only symptoms that are volunteered are worthwhile investigating. Many doctors do not conduct systemic reviews and only ask these questions if other symptoms have been volunteered already in that system.

The past medical history

The past medical history (PMH) in this case has three components: the diagnosis, the evidence, and the management. The management may be omitted if it is mentioned elsewhere, e.g. if carbimazole is in the drug history together with its indication of thyrotoxicosis.

PMH

> *Thyrotoxicosis discovered 6 months ago*
>
> Outline evidence: anxiety, weight loss, abnormal thyroid function tests in Osler Hospital by Dr Miller.
>
> Management: taking carbimazole, 5mg daily.

'Anxiety, weight loss, abnormal thyroid function tests' outlines the evidence for the thyrotoxicosis. Knowing the doctor responsible and the institution would allow the details to be checked, if necessary. In many cases, patients are not able to provide these details and they would have to be extracted from the records, in which case it is helpful to name the hospital or primary care centre or doctor responsible.

A comprehensive past medical history in this format could be written immediately after any consultation, in hospital or primary care with results and dates given to the patient. This would be more reliable than the next doctor having to do so, but this is not customary. This information can be added to the problem-structuring note No. 2. This can be set out in different formats; in this case, it is set out in subheading style, which is in effect a draft of the 'next' past medical history. This problem-structuring approach can also be used to draft discharge summaries on a hospital computer network, which can be updated during the patient's stay and printed out when the patient leaves hospital.[1]

The family history

The family history (FH) (Table 2.3) rarely contains features that form powerful leads. In general, there will be risk factors in the FH. For example, the fact that the patient's mother had type 2 diabetes mellitus means that there is an increased risk of the patient developing type 2 diabetes mellitus. This may have no immediate bearing on the current problems (but she should be checked for diabetes if only to exclude its presence so far). The patient could also be reminded to adopt a healthy diet and lifestyle. The new additions to the problem-structuring note (Box 2.2) are in **bold**.

Table 2.3 FH		
Father		Aged 56—hypertension
Mother		Aged 55—diabetes (onset at 50)
Siblings	male	Aged 34—alive and well
		Aged 26—alive and well
	female	Aged 30—alive and well
Children		None

Box 2.2 Problem-structuring note No. 2

Outline findings: female. Aged 29. Severe sore throat for 2 days, getting worse. Taking carbimazole for 6 months. Sudden loss of consciousness after getting up from chair, recovery within a minute. PMH of thyrotoxicosis (anxiety, weight loss, abnormal thyroid function tests in Osler Hospital) treated with carbimazole. FH of type 2 diabetes mellitus.

Viral pharyngitis?
Outline evidence: severe sore throat for 2 days, getting worse (19/10/13).

Management: paracetamol 500mg 6 hourly PRN. Examine throat. Request WCC: ↓neutrophils, ↑lymphocytes?

Acute bacterial (or follicular) tonsillitis? (mainly streptococcal)
Outline evidence: severe sore throat for 2 days, getting worse (19/10/13).

Management: paracetamol 500mg 6 hourly PRN. Examine throat. Request WCC: ↑neutrophils?

Glandular fever (infectious mononucleosis due to Epstein–Barr virus)?
Outline evidence: severe sore throat for 2 days, getting worse (19/10/13). No skin lumps or lumps elsewhere.

Management: paracetamol 500mg 6 hourly PRN. Examine throat. Request WCC: lymphocytes atypical? Paul–Bunnell or Monospot® +ve?

Drug-induced agranulocytosis? (this is what the patient fears)
Outline evidence: severe sore throat for 2 days, getting worse (19/10/13). Taking carbimazole. Bruising on forehead.

Management: paracetamol 500mg 6 hourly PRN. Examine throat. Request WCC: ↓granulocytes (neutrophils, eosinophils, basophils)?

Postural hypotension syncope? Due to dehydration from infection?
Outline evidence: sudden loss of consciousness after getting up from chair, recovery within a minute (19/10/13). Evidence of acute infection.

Management: look for fall in BP when standing. Request U&E. Consider fluids IV to rehydrate.

Thyrotoxicosis now controlled?
Outline evidence: anxiety, weight loss, abnormal thyroid function tests in April 2008. No heat or cold intolerance currently.

Management: examine for tremor, etc. Carbimazole 5mg od. FT4 and TSH normal?

Increased risk of type 2 diabetes mellitus
Outline evidence: FH of type 2 diabetes mellitus.
Management: test urine for sugar. Fasting glucose.

The version of the problem-structuring note in Box 2.2 is in the same format as the 'textbook' page on 'Sore throat' (see ➲ Sore throat, p.31 and ➲ Sore throat, p.320). This makes comparison easier and allows the 'textbook' entries to be used as templates that can be copied into the problem-structuring note.

The drug history

The drug history (DH) is often placed near the end of the history. If the patient is on medication, then it indicates that this is for an active medical condition as opposed to a PMH. Therefore, there is something to be said for documenting the drug history immediately after the PMH so and current conditions can be thought about together.

> **Drug history**
>
> *Paracetamol 1g 6 hourly (for ?viral pharyngitis, etc.)*
> *Carbimazole 5mg daily for thyrotoxicosis (see PMH for evidence)*
> *Alcohol 10 units per week*
> *Non-smoker*
> *No other recreational drugs*

There is nothing to add to the problem-structuring note from the drug history.

The social history

The social history (SH) is always relevant. The activities of daily living can be considered under the heading of domestic, work, and leisure. Imagine what any person has to do from waking up in the morning to going to sleep at night, and consider whether the patient needs support with any of these activities. Fit young adults who are expected to recover completely may miss school, college, or work, and the timing of their return will have to be considered. Patients who are more dependent on others, such as children and the elderly, may need special provisions. Patients with permanent disabilities may need help with most, if not all, activities of daily living.

> **SH**
>
> *Alone in a flat at present (flatmate on holiday for another week)*
> *Parents live 200 miles away*
> *Works as secretary for insurance firm*

The patient has little domestic support and it would be sensible to admit her to be rehydrated until she is in no danger of fainting on discharge. This has been added to the problem-structuring note.

When the history is complete

The findings that will differentiate between the causes of a sore throat (see ➔ Sore throat, p.31) are the appearance of the throat and the white cell count. Generalized lymphadenopathy, splenomegaly, and petechiae on the palate would also occur commonly in glandular fever and uncommonly in the other differential diagnoses.

➔ Postural fall in blood pressure, p.212 shows that a fall in BP on standing would support postural hypotension because it occurs commonly in patients with this diagnosis and rarely in the other causes of syncope. A raised creatinine and urea would support dehydration because this happens often in dehydration, but infrequently in the other causes of postural hypotension.

The diagnostic thoughts so far are represented in the problem-structuring note in Table 2.4.

Table 2.4 Problem-structuring note No. 3

Outline findings: female. Aged 29. Severe sore throat for 2 days, getting worse. Taking carbimazole for 6 months. Sudden loss of consciousness after getting up from chair, recovery within a minute. PMH of thyrotoxicosis (anxiety, weight loss, abnormal thyroid function tests). FH of type 2 diabetes mellitus.

Viral pharyngitis?	Severe sore throat for 2 days, getting worse. (19/10/13)	Paracetamol 500mg 6 hourly PRN. Examine throat. Request WCC: ↓neutrophils, ↑lymphocytes?
Acute bacterial (or follicular) tonsillitis? (mainly streptococcal)	Severe sore throat for 2 days, getting worse. (19/10/13)	Paracetamol 500mg 6 hourly PRN. Examine throat. Request WCC: ↑neutrophils?
Glandular fever (infectious mononucleosis due to Epstein–Barr virus)?	Severe sore throat for 2 days, getting worse. (19/10/13)	Paracetamol 500mg 6 hourly PRN. Examine throat. Request WCC: lymphocytes atypical? Paul–Bunnell or Monospot® +ve?
Drug-induced agranulocytosis? (this is what the patient fears)	Severe sore throat for 2 days, getting worse (19/10/13). Taking carbimazole.	Paracetamol 500mg 6 hourly PRN. Examine throat. Request WCC: ↓granulocytes (neutrophils, eosinophils, basophils)?
Postural hypotension syncope? Due to dehydration from infection?	Sudden loss of consciousness after getting up from chair, recovery within a minute (19/10/13). Evidence of acute infection.	Look for fall in BP when standing. Request U&E. Consider fluids IV to rehydrate.
Thyrotoxicosis now controlled?	Anxiety, weight loss, abnormal thyroid function tests in April 2008. No heat or cold intolerance currently.	Examine for tremor etc. Carbimazole 5mg od. FT4 and TSH normal?
Increased risk of type 2 diabetes mellitus	FH of type 2 diabetes mellitus.	Test urine for sugar. Fasting glucose.
No domestic support	**Alone in flat at present.**	**Consider admission for initial care.**

Interpreting the physical examination

The physical examination tends to be focused. The 'open mind' approach, where findings are discovered and their meaning looked up later, is described at the end of this section. If this book is referred to before the examination, the reader could focus on the appearance of the throat and palpation of the neck to look for findings that may differentiate between the four differential diagnoses suggested by the history. The reader should also focus on the BP to see if there is a postural fall, and tremor and lid lag for inadequately treated thyrotoxicosis.

General
Looks unwell, flushed
No tremor or lid lag
Temperature 38.5°C
Bilaterally swollen tonsils, red with linear creamy patches
Bilateral, tender, multiple lymph node enlargement in neck. No lymph node swelling in axillae or groins

CVS
Pulse 110/min, regular, low volume
BP 110/70 reclining, 90/50 standing
Heart sounds normal
No murmurs

RS
Chest shape and movement normal
Breath sounds normal

AS
Not jaundiced
Liver—1 finger breadth below costal margin
Spleen not palpable

CNS
Conscious and alert
No neck stiffness
Hand and leg coordination normal
Reflexes all normal and symmetrical

The presence of linear patches of creamy pus in fissures on the surface of enlarged tonsils occurs commonly in patients with bacterial tonsillitis, but less commonly in agranulocytosis, viral pharyngitis, and glandular fever (where there is usually a grey mucoid film). This finding changes the order of the differential diagnoses, but they all remain possible. A high temperature and lymph node enlargement around the jaw occur in all the differential diagnoses of a sore throat and is a poor differentiator. There was no tremor and lid lag to suggest inadequately treated thyrotoxicosis.

The fall in BP when the patient stands up always occurs at some point in postural hypotension and uncommonly in its other differential diagnoses.

Therefore, the order of the possible diagnoses has changed; this is shown in the problem-structuring note in Box 2.3. The format has also changed again from a three-column chart to heading and subheadings.

Box 2.3 Problem-structuring note No. 4

Outline findings: female. Aged 29. Severe sore throat for 2 days, getting worse. Taking carbimazole. Sudden loss of consciousness after getting up from chair, recovery within a minute. PMH of thyrotoxicosis. FH of type 2 diabetes mellitus. No tremor, no lid lag, reflexes normal. Large red tonsils, **linear creamy patches.** Fall in BP on standing.

Acute bacterial (or follicular) tonsillitis? (mainly streptococcal)
Outline evidence: severe sore throat for 2 days, getting worse (19/10/13). **Large red tonsils with linear creamy patches.**

Management: paracetamol 500mg 6 hourly PRN. Examine throat. Request WCC: ↑neutrophils?

Glandular fever (infectious mononucleosis due to Epstein–Barr virus)??
Outline evidence: severe sore throat for 2 days, getting worse (19/10/13). **Large red tonsils with linear creamy patches.**

Management: paracetamol 500mg 6 hourly PRN. Examine throat. Request WCC: lymphocytes atypical? Paul–Bunnell or Monospot® +ve?

Viral pharyngitis?? (less probable)
Outline evidence: severe sore throat for 2 days, getting worse (19/10/13). **Large red tonsils with linear creamy patches.**

Management: paracetamol 500mg 6 hourly PRN. Examine throat. Request WCC: ↓neutrophils, ↑lymphocytes?

Drug induced agranulocytosis? (less probable)
Outline evidence: severe sore throat for 2 days, getting worse (19/10/13). On carbimazole. **Large red tonsils with linear creamy patches.**

Management: paracetamol 500mg 6 hourly PRN. Request WCC: ↓granulocytes (neutrophils, eosinophils, basophils)?

Postural hypotension syncope? Due to dehydration from infection?
Outline evidence: sudden loss of consciousness after getting up from chair, recovery within a minute (19/10/13). **Fall in BP on standing.** Evidence of acute infection.

Management: request U&E. Consider fluids IV to rehydrate.

Thyrotoxicosis now controlled?
Outline evidence: anxiety, weight loss, abnormal thyroid tests in April 2008. No heat or cold intolerance. No tremor, no lid lag, reflexes normal.

Management: carbimazole 5mg od. FT4 and TSH normal?

Increased risk of type 2 diabetes mellitus
Outline evidence: FH of type 2 diabetes mellitus.

Management: test urine for sugar. Fasting glucose.

No domestic support
Outline evidence: alone in a flat at present. Parents 200 miles away.
Management: consider admission for initial care.

Interpreting the investigations

Investigations tend to be performed in a focused way like the physical examination. This means that they are done in order to differentiate between diagnostic possibilities created by the history and examination. However, urine testing, full blood count, urea and electrolytes (U&E), and CXR are often done routinely in the same way as aspects of the physical examination, such as the pulse, temperature, and BP. These are done in case that they will reveal a result that is a good diagnostic lead. This is a form of screening, but if the result is abnormal, then it is investigated in the same way as a presenting complaint. In this case, all the tests, except the CXR, were done in order to differentiate between the diagnostic possibilities, and most of the results were helpful.

> **Investigations**
>
> Urine testing: + glucose, no protein, no blood, no ketones
>
> FBC: Hb 12.4g/dL
> WCC 19.3×10^9/L, neutrophils 90%
> No atypical lymphocytes present
>
> Lab blood glucose 8.4mmol/L
> Na$^+$ 141mmol/L, K$^+$ 4.3mmol/L, urea 10.1mmol/L, creatinine 112micromol/L
> TSH, T4—results awaited
>
> Monospot® test—result awaited
> Throat swab—result awaited
>
> CXR normal

The presence of glucose in the urine and the random glucose of 8.4mmol/L is suspicious of diabetes mellitus. The WCC of 19.3×10^9/L with 90% neutrophils occurs commonly in bacterial tonsillitis, but never (by definition) in agranulocytosis. This is also very rare in viral pharyngitis and glandular fever so that all these diagnoses drop out of contention. The raised creatinine and urea are common in dehydration and less common in other causes of postural hypotension.

The problem-structuring note in Table 2.5 shows how the diagnostic opinions and management have changed in the light of these test results.

Medical and surgical sieves

At this point, you can pause and use the medical and surgical sieves from ➔ Medical and surgical sieves, p.14. You can consider whether you have omitted a diagnosis in the social background or environment, the locomotor, nervous, cardiovascular, respiratory, and alimentary systems, the renal system and urinary tract, and the reproductive, endocrine, autonomic, haematological, and immune systems. Within each of these systems, you can consider whether you have forgotten a congenital, infective, traumatic, neoplastic, or degenerative process. If not, you can move on.

Table 2.5 Problem-structuring note No. 5

Outline findings: female. Aged 29. Severe sore throat for 2 days, getting worse. Taking carbimazole. Sudden loss of consciousness after getting up from chair, recovery within a minute. PMH of thyrotoxicosis. FH of type 2 diabetes mellitus. No tremor, no lid lag. Large red tonsils with linear creamy patches. Fall in BP on standing. Urine testing: +ve glucose. Hb 12.4g/dL, WCC 19.310⁹/L, neutrophils 90%, no atypical lymphocytes present. Lab blood glucose 8.4mmol/L. Urea 10.1mmol/L. Creatinine 112micromol/L.

Acute bacterial (or follicular) tonsillitis (causing systemic effects, e.g. dehydration)	Severe sore throat for 2 days, getting worse (19/10/13). Large red tonsils with linear creamy patches. **WCC of 19.3x10⁹/L with 90% neutrophils.**	Paracetamol 500mg 6 hourly PRN. Begin phenoxymethylpenicillin 500mg qds.
Probably not glandular fever (infectious mononucleosis due to Epstein–Barr virus)?	Severe sore throat for 2 days, getting worse (19/10/13). Large red tonsils with linear creamy patches. **WCC of 19.3x10⁹/L with 90% neutrophils.**	Paracetamol 500mg 6 hourly PRN. Examine throat. Await Monospot® result.
Postural hypotension syncope? Due to dehydration from infection?	Sudden loss of consciousness after getting up from chair, recovery within a minute (19/10/13). Fall in BP on standing. Evidence of acute infection.	Fall in BP when standing. Request U&E. Consider fluids IV to rehydrate.
Dehydration from infection?	Fall in BP on standing. Evidence of acute infection. Urea 10.1mmol/L. Creatinine 112**micromol**/L.	Admit. Encourage oral fluids. For fluids IV if unable to drink 2L in 12h.
Thyrotoxicosis now controlled?	Anxiety, weight loss, abnormal thyroid function tests in April 2008. No heat or cold intolerance. No tremor or lid lag. Reflexes normal.	Carbimazole 5mg od. Await result of FT4 and TSH.
Probable type 2 diabetes mellitus	FH of type 2 diabetes mellitus. Urine glucose +ve. No ketones. Random glucose 8.4mmol/L.	Monitor blood sugar before and 2h after meals. Plan glucose tolerance test.
No domestic support	Alone in a flat at present. Parents 200 miles away.	Admit for initial care.

Writing the diagnosis and management

The positive finding summary could be written out as follows:

> *Female. Aged 29. Severe sore throat for 2 days, getting worse. Taking car-bimazole for 6 months. Sudden loss of consciousness after getting up from chair, recovery within a minute. PMH of thyrotoxicosis (anxiety, weight loss, abnormal thyroid function tests). FH of type 2 diabetes mellitus. Large red tonsils with linear creamy patches. Fall in BP on standing. Urine testing: +ve glucose. Hb 12.4g/dL, WCC 19.3×10⁹/L, neutrophils 90%, no atypical lym-phocytes present. Lab blood glucose 8.4mmol/L, urea 10.1mmol/L, creatinine 112 micromol/L.*

The primary diagnosis (that explains the symptoms that led the patient to seek help) can be written as:

> Primary diagnosis:
> • *Probable acute bacterial (or follicular) tonsillitis (causing systemic effects)*

The other diagnoses can be written as:

> Other diagnoses:
> • *Postural hypotension syncope due to dehydration from infection*
> • *Thyrotoxicosis probably now controlled*
> • *Probable type 2 diabetes mellitus*
> • *No domestic support currently*

The initial plan can be written as:

> Plan:
> • *Reassure patient that there is no agranulocytosis and explain other diagnoses*
> • *Start phenoxymethylpenicillin 500mg qds (because of systemic effects)*
> • *Continue paracetamol 1g qds*
> • *Continue carbimazole 5mg od*
> • *Encourage oral fluids (e.g. 2L in 16h)*
> • *Monitor blood glucose before and 2h after meals*
> • *Help patient to contact family*

It should be noted that this traditional way of writing out the findings does not give the reader an indication of the writer's thought process. It does not provide the particular evidence for each diagnosis or specify at which diagnosis each aspect of the management is directed. This is the approach mostly used in discharge summaries when patients are discharged from hospital. In contrast to this, the problem-structuring notes used here do provide this information.

Case presentations

If you are asked to give a case presentation, then in addition to the positive findings, you should mention negative features. These will imply that you have considered other diagnoses, but were unable to find the supportive features (i.e. that you considered those negative findings to differentiate between your probable diagnosis and those you consider improbable). The information that you require for your case presentation will be found in the 'evidence' column of the latest version of your problem-structuring notes. It is customary to give the history of presenting complaint in some detail, as follows in Box 2.4.

Box 2.4 Case presentation of Ms AM

Ms AM is a 29-year old secretary who came to the A&E department with a severe sore throat, sweats and malaise for 2 days. She also lost consciousness briefly in A&E 30 minutes after arriving.

*She was well until last Friday afternoon 18 October when she developed a **sore throat** at work. It was relieved that day by warm drinks and paracetamol, but when she woke this morning, it was very severe. She remembered that she had been told to report sore throats because she was taking carbimazole and to get a white cell count. She was worried that she might have developed a low white cell count because of this drug. She came to A&E because it was a Saturday morning. When she got up from her seat in the waiting room after being called, she felt dizzy, 'blacked out', and fell to the floor, striking her head. She recovered consciousness within a minute.*

There is a past medical history of thyrotoxicosis (as evidenced last April by anxiety, weight loss, abnormal thyroid function tests). There is a family history of type 2 diabetes mellitus. She shares a flat with a friend who is away at present.

On examination, she looked tired and unwell. Her temperature was 38.5. Her pharynx was red with enlarged tonsils, which showed linear creamy patches. There was lymph node enlargement in the angles of the jaw but not elsewhere. Her pulse was 110/min and regular. The BP was 110/70 reclining and 90/50 standing. The heart sounds were normal and there were no murmurs. The chest was clear. The abdomen was soft and there was no splenic enlargement.

Urine testing showed one plus of glucose but no ketones. The white cell count was 19.3×10^9/L, the neutrophils being 90%. There were no atypical lymphocytes present. The laboratory random blood glucose was 8.4mmol/L, the urea was 10.1mmol/L and the creatinine 112micromol/L.

Clinical opinions

After giving a case presentation, you will be asked to give a clinical opinion and expected to provide the (particular) evidence for your diagnoses. You may be asked if you do not volunteer this information first. The opinion could be based on the latest problem-structuring note.

Clinical opinion on Ms AM

The probable diagnosis is acute follicular tonsillitis (causing systemic effects, e.g. dehydration). This is because she has had a severe sore throat for 2d, there were large red tonsils with linear creamy patches and a white cell count of 19.3×10^9/L with 90% neutrophils. This should be treated with benzyl-penicillin IM or Penicillin V orally because of the systemic effects and the symptoms treated with paracetamol.

There is probably no infectious mononucleosis or agranulocytosis because of the raised neutrophils and absence of atypical lymphocytes. She should be reassured about this.

She has suffered postural hypotension syncope because of the sudden loss of consciousness after getting up from chair with recovery within a minute and the fall in BP on standing. She should not be discharged home until this problem has resolved with rehydration.

She is probably dehydrated from infection because of the pulse of 110/min, fall in BP on standing, urea of 10.1mmol/L, and creatinine of 110micromol/L. Fluids need to be encouraged.

The thyrotoxicosis appears to be controlled. The original anxiety and weight loss have resolved and there was no heat or cold intolerance. There was no tremor or lid lag. She should continue on carbimazole 5mg od, pending the result of T4 and TSH measurements.

She probably has type 2 diabetes mellitus because of the FH of this and the random blood sugar of 8.4mmol/L with no urine ketones. She is to have two fasting blood sugars, and her blood sugars monitored before and 2 hours after meals during the admission. A glucose tolerance test will be done if the fasting sugar is not less than 5.6mmol/L or not more than 7.0mmol/L on two occasions.

She has little domestic support because she lives alone in her flat this weekend and her parents live 200 miles away. She will be admitted and kept in hospital until she is well enough to self-care.

The 'open mind' approach

The preceding paragraphs described how diagnostic hypotheses were generated as soon as the presenting complaints had been heard. These were displayed in the problem-structuring notes. This approach requires the history taker to have the knowledge to identify the best leads and to know which items of information will differentiate between the possible diagnoses. Alternatively, it depends on the history taker looking up the information in the OHCD at different stages in the history and examination and when the test results become available.

The other option is to take the history and to examine the patient in a mechanical way, without interpreting the findings as they are discovered. The abnormal findings can then be listed at the end and then looked up in the OHCD. The thought process would then follow the same pattern as that described in the problem-structuring notes.

As the history and examination is being performed and the results become known, differential diagnoses may also occur to the assessor consciously or subconsciously in a passive way. This will depend on the assessor's knowledge, which can be helped by reading this book during private study. This can be done by covering the list of diagnoses, looking at the diagnostic lead above the list, and then reading the suggestive and confirmatory findings. The reader should then try to guess the hidden diagnosis and then see if he or she was correct.

The plan of the remainder of this book

An example of a systems enquiry has been given already in ⊃ The systems enquiry, p.32. The following shows a typical example of the routine physical examination on which the remainder of this book is based.

The 'routine' physical examination

Note the patient's attire, presence of nebulizer masks, sputum pots, medication packets, etc. The general examination is directed mainly at assessing the skin and reticulo-endothelial system (lymph nodes), and the related matters of temperature control and metabolic rate. During the history, the order of questioning could be decided entirely by thought processes (e.g. probing indirectly for a symptom to chase up a diagnostic possibility that comes to mind), but the physical examination is different. It is more efficient to adopt a routine that is smooth and quick, and not to jump about looking for physical signs that might support the diagnostic idea of that moment.

You have already been looking at the patient's face, general appearance, and immediate vicinity (e.g. walking stick, medication packets, etc.) when taking the history. So for the general examination, begin with the hands and work your way up by inspecting (and, when appropriate, palpating) the arms to the shoulders, examine the scalp, ears, eyes, cheeks, nose, lips, take the temperature, examine inside the mouth, then the neck, breasts, axillae, and then the skin of the abdomen, legs, and feet.

Plan of the general examination

Hands, arms, and shoulders

- *Fingernails*
- *Clubbing*
- *Finger nodules*
- *Finger joint deformity*
- *Rashes*
- *Pain and stiffness in the elbow, shoulder, neck.*

Head and neck

- *Neck stiffness*
- *Patchy hair loss*
- *Eardrum redness*
- *Perforated eardrum.*

Eyes, face, and neck

- *Facial redness, general appearance*
- *Red eye*
- *Iritis*
- *Conjunctival pallor*
- *Temperature—high or low*
- *Mouth lesions*
- *Lumps in the:*
  - *Face*
  - *Submandibular region*
  - *Anterior neck*
  - *Anterior triangle of neck*
  - *Posterior triangle*
  - *Supraclavicular region.*

Trunk

- *Breast discharge*
- *Nipple eczema*
- *Breast lumps*
- *Gynaecomastia in male*
- *Axillary lymphadenopathy*
- *Sparse body hair*
- *Hirsutism*
- *Scar pigmentation*
- *Abdominal striae.*

Legs

- *Inguinal and generalized lymphadenopathy*
- *Sacral, leg, and heel sores.*

Cardiovascular system

Think first of cardiac output, and inspect and feel the hands for warmth or coldness. Feel the radial pulse, take the BP, and check the other pulses in the arms and neck. Next think of venous return and look at the jugular venous pressure (JVP). Then examine the heart itself (palpate, percuss, and then listen to it). Finally, examine output and venous return in the legs by feeling skin temperature, pulses, and looking for oedema of the legs, liver, and lungs.

Cardiac output

- *Peripheral cyanosis*
- *Radial pulse*
  - *Rate*
  - *Rhythm (compare cardiac apex rate, if irregular)*
  - *Amplitude*
  - *Vessel wall*
- *Compare pulses for volume and synchrony*
  Radial, brachial, carotid, (femoral, popliteal, posterior, and anterior tibials after the examining the heart)
- *BP standing and lying in right arm, repeat on left.*

Venous return

- *JVP*

The heart

- *Trachea displaced?*
- *Apex beat displaced?*
- *Parasternal heave*
- *Palpable thrill*
- *Auscultation*
  - *Extra heart sounds*
    —Systolic murmurs
    —Diastolic murmurs.

Cardiac output and venous return in the legs

- *Skin temperature*
- *Posterior and anterior tibials, popliteal, femoral*
- *Venous skin changes*
- *Vein abnormalities*
- *Calf swelling*
- *Leg oedema*
- *Sacral oedema*
- *Liver enlargement*
- *Basal lung crackles.*

Respiratory system

Think of general respiratory structure and function. *Inspect* and think of oxygen and carbon dioxide levels, then the ventilation process, which depends on the chest wall and its movement. *Palpate* by feeling for tactile vocal fremitus. *Percuss* and then *auscultate*. Finally, listen for wheezes, thus assessing airways, from small (high-pitched) to large (low-pitched).

General inspection
- *Tremor and muscle twitching*
- *Cyanosis of the tongue and lips*
- *Clubbing.*

Chest inspection
- *Respiratory rate*
- *Distorted chest wall*
- *Poor expansion*
- *Paradoxical movement.*

Palpation
- *Mediastinum*
  - *Position of trachea*
  - *Position of apex beat.*

Tactile vocal fremitus
- *Present or absent (or increased).*

Percussion
- *Hyper-resonant, resonant, normal, dull, or stony dull.*

Auscultation
- *Diminished breath sounds*
- *Bronchial breathing*
- *Crackles*
- *Rubs*
- *Wheezes, high- or low-pitched, or polyphonic during inspiration and expiration.*

Alimentary and genitourinary systems

Think first of metabolic issues related to general nutrition (obese, normal, thin, cachexia) and ensure that the patient is weighed. Check the mucous membranes, e.g. for signs of vitamin deficiency. Look for skin and eye signs of low fluid volume, and then liver disease. Next, turn your mind to anatomical aspects of the gastrointestinal and genitourinary systems together by inspecting, palpating, and auscultating. Finally, perform examinations (when indicated) that need special equipment, and do the urine tests.

Inspection
- *Obesity*
- *Cachexia*
- *Oral lesions*
- *Jaundice*
- *Hepatic skin stigmata*
- *Loss of skin turgor*
- *Low eye tension.*

Palpation
- *Supraclavicular nodes.*

Inspection of the abdomen
- *Abdominal scars*
- *Veins*
- *General distension*
- *Visible peristalsis*
- *Poor movement.*

Palpation
- *General tenderness*
- *Localized tenderness*
- *Hepatic enlargement*
- *Splenic enlargement*
- *Renal enlargement*
- *Abdominal masses.*

Percussion
- *Dull or resonant*
- *Shifting dullness.*

Auscultation
- *Silent abdomen*
- *Tinkling bowel sounds*
- *Bruits.*

Inspection and palpation again

- *Groin lumps (lymph nodes?)*
- *Scrotal masses*
- *Rectal abnormalities*
- *Melaena, fresh blood*
- *Vaginal and pelvic abnormalities*
- *Urine abnormalities.*

Nervous system

If there are no neurological symptoms or signs detected up to this point, then it is customary to perform an abbreviated examination. This is done by commenting on the fact that the patient was conscious and alert, speech was normal, and that there were no cranial nerve abnormalities noted when looking at the face during the history and general examination. Also, you will have been able to note the patient's gait and movements around the hospital bed or consultation room. According to the GALS system, note and record the *Gait*, appearance, and movement of the *A*rms, *L*egs, and *S*pine.

If the patient was not conscious and alert, then the level of consciousness has to be addressed with the Glasgow Coma Scale.

The brief neurological examination consists of checking coordination and reflexes (because this tests the sensory and motor function of the nerves and central connections involved). The findings may be recorded as in Box 2.5.

Box 2.5 Short CNS examination

- Conscious and alert
- Speech normal
- Facial appearance and movement normal
- Finger–nose pointing normal
- Hand tapping and rotating normal
- Heel–toe test normal (ran heel from opposite knee to toe and back)
- Foot tapping (examiner's hand) normal
- Reflexes (Table 2.6)

Table 2.6 Short CNS examination: reflexes

Reflexes	Right	Left
Biceps normal	+	+
Supinators normal	+	+
Triceps normal	+	+
Knees normal	+	+
Ankles normal	+	+
Plantars normally flexor	↓	↓

The full neurological assessment

The system of examination described here is typical. The general approach is to assess the conscious level (if the patient is not conscious and alert, then it will not be possible to conduct a full neurological examination, which needs the patient's cooperation).

The cranial nerve sequence follows in their numbered sequence. Motor function can be assessed next, beginning with inspection for wasting and involuntary movements, and then 'palpation' by testing tone and power. The upper limbs are examined first and then the lower limbs. Sensation is then tested in the upper, then lower limbs, and finally coordination, reflexes, and gait. The order can be changed by addressing the area of abnormality suggested by the history. For example, if the patient complains of difficulty in walking, then it would be sensible to examine gait, then motor and sensory function, and cranial nerves last.

Nervous system
- Conscious level
- Glasgow Coma Score
- Speech.

Cranial nerves
- Absent sense of smell
- Visual field defects
- Decreased acuity.

Ophthalmoscopy
- Corneal opacity
- Lens opacity
- Papilloedema
- Pale optic disc
- Cupped disc
- Hypertensive retinopathy
- Dot and blot haemorrhages
- New vessel formation
- Pale/black retinal patches
- Ptosis
- Pupil
  - Constriction
  - Irregularities
  - Dilatation
- Diplopia
- Nystagmus
- Absent corneal reflex
- Loss of facial sensation
- Deviation of jaw
- Jaw jerk
- Facial weakness
- Deafness
- Loss of taste
- Palatal weakness
- Neck or shoulder weakness
- Paresis of tongue.

Motor function

Upper limbs
- Arm posture
- Hand tremor
- Wasting of hand
- Wasting of arm
- Tone abnormalities.

Weakness of
- Shoulder abduction and addiction
- Elbow flexion
- Elbow extension
- Wrist extension and flexion
- Handgrip
- Finger adduction and abduction
- Thumb abduction and opposition
- Arm incoordination.

Lower limbs
- Limitation of movement
- Wasting
- Fasciculation
- Tone abnormalities.

Weakness of
- Hip flexion
- Knee extension and flexion
- Foot
  - Plantar flexion
  - Dorsiflexion
  - Eversion and inversion
- Bilateral spastic paraparesis
- Spastic hemiparesis.

Sensation

Upper limb sensation
- Hypoaesthesia of
  - Palm
  - Dorsum of hand
  - Lateral arm
  - Ulnar border of arm
- Dissociated sensory loss
- Progressive sensory loss
- Cortical sensory loss.

Lower limb
- Hypoaesthesia of
  - Inguinal area
  - Anterior thigh
  - Shin
  - Lateral foot
- Progressive downward loss
- Dissociated sensory loss
- Multiple areas of loss.

Reflexes
- Brisk or
- Diminished, in biceps, supinator, triceps, knee, ankle, and plantars
- Gait abnormalities.

Mental state examination

Think of the sequence of perception, 'affect', drive and arousal, cognitive processes (check memory of different duration, ability to reason with that memory, and then the nature of beliefs arrived at with such reasoning), and then actions in response to these:

- *Perception*: attentiveness and any hallucination, visual or auditory
- *Mood*: depression or elation
- *Mental: drive* rate of speech, anxiety
- *Cognition*: (6/10 or less correct implies impairment)
- *Orientation*: time to nearest hour, year, address of hospital
- *Short-term memory*: repeat a given name and address, name 2 staff
- *Long-term memory*: own age, date of birth, current monarch, dates of wars
- *Concentration*: count backwards from 20 to 1
- *Beliefs*: patient's perception and insight of health, self-confidence, any extreme convictions
- *Activity*: physical and social activity, employment, physical signs of drug use.

Basic blood and urine test results

First check the patient's name, gender, age, and address to make sure whose sample you are handling and whose results you are interpreting. The following are interpreted in Chapter 11:

Urine testing
- *Microscopic haematuria*
- *Asymptomatic proteinuria*
- *Glycosuria*
- *Raised urine or plasma bilirubin*
  - *Hepatocellular jaundice*
  - *Obstructive jaundice.*

Biochemistry
- *Hypernatraemia*
- *Hyponatraemia*
- *Hyperkalaemia*
- *Hypokalaemia*
- *Hypercalcaemia*
- *Hypocalcaemia*
- *Raised alkaline phosphatase.*

Haematology
- *Low haemoglobin*
- *Microcytic anaemia*
- *Macrocytic anaemia*
- *Normocytic anaemia*
- *Very high ESR or CRP.*

Abnormal chest X-ray appearances

Many CXR appearances may be recognizable immediately as indicating a specific diagnosis, but if not, the following appearances are considered in Chapter 12:

- Area of uniform opacification with a well-defined border
- Rounded opacity (or opacities)
- Multiple 'nodular' shadows and 'miliary mottling'
- Diffuse, poorly defined hazy opacification
- Increased linear markings
- Dark lung/lungs
- Abnormal hilar shadowing
- Upper mediastinal widening
- Abnormal cardiac shadow.

Reference

1. Llewelyn DEH, Ewins DL, Horn J, Evans TGR, McGregor AM (1988). Computerised updating of clinical summaries: new opportunities for clinical practice and research. *BMJ* 297, 1504–6.

General and endocrine symptoms and physical signs

General principles 62
Fingernail abnormality 64
Clubbing 66
Terry's lines: dark pink or brown bands on nails 68
Vasculitic nodules on fingers 69
Hand arthropathy 70
Lumps around the elbow 71
Neck stiffness 72
Hair loss in a specific area 74
Diffuse hair loss 75
External ear abnormalities 76
Painful ear 78
Discharging ear 80
Striking facial appearance 82
Proptosis of eye(s) or exophthalmos 84
Red eye 86
Iritis (anterior uveitis) 88
Clinical anaemia 90
Fever 91
Low body temperature 91
Mouth lesions 92
Red pharynx and tonsils 93
'Parotid' swelling 94
Lump in the face (non-parotid lesion) 95
Submandibular lump—not moving with tongue protrusion or on swallowing 96
Anterior neck lump—moving with tongue protrusion and swallowing 98

Neck lump—moving with swallowing but not with tongue protrusion 99
Bilateral neck mass—moving with swallowing but not with tongue protrusion 100
Solitary thyroid nodule 101
Lump in anterior triangle of neck 102
Lump in posterior triangle of neck 103
Supraclavicular lump(s) 104
Galactorrhoea 105
Nipple abnormality 106
Breast lump(s) 107
Gynaecomastia 108
Axillary lymphadenopathy 110
Hirsutism in a female 111
Abdominal striae 112
Obesity 113
Pigmented creases and flexures (and buccal mucosa) 114
Spider naevi 115
Thin, wasted, cachectic 116
Purpura 118
Generalized lymphadenopathy 120
Localized groin lymphadenopathy 122
Pressure sores 122

General principles

The findings are discussed in a sequence of the general examination. You will have been looking at the patient's face during the history. Begin with the fingernails and joints, backs and fronts of hands, arms, elbows, moving up to the neck and scalp, then down to the face, mouth, the throat, the breasts, axillae, trunk, and groin. Note any skin abnormalities.

Findings with endocrine causes

- Diffuse hair loss, p.75
- Striking facial appearance, p.82
- Proptosis of eye(s) or exophthalmos, p.84
- Low body temperature, p.91
- Solitary thyroid nodule, p.101
- Galactorrhoea, p.105
- Gynaecomastia, p.108
- Hirsutism in a female, p.111
- Abdominal striae, p.112
- Obesity, p.113
- Pigmented creases and flexures (and buccal mucosa), p.114

Fingernail abnormality

Classify fingernail changes by 'naming' them first. Some have few causes and are good diagnostic leads.

Classification	
Clubbing **due to many causes (see ⊃ Clubbing, p.66)**	*Confirmed by*: angle lost between nail and finger (no gap when nails of same finger on both hands apposed, bogginess of nail bed, increased nail curvature, both longitudinally and transversely, and drumstick finger appearance).
Terry's lines **due to many causes (see ⊃ Terry's lines: dark pink or brown bands on nails, p.68)**	*Confirmed by*: nail tips having dark pink or brown bands.
Nail fold infarcts **due to vasculitis due to many causes (see ⊃ Vasculitic nodules on fingers, p.69)**	*Confirmed by*: dark blue-black areas in nail fold.
Koilonychia **due to iron deficiency anaemia (occasionally ischaemic heart disease or syphilis)**	*Suggested by*: spoon-shaped nails. *Confirmed by*: ↓Hb, ↓ferritin from iron deficiency (basal or exercise **ECG** for ischaemic heart disease; **serology** for syphilis).
Onycholysis **due to psoriasis, hyperthyroidism**	*Suggested by*: nail thickened, dystrophic, and separated from the nail bed. *Confirmed by*: clinical appearance and evidence of cause, e.g. skin changes of psoriasis or ↑**FT4** ± ↑**FT3** and ↓**TSH.**
Beau's lines **due to any period of severe illness**	*Suggested by*: transverse furrows. *Confirmed by*: history of associated condition.
Longitudinal lines **due to lichen planus, alopecia areata, Darier's disease**	*Suggested by*: transverse furrows (ending in triangular nicks and nail dystrophy in Darier's disease).
Onychomedesis **due to any period of severe illness**	*Suggested by*: shedding of nail. *Confirmed by*: history of associated condition.

Muehrcke's lines **due to** **hypoalbuminaemia**	*Suggested by:* paired, white, parallel, transverse bands. *Confirmed by:* serum albumin <20g/L.
Nail pitting **due to psoriasis or** **alopecia areata**	*Suggested by:* small holes in nail. *Confirmed by:* rash on extensor surfaces with silvery scales (psoriasis) or circumscribed areas of hair loss (alopecia areata).
Splinter haemorrhages **due to infective** **endocarditis (sometimes** **due to manual labour)**	*Suggested by:* fine, longitudinal, haemorrhagic streaks under the nail. *Confirmed by:* history of manual labour (or fever, changing heart murmurs, and bacterial growth on several **blood cultures**).
Chronic paronychia **due to chronic infection** **of nail bed**	*Suggested by:* red, swollen, and thickened skin in nail fold. *Confirmed by:* response to antibiotics (erythromycin for bacterial infection or nystatin for fungal infection).
Mees' lines **due to arsenic poisoning** **or renal failure, Hodgkin's** **disease, heart failure**	*Suggested by:* single, white, transverse bands. *Confirmed by:* presence of associated conditions.
'Yellow' nails **due to lymphoedema,** **bronchiectasis,** **hypoalbuminaemia**	*Suggested by:* colour! *Confirmed by:* presence of associated condition.

Clubbing

Present when the angle is lost between nail and finger (no gap when nails of same finger on each hand apposed). Initial investigations: FBC, ESR/CRP, CXR. Subsequent tests depend on other evidence below and the possibilities suggested.

Main differential diagnoses and typical outline evidence, etc.	
Subacute bacterial endocarditis	*Suggested by:* general malaise, weight loss, pallor, low-grade fever, changing heart murmurs ± past medical history (PMH) of valve or congenital heart disease. **FBC**: ↓Hb, ↑WBC, ↑↑**ESR**, ↑↑**CRP**. *Confirmed by:* growth of organism, e.g. *Streptococcus viridians* after **serial blood cultures** ± endocardial vegetations on **transoesophageal echocardiography.** *Finalized by the predictable outcome of management,* e.g. treatment on high index of suspicion, hospital admission, avoidance of antibiotics before blood cultures, initial benzylpenicillin and gentamicin IV for 4wk with gentamicin levels.
Cyanotic congenital heart disease	*Suggested by:* long past history, central cyanosis. *Confirmed by:* **echocardiogram** appearances. *Finalized by the predictable outcome of management,* e.g. O_2 therapy, treatment of heart failure and infection, surgical intervention.
Bronchial carcinoma	*Suggested by:* malaise, increased cough, weight loss, haemoptysis. Smoking history. Opacity (suggestive of mass ± pneumonia ± effusion) on **CXR** and **CT scan**. *Confirmed by:* **bronchoscopy** appearances and histology. *Finalized by the predictable outcome of management,* e.g. control of pain and infection. Non-small cell tumours: excision, radiotherapy, or combined radiotherapy and chemotherapy depending on staging. Small cell tumours: chemotherapy or palliative radiotherapy.
Bronchiectasis	*Suggested by:* chronic cough, productive of copious purulent, often rusty-coloured sputum. *Confirmed by:* **CXR** and **CT scan**: thickened 'tram line' (dilated) bronchi. **Bronchoscopy** appearances. *Finalized by the predictable outcome of management,* e.g. postural drainage, antibiotics according to sputum culture and sensitivity, bronchodilators (e.g. nebulized salbutamol), steroids (e.g. prednisolone), surgerical removal of affected segments.
Lung abscess	*Suggested by:* cough, very ill, spiking fever, PMH of lung disease. *Confirmed by:* **CXR**: mass containing fluid level (air above pus). *Finalized by the predictable outcome of management,* e.g. antibiotics according to sputum culture and sensitivity for up to 6wk, aspiration, and antibiotic instillation, surgical excision.

Empyema	*Suggested by:* cough, being very ill, fever, stony dull over one lung.
	Confirmed by: neutrophilia. **CXR**: long opacity on one view. Aspiration of pus, culture and sensitivity.
	Finalized by the predictable outcome of management, e.g. antibiotics, chest drain.
Fibrosing alveolitis	*Suggested by:* cough, fine crackles, especially bases.
	Confirmed by: **CXR + HRCT**: bilateral diffuse nodular shadows or honeycombing (late finding).
	Finalized by the predictable outcome of management, e.g. oral steroids (e.g. prednisolone) for up to 4mo, immunosuppressants (e.g. azathioprine), or both.
Hepatic cirrhosis	*Suggested by:* long history of liver disease, e.g. due to high alcohol intake, ascites, U&E and CXRs, prominent abdominal veins. In males: spider naevi, gynaecomastia.
	Confirmed by: ↓**serum albumin**, abnormal **liver function tests. (LFTs) and liver biopsy** findings.
	Finalized by the predictable outcome of management, e.g. no alcohol, low-salt diet if ascites, vitamin K **if** ↑ **prothrombin time**, anti-flu and pneumococcal vaccination, colestyramine if pruritus.
Crohn's disease	*Suggested by:* history of chronic diarrhoea and abdominal pain, low weight.
	Confirmed by: **colonoscopy and biopsy, barium enema,** and **barium meal and follow-through.**
	Finalized by the predictable outcome of management, e.g. oral prednisolone if mild, IV if severe, immunosuppressants (e.g. methotrexate), immunotherapy (e.g. infliximab).
Ulcerative colitis	*Suggested by:* history of intermittent diarrhoea with blood and mucus, low weight.
	Confirmed by: **colonoscopy** and **biopsy.**
	Finalized by the predictable outcome of management, e.g. prednisolone PO + mesalazine, prednisolone enema; hydrocortisone IV if severe followed by prednisolone PO and sulfasalazine ± surgery.
Normal variant or familial clubbing	*Suggested by:* incidental finding with no symptoms or signs of any other illness that could act as a pathological cause and± family history.
	Confirmed by: FBC, U&E, and CXR showing no findings that could explain clubbing.
	Finalized by the predictable outcome of management, e.g. reassurance and follow up resulting in no subsequent explanatory illness.

Terry's lines: dark pink or brown bands on nails

Initial investigations: FBC, LFT, CXR, ESR/CRP. Subsequent tests depend on other evidence:

Main differential diagnoses and typical outline evidence, etc.	
Hepatic cirrhosis	*Suggested by:* long history of liver disease, e.g. due to high alcohol intake, ascites, prominent abdominal veins. In males: spider naevi, gynaecomastia. *Confirmed by:* ↓**serum albumin**, abnormal **LFTs. Liver biopsy** findings. *Finalized by the predictable outcome of management,* e.g. no alcohol, low salt diet if ascites, vitamin K **if ↑ prothrombin time**, anti-flu and pneumococcal vaccination, colestyramine for pruritus.
Congestive cardiac failure	*Suggested by:* dyspnoea, orthopnoea, paroxysmal nocturnal dyspnoea (PND), ↑JVP, gallop rhythm, basal inspiratory crackles, ankle oedema. *Confirmed by:* **CXR** and **echocardiography.** *Finalized by the predictable outcome of management,* e.g. diuretics (e.g. furosemide), ACE inhibitors (e.g. ramipril), β-blockers (e.g. bisoprolol), spironolactone, and digoxin.
Diabetes mellitus (DM)	*Suggested by:* thirst, polydipsia, polyuria, fatigue, family history. *Confirmed by:* **fasting blood glucose** ≥7.0mmol/L on two occasions OR fasting, random or 2h GTT glucose ≥11.1mmol/L once only with symptoms or HbA1c > 48mmol/mol (6.5%). *Finalized by the predictable outcome of management,* e.g. diabetic diet, lifestyle advice, e.g. exercise, no smoking. Insulin for type 1 diabetes mellitus. Metformin, sulphonylureas, gliptins and GLP-1 agonists, SGLT2 inhibitors, insulin for type 2 DM.
Cancer somewhere	*Suggested by:* weight loss and anorexia with symptoms developing over months, bone pain. *Confirmed by:* careful history, examination, **CXR, FBC, ESR,** and follow-up.
Old age	*Suggested by:* age >75y. *Confirmed by:* no other illness discovered on follow-up.

Vasculitic nodules on fingers

Nodules and dark lines in nail folds are focal areas of infarction, which suggest local vasculitis. Initial investigations: FBC, ESR/CRP. Subsequent tests depend on other evidence:

Main differential diagnoses and typical outline evidence, etc.	
Systemic lupus erythematosus (SLE)	*Suggested by:* swelling of distal interphalangeal (IP) joints, any other large joints, malar rash, pleural effusion, especially in Afro-Caribbean females. Multisystem dysfunction.
	Confirmed by: **FBC**: ↓Hb, ↓WBC. ↑**ESR** or ↑**CRP. Anti-nuclear antibody** +ve, especially if directed at **double-stranded DNA.**
	Finalized by the predictable outcome of management, e.g. NSAIDs for mild disease, topical steroids, sunblocks for rashes, antimalarials, e.g. hydroxychloroquine for joint pain. For systemic disease and renal disease: oral steroids and immunosuppressants. Plasmapharesis for severe cases.
Subacute bacterialendocarditis ('Osler nodes')	*Suggested by:* general malaise, weight loss, pallor, low-grade fever, changing heart murmurs ± PMH of valve or congenital heart disease. **FBC**: ↓Hb, ↑WCC. ↑↑ESR, ↑↑**CRP**.
	Confirmed by: growth of organism, e.g. *Streptococcus viridians* after **serial blood cultures** ± endocardial vegetations on **transoesophageal echocardiography.**
	Finalized by the predictable outcome of management, e.g. avoidance of antibiotics before blood cultures, initial benzylpenicillin and gentamicin IV pending culture results.

Hand arthropathy

Look at the finger joints (IP joints), the knuckles (the metacarpophalangeal or MCP joints), and compare. Finally, look at the wrist. Initial investigations: FBC, RF, ANA, X-ray hands. Subsequent tests depend on other evidence:

Main differential diagnoses and typical outline evidence, etc.	
Primary (post-menopausal) osteoarthrosis	*Suggested by:* Heberden's nodes (paired bony nodes on terminal IP joints). *Confirmed by:* **X-ray** appearances of affected joints. *Finalized by the predictable outcome of management,* e.g. analgesics and NSAIDs if not contraindicated + gastric acid reduction, e.g. proton pump inhibitor (PPI).
Rheumatoid arthritis (RA)	*Suggested by:* swelling and deformity of phalangeal joints (with ulnar deviation), of wrist, and 'rheumatoid nodules'. *Confirmed by:* +ve **rheumatoid factor. X-ray** appearances of affected joints. *Finalized by the predictable outcome of management,* e.g. physiotherapy and occupational therapies, analgesics, and NSAIDs + gastric acid reduction (e.g. PPI), low- dose prednisolone, disease-modifying drugs (DMARDs) (e.g. methotrexate), immunotherapy, e.g. infliximab.
Psoriatic arthropathy	*Suggested by:* swelling and deformity of distal (or all) IP joints. **X-ray** appearances of affected joints. *Confirmed by:* dry rash with silvery scales (especially near elbow extensor surface). *Finalized by the predictable outcome of management,* e.g. NSAIDs, e.g. diclofenac + gastric acid reduction (e.g. PPI), DMARDS, e.g. methotrexate, leflunomide; immunotherapy e.g. infliximab.
SLE	*Suggested by:* swelling and deformity of all (or distal) IP joints, butterfly facial rash, signs of pleural/pericardial effusion, renal impairment. *Confirmed by:* +ve **anti-nuclear factor,** ↑ double stranded **DNA antibodies.** *Finalized by the predictable outcome of management,* e.g. NSAIDs for mild disease, sunblocks and topical steroids for rashes, antimalarials, e.g. hydroxychloroquine for joint pain, for systemic or renal disease, oral steroids and immunosuppressants. Plasmapharesis for severe cases.

Lumps around the elbow

Inspect and palpate with care so as not to hurt the patient. Initial investigations: FBC, RF, Pl urate, X-ray elbow. Subsequent tests depend on other evidence:

Main differential diagnoses and typical outline evidence, etc.	
Osteoarthritis	*Suggested by:* joint deformity, intermittent pain and swelling, paired Heberden's nodes over distal I-P joints in primary osteoarthritis. *Confirmed by:* clinical appearance if gross. If mild, **X-ray** showing loss of joint space (due to atrophy of cartilage) and −ve **rheumatoid factor.** *Finalized by the predictable outcome of management,* e.g. analgesics and NSAIDs + gastric acid reduction, e.g. PPI.
Rheumatoid nodules	*Suggested by:* mobile subcutaneous nodule. *Confirmed by:* history or joint changes of rheumatoid arthritis and +ve **rheumatoid factor.** *Finalized by the predictable outcome of management,* e.g. physiotherapy and occupational therapies, analgesics and NSAIDs + gastric acid reduction (e.g. PPI), low dose prednisolone, DMARDs (e.g. methotrexate), immunotherapy, e.g. infliximab.
Xanthomatosis	*Suggested by:* pale subcutaneous plaques attached to underlying tendon. *Confirmed by:* **hyperlipidaemia** on blood testing. *Finalized by the predictable outcome of management,* e.g. treatment of hyperlipidaemia, excision or electrocautery if unsightliness remains.
Gouty tophi	*Suggested by:* irregular hard nodules, risk factors or PMH of gout. *Confirmed by:* ↑**plasma urate. Biopsy:** urate crystals present. *Finalized by the predictable outcome of management,* e.g. allopurinol, local excision of tophi if required.

Neck stiffness

Distinguish between limited range of neck movement and neck stiffness throughout range of movement. Initial investigations: FBC, X-ray neck. (Other tests in **bold**:)

- Limited neck range of movement.

Main differential diagnoses and typical outline evidence, etc.	
Chronic cervical spondylosis with osteophytes	*Suggested by:* no fever or associated symptoms. *Confirmed by:* limitation in range of neck movement, but no stiffness within free range of movement. **WCC** normal, no fever, no neurological signs, **neck X-ray** appearance. *Finalized by the predictable outcome of management,* e.g. analgesics, muscle relaxants, and NSAIDs (if no contraindication) + gastric acid reduction (e.g. PPI), intermittent cervical collar, physiotherapy.

- Neck stiffness throughout range of movement.

Bacterial meningitis	*Suggested by:* gradual headache over days, photophobia, vomiting. Fever, ↑neutrophil count. Petechial rash (in meningococcal meningitis). *Confirmed by:* **lumbar puncture**: turbid CSF, ↑CSF neutrophil count with ↓glucose. Bacteria on microscopy. Growth of bacteria on culture of CSF. *Finalized by the predictable outcome of management,* e.g. ABC (airway, breathing, circulation) benzylpenicillin IV/IM while awaiting transport to hospital (cefotaxime for penicillin allergic patients), gain IV access, contact tracing, and treatment.
Viral meningitis	*Suggested by:* gradual headache over days. Fever, ↑lymphocyte count, normal neutrophil count. *Confirmed by:* **lumbar puncture**: clear CSF. ↑CSF lymphocyte count with normal glucose. No bacteria on microscopy. No growth of bacteria on CSF culture. *Finalized by the predictable outcome of management,* e.g. analgesia, reassurance that illness is self-limiting; if features suspicious of encephalitis, aciclovir.
Meningism due to viral infection	*Suggested by:* gradual headache over days. Fever, ↑lymphocyte count, normal neutrophil count. *Confirmed by:* **lumbar puncture**: clear CSF. Normal CSF white cell count. No bacteria on microscopy. No growth of bacteria on CSF culture. *Finalized by the predictable outcome of management,* e.g. analgesia, reassurance that illness is self-limiting.

Subarachnoid haemorrhage	*Suggested by:* sudden onset of headache over seconds. Variable degree of consciousness. No fever. Normal WCC.
	Confirmed by: **CT or MRI brain scan appearance. Lumbar puncture:** bloodstained CSF that does not clear in successive bottle collection (may be negative if <2h after the bleed, or presence of xanthochromia in CSF (12h to 2wk after the haemorrhage).
	Finalized by the predictable outcome of management, e.g. discussion with neurosurgeons, regular monitoring of vital signs and Glasgow coma scale. If no rebleeding, clipping of an aneurysm ± clot evacuation if surgically feasible.
Acute cervical spondylitis	*Suggested by:* gradual neck pain (occasionally a headache) over hours or days. Immobile neck. Usually past history of similar episodes. No fever.
	Confirmed by: above history.
	Finalized by the predictable outcome of management, e.g. analgesics and NSAIDs if not contraindicated + prophylactic gastric acid reduction (e.g. PPI), cervical collar, physiotherapy.
Posterior fossa tumour	*Suggested by:* headache, papilloedema.
	Confirmed by: **CT or MRI scan** appearances.
	Finalized by the predictable outcome of management, e.g. analgesia, dexamethasone to reduce brain oedema, treatment of seizures with anti-epileptics, assessment for resection or palliative surgery, palliative radiotherapy.
Anxiety with semi-voluntary resistance	*Suggested by:* improvement with reassurance or temporary distraction.
	Confirmed by: resolution after rest and observation.
	Finalized by the predictable outcome of management, e.g. analgesia, reassurance.

Hair loss in a specific area

Examine overall and then gently part hair to examine scalp. Use magnifying glass if hair is abnormal. Initial investigations: FBC, ferritin, TSH.

Main differential diagnoses and typical outline evidence, etc.

Alopecia areata	*Suggested and confirmed by:* well-circumscribed loss with exclamation mark hairs. *Finalized by the predictable outcome of management,* e.g. reassurance, advice not to scratch, local triamcinolone if slow to resolve.
Alopecia totalis	*Suggested by:* total hair loss on head. *Finalized by the predictable outcome of management:* treatment of underlying problems (e.g. stress, iron deficiency, hypothyroidism), use of wig, local minoxidil for androgenic alopecia.
Polycystic ovary syndrome	*Suggested by:* bitemporal recession and occipital thinning. Hirsutism on trunk. Onset near puberty. Obesity. *Confirmed by:* ↑**testosterone** and ↓**SHBG**. ↑**LH**, **ovarian US scan.** *Finalized by the predictable outcome of management:* metformin to reduce insulin resistance, combined oestrogen 'pill' to ↑SHBG and ↓free androgen, combined with cyproterone for hirsutism. Clomifene to induce ovulation.
Testosterone-secreting ovarian tumour	*Suggested by:* bitemporal recession and occipital thinning. Rapid onset over months. *Confirmed by:* ↑↑**testosterone** and ↓**LH**, **ovarian US scan**, and **laparoscopy** appearance. *Finalized by the predictable outcome of management:* resection of tumour.

Scarring after tinea, discoid lupus, pseudopelade of Brocq, folliculitis decalvans, pseudofolliculitis barbe, dissecting cellulitis, lichen planopilaris, scleroderma, morphea, amyloidosis, lymphoma, sarcoidosis.

Diffuse hair loss

Examine trunk, pubic, and limb hair too (alopecia universalis). Initial investigations: FBC, ferritin.

Main differential diagnoses and typical outline evidence, etc.	
Cytotoxic drugs	*Suggested by:* mainly head hair loss. History of recent cytotoxic drugs.
	Confirmed by: improvement after stopping cytotoxic drug.
	Finalized by the predictable outcome of management, e.g. explanation and temporary wig while awaiting recovery.
Iron deficiency	*Suggested by:* mainly head hair loss. Koilonychia, pallor of conjunctivae.
	Confirmed by: ↓Hb, ↓MCV, ↓MCHC, **↓ferritin.** Improvement if iron stores restored.
	Finalized by the predictable outcome of management: iron replacement, e.g. ferrous sulfate, investigation and treatment of the underlying cause.
Severe illness	*Suggested by:* mainly head hair loss. History of recent severe illness.
	Confirmed by: improvement with restoration of health.
	Finalized by the predictable outcome of management, e.g. treatment of underlying illness.
Hypogonadism	*Suggested by:* loss of hair from axilla, pubic area.
	Confirmed by: **↓testosterone** or **↓oestrogen** with **↑FSH** and **↑LH** in primary gonadal failure; normal or ↓LH, normal or ↓FSH if 2° to pituitary disease.
	Finalized by the predictable outcome of management, e.g. cyclical oestrogen in female or testosterone replacement therapy in male (IM, gel, patch or implant, provided prostatic-specific antigen normal).
Recent pregnancy	*Suggested by:* mainly head hair loss. Recent pregnancy.
	Confirmed by: improvement after delivery.
	Finalized by the predictable outcome of management, e.g. explanation and reassurance but no active treatment.

External ear abnormalities

Inspect the pinna for scars and other abnormalities. Examine the auditory meatus by first pulling the pinna up and back to straighten the cartilaginous bend. (In infants, pinna is pulled back and down.) Swab any discharge and remove any wax. Initial investigations: swab, culture, and sensitivity.

Main differential diagnoses and typical outline evidence, etc.

Congenital anomalies	*Suggested by:* malformed pinna, accessory tags, auricles, and pre-auricular pit, sinus, or fistula and microtia (no pinna ± atresia of ear canal). *Confirmed by:* above clinical appearances. **CT and MRI scans** to exclude other associated abnormalities.
Infected pre-auricular sinus	*Suggested by:* a small dimple anterior to tragus with a discharge. *Confirmed by:* deep tract that lies close to the facial nerve. Swab, culture, and sensitivity. *Finalized by the predictable outcome of management,* e.g. antibiotics according to culture and sensitivity, excision if recurrent infection.
Chondrodermatitis nodularis chronica helicis	*Suggested by:* painful nodular lesions on the upper margin of the pinna in men (helical rim) or antihelix (in women), pain wakes patient up at night. *Confirmed by:* clinical appearance. *Finalized by the predictable outcome of management,* e.g. avoid pressure (lying on other side), local triamcinolone, or excision.
Pinna haematoma resulting in a 'cauliflower' ear	*Suggested by:* history of blunt trauma. *Confirmed by:* appearance of bleeding in the subperichondrial plane that elevates the perichondrium to form a haematoma. *Finalized by the predictable outcome of management,* e.g. aspiration with a wide-bore needle followed by firm pressure dressing; or failing this, incision and drainage.
Exostosis (localized bony hypertrophy) may cause buildup of wax or debris or conductive deafness	*Suggested by:* palpable bony projections in the ear canals, accumulated wax difficult to clear ± history of frequent swimming in cold water. *Confirmed by:* sessile, smooth, often multiple, bilateral bony overgrowths of the ear canals. *Finalized by the predictable outcome of management,* e.g. no treatment or if wax accumulation, surgical removal of exostoses.

Wax (cerumen)— may cause conductive deafness if it impacts	*Suggested by:* hearing difficulty, irritation in the ear, dark brown, shiny, soft mass. *Confirmed by:* improvement in hearing after removal. *Finalized by the predictable outcome of management,* e.g. slightly warm olive oil drops, ear syringing, or suctioning.
Foreign bodies in the ear	*Suggested by:* visible foreign body and inflammation (in a child or patient with learning difficulties). *Confirmed by:* retrieval of foreign body. *Finalized by the predictable outcome of management,* e.g. removal by gentle syringing or forceps, a button battery needs to be removed immediately or if an insect, apply some olive oil first.

Painful ear

Consider referred pain from neck (C3, C4, and C5), throat, and teeth, and examine these too. Insert the largest comfortable aural speculum gently. Initial investigations: swab, culture, and sensitivity.

Main differential diagnoses and typical outline evidence, etc.	
Otitis externa (swimmer's ear) due to eczema, psoriasis, trauma, Pseudomonas, fungal infection	*Suggested by:* itching, irritation, pain, discharge, and tragal tenderness, recent ear syringing. *Confirmed by:* acute inflammation of the skin of the meatus, **culture of swab**, intact tympanic membrane. *Finalized by the predictable outcome of management,* e.g. analgesics, if mild—antibiotics and steroid drops; if severe, clearing of debris and keeping ear dry, ear canal dressing with ribbon gauze impregnated with antiseptic and changed daily and no swimming.
Malignant necrotizing otitis externa	*Suggested by:* pain, discharge, and tragal tenderness in a diabetic, elderly, or immunosuppressed person, facial palsy. *Confirmed by:* **X-ray** showing local bone erosion, isotope bone scan, and **white cell scan.** *Finalized by the predictable outcome of management,* e.g. aural toilet, local and systemic antibiotics; surgical debridement if severe.
Furunculosis (staphylococcal abscess in hair follicle) often diabetic	*Suggested by:* acutely painful throbbing ear, pain worse on moving the pinna or pressing on tragus. *Confirmed by:* appearance of a boil in the meatus. *Finalized by the predictable outcome of management,* e.g. insertion of wick soaked in ichthammol to ease pain, analgesics, and oral antibiotics.
Bullous myringitis (associated with influenza infection or Mycoplasma pneumoniae)	*Suggested and confirmed by:* extremely painful haemorrhagic blisters on the drum and deep meatal skin, and fluid behind the drum. *Finalized by the predictable outcome of management,* e.g. analgesia alone.
Barotrauma (aerotitis)	*Suggested by:* history of ear pain during descent in an aircraft or diving. *Confirmed by:* relief by decompression (e.g. holding nose and swallowing). *Finalized by the predictable outcome of management,* e.g. repeated Valsalva manoeuvre to open up the Eustachian tube, with use of topical nasal decongestants; myringotomy if intractible.

Temporomandibular joint dysfunction	*Suggested by:* earache, facial pain, and joint clicking or popping related to malocclusion, teeth-grinding, or joint derangement.
	Confirmed by: tenderness exacerbated by lateral movement of the open jaw, or trigger points in the pterygoids.
	Finalized by the predictable outcome of management: simple analgesics, e.g. paracetamol, NSAIDs, muscle relaxants and correction of malocclusive bite.

Discharging ear

Examine the tympanic membrane quadrants in turn. Note colour, translucency, and any bulging or retraction of the membrane. Note size, position, and site (marginal or central) of any perforations. Drum movement during a Valsalva manoeuvre also depends on a patient's Eustachian tube. Initial investigations: swab, culture, and sensitivity.

Main differential diagnoses and typical outline evidence, etc.	
Acute otitis media (due to *Pneumococcus*, *Haemophilus*, *Streptococcus*, and *Staphylococcus*, occasionally complicated by mastoiditis)	*Suggested by:* rapid onset over hours of throbbing and severe pain and fever, irritability, anorexia, or vomiting after an upper respiratory tract infection. *Confirmed by:* bulging red drum or profuse purulent discharge for 48h after drum perforates. Swab, culture and sensitivity. *Finalized by the predictable outcome of management,* e.g. analgesics, antibiotics if symptoms persist after 24h, myringotomy if bulging persists.
Otitis media with effusion (serous, secretory, or glue ear) usually in young children	*Suggested by:* gradual onset over weeks or months of deafness and intermittent ear pain. *Confirmed by:* loss of drum's light reflex or retraction relieved by grommets. *Finalized by the predictable outcome of management,* e.g. advise that it may improve spontaneously; treatment of predisposing conditions, e.g. allergic rhinitis, cleft palate; insertion of grommets ± adenoidectomy if persistence.
Chronic suppurative otitis media (may lead to cholesteatoma, petrositis, labyrinthitis, facial palsy, meningitis, intracranial abscess)	*Suggested by:* offensive purulent discharge, hearing loss, but no pain. *Confirmed by:* central drum perforation, swab, culture and sensitivity. *Finalized by the predictable outcome of management,* e.g. local and systemic antibiotics based on culture and sensitivity; regular aural toilet; myringoplasty and cortical mastoidectomy if severe.
Cholesteatoma (locally destructive stratified squamous epithelium)	*Suggested by:* foul discharge, deafness, headache, ear pain, facial paralysis, and vertigo. *Confirmed by:* continuing mucopurulent discharge, swab, culture, and sensitivity, pearly white soft matter (keratin) in attic or posterior marginal perforation. *Finalized by the predictable outcome of management,* e.g. if early retraction pocket, clean and remove keratin; if advanced, mastoid surgery.

Chronic otitis externa	*Suggested by:* watery discharge, itching, bilateral symptoms, painless and relapsing.
	Confirmed by: erythema and weeping of meatus.
	Finalized by the predictable outcome of management, e.g. keeping ears dry, regular aural toilets, avoidance of local antibiotic drops, oral antibiotics when indicated according to culture and sensitivity.
Auditory canal trauma	*Suggested by:* bloody discharge.
	Confirmed by: history of trauma, laceration, and erythema.
	Finalized by the predictable outcome of management, e.g. analgesics, stopping bleeding with pressure + dressing, suturing if needed.
CSF otorrhoea	*Suggested by:* history of head or facial trauma or surgery.
	Confirmed by: halo sign on filter paper.
	Finalized by the predictable outcome of management, e.g. observation, prophylactic antibiotics.

Striking facial appearance

Best recognized when meeting patient for the first time, but there is a wide normal variation. Initial investigations: TSH, ±FT4.

Main differential diagnoses and typical outline evidence, etc.	
Parkinson's disease	*Suggested by:* rigidity, lack or slowness of movements, reduced or absence of arm swing on walking, mask-like (akinetic) face ± hand or head tremor. *Confirmed by:* response to dopaminergic drugs. **CT and MRI scans** to eliminate other diagnoses. (Failure to respond to levodopa indicates no idiopathic Parkinson's disease.) *Finalized by the predictable outcome of management,* e.g. initially dopamine-releasing agents (e.g. amantadine), monoamine oxidase inhibitors (e.g. selegiline), or anticholinergics (e.g. trihexyphenidyl). In later severe disease, levodopa or dopamine agonists.
Huntington's chorea (or drug effect)	*Suggested by:* choreiform—jerky, purposeless facial movement or athetosis (writhing facial movement), tongue protrusion, and a bizarre gait. *Confirmed by:* family history or response to withdrawal of drug or dose reduction (if due to drug effect); also **genetic studies.** *Finalized by the predictable outcome of management,* e.g. symptomatic, e.g. tetrabenazine and haloperidol to reduce involuntary movements.
Bilateral upper or lower motor neurone lesion (due to motor neurone disease, cerebrovascular disease, myasthenia gravis)	*Suggested by:* paucity of movement of face, muscle weakness, and fasciculation. *Confirmed by:* other features of cause and **MRI** or **CT scan**. *Finalized by the predictable outcome of management,* e.g. physiotherapy, occupational, and speech therapies, psychological support.
Thyrotoxicosis due to Graves' disease, single or multiple toxic nodules	*Suggested by:* anxious-looking, thin, lid retraction and lag, tremor, hyperreflexia, diffuse goitre in Graves', visible or palpable nodules(s) if toxic nodules. *Confirmed by:* ↓**TSH** and ↑**T3** or ↑**T4** or both. **Thyroid antibodies** +ve if Graves'. **US scan or isotope scan** appearance if thyroid antibody –ve and hidden nodule suspected. *Finalized by the predictable outcome of management,* e.g. propranolol 40–80mg 8 hourly to control symptoms, carbimazole 40mg od reduced to 5–15mg od over 1–3mo period depending on TFT results; continued for 6–18mo; radioiodine therapy if hot nodule(s) or relapse of Graves' disease after full course.

Hypothyroidism	*Suggested by:* puffy face, obesity, cold intolerance, tiredness, constipation, bradycardia.
	Confirmed by: ↑**TSH, ↓FT4.**
	Finalized by the predictable outcome of management, e.g. initially levothyroxine 50 micrograms od; if elderly or if angina, 25 micrograms od, checking TFT after 4–8wk and adjust dose accordingly.
Acromegaly	*Suggested by:* large, wide face, embossed forehead, jutting jaw (prognathism) widely spaced teeth, and large tongue. Skull X-ray showing bony abnormalities. Hand X-ray showing typical tufts on terminal phalanges.
	Confirmed by: ↑**IGF,** failure to suppress GH to <2mU/L with **oral GTT. MRI or CT head scan** showing enlarged pituitary fossa.
	Finalized by the predictable outcome of management, e.g. somatostatin or transsphenoidal hypophysectomy with or without radiotherapy.
Glucocorticoid steroid therapy	*Suggested by:* truncal obesity, purple striae, bruising, moon face, and buffalo hump.
	Confirmed by: drug history: taking high dose of glucocorticoid.
	Finalized by the predictable outcome of management, e.g. stopping medication if appropriate.
Cushing's disease (ACTH driven)	*Suggested by:* truncal obesity, purple striae, bruising, moon face, and buffalo hump. Pigmented creases (suggest ↑ACTH, especially in ectopic ACTH from a carcinoma or carcinoid tumour). ↑**24h urinary free cortisol**.
	Confirmed by: 2x ↑**midnight cortisol** and ↑**midnight ACTH** and failure to suppress cortisol after dexamethasone 0.5mg 6 hourly for 48h (but does suppress after 2mg 6 hourly for 48 hours) and bilaterally large adrenals on **CT or MRI scan**.
	Finalized by the predictable outcome of management, e.g. initial control with metyrapone until response to surgery. Removal of pituitary adenoma or bilateral adrenalectomy if source not identified.
Cushing's syndrome due to adrenal adenoma or carcinoma	*Suggested by:* truncal obesity, purple striae, and bruising. No pigmentation in skin creases. ↑**24h urinary free cortisol**.
	Confirmed by: 2x ↑**midnight cortisol** and ↓**midnight ACTH** and failure to suppress cortisol after **dexamethasone suppression test** 0.5mg 6 hourly for 48h and after 2mg 6 hourly for 48h, and unilateral large adrenal on **CT or MRI scan**.
	Finalized by the predictable outcome of management, e.g. initial control with metyrapone until surgical treatment successful. Adrenalectomy for adenoma and carcinoma, also radiotherapy.

Proptosis of eye(s) or exophthalmos

Prominent eye suggested by sclera showing between the cornea and upper lid margin (may also be due to lid retraction due to sympathetic over-activity or lung disease). If in doubt, look down on eyes from above. (In myopia there is a large eyeball but the sclera is not visible.) Initial investigations: TSH±FT4, CT orbit.

Main differential diagnoses and typical outline evidence, etc.	
Ophthalmic Graves' disease (± thyrotoxicosis)	*Suggested by:* bilateral (usually) exophthalmos, goitre, pretibial myxoedema, and lid retraction. Eyes not closing during sleep if severe. *Confirmed by:* ↑titre of thyroid antibodies (with ↓TSH, and ↑FT4 or ↑T3). **CT scan** appearance. *Finalized by the predictable outcome of management,* e.g. if mild, dark glasses, eye lubricants before bed or artificial tears during day; in severe cases, steroids PO or IV, external radiation or orbital decompression +treatment of thyrotoxicosis.
Orbital cellulitis (medical emergency)	*Suggested by:* pain, fever, unilateral lid swelling, decreased vision, and double vision. Neurological signs in advanced disease. *Confirmed by:* **CT or MRI scan** appearance, and response to antibiotics. *Finalized by the predictable outcome of management,* e.g. antibiotics IV in hospital.
Cortico-cavernous fistula	*Suggested by:* unilateral engorgement of eye surface vessels, lid and conjunctiva, pulsatile with bruit over eye. *Confirmed by:* **CT or MRI scan** appearance. *Finalized by the predictable outcome of management,* e.g. pain control, endovascular closure.
Orbital tumours— rarely 1°, often 2°, especially reticulosis	*Suggested by:* unilateral proptosis and displacement of the eyeball. Lymph node, liver or spleen enlargement. *Confirmed by:* **CT or MRI scan** appearance. *Finalized by the predictable outcome of management,* e.g. pain control and treatment of eye infection, surgical decompression.

Red eye

Gritty pain suggests external cause. Aching pain suggests internal cause. Light sensitivity always accompanies inflammation in the eye. Fluorescein (Fl) yellow dye glows green with a blue examination light and stains all epithelial breaks. Initial investigations: Fl stain, swab, culture, and sensitivity.

Main differential diagnoses and typical outline evidence, etc.	
Spontaneous subconjunctival haemorrhage	*Suggested by:* painless bright red area on conjunctiva (oxygenated blood) and no light sensitivity. *Confirmed by:* clinical appearance and resolution over days. No Fl staining of cornea (not done often). *Finalized by the predictable outcome of management,* e.g. no direct treatment but treatment of associated sustained hypertension.
Conjunctivitis due to bacterial infection	*Suggested by:* red sticky eyes, dilated blood vessels on the eyeball and the tarsal (lid) conjunctiva with a purulent discharge ± bilateral ± gritty pain. *Confirmed by:* clinical appearance. Not light-sensitive and no Fl stain of cornea. *Finalized by the predictable outcome of management,* e.g. antibacterial eye drops, treat any underlying cause, e.g. dry eyes, blepharitis.
Conjunctivitis due to viral infection	*Suggested by:* red eyes with dilated vessels on the eyeball only, ± in one quadrant around the cornea with a watery 'tap running' discharge. Gritty pain ± impaired vision. *Confirmed by:* Fl stain showing dendritic (branching) pattern and resolution with topical antiviral. *Finalized by the predictable outcome of management,* e.g. aciclovir if herpetic infection.
Conjunctivitis due to allergy	*Suggested by:* red eyes with pink swollen conjunctiva and white stringy mucoid discharge, usually bilateral, episodic, and seasonal. *Confirmed by:* no Fl stain, and no visual loss and resolution with sodium cromoglycate (over 6wk) or steroid eye drops. *Finalized by the predictable outcome of management,* e.g. advice to avoid allergens, topical sodium cromoglicate with oral antihistamine.
Giant papillary conjunctivitis	*Suggested by:* patient wearing soft contact lens, history of eye surgery. Eye red, itchy, and watery. *Confirmed by:* cobblestone appearance of conjunctiva. *Finalized by the predictable outcome of management,* e.g. removal of irritating sutures, suspension of contact lens use until recovery. Advice about lens hygiene and minimizing wearing time.

Corneal ulcer (ulcerative keratitis) **due to abrasion or Herpes simplex, Pseudomonas, Candida, Aspergillus, protozoa**	*Suggested by:* painful, watering, light-sensitive, deeply red eye with yellowish abscess in the cornea, purulent discharge, and blurring of vision. *Confirmed by:* slit lamp examination after **fluorescein instillation** showing hypopyon (pus in the eye). Dendritic staining pattern in herpes. *Finalized by the predictable outcome of management,* e.g. analgesics, cycloplegic eye drops (e.g. cyclopentolate) to ease pain, aciclovir in herpetic infections, eye patching for at least 24h (and no steroid eye drops until a herpes infection excluded).
Episcleritis	*Suggested by:* localized red eye with superficial vessel dilatation, mild pain, no visual loss or light sensitivity, history of recurrent episodes. *Confirmed by:* one drop of phenylephrine 2.5% causing a blanching of the lesion. *Finalized by the predictable outcome of management,* e.g. unless mild and settles spontaneously, steroid eye drops and NSAIDs.
Scleritis associated with RA, SLE	*Suggested by:* localized area of dark red, dilated superficial and deep vessel on the sclera with aching pain and tenderness. Features of associated illness. *Confirmed by:* failure to blanch with one drop of 2.5% phenylephrine. *Finalized by the predictable outcome of management,* e.g. urgent referral for monitoring of progress ± systemic steroids.
Acute closed-angle glaucoma	*Suggested by:* severely painful red eye with marked visual loss, accompanied by nausea and vomiting ± history of haloes around lights and severe headache with blurred vision. *Confirmed by:* dull grey cornea, non-reacting and irregular pupil with **raised ocular pressures**. *Finalized by the predictable outcome of management,* e.g. analgesics and antiemetics, β-blocker drops, e.g. timolol; oral acetazolamide; laser iridotomy to prevent recurrence.
Iritis or anterior uveitis	*Suggested by:* redness around cornea, haze in front of iris, and severe photophobia. *Confirmed by:* small, non-reacting and irregular pupil, **slit lamp examination** showing flare, cells and hypopyon (pus in eye). *Finalized by the predictable outcome of management,* e.g. topical steroids but systemic steroids and immunosuppressants if severe.

Iritis (anterior uveitis)

Redness in cornea next to iris (circumcorneal injection) with muddy appearance of fluid in front of iris. The eye is painful, red, and watering with photophobia and blurred vision. All cases are referred for specialist ophthalmic management and follow-up to prevent long-term damage with adhesions and glaucoma. Initial investigations: slit-lamp examination, swab, culture, and sensitivity, RF, CXR.

Main differential diagnoses and typical outline evidence, etc.

Trauma (usually surgical)	*Suggested by:* history of impact accident, recent surgery. *Confirmed by:* **slit-lamp examination** showing blood in the front of the eye and 'D'-shaped distortion of the pupil if torn from its base or perforation if the pupil is pointing. *Finalized by the predictable outcome of management*, e.g. symptomatic: analgesia, dark glasses, surgical follow-up.
Infection: herpes simplex, zoster, TB, syphilis, leprosy, protozoa, fungi	*Suggested by:* general malaise, fever, leucocytosis. *Confirmed by:* **bacteriological culture** of eye swab or **viral immunology**. *Finalized by the predictable outcome of management*, e.g. symptomatic: analgesia, dark glasses, treatment according to virology or culture and sensitivity, surgical follow-up.
Autoimmune diseases: ankylosing spondylitis, Reiter's disease, juvenile chronic arthritis, immune ocular disease	*Suggested by:* arthritis, anaemia, no obvious fever, raised ESR. *Confirmed by:* **immunology** (seronegative for Rheumatoid factor). **Protein electrophoresis**. *Finalized by the predictable outcome of management*, e.g. symptomatic: analgesia, dark glasses, specialist management with oral steroids and immunosuppressive agents.
Sarcoidosis	*Suggested by:* history of dry cough, breathlessness, malaise, fatigue, weight loss, enlarged lacrimal glands, erythema nodosum. Raised serum ACE. *Confirmed by:* **CXR** appearances (e.g. bilateral lymphadenopathy), **tissue biopsy** showing non-caseating granuloma. **Slit-lamp examination** showing large keratic precipitates. *Finalized by the predictable outcome of management*, e.g. analgesia, NSAIDs for pain and erythema nodosum; oral steroids and immunosuppressive agents if severe.

Ulcerative colitis	*Suggested by:* history of diarrhoea with mucus and blood.
	Confirmed by: **colonoscopy** appearance and **biopsy** histology.
	Finalized by the predictable outcome of management, e.g. prednisolone PO + mesalazine, prednisolone retention enemas; if severe: hydrocortisone IV followed by prednisolone PO and sulfasalazine; surgery.
Crohn's disease	*Suggested by:* history of abdominal pain, diarrhoea, weight loss.
	Confirmed by: **colonoscopy, barium enema** and **meal** and follow-through.
	Finalized by the predictable outcome of management, e.g. prednisolone for 2wk for mild attacks. Steroids IV in severe cases. Immunosuppressants (e.g. methotrexate), immunotherapy (e.g. infliximab).

Clinical anaemia

Subconjunctival pallor (± face, nail, and hand pallor). Initial investigations: FBC.

Main differential diagnoses and typical outline evidence, etc.	
Microcytic due to iron deficiency, thalassaemia, etc (see ➋ Microcytic anaemia, p.567)	*Suggested by:* history of blood loss or family history of haemoglobinopathy (especially in Mediterranean origin) and sideroblastic anaemia. *Confirmed by:* **FBC**: ↓Hb and ↓MCV.
Macrocytic (see ➋ Macrocytic anaemia, p.568)	*Suggested by:* family history of pernicious anaemia, hypothyroidism, antifolate, and cytotoxic drugs or alcohol. *Confirmed by:* **FBC**: ↓Hb and ↑MCV, ↑TSH. **Film:** hypersegmented polymorphs in B12 deficiency.
Normocytic (see ➋ Normocytic anaemia, p.570)	*Suggested by:* history of chronic intercurrent illness, e.g. chronic renal failure, anaemia of chronic disease, etc. *Confirmed by:* **FBC**: ↓Hb and normal MCV.
Hypoplastic or aplastic anaemia	*Suggested by:* gradual onset without blood loss and potentially causal medication. *Confirmed by:* **FBC**: ↓Hb and normal MCV and **bone marrow biopsy:** atrophic. *Finalized by the predictable outcome of management,* e.g. stopping potential causative drugs. If persistent and severe, blood and platelet transfusion, combination immunosuppressants and bone marrow transplantation.
Leukaemia	*Suggested by:* gradual onset and enlarged spleen or lymph node (rapid deterioration in acute leukaemia). *Confirmed by:* **FBC**: ↓Hb and normal MCV, ↑↑WCC. **Bone marrow biopsy**: replacement by leukaemic cells. *Finalized by the predictable outcome of management,* e.g. blood and platelet transfusions, chemotherapy, and bone marrow transplantation.

Fever

Temperature >37°C. Fever is not a 'good lead'. The causes suggested here are broad. The approach is to listen carefully and examine for better diagnostic leads. Initial tests: FBC, MSU, blood cultures, viral and autoimmune serology:

Main differential diagnoses and typical outline evidence, etc.	
Infection	*Suggested by:* low grade or high fever with ↑WCC and usually symptoms and signs pointing to a focus.
	Confirmed by: **serology ± cultures** of blood and other body fluids.
Thrombus, tissue necrosis, neoplasm, autoimmune diseases, drugs	*Suggested by:* low-grade fever, history of severe illness, or trauma. WCC normal.
	Confirmed by: specific tests, e.g. **CXR, Doppler US scan of leg veins.**

Low body temperature

Temperature <35°C—but confirm with low reading thermometer—it could be lower. Also confirm with rectal temperature. Initial investigations: FBC, TSH, FT4.

Main differential diagnoses and typical outline evidence, etc.	
True hypothermia due to prolonged exposure to cold or hypothyroidism	*Suggested by:* history of immersion or cold weather exposure. Temperature <35°C with low reading rectal thermometer.
	Confirmed by: temperature chart using low reading rectal thermometer.
	Finalized by the predictable outcome of management, e.g. rewarming patient slowly, e.g. 0.5°C/h (faster may be fatal). Ventilation, IV access, antibiotics, and bladder catheterization. Liaise with social services to prevent recurrence.

Mouth lesions

Examine lips, buccal mucosa, teeth, tongue, tonsils, and pharynx. Initial investigations: FBC.

Main differential diagnoses and typical outline evidence, etc.	
Local aphthous ulcers	*Suggested by:* red, painful ulcer with associated lymph node enlargement.
	Confirmed by: spontaneous resolution within days.
	Finalized by the predictable outcome of management, e.g. topical oral analgesic ointment.
Local infection and gingivitis	*Suggested by:* vesicles in herpes simplex, creamy white plaques in oral candidiasis.
	Confirmed by: spontaneous resolution or within days of oral antiseptic or antifungal treatment.
	Finalized by the predictable outcome of management, e.g. oral antiseptic or antifungal.
Carious teeth	*Suggested by:* intermittent toothache, broken and/or severely discoloured teeth.
	Confirmed by: formal dental examination.
	Finalized by the predictable outcome of management, e.g. oral antiseptic, dental treatment.
Traumatic ulceration	*Suggested by:* jagged ulcers or lacerations.
	Confirmed by: history of trauma, injury, ill-fitting dentures, shallow, painful ulcers.
	Finalized by the predictable outcome of management, e.g. referral for dental assessment.
Vitamin deficiency e.g. B$_{12}$, riboflavin, nicotinic acid	*Suggested by:* atrophic glossitis, fissured tongue; 'raw beef' in B$_{12}$ deficiency, magenta in riboflavin deficiency.
	Confirmed by: response to vitamin supplements.
	Finalized by the predictable outcome of management, e.g. treat underlying conditions, e.g. malabsorption, refer to dietitian, advise well-balanced diet and vitamin supplements.
Hereditary haemorrhagic telangiectasia	*Suggested by:* telangiectasia on the face, around the mouth, on the lips and tongue, epistaxis, anaemia.
	Confirmed by: family history and examination of relatives.
Peutz–Jegher's syndrome (associated with intestinal polyps)	*Suggested by:* peri-oral pigmentation (not the tongue).
	Confirmed by: finding polyps on **colonoscopy**.
	Finalized by the predictable outcome of management, e.g. referral for long-term follow-up with colonoscopy and removal of any suspect lesions.

Red pharynx and tonsils

Initial investigations: FBC.

Main differential diagnoses and typical outline evidence. etc.	
Viral pharyngitis	*Suggested by:* sore throat, pain on swallowing, fever, cervical lymphadenopathy, and injected fauces. ↑lymphocytes, normal, or ↓leucocytes. *Confirmed by:* –ve **throat swab** for bacterial culture, dehydration: resolution within days. *Finalized by the predictable outcome of management,* e.g. gargles/lozenges, paracetamol, etc.
Acute follicular tonsillitis (streptococcal)	*Suggested by:* severe sore throat, pain on swallowing, fever, enlarged tonsils with white patches (like strawberries and cream). Cervical lymphadenopathy, especially in angle of jaw. Fever, ↑leucocytes in WCC. *Confirmed by:* **throat swab** for culture and sensitivities of organisms. *Finalized by the predictable outcome of management,* e.g. analgesic, antibiotics, e.g. phenoxymethylpenicillin or cephalosporin or co-amoxiclav.
Infectious mononucleosis (glandular fever) due to Epstein–Barr virus	*Suggested by:* very severe throat pain with enlarged tonsils covered with grey mucoid film. Petechiae on palate. Profound malaise. Generalized lymphadenopathy, splenomegaly. *Confirmed by:* ↑atypical lymphocytes in WBC. **Paul–Bunnell** or **Monospot®** test +ve. **Viral titres**. *Finalized by the predictable outcome of management,* e.g. gargles/lozenges, analgesics, e.g. paracetamol (amoxicillin causes rash, aspirin may cause Reye syndrome).
Candidiasis of buccal or oesophageal mucosa	*Suggested by:* painful dysphagia, white plaque, history of immunosuppression/diabetes/recent antibiotics. *Confirmed by:* **oesophagoscopy** showing erythema and plaques, **brush cytology ± biopsy** showing spores and hyphae. *Finalized by the predictable outcome of management,* e.g. analgesics, antifungal lozenges or solutions, e.g. nystatin suspension or oral fluconazole.
Agranulocytosis e.g. antithyroid drugs	*Suggested by:* sore throat, history of taking a drug (e.g. carbimazole) or contact with noxious substance. *Confirmed by:* low or absent neutrophil count. *Finalized by the predictable outcome of management,* e.g. stopping offending drug, broad-spectrum antibiotics IV or PO, if febrile.
Also with oropharyngeal ulceration;	Herpes zoster infection, herpes simplex infection, local herpangina, aphthous ulceration, etc.
without oropharyngeal ulceration	Reflux oesophagitis, epiglottitis, blood dyscrasia, etc.

'Parotid' swelling

Swelling between anterior border of masseter muscle (teeth clenched) to lower half of ear and from zygoma to angle of jaw. Initial investigations: FBC.

Main differential diagnoses and typical outline evidence, etc.	
Parotid duct obstruction (usually due to stone)	*Suggested by:* intermittent infection or no discharge from duct. *Confirmed by:* **plain X-ray** showing radio-opaque stone or **sialography** to show filling defect. *Finalized by the predictable outcome of management,* e.g. analgesia, surgical stone removal.
Parotid tumour	*Suggested by:* no obvious features of alterative non-malignant or infective condition. *Confirmed by:* urgent surgical referral for **biopsy** or exploration. *Finalized by the predictable outcome of management,* e.g. surgical excision.
Mumps parotitis	*Suggested by:* acute painful swelling of whole gland(s), contact with other cases. *Confirmed by:* bilateral swelling or associated pancreatitis or orchitis (rising mumps **viral titre**). *Finalized by the predictable outcome of management,* e.g. analgesia, fluids, etc.
Suppurative parotid infection	*Suggested by:* hot, tender, fluctuant swelling with high fever. No discharge from duct orifice. *Confirmed by:* WBC: ↑neutrophils response to antibiotics, drainage. *Finalized by the predictable outcome of management,* e.g. referral for surgery.
Non-suppurative parotitis from ascending infection along parotid duct	*Suggested by:* unilateral swelling, oral sepsis or poor general condition, fever. *Confirmed by:* WCC: ↑neutrophils, resolution with antibiotics. *Finalized by the predictable outcome of management,* e.g. analgesia, broad-spectrum antibiotics.
Parotid Sjögren's syndrome	*Suggested by:* dry mouth and eyes with no tears. *Confirmed by:* **rheumatoid factor** +ve, **anti Ro (SSA)** and **anti-La (SSB)** +ve. *Finalized by the predictable outcome of management,* e.g. oral lubricants (e.g. gelatin lozenge) and eye lubricant (e.g. methylcellulose).
Parotid sarcoidosis	*Suggested by:* history of dry cough, enlarged lacrimal glands, erythema nodosum, ↑serum ACE. *Confirmed by:* **CXR** appearances (e.g. bilateral lymphadenopathy) and **tissue biopsy** showing non-caseating granuloma. *Finalized by the predictable outcome of management,* e.g. oral lubricants, e.g. gelatin lozenge, NSAID if associated polyarthalgia; oral steroids if associated hypercalcaemia, or lung, heart, neurological involvement.

Lump in the face (non-parotid lesion)

Main differential diagnoses and typical outline evidence, etc.

Pre-auricular lymph node inflammation	*Suggested by:* tender, nodular swelling in front of ear. *Confirmed by:* above clinical features, spontaneous resolution, histology. *Finalized by the predictable outcome of management,* e.g. resolution on follow up in days; if not excision biopsy.
Pre-auricular lymphoma	*Suggested by:* non-tender, nodular swelling in front of ear. *Confirmed by:* **biopsy.** *Finalized by the predictable outcome of management,* e.g. surgical excision.
Basal cell carcinoma	*Suggested by:* painless ulcer with rolled edge. *Confirmed by:* **biopsy** appearance. *Finalized by the predictable outcome of management,* e.g. surgical excision.
Sebaceous cyst	*Suggested by:* fluctuant swelling with central punctum. *Confirmed by:* **incision** and content evacuation. *Finalized by the predictable outcome of management,* e.g. no treatment, antibiotics if infected, surgical excision if persistent.
Subcutaneous abscess	*Suggested by:* tender fluctuant swelling. *Confirmed by:* **incision** when pointing. *Finalized by the predictable outcome of management,* e.g. incision ± antibiotic.
Dental abscess	*Suggested by:* tenderness of underlying tooth (tap gently). *Confirmed by:* **dental exploration**. *Finalized by the predictable outcome of management,* e.g. dental surgery.
Skin melanoma	*Suggested by:* painless swelling with pigment and red edge. *Confirmed by:* **wide excision biopsy** and histology. *Finalized by the predictable outcome of management,* e.g. surgical excision.

Submandibular lump—not moving with tongue protrusion or on swallowing

Below the mandible and above the digastric muscle. Initial investigations: FBC.

Main differential diagnoses and typical outline evidence, etc.	
Mumps sialitis	*Suggested by:* acute painful swelling of whole gland(s), contact with others cases.
	Confirmed by: bilateral swelling or associated pancreatitis or orchitis. (↑**mumps titre** if in doubt.)
	Finalized by the predictable outcome of management, e.g. analgesia, maintain hydration.
Non-suppurative sialitis from ascending infection along duct	*Suggested by:* unilateral swelling, oral sepsis, or poor general condition.
	Confirmed by: discharge from duct orifice. Resolution with antibiotics.
	Finalized by the predictable outcome of management, e.g. rehydration, antibiotics, oral hygiene, lemon drops to stimulate saliva production, surgical drainage if intractable.
Suppurative salivary infection	*Suggested by:* hot, tender, fluctuant swelling with high fever. No discharge from duct orifice.
	Confirmed by: **US scan** appearance.
	Finalized by the predictable outcome of management, e.g. incision and drainage ± antibiotics.
Salivary duct obstruction (usually due to stone)	*Suggested by:* intermittent infection or no discharge from duct.
	Confirmed by: **US scan,** response to stomaplasty.
	Finalized by the predictable outcome of management, e.g. rehydration, analgesia, and antibiotics if fever and ↑WCC, awaiting spontaneous passage of small stone; surgical removal if large.
Salivary Sjögren's syndrome	*Suggested by:* dry mouth and eyes with no tears.
	Confirmed by: **rheumatoid factor** +ve, **anti-Ro (SSA)** and **anti-La (SSB)** +ve.
	Finalized by the predictable outcome of management, e.g. oral lubricants (e.g. gelatin lozenge) and eye lubricant (e.g. methylcellulose).
Salivary sarcoidosis	*Suggested by:* dry cough, enlarged lacrimal glands, and erythema nodosum.
	Confirmed by: **CXR** appearances (e.g. bilateral lymphadenopathy) and tissue biopsy showing non-caseating granuloma.
	Finalized by the predictable outcome of management, e.g. oral lubricants (e.g. gelatin lozenge), NSAID if associated polyarthalgia; oral steroids if associated hypercalcaemia, or lung, heart, neurological involvement.

Salivary tumour due to adenocarcinoma, squamous cell tumour, etc.	*Suggested by:* no obvious features of alternative non-malignant or infective condition. *Confirmed by:* **biopsy or surgical exploration**. *Finalized by the predictable outcome of management*, e.g. surgical excision.
Submandibular lymph node inflammation	*Suggested by:* tender, solid, nodular swelling between rami of mandible, especially <20y of age. *Confirmed by:* above clinical features or **US scan**. *Finalized by the predictable outcome of management*, e.g. resolution within days.
Submandibular lymph node malignancy	*Suggested by:* non-tender, solid nodular swelling between rami of mandible, especially age >20y. *Confirmed by:* **US scan, biopsy** appearance. *Finalized by the predictable outcome of management*, e.g. surgical excision.
Ranula	*Suggested by:* transilluminable cyst lateral to midline, with domed, bluish discoloration in floor of mouth lateral to frenulum. *Confirmed by:* clinical appearance, **US scan**, and histology after excision. *Finalized by the predictable outcome of management*, e.g. surgical excision.
Submental dermoid	*Suggested by:* midline cyst and age <20 years. *Confirmed by:* **histology** after excison. *Finalized by the predictable outcome of management*, e.g. surgical excision.

Anterior neck lump—moving with tongue protrusion and swallowing

Suggests extrathyroid tissue. Initial investigations: ultrasound (US) scan.

Main differential diagnoses and typical outline evidence, etc.	
Thyroglossal cyst	*Suggested by:* fluctuant, cystic lump in midline or just to the left.
	Confirmed by: **US scan** shows cystic lesion, **radioisotope scan** (cyst is cold), **CT scan, histology** of excised tissue.
	Finalized by the predictable outcome of management, e.g. surgical excision showing cyst.
Ectopic thyroid tissue	*Suggested by:* solid lump in midline or just laterally.
	Confirmed by: **US scan** shows non-cystic lesion, **radioisotope scan:** nodule taking up iodine, **CT scan, histology** of excised tissue.
	Finalized by the predictable outcome of management, e.g. surgical excision.

Neck lump—moving with swallowing but not with tongue protrusion

Suggests a goitre (or something attached to thyroid gland). The following are preliminary diagnoses (see also ➲ Bilateral neck mass—moving with swallowing but not with tongue protrusion, p.100). Initial investigations: TSH, FT4.

Main differential diagnoses and typical outline evidence, etc.	
Thyrotoxic goitre	*Suggested by:* sweating, fine tremor, tachycardia, weight loss, lid lag. *Confirmed by:* ↑FT4 ± ↑FT3 and ↓↓TSH. **US scan** appearance, **isotope scan** appearance. *Finalized by the predictable outcome of management,* e.g. propranolol to control symptoms, carbimazole 40mg od reduced to 5–15mg over 1–3mo period. FBC before starting treatment, warning about agranulocytosis, sore throat.
Hypothyroid goitre	*Suggested by:* cold intolerance, tiredness, constipation, bradycardia. *Confirmed by:* ↑TSH, ↓FT4. **US scan ± thyroid antibodies** +ve. *Finalized by the predictable outcome of management,* e.g. levothyroxine 25–50 micrograms od. Regular checks on TFT to keep in normal range.
Euthyroid goitre	*Suggested by:* absence of sweating, fine tremor, weight change, cold intolerance, tiredness, lid lag; normal bowel habit, normal pulse rate. *Confirmed by:* normal FT4, and normal TSH. *Finalized by the predictable outcome of management,* e.g. no treatment or surgery if causing symptoms of compression in neck or thoracic inlet.

Bilateral neck mass—moving with swallowing but not with tongue protrusion

(Central mass crossing the midline.) Initial investigations: TSH, FT4, ultrasound scan of goitre.

Main differential diagnoses and typical outline evidence, etc.	
Graves' disease	*Suggested by:* clinical thyrotoxicosis, exophthalmos, pretibial myxoedema. No nodules. *Confirmed by:* ↑**FT4** or ↑**FT3** and ↓**TSH** and **TSH receptor antibody** +ve. Diffusely increased uptake on **thyroid isotope scan**. *Finalized by the predictable outcome of management,* e.g. propranolol 40–80mg 8 hourly to control symptoms. Carbimazole 40mg od reduced to 5–10mg over 1–3mo with monthly TFT. FBC before starting. Written warning for agranulocytosis causing sore throat. Radioiodine or thyroidectomy offered if relapse after 6–18mo carbimazole.
Hashimoto's thyroiditis	*Suggested by:* clinically euthyroid or hypothyroid (or rarely transient thyrotoxicosis). Multiple nodules in large gland. *Confirmed by:* ↑**FT4** transiently then ↓**FT4** and ↑**TSH**, ↑↑**thyroid antibody titre**. Diffuse poor uptake on **thyroid isotope scan**. *Finalized by the predictable outcome of management,* e.g. analgesic, oral steroid if persistent pain. Thyroxine if TSH persistently.
'Simple' goitre	*Suggested by:* clinically euthyroid. Not nodular. *Confirmed by:* **FT4** and **FT3** normal, **TSH** normal and **thyroid antibodies** –ve. *Finalized by the predictable outcome of management,* e.g. reassurance, no change with no treatment.
Toxic multinodular goitre	*Suggested by:* multiple nodules and clinically thyrotoxic. *Confirmed by:* ↑**FT4** or ↑**FT3**, and ↓**TSH** and nodules on **US scan or thyroid isotope scan**. *Finalized by the predictable outcome of management,* e.g. carbimazole (±β-blocker for symptoms), radioiodine (but not used if compression of adjacent structures in the neck and thoracic inlet); surgery instead.
Non-toxic multinodular goitre	*Suggested by:* multiple nodules, clinically euthyroid. *Confirmed by:* **FT4** or **FT3** normal, **TSH** normal. Nodules on **US scan or thyroid isotope scan**. *Finalized by the predictable outcome of management,* e.g. of surgery if symptomatic.
Thyroid enzyme deficiency (rare)	*Suggested by:* presentation in childhood, clinically hypothyroid or euthyroid. Smooth goitre, not nodular. *Confirmed by:* ↓**FT4** and ↓**TSH** but with abnormal (high or low) radioiodine uptake. Thyroid antibodies –ve. *Finalized by the predictable outcome of management,* e.g. thyroxine replacement.

Solitary thyroid nodule

Initial investigations: TSH, FT4, ultrasound scan of thyroid.

Main differential diagnoses and typical outline evidence, etc.	
Autonomous toxic thyroid nodule	*Suggested by:* single nodule and 'clinically thyrotoxic': weight loss, frequent bowel movement, tachycardia, sweats, tremor. *Confirmed by:* ↑**FT4** or ↑**FT3**, ↓**TSH**, and single, hot nodule thyroid isotope (iodine or technetium) scan. *Finalized by the predictable outcome of management,* e.g. radioactive iodine therapy (treatment of choice) controlling symptoms with β-blocker ± carbimazole until euthyroid.
Thyroid carcinoma: papillary 60%, follicular 25%, medullary 5%, lymphoma 5%, anaplastic <1%	*Suggested by:* single nodule and clinically euthyroid. *Confirmed by:* normal **FT4** or **FT3**, normal **TSH**, and single, cold nodule **thyroid isotope scan**. Solid on **US scan**. Malignant cells on **needle aspiration** or **excision**. *Finalized by the predictable outcome of management,* e.g. total thyroidectomy, radioactive iodine for residual tissue and any tumour with follow-up scans and serum thyroglobulin, and eradication of any recurrence.
Thyroid adenoma	*Suggested by:* single nodule and clinically euthyroid. *Confirmed by:* normal **FT4** or **FT3**, normal **TSH**, and single, cold nodule **thyroid isotope scan**. Solid on **US thyroid scan**. No malignant cells on **needle aspiration** or **excision**. *Finalized by the predictable outcome of management,* e.g. partial thyroidectomy.
Thyroid cyst	*Suggested by:* single nodule and clinically euthyroid. *Confirmed by:* normal **FT4** or **FT3**, normal **TSH**, and single, cold nodule **thyroid isotope scan**. Cyst on **US scan**. Disappears on **needle aspiration** and no malignant cells then or if removed. *Finalized by the predictable outcome of management,* e.g. needle aspiration and surgery if persistent recurrence.

Lump in anterior triangle of neck

Below digastric and anterior to sternomastoid muscles. Initial investigations: FBC, ultrasound scan.

Main differential diagnoses and typical outline evidence, etc.

Lymph node inflammation	*Suggested by:* tender, solid nodular swelling.
	Confirmed by: above clinical features, **CT scan**.
	Finalized by the predictable outcome of management, e.g. reassurance, follow-up until resolved ± treatment of underlying cause.
Acute abscess	*Suggested by:* hot, tender, fluctuant swelling with high fever, WCC: ↑neutrophils.
	Confirmed by: clinical features and discharge of pus after incision.
	Finalized by the predictable outcome of management, e.g. incision ± antibiotics.
Tuberculosis ('cold') abscess	*Suggested by:* fluctuant swelling with low grade or no fever.
	Confirmed by: acid-fast bacilli (AFB) on microscopy or culture and sensitivity of **aspirate**.
	Finalized by the predictable outcome of management, e.g. provisional treatment with isoniazid, pyrazinamide, rifampicin and ethambutol for 2mo ±pyridoxine pending result of culture and sensitivity; contact tracing.
Branchial cyst	*Suggested by:* fluctuant swelling at anterior border of sternomastoid muscle, <20y of age.
	Confirmed by: **US scan**, **CT scan**, surgical anatomy, appearance and *histology* on excision.
	Finalized by the predictable outcome of management, e.g. surgical excision.
Cystic hygroma	*Suggested by:* fluctuant swelling that transilluminates well, <20y of age.
	Confirmed by: **US scan**, **CT scan**, surgical anatomy, appearance and histology on **excision**, or regression with sclerosant.
	Finalized by the predictable outcome of management, e.g. surgical excision.
Pharyngeal pouch	*Suggested by:* intermittent, fluctuant swelling (usually on left) and dysphagia.
	Confirmed by: **barium swallow** fills pouch.
	Finalized by the predictable outcome of management, e.g. surgical excision.
Carotid body tumour (chemodectoma)	*Suggested by:* mobile, arising from carotid bifurcation (upper third of sternomastoid), soft, and gently pulsatile.
	Confirmed by: **US scan**, **CT scan**, surgical anatomy, appearance and histology after excision.
	Finalized by the predictable outcome of management, e.g. surgical excision.
Hodgkin's or non-Hodgkin's lymphoma	*Suggested by:* non-tender, solid nodular swelling between rami of mandible, especially >20y of age ± fever, weight loss. Chest pain with alcohol in Hodgkin's.
	Confirmed by: **US scan**, **CT scan**, **biopsy** with or without or excision.
	Finalized by the predictable outcome of management, e.g. radiotherapy or chemotherapy depending on the stage of disease.

Lump in posterior triangle of neck

Behind sternomastoid and in front of trapezius. Initial investigations: FBC, ultrasound scan.

Main differential diagnoses and typical outline evidence, etc.	
Acute abscess	*Suggested by:* hot, tender fluctuant swelling with high fever, WCC: ↑neutrophils. *Confirmed by:* clinical features and discharge of pus after incision. *Finalized by the predictable outcome of management:* incision ± antibiotics.
Cystic hygroma	*Suggested by:* fluctuant swelling that transilluminates well, <20y of age. *Confirmed by:* **US scan, CT scan**, surgical anatomy, appearance and histology on excision, or regression with sclerosant. *Finalized by the predictable outcome of management,* e.g. surgical excision.
Lymph node inflammation	*Suggested by:* tender, solid nodular swelling. *Confirmed by:* above clinical features, **US scan**. *Finalized by the predictable outcome of management,* e.g. reassurance, follow-up until resolved.
Hodgkin's or non-Hodgkin's lymphoma	*Suggested by:* non-tender, solid nodular swelling. Chest pain with alcohol in Hodgkin's. *Confirmed by:* **US scan, CT scan, biopsy** with or without or excision. *Finalized by the predictable outcome of management,* e.g. plan radiotherapy or chemotherapy depending on stage of disease.
Metastasis in lymph node	*Suggested by:* non-tender, solid nodular swelling. *Confirmed by:* **US scan, CT scan, biopsy** ± excision. *Finalized by the predictable outcome of management,* e.g. plan radiotherapy or chemotherapy depending on stage of disease.
Tuberculous ('cold') abscess	*Suggested by:* non-tender, cystic swelling >50y of age. *Confirmed by:* **US scan, CT scan, aspiration** biopsy or excision, culture of AFB. *Finalized by the predictable outcome of management,* e.g. provisional treatment with isoniazid, pyrazinamide, rifampicin and ethambutol for 2mo ±pyridoxine pending result of culture and sensitivity; contact tracing.

Supraclavicular lump(s)

Initial investigations: ultrasound scan.

Main differential diagnoses and typical outline evidence, etc.

Lymph node inflammation	*Suggested by:* tender, solid nodular swelling, especially <20y of age. *Confirmed by:* clinical features. **US scan**: solid lesion. *Finalized by the predictable outcome of management,* e.g. reassurance, follow-up to ensure resolution.
Lymphoma	*Suggested by:* rubbery, matted nodes. Confirmed by: lymph node **biopsy**. *Finalized by the predictable outcome of management,* e.g. radiotherapy or chemotherapy depending on stage.
Lymph node secondary to gastric or lung carcinoma	*Suggested by:* rock-hard, fixed nodes, Virchow's node in left supraclavicular fossa (Troisier's sign). Confirmed by: lymph node **biopsy, gastroscopy, bronchoscopy**. *Finalized by the predictable outcome of management,* e.g. radiotherapy or chemotherapy depending on primary source and stage.
Aneurysm of subclavian artery	*Suggested by:* pulsatile cyst. *Confirmed by:* **US scan** and **MRI scan** or **angiography.** *Finalized by the predictable outcome of management,* e.g. surgical excision and repair.

Galactorrhoea

Spontaneous or expressible milky fluid. Initial investigations: prolactin, TSH, FT4, pregnancy test.

Main differential diagnoses and typical outline evidence, etc.	
1° hyperprolactinaemia	*Suggested by:* infertility, oligomenorrhoea, or amenorrhoea. *Confirmed by:* ↑**prolactin** and normal **TSH** and **T4**. **Pituitary CT or MRI scan**: normal. *Finalized by the predictable outcome of management:* dopamine agonists, e.g. long-term bromocriptine or cabergoline.
Prolactinoma	*Suggested by:* infertility, oligomenorrhoea, or amenorrhoea. In large tumours, field defects and loss of secondary sexual characteristics. *Confirmed by:* ↑**prolactin** and normal **TSH** and **T4**. Micro- or macro-adenoma on **pituitary CT or MRI scan.** *Finalized by the predictable outcome of management,* e.g. dopamine agonist, e.g. bromocriptine and cabergoline. Surgical intervention if intolerance to medical treatment or presence of field defect or other pressure effects.
Pregnancy	*Suggested by:* amenorrhoea, frequency of urine in woman of childbearing age. *Confirmed by:* **pregnancy test** +ve. *Finalized by the predictable outcome of management,* e.g. progression of pregnancy.
1° hypothyroidism	*Suggested by:* cold intolerance, tiredness, constipation, bradycardia. *Confirmed by:* ↑**TSH**, ↓**FT4**. *Finalized by the predictable outcome of management,* e.g. levothyroxine, e.g. 50 micrograms od. Check TFT after 1–2mo and titrate dose.
Drugs	*Suggested by:* taking chlorpromazine and other major tranquilizers, metoclopramide, domperidone. *Confirmed by:* ↑**prolactin**, resolution and lowering of prolactin after stopping suspect drug. *Finalized by the predictable outcome of management,* e.g. stop causative drug.
'Idiopathic galactorrhoea'	*Suggested by:* galactorrhoea, no other findings. *Confirmed by:* normal **prolactin**. *Finalized by the predictable outcome of management,* e.g. short course (e.g. 4wk) of dopamine agonists, e.g. cabergoline.

Nipple abnormality

Initial investigations: swab of discharge, culture, and sensitivity.

Main differential diagnoses and typical outline evidence, etc.	
Paget's disease of nipple with underlying carcinoma	*Suggested by:* breast nipple 'eczema'. *Confirmed by: in situ* malignant change on histological examination of **skin scrapings**. *Finalized by the predictable outcome of management,* e.g. surgical excision or mastectomy combined with endocrine therapy and chemotherapy.
Duct ectasia and chronic infection	*Suggested by:* green or brown nipple discharge. *Confirmed by:* chronic inflammation on **histology** of excised ducts. *Finalized by the predictable outcome of management,* e.g. analgesics for breast pain, surgical excision of lumps, antibiotics for infection.
Duct papilloma	*Suggested by:* bleeding from nipple. *Confirmed by:* excision of affected ducts. Benign histology of **excised ducts**. *Finalized by the predictable outcome of management,* e.g. surgical referral for excision of affected ducts.
Mammillary fistula	*Suggested by:* discharge from para-areolar region aged 30–40. *Confirmed by:* benign **histology** of excised ducts. *Finalized by the predictable outcome of management,* e.g. surgical excision of affected ducts.

Breast lump(s)

Initial investigations: mammography, ultrasound, and fine needle aspiration.

Main differential diagnoses and typical outline evidence, etc.	
Benign fibrous mammary dysplasia	*Suggested by:* generally painful breast lumpiness, greatest near axilla. Cyclically related to periods. *Confirmed by:* relief on **aspiration** of cysts, diuretics or oestrogen suppression. *Finalized by the predictable outcome of management,* e.g. aspiration of cysts.
Fibroadenoma	*Suggested by:* smooth and mobile lump ('breast mouse'), usually in ages 15–30y. *Confirmed by:* appearance on **mammogram** confirmed by benign **histology** after excision. *Finalized by the predictable outcome of management,* e.g. surgical excision of adenoma.
Cyst(s)	*Suggested by:* spherical, fluctuant lump, single or multiple, painful before periods. *Confirmed by:* cysts on **mammography**, benign tissue after excision. *Finalized by the predictable outcome of management,* e.g. surgical excision of cyst.
Acute or chronic abscess	*Suggested by:* fluctuant lump, hot and tender, acute presentation often in puerperium, chronic after antibiotics. *Confirmed by:* response to drainage, exision of chronic abscess, and **histology** to exclude carcinoma. *Finalized by the predictable outcome of management,* e.g. surgical drainage.
Fat necrosis or sclerosing adenosis	*Suggested by:* firm, solitary localized lump. *Confirmed by:* appearance on mammogram and benign **histology** after excision. *Finalized by the predictable outcome of management,* e.g. surgical excision of affected tissue.
Carcinoma infiltrating ductal cancer or invasive lobar cancers	*Suggested by:* fixed, irregular, hard, painless lump, nipple retraction, fixed to skin (peau d'orange) or muscle, and local, hard or firm, fixed nodes in axilla. *Confirmed by:* **mammography** showing ill-defined, spiculate borders, faint linear or irregular calcification, and abnormal adjacent structures. Malignant histology after **breast aspiration** or **excision**. *Finalized by the predictable outcome of management,* e.g. surgical excision.

Gynaecomastia

This is usually reported by the patient or sometimes discovered during the general examination. Breast swelling in males is a palpable disc of firm tissue. If there is no disc, it suggests fatty tissue only. Initial investigations: LH, FSH, plasma testosterone, oestrogens.

Main differential diagnoses and typical outline evidence, etc.	
Immature testis	*Suggested by:* adolescence and no testicular lump. *Confirmed by:* normal testosterone, oestrogen and LH levels normal, **US scan of testis**. *Finalized by the predictable outcome of management,* e.g. resolution after explanation and reassurance that spontaneous resolution can be expected over months.
Digoxin, spironolactone	*Suggested by:* taking of drug and no testicular lump. *Confirmed by:* improvement when suspect drug stopped.
High alcohol intake	*Suggested by:* high alcohol intake and no testicular lump. *Confirmed by:* improvement when alcohol stopped.
Hepatic cirrhosis	*Suggested by:* long history of high alcohol intake (usually), spider naevi, abnormal liver size (large or small) and consistency (fatty or hard). *Confirmed by:* **LFT** abnormal, ↓**LH**, ↑**oestrogens**, ↓**testosterone**. *Finalized by the predictable outcome of management,* e.g. dietary and alcohol advice, avoidance of sedatives and opiates. Vitamin K *if* ↑*prothrombin time*. Colestyramine for pruritus. Spironolactone ± furosemide for oedema, ascites. Interferon alfa to delay development of hepatoma.
Testicular tumours	*Suggested by:* scrotal mass ± pain, tenderness if haemorrhage occurs (sometimes in undescended testis). *Confirmed by:* **testicular US scan**, inguinal exploration, ↑**alpha-fetoprotein**, ↑β-**hCG**. *Finalized by the predictable outcome of management,* e.g. orchidectomy, radiotherapy or chemotherapy. (Seminomas are radiosensitive, teratomas sensitive to combination chemotherapy.)
Hypogonadism (1° testicular disease, or 2° to low LH from pituitary defect or tumour)	*Suggested by:* sparse pubic hair, no drug or alcohol history, poor libido. *Confirmed by:* **low testosterone**, ↑**LH** (in primary testicular disease), ↓**LH** or normal (if secondary to pituitary diseases). *Finalized by the predictable outcome of management,* e.g. testosterone replacement therapy IM, gel, patch, or depot injection.

Bronchial carcinoma	*Suggested by:* smoking history, haemoptysis, weight loss, clubbing.
	Confirmed by: **CXR, bronchoscopy** with biopsy.
	Finalized by the predictable outcome of management, e.g. surgical resection combined with radiotherapy or chemotherapy.
Klinefelter's syndrome	*Suggested by:* poor sexual development, infertility, eunuchoid.
	Confirmed by: **47, XXY karyotype**.
	Finalized by the predictable outcome of management, e.g. testosterone replacement therapy IM, gel, patch, or depot injection.
Obesity	*Suggested by:* no breast tissue, only mammary fat.
	Confirmed by: improvement with weight loss.
	Finalized by the predictable outcome of management, e.g. lifestyle changes; diet and exercise, drug and surgical treatment, e.g. gastric banding, if intractable and life-threatening.

Axillary lymphadenopathy

Axillary lymphadenopathy ± tenderness. Initial investigations: FBC, CRP, ESR, lymph node biopsy.

Main differential diagnoses and typical outline evidence, etc.	
Reaction to infection, e.g. viral prodrome, HIV infection, etc.	*Suggested by:* tender, solid nodular swelling(s). *Confirmed by:* clinical features. *Finalized by the predictable outcome of management, e.g.* identifying underlying cause and treating it if necessary.
Infiltration by tumour, e.g. breast	*Suggested by:* non-tender, solid nodular swelling(s). *Confirmed by:* excision biopsy. *Finalized by the predictable outcome of management, e.g.* identifying underlying cause and treating it if necessary.
Reticulosis or primary tumour	*Suggested by:* non-tender, solid nodular swelling(s). *Confirmed by:* excision biopsy. *Finalized by the predictable outcome of management, e.g.* identifying underlying cause and treating it if necessary.
Drug effect	*Suggested by:* drug history, e.g. phenytoin, retroviral drugs. *Confirmed by:* improvement when drug withdrawn. *Finalized by the predictable outcome of management, e.g.* stopping suspect drug.

Hirsutism in a female

Upward extension of pubic hair in female. Hirsute upper lip, sideburns, chin.
Initial investigations: plasma LH, FSH, testosterone, SHBG, ultrasound scan
ovaries.

Main differential diagnoses and typical outline evidence, etc.	
Racial skin sensitivity	*Suggested by:* family history, normal menstrual periods (and fertility if applicable). *Confirmed by:* **LH** normal, **testosterone** normal. *Finalized by the predictable outcome of management,* e.g. explanation, recommend cosmetic measures.
Polycystic ovary syndrome	*Suggested by:* gradual increase in hirsutism since puberty, thin head hair, irregular periods, infertility. *Confirmed by:* ↑**testosterone**, ↓**SHBG**, ↑**LH** (tests done in follicular phase of menstrual cycle). **US scan** showing cystic ovaries. *Finalized by the predictable outcome of management,* e.g. metformin to reduce insulin resistance, combined oestrogen 'pill' to ↓SHBG and ↓free androgen, with cyproterone for hirsutism. Clomiphene to induce ovulation.
Ovarian or adrenal carcinoma	*Suggested by:* change in hair pattern over months, voice deepening, breast atrophy, no periods, cliteromegaly. *Confirmed by:* ↓**LH** and ↑↑**testosterone**. **US scan** and laparoscopy findings. *Finalized by the predictable outcome of management,* e.g. surgical removal of adrenal or ovary-containing tumour.
Cushing's disease (ACTH driven)	*Suggested by:* truncal obesity, purple striae, bruising, moon face, and buffalo hump. Pigmented creases (suggest ↑ACTH, especially in ectopic ACTH from a carcinoma or carcinoid tumour). ↑**24h urinary free cortisol**. *Confirmed by:* 2x ↑**midnight cortisol** and ↑**midnight ACTH** and failure to suppress cortisol after dexamethazone 0.5mg 6 hourly for 48h (but does suppress after 2mg 6 hourly for 48 hours) and bilaterally large adrenals on **CT or MRI scan.** *Finalized by the predictable outcome of management,* e.g. initial control with metyrapone until response to surgery. Removal of pituitary adenoma or bilateral adrenalectomy if source not identified.
Cushing's syndrome due to adrenal adenoma or carcinoma	*Suggested by:* truncal obesity, purple striae, and bruising. No pigmentation in skin creases. ↑**24h urinary free cortisol**. *Confirmed by:* 2x ↑**midnight cortisol** and ↓**midnight ACTH** and failure to suppress cortisol after **dexamethasone suppression test** 0.5mg 6 hourly for 48h and after 2mg 6 hourly for 48h, and unilateral large adrenal on **CT or MRI scan.** *Finalized by the predictable outcome of management,* e.g. initial control with metyrapone until surgical treatment successful. Adrenalectomy for adenoma and carcinoma, also radiotherapy.

Abdominal striae

White striae are healed pink or purple striae. Initial investigations: pregnancy test, 24 hour urinary free cortisol.

- Pink striae

Main differential diagnoses and typical outline evidence, etc.	
Pregnancy	*Suggested by:* no periods and obvious pregnant uterus. *Confirmed by:* **pregnancy test** +ve and **US scan abdomen/pelvis**. *Finalized by the predictable outcome of management,* e.g. progress of pregnancy.
Simple obesity	*Suggested by:* large abdomen and usually rapid weight increase. *Confirmed by:* above clinical findings. *Finalized by the predictable outcome of management,* e.g. lifestyle changes, diet, and exercise.

- Purple striae

Main differential diagnoses and typical outline evidence, etc.	
Glucocorticoid steroid therapy	*Suggested by:* truncal obesity, purple striae, bruising, moon face, and buffalo hump. *Confirmed by:* drug history: taking high dose of glucocorticoid. *Finalized by the predictable outcome of management,* e.g. stopping medication if appropriate.
Cushing's disease (ACTH driven)	*Suggested by:* truncal obesity, purple striae, bruising, moon face, and buffalo hump. Pigmented creases (suggest ↑ACTH, especially in ectopic ACTH from a carcinoma or carcinoid tumour). **↑24h urinary free cortisol**. *Confirmed by:* 2x **↑midnight cortisol** and **↑midnight ACTH** and failure to suppress cortisol after dexamethasone 0.5mg 6 hourly for 48h (but does suppress after 2mg 6 hourly for 48 hours) and bilaterally large adrenals on **CT** or **MRI scan**. *Finalized by the predictable outcome of management,* e.g. initial control with metyrapone until response to surgery. Removal of pituitary adenoma or bilateral adrenalectomy if source not identified.
Cushing's syndrome due to adrenal adenoma or carcinoma	*Suggested by:* truncal obesity, purple striae, and bruising. No pigmentation in skin creases. **↑24h urinary free cortisol**. *Confirmed by:* 2x **↑midnight cortisol** and **↓midnight ACTH** and failure to suppress cortisol after **dexamethasone suppression test** 0.5mg 6 hourly for 48h and after 2mg 6 hourly for 48h, and unilateral large adrenal on **CT** or **MRI scan**. *Finalized by the predictable outcome of management,* e.g. initial control with metopirone until surgical treatment successful. Adrenalectomy for adenoma and carcinoma, also radiotherapy.

Obesity

Definition: BMI >30kgm^{-2}. Initial investigations: TSH, FT4, 24h urinary free cortisol.

Main differential diagnoses and typical outline evidence, etc.	
Simple obesity	*Suggested by:* limb and truncal obesity.
	Confirmed by: TSH and FT4 normal. 24h urinary cortisol normal.
	Finalized by the predictable outcome of management, e.g. lifestyle changes, dieting, and exercise. Medical and surgical treatment for appropriate candidates.
Hypothyroidism	*Suggested by:* cold intolerance, tiredness, ↑constipation, bradycardia.
	Confirmed by: **↑TSH, ↓FT4**.
	Finalized by the predictable outcome of management, e.g. levothyroxine 50 micrograms/d, assessing clinically and TSH after 4–8wk, aiming TSH to be normal (not suppressed). For elderly or in angina, beginning with half the dose of levothyroxine.
Cushing's disease (ACTH driven)	*Suggested by:* truncal obesity, purple striae, bruising, moon face, and buffalo hump. Pigmented creases (suggest ↑ACTH, especially in ectopic ACTH from a carcinoma or carcinoid tumour). **↑24h urinary free cortisol**.
	Confirmed by: 2x **↑midnight cortisol** and **↑midnight ACTH** and failure to suppress cortisol after dexamethasone 0.5mg 6 hourly for 48h (but does suppress after 2mg 6 hourly for 48h) and bilaterally large adrenals on **CT or MRI scan**.
	Finalized by the predictable outcome of management, e.g. initial control with metyrapone until response to surgery. Removal of pituitary adenoma or bilateral adrenalectomy if source not identified.
Cushing's syndrome due to adrenal adenoma or carcinoma	*Suggested by:* truncal obesity, purple striae, and bruising. No pigmentation in skin creases. **↑24h urinary free cortisol**.
	Confirmed by: 2x **↑midnight cortisol** and **↓midnight ACTH** and failure to suppress cortisol after **dexamethasone suppression test** 0.5mg 6 hourly for 48h and after 2mg 6 hourly for 48h, and unilateral large adrenal on **CT or MRI scan**.
	Finalized by the predictable outcome of management, e.g. initial control with metyrapone until surgical treatment successful. Adrenalectomy for adenoma and carcinoma, also radiotherapy.

Pigmented creases and flexures (and buccal mucosa)

Suggests excess ACTH secretion. Initial investigations: U&E, 9a.m. fasting cortisol, 24h urinary free cortisol.

Main differential diagnoses and typical outline evidence, etc.	
Addison's disease = 1° adrenal failure due to autoimmune destruction or TB	*Suggested by:* fatigue, ↓BP, and postural drop. *Confirmed by:* ↓9a.m. cortisol with poor response to **Synacthen® stimulation test** and ↑**ACTH**. *Finalized by the predictable outcome of management,* e.g. hydrocortisone (e.g. 10mg a.m. and 5mg p.m.) and fludrocortisone 50–200 micrograms. Supply of steroid deficiency warning card. Hydrocortisone IM if oral therapy not possible.
Cushing's disease (ACTH-driven)	*Suggested by:* truncal obesity, purple striae, bruising, moon face, and buffalo hump. Pigmented creases (suggest ↑ACTH, especially in ectopic ACTH from a carcinoma or carcinoid tumour). ↓**24h urinary free cortisol**. *Confirmed by:* 2x ↑**midnight cortisol** and failure to suppress cortisol after dexamethasone 0.5mg 6 hourly for 48h, and ↑**midnight ACTH** and bilaterally large adrenals on **CT** or **MRI scan**. *Finalized by the predictable outcome of management,* e.g. initial control with metyrapone until response to surgery. Removal of pituitary adenoma or bilateral adrenalectomy if source not identified.
Ectopic ACTH secretion	*Suggested by:* general weakness, proximal myopathy, usually evidence of lung cancer or other malignancy. *Confirmed by:* ↓serum potassium, 2x ↑**midnight cortisol**, and ↑**ACTH**. *Finalized by the predictable outcome of management,* e.g. metopirone to reduce cortisol production. Surgical treatment if tumour source of ACTH can be localized or bilateral adrenalectomy if tumour source cannot be localized.

Spider naevi

Red, pinhead-sized spots with radiating blood vessels that empty when centre pressed by pinhead-sized object. Initial investigations: pregnancy test, LFTs.

Main differentials, typical outline evidence & initial management	
Normal	*Suggested by:* small numbers on chest (<3), usually in a young woman on chest and upper back.
	Confirmed by: no increase with time.
	Finalized by the predictable outcome of management, e.g. no change if left alone, explanation, and reassurance.
Taking oestrogens	*Suggested by:* small numbers on chest in a young woman on pill.
	Confirmed by: decrease when pill stopped in due course (no urgency).
	Finalized by the predictable outcome of management, e.g. after stopping.
Pregnancy	*Suggested by:* moderate numbers in a pregnant woman.
	Confirmed by: decrease when pregnancy over.
	Finalized by the predictable outcome of management, e.g. explanation and reassurance only.
Liver failure	*Suggested by:* large numbers on chest, also on neck and face, jaundice, features of liver failure.
	Confirmed by: **↓albumin, ↑prothrombin time.**
	Finalized by the predictable outcome of management, e.g. explanation, no alcohol, dietary advice, vitamin K **if** ↑prothrombin time, low-salt diet if ascites, anti-flu and pneumococcal vaccination, colestyramine for pruritus.

Thin, wasted, cachectic

Initial investigations: FBC, TSH, FT4.

Main differential diagnoses and typical outline evidence, etc.

Low calorie intake, e.g. anorexia nervosa, alcoholism, drug abuse, any prolonged systemic illness, e.g. severe COPD	*Suggested by:* dietary history. *Confirmed by:* dietitian's assessment, as inpatient if necessary. *Finalized by the predictable outcome of management*, e.g. controlled balanced diet with food chart to document intake, twice weekly weighing.
Thyrotoxicosis	*Suggested by:* normal or increased appetite plus weight loss despite adequate intake, frequent loose bowel movement, lid retraction and lag, sweats, tachycardia. *Confirmed by:* ↓TSH, ↑FT4 and/or ↑FT3. *Finalized by the predictable outcome of management*, e.g. propranolol to control symptoms, antithyroid drugs, e.g. carbimazole; radioiodine for hot nodules or radioiodine or surgery if relapse after 6–18mo course.
AIDS	*Suggested by:* signs of opportunistic infection, e.g. oral candidiasis, oral hairy leukoplakia, Kaposi's sarcoma, lymphadenopathy. *Confirmed by:* detection of **HIV antibodies** in serum, **HIV RNA** in plasma. *Finalized by the predictable outcome of management*, e.g. chemotherapy using anti-retroviral therapy, chemoprophylaxis against opportunistic infections, e.g. TB, and general and sexual health advice.
Malignancy	*Suggested by:* progressive weight loss and malaise, poor appetite. *Confirmed by:* metastases in liver on **US scan**, bone 2° on **plain X-rays**, 1°tumour on **upper or lower GI endoscopy, bronchoscopy,** etc. *Finalized by the predictable outcome of management*, e.g. surgery or chemotherapy or radiotherapy, depending on nature of primary source and staging of disease.
TB	*Suggested by:* cough, night sweats, haemoptysis, CXR: abnormal shadowing. *Confirmed by:* **AFB in sputum** on microscopy, **mycobacteria on culture**, response to antibiotics. *Finalized by the predictable outcome of management*, e.g. provisional treatment with isoniazid, pyrazinamide, rifampicin and ethambutol for 2mo pending result of culture and sensitivity. Pyridoxine if malnourished; contact tracing.

Purpura

Covers a spectrum from small pinpoint petechiae to large areas of 'bruising' in skin; do not blanch when compressed. Initial investigations: FBC, ESR, clotting (PT/INR).

Main differential diagnoses and typical outline evidence, etc.	
Thrombocytopenia due to autoimmune process or idiopathic (ITP), SLE	*Suggested by:* petechiae, haemorrhagic manifestations, e.g. epistaxis, and history of associated condition, e.g. viral illness. *Confirmed by:* ↓**platelet count** but RBC and WCC normal. No splenomegaly and normal bone marrow examination; **platelets antibodies** +ve. *Finalized by the predictable outcome of management,* e.g. for mild cases (e.g. platelets >20x10⁹ or no haemorrhagic manifestations): observation only. Otherwise, oral steroids over 2wk, then tapered over months ± immunoglobulin, immunosuppressants, and splenectomy.
Pancytopenia due to aplastic anaemia, hypersplenism, myelodysplasia, disseminated intravascular coagulation	*Suggested by:* petechiae and history of associated condition. *Confirmed by:* ↓**platelet count**, ↓WCC, ↓Hb. *Finalized by the predictable outcome of management,* e.g. prompt treatment of infections, prophylactic antibiotics, and antifungal agents, ± oral steroids and immunoglobulin IV.
Platelet dysfunction due to aspirin, NSAIDs, renal failure	*Suggested by:* bruising and drug history. *Confirmed by:* reduced bruising when suspected drug stopped or other cause removed. *Finalized by the predictable outcome of management,* e.g. stopping suspected drug or treating potential cause.
Congenital vasculopathy due to Osler–Weber–Rendu syndrome, etc.	*Suggested by:* bruising from punctiform malformations on mucous membranes. Nose bleeds, gastrointestinal (GI) bleeding. *Confirmed by:* clinical findings, and normal **platelet count** and **clotting**. *Finalized by the predictable outcome of management,* e.g. topical oestrogen.

Acquired vasculopathy **senile changes, autoimmune vasculitis (Henoch–Schönlein), steroids, scurvy**	*Suggested by:* bruising into associated thin skin with atrophied subcutaneous tissue. *Confirmed by:* normal **platelet count** and **clotting**. *Finalized by the predictable outcome of management,* e.g. protection of skin from mechanical injury, treatment directed at cause, e.g. oral steroids for autoimmune conditions.
Acquired coagulopathy **due to liver disease, vitamin K deficiency, DIC**	*Suggested by:* bruising and history of associated condition. *Confirmed by:* prolonged **prothrombin time**. *Finalized by the predictable outcome of management,* e.g. protection of skin and joints from injury, treatment directed at cause, e.g. vitamin K injections for vitamin K deficiency.
Congenital coagulopathy **e.g. Von Willebrand's disease**	*Suggested by:* lifelong bruising and bleeding (after tooth extraction, heavy periods). *Confirmed by:* abnormal platelets function (count normal) and **prolonged activated partial thromboplastin time (APTT)**. *Finalized by the predictable outcome of management,* e.g. protection of skin and joints from injury, avoidance of NSAIDs. In Von Willebrand's, vasopressin for mild bleeding; Rich Factor VIII prior to surgery.
Drug effect	*Suggested by:* drug history, e.g. warfarin, steroids. *Confirmed by:* improvement or drug withdrawal. *Finalized by the predictable outcome of management,* e.g. stopping suspected drugs.

Generalized lymphadenopathy

Initial investigations: FBC, CRP, ESR, Paul–Bunnell test, Mantoux test, CXR, U/S scan.

Main differential diagnoses and typical outline evidence, etc.

Infectious mononucleosis (glandular fever) due to Epstein–Barr virus	*Suggested by:* very severe throat pain with enlarged tonsils covered with creamy membrane. Petechiae on palate. Profound malaise. Generalized lymphadenopathy, splenomegaly. *Confirmed by:* **Paul–Bunnel test** +ve. **Viral titres**: ↑Epstein–Barr titres. *Finalized by the predictable outcome of management*, e.g. paracetamol, avoid antibiotics (amoxicillin may cause rash).
Hodgkin's lymphoma	*Suggested by:* anaemia, splenomegaly, multiple lymph node enlargement. *Confirmed by:* **lymph node histology** showing Reed–Sternberg cells. *Finalized by the predictable outcome of management*, e.g. radiotherapy for the early stage, for the more advanced chemotherapy (MOPP) alone or combined with radiotherapy.
Non-Hodgkin's lymphoma	*Suggested by:* anaemia, multiple lymph node enlargement. *Confirmed by:* **lymph node histology** with no Reed–Sternberg cells. *Finalized by the predictable outcome of management*, e.g. radiotherapy for localized disease, chlorambucil for systemic disease.
Chronic myeloid leukaemia (CML)	*Suggested by:* splenomegaly, variable hepatomegaly, bruising, anaemia. *Confirmed by:* presence of **Philadelphia chromosome**, ↑**WCC**, e.g. >100x10⁹/L. *Finalized by the predictable outcome of management*, e.g. allopurinol, imatinib, HLA typing, sibling-matched allogenic transplantation in the chronic phase.
Chronic lymphocytic leukaemia (CLL)	*Suggested by:* anorexia, weight loss, enlarged, rubbery, non-tender lymph nodes. Hepatomegaly, late splenomegaly. Bruising, anaemia. *Confirmed by:* **FBC:** marked lymphocytosis. **Bone marrow** infiltration with leukaemic cells. *Finalized by the predictable outcome of management*, e.g. monitoring of asymptomatic patients, chemotherapy for the symptomatic, allogenic, or autologous stem cell transplantation.

Acute myeloid leukaemia (AML)	*Suggested by:* generalized lymphadenopathy in adult patient, previous cytotoxics for myelodysplasia, variable hepatomegaly, bruising, anaemia.
	Confirmed by: blast cells in **bone marrow biopsy**.
	Finalized by the predictable outcome of management, e.g. explanation and counselling, prompt treatment of infection, supportive transfusions, allopurinol to prevent hyperuricaemia, plan for need of cranial irradiation and intrathecal chemotherapy, cytotoxics, stem cell transplantation.
Acute lymphoblastic leukaemia (ALL)	*Suggested by:* generalized lymphadenopathy in childhood or Down's patient, variable hepatomegaly, bruising, anaemia.
	Confirmed by: presence of **immunological marker** of common (CD10), T-cell, β-cell, null-cell, associated **chromosomal abnormalities**.
	Finalized by the predictable outcome of management, e.g. explanation and counselling, prompt treatment of infection, supportive transfusions, allopurinol to prevent hyperuricaemia, cranial irradiation and intrathecal chemotherapy, cytotoxics, stem cell transplantation.
Sarcoidosis	*Suggested by:* dry cough, breathlessness, malaise, fatigue, weight loss, enlarged lacrimal glands, erythema nodosum.
	Confirmed by: **CXR** appearances (e.g. bilateral lymphadenopathy) and **tissue biopsy** showing non-caseating granuloma.
	Finalized by the predictable outcome of management, e.g. observation if asymptomatic, then NSAIDs for pains and erythema nodosum; if symptoms not mild or progression, oral steroids and immunosuppressive agents.
Drug effect	*Suggested by:* drug history, e.g. phenytoin, retroviral drug.
	Confirmed by: improvement when drug withdrawn.
	Finalized by the predictable outcome of management, e.g. stopping suspected drug(s).

Localized groin lymphadenopathy

Non-specific finding. Initial investigations: FBC.

Main differential diagnosis and typical outline evidence, etc.	
Infection somewhere in lower limb or pelvis (usually in past and node remained large)	*Suggested by:* enlarged nodes confined to groins. *Confirmed by:* local infection in foot or leg, or no symptoms or signs of generalized condition. *Finalized by the predictable outcome of management,* e.g. antibiotics if bacterial infection not resolving within days.

Pressure sores

Blisters or ulcers on heel or sacrum. Initial investigations: FBC, U&E.

Main differential diagnoses and typical outline evidence, etc.	
Prolonged contact	*Suggested by:* history ± sensory loss, e.g. spinal cord injury, cerebrovascular accident. *Confirmed by:* response to frequent turning, dressings, and wound care. *Finalized by the predictable outcome of management,* e.g. frequent turning, dressings, and wound care. Swab wound and treat specific infections, e.g. MRSA.
Poor nutrition	*Suggested by:* weight falling, **↓Hb**, **↓total protein**, **↓potassium**. *Confirmed by:* formal dietary assessment, response to improved nutrition. *Finalized by the predictable outcome of management,* e.g. controlled diet, food diary, weighing 2x weekly, monitor FBC, serum protein, potassium, etc.

Skin symptoms and physical signs

Diagnosis in dermatology 124
Brown macule 126
Red macule 128
Pale macule 129
Papules 130
Nodules 134
Blisters 138
Erythema 142
Purpura and petechiae 146
Pustules 148
Hyperkeratosis, scales, and plaques 150
Itchy scalp 154
Itchy skin with lesions but no wheals 156
Itch with wheals 160
Itch with no skin lesion 161
Skin ulceration 162
Photosensitive rash 164
Pigmented moles 166
A tumour on the skin 168
Hyperpigmented skin 170
Hypopigmented skin 172

Diagnosis in dermatology

Diagnosis is based on pattern recognition in a far more direct way in dermatology than in other specialties. The diagnosis becomes final with the response of the problem to treatment or by its long-term progress. Biopsy and histology are also used widely, especially when malignancy is suspected or the treatment involves prolonged use of toxic drugs. Identify one aspect of the skin appearance so that it can be used as a diagnostic lead, and scan the pages showing diagnoses linked to that lead to see if you can recognize the remainder of a pattern compatible only with one condition. By seeing many patients, you will learn to 'recognize' conditions more readily.

Brown macule

Flat, well-demarcated area of brown skin of any size. Main test is photography to assess change or biopsy usually to exclude malignancy. Initial investigations (other tests in **bold** below): FBC, digital photography of lesion.

Main differential diagnoses and typical outline evidence, etc.	
Flat mole (junctional naevus) (distinguish from malignant melanoma)	*Suggested by:* little variability of brown pigmentation, smooth outline—not irregular, multiple, no symmetry of lesions, not raised, or surrounded by erythema. *Confirmed by:* no change over weeks to months, benign **biopsy** appearance.
Freckles and solar lentigines	*Suggested by:* small (<5mm), pale brown, asymmetrical macules, especially on face, red-haired, increased prominence after exposure to sun, asymmetrically distributed. *Confirmed by:* no change over months to years. *Finalized by the predictable outcome of management,* e.g. good response to cryotherapy.
Chloasma	*Suggested by:* appearance of large (>5mm) areas of pigmentation during pregnancy. *Confirmed by:* resolution in months following delivery. *Finalized by the predictable outcome of management,* e.g. sunscreens, and camouflage cosmetics.
Café-au-lait spot often (esp. if >6 in no. and >5mm diameter) associated with neurofibromatosis	*Suggested by:* one or more light brown, flat, sharply demarcated, evenly pigmented oval macules. *Confirmed by:* no change over months to years.
Pseudo-acanthosis nigricans (benign, no association with malignancy)	*Suggested by:* dark spots on the skin in the flexures, e.g. axillae of obese people, type 2 diabetics, or acromegalics. *Confirmed by:* no change over months or years. Diagnosis of underlying condition. *Finalized by the predictable outcome of management,* e.g. treating underlying condition resulting in resolution.
Acanthosis nigricans (may be associated with malignancy, diabetes mellitus or malignancy)	*Suggested by:* skin thickening and pigmentation over months or years. *Confirmed by:* presence of pigmented, velvety, and papillomatous skin lesion of flexures, neck, nipples, and umbilicus. *Finalized by the predictable outcome of management,* e.g. improvement after weight reduction, and after treating underlying conditions.

Berloque dermatitis	*Suggested by:* red-brown macules on neck after exposure to sunlight. *Confirmed by:* history of bergamot-containing cosmetics applied to same area. *Finalized by the predictable outcome of management,* e.g. sunblock and avoidance of exposure to sun.
Plant chemical hyperphotosensitivity	*Suggested by:* red-brown macules on arms, hands, and face (blistering first) after exposure to sunlight. *Confirmed by:* history of cutting plants (e.g. giant hogweed) without skin covering. *Finalized by the predictable outcome of management,* e.g. sunblock and avoidance of exposure to sun and exposure to certain plants.
Hutchinson's freckle (with risk of progression to malignant melanoma)	*Suggested by:* large, irregular macule developed from smaller one with variable expansion, regression, or coalescence to form irregular pigmented areas up to 10cm in diameter. *Confirmed by:* history and appearance and no change over time (biopsy to exclude malignancy if there is change).
Peutz–Jegher's syndrome (with risk of colonic and other neoplasms)	*Suggested by:* small (<5mm) macules on the lips, in the mouth, and around the eyes and nose; also around the anus, hands, and feet. Present since infancy or childhood and fade with age. *Confirmed by:* presence of *polyposis coli* on **colonoscopy**. *Finalized by the predictable outcome of management,* e.g. colectomy.

Red macule

Flat, well-demarcated area of red skin. Main test is photography to assess change or biopsy, usually to exclude malignancy. Initial investigations (other tests in **bold** below): digital photography of lesion.

Main differential diagnoses and typical outline evidence, etc.	
Drug reaction or allergy (e.g. due to penicillins, cephalosporins, anti-epileptics)	*Suggested by:* red macular (or papular) rash up to 2wk after taking drug ± itching, burning, uniform pigmentation, symmetrical, on lower face or trunk ± fever, eosinophilia. *Confirmed by:* resolution when drug removed and no recurrence if avoided. *Finalized by the predictable outcome of management,* e.g. emollient, antihistamines, withdrawal of most recently used drugs, e.g. antibiotics.
Viral exanthema from unknown agent	*Suggested by:* red, non-itchy rash with uniform pigmentation. Related systemic symptoms. *Confirmed by:* appearance, spontaneous resolution. *Finalized by the predictable outcome of management,* e.g. antipyretic.
Measles	*Suggested by:* red, non-itchy rash with uniform pigmentation. Related systemic symptoms. *Confirmed by:* appearance, spontaneous resolution, consistent with an incubation period of 10–14 days. *Finalized by the predictable outcome of management,* e.g. antipyretic.
Rubella (in pregnant mothers complicated by congential malformation)	*Suggested by:* red, non-itchy rash with uniform pigmentation. Related systemic symptoms. *Confirmed by:* appearance, spontaneous resolution, consistent with an incubation period of 14–21 days. *Finalized by the predictable outcome of management,* e.g. antipyretic.

Pale macule

Flat, well-demarcated, pale area. Initial investigations (other tests in **bold** below): digital photography of lesion.

Main differential diagnoses and typical outline evidence, etc.	
Post-inflammatory hypopigmentation	*Suggested by:* history of preceding red macule. *Confirmed by:* resolution when drug removed and no recurrence if avoided. *Finalized by the predictable outcome of management,* e.g. resolution after withdrawal of most recent drugs, especially antibiotics.
Vitiligo	*Suggested by:* FH, non-itchy, white patches of the skin, usually sun-exposed areas, premature greying of hair, and symptoms of other associated autoimmune disorders, e.g. thyroid problems, pernicious anaemia, alopecia areata, and diabetes mellitus. *Confirmed by:* typical appearance, +ve **autoimmune profile**, **skin biopsy** shows absence of melanocytes. *Finalized by the predictable outcome of management,* e.g. treating underlying conditions, sunscreens, and use of cosmetics. Counselling in depressed patients (because of appearance), topical steroids, psoralen and UVA (PUVA), or depigmentation of normal skin to match affected one.
Pityriasis versicolor	*Suggested by:* history of excessive sweating or immunosupression. Appearance of well-defined, scaly, pale brownish, and uneven patches, usually on upper back and chest. *Confirmed by:* **microscopy, culture**, and **Wood's light examination** of skin scrapings show presence of *Pityrosporum orbiculare*. *Finalized by the predictable outcome of management,* e.g. good response to local application of selenium sulphide or ketoconazole shampoos, and to systemic antifungals, e.g. itraconazole if severe.
Pityriasis alba	*Suggested by:* young age, excessive dry skin, abrasive clothing, stress, and atopy. Skin lesions itchy and more apparent in summer. *Confirmed by:* presence of superficial, pale, slightly scaly, brown macules with irregular margins on face, neck, arms, and trunk, and the rash quickly becoming red in the sun. *Finalized by the predictable outcome of management,* e.g. moisturizing creams, topical steroids, and oral antihistamines, e.g. chlorphenamine.

Papules

Raised lesion, <5mm diameter. Initial investigations (other tests in **bold** below): digital photography of lesion.

Main differential diagnoses and typical outline evidence, etc.	
Acne	*Suggested by:* young teen, oily skin. *Confirmed by:* multiple comedones, open (blackhead spots) or closed (whitehead spots), in addition to papules and pustules, cysts, and scarring depending on severity. *Finalized by the predictable outcome of management,* e.g. response to washing the face gently with a cleanser. Topical and/or systemic treatments for weeks, months, or years.
Scabies	*Suggested by:* severe itching, especially at night ± other members of family affected. *Confirmed by:* presence of burrows on sides of fingers, wrists, ankles, and nipples. **Microscopic examination**. *Finalized by the predictable outcome of management,* e.g. malathion lotion applied on the whole body for 24h, repeated after 2wk and treatment of all close contacts, washing clothes and bedding.
Viral wart	*Suggested by:* history of contacts, use of swimming baths, immunosuppressant. *Confirmed by:* presence of dome- or flat-topped papules on hand, leg, and face, usually multiple. *Finalized by the predictable outcome of management,* e.g. topical salicylic acid, cryotherapy, cautery, or curettage if no spontaneous resolution.
Molluscum contagiosum	*Suggested by:* affecting children or young adults, and history of contacts. *Confirmed by:* dome-shaped, umbilicated papules; if squeezed, produce a cheesy material. *Finalized by the predictable outcome of management,* e.g. expressing contents with forceps, curettage, or cryotherapy if no spontaneous resolution.
Orf	*Suggested by:* history of contact with sheep, e.g. farmers, vets. Bottle-feeding of a lamb. Presence of affected sheep. *Confirmed by:* solitary, rapidly growing, red papule, usually on a finger. *Finalized by the predictable outcome of management,* e.g. if no spontaneous resolution, topical and systemic antibiotics for systemic infections.
Campbell-de-Morgan spots	*Suggested by:* small, bright red non-blanching papules on trunk of elderly or middle-aged people. Can be associated with chemical exposure, pregnancy, and prolactinoma. *Confirmed by:* no change for months. *Finalized by the predictable outcome of management,* e.g. if no change over time, excision by cauterization.

Skin tags	*Suggested by:* elderly or middle-aged, often obese. *Confirmed by:* pedunculated, usually neck, axilla, eyelids. *Finalized by the predictable outcome of management,* e.g. excision or cryotherapy.
Milia	*Suggested by:* age, usually a child. Mostly on face as small, white papules. *Confirmed by:* above typical appearance. *Finalized by the predictable outcome of management,* e.g. spontaneous resolution with no specific treatments.
Insect bite	*Suggested by:* history. *Confirmed by:* presence of a localized papule or blister, or a generalized allergic reaction. A sting mark in the centre. *Finalized by the predictable outcome of management,* e.g. if anaphylactic reaction, adrenaline and oxygen; carrying adrenaline auto-injector for future events. For local irritation, ice pack, and antihistamines.
Early seborrhoeic wart	*Suggested by:* patient is elderly or middle-aged. Pigmented, raised spot. *Confirmed by:* multiple lesions, mostly on trunk and face. Lesions have a 'stuck-on' appearance with keratin plugs and well-defined edges. *Finalized by the predictable outcome of management,* e.g. liquid nitrogen or cryotherapy.
Xanthomata	*Suggested by:* yellowish papules on the hands, tendons, and eyelids. *Confirmed by:* raised **fasting lipids**. *Finalized by the predictable outcome of management,* e.g. treating underlying hyperlipidaemia ± cauterization or excision.
Guttate psoriasis	*Suggested by:* +ve FH. Sudden onset. History of a throat infection. *Confirmed by:* acute, symmetrical eruption of 'drop-like' and slightly scaly lesions on trunk and limbs. *Finalized by the predictable outcome of management,* e.g. antibiotics for streptococcal infections, topical agents (e.g. emollients), steroids, vitamin D analogues, dithranol. Systemic treatment, e.g. PUVA, methotrexate.
Lichen planus	*Suggested by:* very itchy, polygonal, flat-topped, violaceous papules affecting flexor surfaces, palms, soles, membrane, and genitalia. Recurrent and can affect mucous membranes like inside of mouth. *Confirmed by:* typical appearance of the rash. If necessary, **skin biopsy** with the typical telltale appearance under the microscope. *Finalized by the predictable outcome of management,* e.g. spontaneous resolution, response to topical steroids, oral antihistamines. Mouthwashes for the oral lesions. Systemic oral steroids or PUVA if severe.

Main differential diagnoses and typical outline evidence, etc.

Pityriasis lichenoides chronica	*Suggested by:* chronic nature, scattered, small papules on limbs and trunk. *Confirmed by:* papules topped by a fine, single scale. *Finalized by the predictable outcome of management,* e.g. antibiotics for associated infections, antihistamines for itching ± local steroids, or tacrolimus ointments, or UV treatment.
Prickly heat	*Suggested by:* history of travel to a high temperature area. *Confirmed by:* tiny red papules improving when back to colder environment. *Finalized by the predictable outcome of management,* e.g. cool bathing and avoidance of excessive temperatures.
Keratosis pilaris	*Suggested by:* papule in child or young adults, better during summer, worse in winter. *Confirmed by:* tiny, follicular, hyperkeratotic, non-itchy papules with erythema on upper arms with a typical gooseflesh or sandpaper appearance. *Finalized by the predictable outcome of management,* e.g. abrasive pad to smooth skin, exposure to sun; local treatment, high potency steroids, urea, and topical retinoids if severe.
Blue naevus	*Suggested by:* solitary, blue, small papule on the dorsum of the foot or hand. *Confirmed by:* colour is a shade of blue. **Excision** and **histology**. *Finalized by the predictable outcome of management,* e.g. excisional biopsy.
Basal cell carcinoma	*Suggested by:* history of chronic solar damage, in white-skinned, most commonly face and neck. Nodular, domed-shaped, necrozing in the centre, producing an ulcer with rolled edges. *Confirmed by:* **excision** and **histology**. *Finalized by the predictable outcome of management,* e.g. cryotherapy, excision, or radiotherapy.
Malignant melanoma	*Suggested by:* FH, fair skin, multiple moles. The mole itself is asymmetrical in shape, has an irregular border, is deep black or two colours and >7mm in diameter. *Confirmed by:* **excision** and **histology**. *Finalized by the predictable outcome of management,* e.g. excisional biopsy.

Darier's disease	*Suggested by:* usually teenagers or young adults, other members of the family may be affected, unpleasant smell from patient. *Confirmed by:* itchy, scaly, waxy, greasy papules, commonly affect the chest. *Finalized by the predictable outcome of management,* e.g. avoiding sun exposure, heat and humidity. Moisturizers and sunscreens. Tretinoin 0.1% cream under occlusion or a potent topical steroid.
Acanthosis nigricans	*Suggested by:* skin thickening and pigmentation over months or years. *Confirmed by:* presence of pigmented, velvety, and papillomatous skin lesion of flexures, neck, nipples, and umbilicus, ± underlying disease, e.g. diabetes mellitus, acromegaly and malignancy. *Finalized by the predictable outcome of management,* e.g. weight reduction and treating underlying conditions.
Pseudoxanthoma elasticum	*Suggested by:* grouped, yellowish papules, mainly affecting neck and axillae. *Confirmed by:* presence of loose, wrinkled, and yellow skin. Involvement of arteries, e.g. presence of retinal angioid streaks. *Finalized by the predictable outcome of management,* e.g. reducing cardiovascular risk factors.
Tuberous sclerosis	*Suggested by:* presence of skin lesions in a patient, usually a child with learning difficulties and epilepsy. *Confirmed by:* multiple, red-yellow papules on face, especially on the nasal area and cheeks. *Finalized by the predictable outcome of management,* e.g. genetic counselling, laser treatment for papules.

Nodules

Raised lesions >5mm diameter ± fixed to skin. Best viewed with magnifying glass. Patients usually report lesions because of unsightliness. Initial investigations (other tests in **bold** below): digital photography of lesion.

Main differential diagnoses and typical outline evidence, etc.	
Sebaceous cyst	*Suggested by:* a smooth, spherical, dermal nodule, usually on back of head and neck. *Confirmed by:* slowly growing over time. Sometimes a visible pole that periodically drains. *Finalized by the outcome of management,* e.g. excision if distressing.
Lipoma	*Suggested by:* soft, ill-defined lesion. *Confirmed by:* sometimes multiple in nature, soft consistency. *Finalized by the predictable outcome of management,* e.g. excision if annoying.
Basal cell carcinoma	*Suggested by:* history of chronic solar damage, white-skinned, most commonly face and neck. Nodular, domed-shaped, necrozing in the centre, producing an ulcer with rolled edges. *Confirmed by:* **histology.** *Finalized by the predictable outcome of management,* e.g. cryotherapy, excision, or radiotherapy.
Warts	*Suggested by:* soft, ill-defined lesion. *Confirmed by:* sometimes multiple in nature, soft consistency. *Finalized by the predictable outcome of management,* e.g. excision if annoying.
Xanthoma	*Suggested by:* yellowish papules on the hands, tendons, and eyelids. *Confirmed by:* ↑**fasting lipids.** *Finalized by the predictable outcome of management,* e.g. treating underlying hyperlipidaemia ± cauterization or excision.
Acne	*Suggested by:* young teen, oily skin. *Confirmed by:* multiple comedones; open (blackhead spots) or closed (whitehead spots), in addition to papules and pustules, cysts, and scarring, depending on severity. *Finalized by the predictable outcome of management,* e.g. washing face gently with cleanser but persistence for weeks, months or years. Topical and/or systemic treatment if severe.
Dermatofibroma	*Suggested by:* solitary or multiple nodules—exposed sites in limbs. History of minor injury, thorn pricks, or an insect bite, may be some FH. *Confirmed by:* can hold the lesion between two fingers; feels like hard lump in dermis with the surface looking as if sucked in. *Finalized by the predictable outcome of management,* e.g. excision biopsy.

Squamous cell carcinoma	*Suggested by:* background of solar damage. History of cumulative, previous skin lesion like Bowen's disease. A crusted, thick, eroded nodule, usually on exposed sites. *Confirmed by:* **biopsy histology**. *Finalized by the predictable outcome of management*, e.g. excisional biopsy, radiotherapy.
Keratoacanthoma	*Suggested by:* history of prolonged sun exposure, suggested by rapidly growing tumour reaching a larger size, present on face, ears, or dorsa of hands. *Confirmed by:* rapid growth for almost 2mo, followed by a static phase, and then involution—each stage lasting about 2mo. **Biopsy result.** *Finalized by the predictable outcome of management*, e.g. curettage and histology.
Gouty tophi	*Suggested by:* history of recurrent joint pain. Cutaneous nodules with stretched over and normal texture skin, on the fingers usually, occasionally the ear. *Confirmed by:* **aspiration from tophi**—uric acid crystals. *Finalized by the predictable outcome of management*, e.g. analgesics, allopurinol ± excision of tophus.
Chondrodermatitis nodularis helicis externa	*Suggested by:* pressure effect on ear, especially when sleeping. Waking patient up from sleep due to pain. *Confirmed by:* small, crusted nodule on the external ear. *Finalized by the predictable outcome of management*, e.g. sleeping on the other side. Local injection of triamcinolone or excision.
Rheumatoid nodules	*Suggested by:* previously well-documented history of rheumatoid disease. *Confirmed by:* presence of painless, small lumps under the skin and over pressure points (e.g. elbow), knuckles nodule typical on elbow. Multiple joint swelling and deformities. **Rheumatoid factor** +ve. *Finalized by the predictable outcome of management*, e.g. analgesics, NSAIDs, avoiding irritating trauma, local steroid injections, or excision of nodules.
Heberden's nodes	*Suggested by:* history of chronic osteoarthritis. *Confirmed by:* presence of painless, small nodes (bony growths) on the terminal interphalangeal joints.
Pyogenic granuloma	*Suggested by:* rapidly growing, vascular nodule, easily bleeds. *Confirmed by:* excision **biopsy, histology**. *Finalized by the predictable outcome of management*, e.g. 'shave biopsy', curettage and electrocautery.
Malignant melanoma	*Suggested by:* FH, fair skin, multiple moles, by mole being asymmetrical in shape, irregular border, deep black or two colours, and >7mm in diameter. *Confirmed by:* excision + **histology** of lesion *Finalized by the predictable outcome of management*, e.g. excisional biopsy, etc.

Main differential diagnoses and typical outline evidence, etc.

Erythema nodosum	*Suggested by:* red, tender, deeply placed nodules, usually on the shin. Multiple and bilateral. Associated fever and joint pain. Can be idiopathic or associated with infection or inflammatory bowel disease. *Confirmed by:* ↑**ESR; CXR**: bilateral, hilar lymphadenopathy. *Finalized by the predictable outcome of management,* e.g. analgesics, NSAIDs with or without systemic steroids.
Polyarteritis nodosa	*Suggested by:* tender nodules, fever, joint pain, neuropathic symptoms. *Confirmed by:* ↑**ESR, +ve autoimmune profile, +ve p-ANCA**. *Finalized by the predictable outcome of management,* e.g. analgesics, NSAIDs.
Lepromatous leprosy	*Suggested by:* multiple pale nodules on face, ears, and other places. *Confirmed by:* **microbiology, biopsy.** *Finalized by the predictable outcome of management,* e.g. combination of rifampicin, clofazimine, and dapsone for 2y.
2° syphilis	*Suggested by:* history of ulcers in genitalia. Nodular scaly lesion on hands and soles. Constitutional symptoms. *Confirmed by:* **serological tests, microbiology.** *Finalized by the predictable outcome of management,* e.g. benzylpenicillin IM.
Lupus vulgaris	*Suggested by:* slow onset over months to years, hyperkeratotic, crusted nodule, usually at the site of accidental inoculation. *Confirmed by:* +ve **tuberculin test**. +ve **microbiology** for mycobacterium. *Finalized by the predictable outcome of management,* e.g. antituberculosis combination treatment. Surgical excision for early lesions.
Fish tank or swimming pool granuloma	*Suggested by:* occupation or hobbies bring the patient in contact with fish, or history of trauma treated in the past with antibiotics with no response. *Confirmed by:* +ve **microbiology** tests for mycobacterium. *Finalized by the predictable outcome of management,* e.g. antibiotics as per culture and sensitivity.

Blisters

Blisters <0.5cm diameter are vesicles, blisters >0.5cm are bullae. Initial investigations (other tests in **bold** below): digital photography of lesion.

Main differential diagnoses and typical outline evidence, etc.	
Skin friction	*Suggested by:* presence of blister friction marks on skin and a possible bruising.
	Confirmed by: history of traumatic friction.
	Finalized by the predictable outcome of management, e.g. keep clean, intact. If bursts, get rid of remaining fluid, then apply clean dressing.
Thermal burns	*Suggested by:* presence of blister possibly with some erythema.
	Confirmed by: history of burn.
	Finalized by the predictable outcome of management, e.g. to relieve pain with waterproof antiseptic dressing (to prevent transpiration from damaged cells). Assess the degree of burn and treat accordingly.
Leg oedema	*Suggested by:* blister in the presence of swollen legs.
	Confirmed by: presence of severe pitting oedema, resolution when oedema treated.
	Finalized by the predictable outcome of management, e.g. diuretics, treat associated infections and the underlying cause of oedema if any.
Chemical burns	*Suggested by:* presence of blisters, possibly with traces of chemical.
	Confirmed by: history of contact with chemical.
	Finalized by the predictable outcome of management, e.g. pain control, assessment of degree of the burn, and treat accordingly.
Insect bites	*Suggested by:* history of contact with insect.
	Confirmed by: site of sting surrounded by redness.
	Finalized by the predictable outcome of management, e.g. paracetamol and antihistamines.
Chicken pox	*Suggested by:* contact with a case of chickenpox, a prodromal illness for 1–2d before the appearance of a rash.
	Confirmed by: erythematous lesions, rapidly changing to vesicles, then pustules, followed by crusts after 2–3d. Lesions itchy.
	Finalized by the predictable outcome of management, e.g. antipyretics, antihistamines, and calamine lotion to ease itching and irritability.
Herpes simplex	*Suggested by:* presence of contacts and occurring at a similar site each time, usually lips, face, or genitals, associated respiratory infection ('cold sore'). Lesions recurring.
	Confirmed by: presence of vesicles on the mouth or genitalia. Painful, later crusting with local lymphadenopathy.
	Finalized by the predictable outcome of management, e.g. paracetamol for pain. Aciclovir cream applied five times daily for recurrent mild facial and genital infections. Aciclovir orally for more severe infections. Confirmed genital herpes in a pregnant woman at the time of delivery is an indication for Caesarean section.

Herpes zoster	*Suggested by:* pain, tenderness and paraesthesia in the affected area before the appearance of the rash.
	Confirmed by: presence of typical lesions, which are usually unilateral.
	Finalized by the predictable outcome of management, e.g. for mild causes—analgesics, rest; local calamine lotion for more severe cases; and if seen within 72h of the rash appearance, give aciclovir 800mg five times daily for 1wk.
Herpetic whitlow	*Suggested by:* a painful lesion on finger, usually in a nurse or a dentist attending a patient with herpetic lesion, or in sportsmen like wrestlers (direct inoculation).
	Confirmed by: presence of a painful vesicular lesion on a finger.
	Finalized by the predictable outcome of management, e.g. paracetamol for pain. Aciclovir cream or tablets, depending on severity.
Hand, foot, and mouth disease	*Suggested by:* presence of prodromal symptoms before the appearance of lesions restricted to the feet, hands, and mouth in a child or an adult.
	Confirmed by: presence of vesicles surrounded by an intense skin erythema on the palms, soles, and in the mouth.
	Finalized by the predictable outcome of management, e.g. analgesia, and the self-limiting nature of the condition.
Pompholyx	*Suggested by:* history of atopy, stress, allergic reactions to fungal infections elsewhere.
	Confirmed by: presence of persistent, itchy, clear blisters on fingers, sometimes palms.
	Finalized by the predictable outcome of management, e.g. symptomatic treatments.
Acute eczema: contact dermatitis or atopic	*Suggested by:* acute onset affecting a particular site, suggesting contact with certain objects. History of occupation, hobbies, or nickel sensitivity can suggest a clue.
	Confirmed by: presence of vesicles, and sometimes large blisters with erythema, oedema, papules, and vesicles seen on the affected part.
	Finalized by the predictable outcome of management, e.g. avoid contact with allergens, if possible; moisturizers, creams, and topical steroids. Topical or systemic antibiotic if there is infection.
Pemphigus	*Suggested by:* presence of superficial blisters on the scalp, face, back, chest, and flexures. These may be preceded by mouth erosions several weeks or months before. History of other autoimmune disease like hypothyroidism or myasthenia gravis.
	Confirmed by: presence of **IgG auto-antibodies** to epidermal components. Direct **immunofluorescence studies** show deposition of IgG antibodies in epidermis.
	Finalized by the predictable outcome of management, e.g. high dose of prednisolone PO (e.g. 1–1.5mg/kg/d) ± azathioprine or cyclophosphamide.

Main differential diagnoses and typical outline evidence, etc.

Pemphigoid	*Suggested by:* tense, large blisters, arising on a red or a normal-looking skin, usually in an elderly patient, on the limbs, trunk and flexures, and very rarely, in the mouth. *Confirmed by:* specific **IgG antibodies** to the antigens BP230 and BP180 in subepidermal area. **Direct immunofluorescence studies** showing IgG and C3 antibodies in subepidermal area. *Finalized by the predictable outcome of management,* e.g. usually a low dose of prednisolone PO, e.g. 30–60mg daily with or without azathioprine.
Dermatitis herpetiformis associated with gluten enteropathy	*Suggested by:* a young adult male with gluten sensitivity, with small symmetrical, very itchy blisters on the extension surfaces. *Confirmed by:* **direct immunofluorescence** studies showing depositions and IgA antibodies in the dermis. *Finalized by the predictable outcome of management,* e.g. use of local and systemic antibiotics.
Bullous impetigo	*Suggested by:* presence of extensive, non-itchy golden or brown blisters, on face and limbs in children and adults. *Confirmed by:* **isolation of *Staphylococcus*** in the blister fluid. *Finalized by the predictable outcome of management,* e.g. use of local and systemic antibiotics.
Bullous drug eruption	*Suggested by:* use of a drug in the preceding 2–3 wk, e.g. barbiturates, furosemide. *Confirmed by:* accurate prescribing records of potential causal drug. +ve **patch or intradermal tests.** *Finalized by the predictable outcome of management,* e.g. withdrawal of the causative drug. Emollients and/or topical steroids.
Erythema multiforme a severe form involving mucous membranes called Stevens–Johnson syndrome	*Suggested by:* presence of a potential cause like drug or infection. *Confirmed by:* presence of red rings with a central pale or purple area, giving the appearance of an 'iris' or a target lesion which then blisters. *Finalized by the predictable outcome of management,* e.g. identification and treatment of the underlying cause. Symptomatic treatment for mild cases and hospital admission, for sever ones.
Pemphigoid gestationis	*Suggested by:* presence of similar bullae lesions during previous pregnancies, subsided after delivery. *Confirmed by:* presence of intensely itchy bullae associated with pregnancy. *Finalized by the predictable outcome of management,* e.g. prednisolone PO, e.g. 30–60mg daily.

Porphyrias	*Suggested by:* presence of other affected members in the family. Lesions consist of painful red blistering eruptions.
	Confirmed by: presence of **porphyrins in blood and urine**, **gene studies**.
	Finalized by the predictable outcome of management, e.g. avoid sun exposure, alcohol, or aggravating drugs. Correct iron deficiency if present.
Toxic epidermal necrolysis	*Suggested by:* severe bullous eruption when taking an anticonvulsant, antibiotic, or allopurinol.
	Confirmed by: associated severe epidermal loss.
	Finalized by the predictable outcome of management, e.g. hospital admission, usually on an ITU ward.
Epidermolysis bullosa	*Suggested by:* blistering of skin after minimal trauma.
	Confirmed by: **genetic studies** (mapped to chromosomes 12 and 17). Prenatal diagnosis.
	Finalized by the predictable outcome of management, e.g. avoidance of trauma, supportive measures, and treatment of infection.

Erythema

Reddening of the skin that blanches on pressure. Initial investigations (other tests in **bold** below): digital photography of lesion.

Main differential diagnoses and typical outline evidence, etc.

Cellulitis	*Suggested by:* painful red area on a limb, fever. An underlying condition, e.g. diabetes mellitus. *Confirmed by:* swelling, redness, localized pain, malaise. *Finalized by the predictable outcome of management,* e.g. antibiotic effective against *Streptococcus* or *Staphylococcus*, e.g. benzylpenicillin, etc. and flucloxacillin may be IV initially.
Gout	*Suggested by:* severe joint redness, pain, and swelling, usually in one joint, commonly that of the big toe. *Confirmed by:* ↑**serum uric acid** and the presence of urate crystals in **joint fluid aspirate**. *Finalized by the predictable outcome of management,* e.g. indometacin or, if contraindicated, colchicine to a maximum of 6mg until pain disappears or side-effects appear. Long term allopurinol.
Thermal burn	*Suggested by:* presence of blister, possibly with some erythema. *Confirmed by:* history of burn. *Finalized by the predictable outcome of management,* e.g. relieve pain with sterile, waterproof dressing to prevent transpiration from damaged cells. Assess the degree of burn and treat accordingly.
Chemical burn	*Suggested by:* the presence of blisters, possibly with traces of chemical. *Confirmed by:* history of chemical burn. *Finalized by the predictable outcome of management,* e.g. pain control with sterile, waterproof dressing to prevent transpiration from damaged cells, assessment of degree of the burn, and treat accordingly.
Sunburn	*Suggested by:* history of exposure to sun. *Confirmed by:* redness of exposed area. *Finalized by the predictable outcome of management,* e.g. no more sun. Soothing ointments; antihistamine if heat and cold intolerance due to loss of temperature regulation.
Drug eruption	*Suggested by:* intake of a drug in the preceding 2–3wk. *Confirmed by:* accurate prescribing records. **Patch skin testing.** *Finalized by the predictable outcome of management,* e.g. withdrawal of causative drug. Emollients and/or topical steroids.
Fixed drug eruptions	*Suggested by:* appearance of the rash at the same place every time the same drug taken. *Confirmed by:* **patch skin testing.** *Finalized by the predictable outcome of management,* e.g. avoiding the causative drug.
Viral toxic erythema	*Suggested by:* systemic symptoms with no obvious focus of infection in a child. *Confirmed by:* resolution when systemic symptoms resolve. *Finalized by the predictable outcome of management,* e.g. symptomatic treatment.

Rosacea	*Suggested by:* facial erythema in middle-aged males or females. *Confirmed by:* presence of flushes, erythema, telangiectasis, papules, and pustules. Sometimes the presence of **rhinophyma** (a red, lobulated nose). No comedones as in acne. *Finalized by the predictable outcome of management,* e.g. topical metronidazole 0.75% cream twice daily or tetracycline PO for 3–4wk, reduced dose for 2–3mo.
Palmar erythema	*Suggested by:* associated evidence of liver cirrhosis, pregnancy, and polycythaemia. *Confirmed by:* resolution with underlying condition. *Finalized by the predictable outcome of management,* e.g. treatment of underlying cause.
Drug phototoxicty	*Suggested by:* taking a drug and rash in areas exposed to sunlight. *Confirmed by:* disappearance of the rash after discontinuing the offending drug. *Finalized by the predictable outcome of management,* e.g. discontinuation of the offending drug. Emollients and/or topical steroids.
Erythema multiforme due to sarcoidosis	*Suggested by:* red, tender, deeply placed nodules, usually on the shin. Multiple and bilateral. Associated facet and joint pain. *Confirmed by:* ↑**ESR**; **CXR**: bilateral, hilar lymphadenopathy. *Finalized by the predictable outcome of management,* e.g. analgesics, NSAIDs ± systemic steroids.
Systemic lupus erythematosus (SLE)	*Suggested by:* facial butterfly eruptions commonly in females, with evidence of multisystem involvement. *Confirmed by:* **antinuclear auto-antibodies**. *Finalized by the predictable outcome of management,* e.g. sunscreens if multisystemic disease, steroids with or without immunosuppressive agents.
Erythema ab igne	*Suggested by:* history of an erythema on the shin of an elderly patient who sits before an open fire. *Confirmed by:* improving when avoiding sitting in front of a fire. *Finalized by the predictable outcome of management,* e.g. stop causative behaviour.
Livedo reticularis	*Suggested by:* cyanotic, net-like discoloration skin of legs. *Confirmed by:* presence of an underlying cause, e.g. exposure to cold, SLE, and polycythaemia. *Finalized by the predictable outcome of management,* e.g. treat underlying cause.
HIV seroconversion	*Suggested by:* fever, malaise, nausea, and vomiting with lymphadenopathy, erythematous rash in a homosexual or IV drug-user. *Confirmed by:* detection of **P24 antigen or HIV RNA by PCR**. *Finalized by the predictable outcome of management,* e.g. of underlying disease.

Main differential diagnoses and typical outline evidence, etc.

Erythema nodosum (sarcoid, tuberculosis (TB), drugs, Streptococcus)	*Suggested by:* presence of tender, reddish-blue nodules, usually on the calves and shins, and presence of an underlying condition, e.g. bacterial, viral, fungal, drugs, and systemic disease. *Confirmed by:* **skin biopsy.** *Finalized by the predictable outcome of management,* e.g. pain relief by analgesics or NSAIDs.
Erythema induratum (TB: Bazin's disease)	*Suggested by:* presence of red, indurated lesions on the lower legs. *Confirmed by:* **biopsy** of lesion. *Finalized by the predictable outcome of management,* e.g. analgesia. Treat underlying cause.
Erythema chronicum migrans (Lyme disease)	*Suggested by:* slowly expanding erythematous ring at the site of a tic bite, on a limb usually ± multisystem symptoms. *Confirmed by:* **serology.** *Finalized by the predictable outcome of management,* e.g. doxycyline for 2–3wk. In children below 8y and in pregnancy: amoxicillin for a similar period.

Purpura and petechiae

Purplish lesions resulting from free red blood cells in the skin. They do not blanch on pressure. Purpurae are large (>5mm) and imply clotting defects or blood vessel fragility; petechiae are small (<5mm) and imply platelet defects or vasculitis. Initial investigations (other tests in **bold** below): digital photography of lesion, FBC, U&E, LFT.

Main differential diagnoses and typical outline evidence, etc.	
Trauma	*Suggested by:* history. *Confirmed by:* lesions matching site of trauma. *Finalized by the predictable outcome of management,* e.g. symptomatic treatment.
Senile purpura	*Suggested by:* elderly patient. *Confirmed by:* atrophic small veins and skin. No treatment, just reassurance.
Liver disease	*Suggested by:* jaundice, hepatomegaly, etc. *Confirmed by:* abnormal **LFT and ultrasound (US) scan of liver.** *Finalized by the predictable outcome of management,* e.g. treat underlying condition.
Raised venous pressure, e.g. vomiting	*Suggested by:* history of vomiting, etc. *Confirmed by:* presence of purpuric spot, usually around the eyes. *Finalized by the predictable outcome of management,* e.g. spontaneous resolution.
Drugs (steroids, warfarin, aspirin)	*Suggested by:* intake of drugs. *Confirmed by:* disappearance when drug stopped. *Finalized by the predictable outcome of management,* e.g. resolution after discontinuation of the causative agent.
Vasculitis (Henoch–Schönlein, connective tissue)	*Suggested by:* purpurae on buttock and extensor surfaces, typically in a young male. Associated features of cause, e.g. proteinuria, hypertension, and abdominal pain of Henoch–Schönlein syndrome. *Confirmed by:* typical appearance of the rash. *Finalized by the predictable outcome of management,* e.g. treatment of underlying cause, e.g. with systemic steroids.
Thrombocytopaenia (e.g. idiopathic thrombocytopaenic purpura (ITP), drug-induced, bone marrow replacement, aplastic anaemia)	*Suggested by:* features of the underlying cause. *Confirmed by:* FBC: ↓platelets, etc. *Finalized by the predictable outcome of management,* e.g. resolution after treating the underlying condition.

Renal failure	*Suggested by:* symptoms and signs of renal impairment. *Confirmed by:* ↑**urea**, ↑**creatinine.** *Finalized by the predictable outcome of management, e.g.* of underlying condition.
Endocarditis	*Suggested by:* presence of fever, general malaise, heart murmur. *Confirmed by:* +ve **blood cultures** and an abnormal **echocardiogram**. *Finalized by the predictable outcome of management, e.g.* benzylpenicillin IV + gentamicin.
Paraproteinaemia	*Suggested by:* back pain, loss of appetite, high temperature. *Confirmed by:* paraprotein on **electrophoresis.** *Finalized by the predictable outcome of management, e.g.* treatment of underlying cause.
Clotting disorder (haemophilia A and B)	*Suggested by:* easy bleeding into muscles and joints, and delayed clotting. *Confirmed by:* **clotting screen**. *Finalized by the predictable outcome of management, e.g.* vitamin K; treatment of clotting defect.
Meningoccocal septicaemia	*Suggested by:* rapidly progressive disease with headaches, neck stiffness, vomiting, and photophobia. *Confirmed by:* **blood culture** and **lumbar puncture.** *Finalized by the predictable outcome of management, e.g.* benzylpenicillin IM.
Vitamin K deficiency	*Suggested by:* disorder in a patient with malnutrition or malabsorption, gastrointestinal (GI) bleeding. *Confirmed by:* reversal of bleeding when supplied with vitamin K. *Finalized by the predictable outcome of management, e.g.* vitamin K replacement.
Vitamin C deficiency	*Suggested by:* anorexia, cachexia, gingivitis, loose teeth, and halitosis; pregnancy, poverty, odd diet. *Confirmed by:* low **vitamin C level.** *Finalized by the predictable outcome of management, e.g.* vitamin C supplement.
Disseminated intravascular coagulation (DIC)	*Suggested by:* severe bruising and failure to clot after starting to bleed. Features of a severe underlying condition such as malignancy, sepsis, trauma, and obstetric emergencies. *Confirmed by:* **FBC**: ↓platelets, ↑**PT**, ↑**APTT**, ↓**fibrinogen**. *Finalized by the predictable outcome of management, e.g.* treatment of the cause, and replacement of platelets and clotting factors.

Pustules

A well-defined, pus-filled lesion. Initial investigations (other tests in **bold** below): digital photography of lesion.

Main differential diagnoses and typical outline evidence, etc.	
Impetigo	*Suggested by:* presence of easily ruptured vesicles, leaving yellow crusted exudates, usually affect the face and extremities.
	Confirmed by: typical look and site of lesion.
	Finalized by the predictable outcome of management, e.g. local or systemic antibiotics, depending on severity.
Folliculitis	*Suggested by:* lesions being in hair-baring areas—in women, there might be a history of hair removal by shaving or waxing.
	Confirmed by: **swab**: isolation S. aureus.
	Finalized by the predictable outcome of management, e.g. local or systemic antibiotics.
Sycosis barbae	*Suggested by:* folliculitis in the beard area.
	Confirmed by: **swab** isolation of S. aureus.
	Finalized by the predictable outcome of management, e.g. local or systemic antibiotics.
Herpes simplex	*Suggested by:* presence of contacts and occurring at a similar site each time, usually lips, face, or genitals, and sometimes the presence of a respiratory infection, therefore called a 'cold sore'. Lesions recurring.
	Confirmed by: presence of painful vesicles on the mouth or genitalia.
	Finalized by the predictable outcome of management, e.g. paracetamol for pain. Aciclovir cream applied five times daily for recurrent mild facial and genital infections, and aciclovir PO for more severe infections. Confirmed genital herpes in a pregnant woman at the time of delivery is an indication for Caesarean section.
Herpes zoster	*Suggested by:* pain, tenderness, and paraesthesia in the affected area before the appearance of the rash.
	Confirmed by: presence of typical lesions which are normally unilateral.
	Finalized by the predictable outcome of management, e.g. for mild causes—analgesics, rest, local calamine lotion; for more severe cases and if seen within 72h of the rash appearance, give aciclovir 800mg five times daily for 1wk.
Acne vulgaris	*Suggested by:* presence of comedones, open (blackheads) or closed (whiteheads), papules, pustules, cysts, or scars depending on severity. Comedones appear first at around the age of 12y, then evolve into the different other lesion.
	Confirmed by: typical features of the skin lesions.
	Finalized by the predictable outcome of management, e.g. for mild acne, use local treatments (e.g. benzoyl peroxide cream or gel bd, tretinoin cream or gel) or local antibiotic gels like Zineryt®, with or without oral antibiotic, e.g. minocycline.

Rosacea	*Suggested by:* facial erythema in middle-aged males or females.
	Confirmed by: flushes, erythema, telangiectasis, papules and pustules ± rhinophyma (a red lobulated nose). No comedones as in acne.
	Finalized by the predictable outcome of management, e.g. topical metronidazole or tetracycline PO for 3–4wk with lower dose for 2–3mo.
Hydranitis suppurativa	*Suggested by:* pustules in axilla, groin.
	Confirmed by: recurrent problem.
	Finalized by the predictable outcome of management, e.g. local or systemic antibiotics.
Candidiasis	*Suggested by:* itchy, symmetrical with 'satellite' pustules outside the outer edge of the skin rash. Underlying conditions, e.g. diabetes mellitus, AIDS or Cushing's.
	Confirmed by: **swabs and skin scrapings.**
	Finalized by the predictable outcome of management, e.g. local clotrimazole or miconazole for 2–4wk. Systemic treatment such as fluconazole for non-responding cases.
Localized pustular psoriasis	*Suggested by:* chronic nature of the illness in an elderly patient with psoriasis elsewhere.
	Confirmed by: presence of pustules surrounded by a scaly, erythematous skin on the palms and soles.
	Finalized by the predictable outcome of management, e.g. moderate to potent strength topical steroid.
Generalized pustular psoriasis	*Suggested by:* acute onset with fever, malaise, and general ill health with a psoriatic rash.
	Confirmed by: presence of sheets of small, yellowish pustules, on an erythematous background, which may spread rapidly.
	Finalized by the predictable outcome of management, e.g. rehydration IV with or without antibiotics + local measures.
Dermatitis herpetiformis associated with gluten enteropathy	*Suggested by:* a young adult male with gluten sensitivity, with small, symmetrical, very itchy blisters in the extensor surfaces.
	Confirmed by: **direct immunofluorescence** studies showing depositions and IgA antibodies in the dermis.
	Finalized by the predictable outcome of management, e.g. local and systemic antibiotics.
Pseudomonas infection	*Suggested by:* history of long-term treatment of acne (if lesions are on face) or history of exposure to contaminated baths or whirlpools (if lesions are on body).
	Confirmed by: **swabs + isolation of organism, culture and sensitivity**.
	Finalized by the predictable outcome of management, e.g. with appropriate antibiotic based on culture and sensitivity.
Drug reactions	*Suggested by:* intake of a potentially causative drug in the preceding 2–3wk.
	Confirmed by: accurate prescribing records. Patch test.
	Finalized by the predictable outcome of management, e.g. withdrawal of the causative drug. Emollients and/or topical steroids.

Hyperkeratosis, scales, and plaques

Hyperkeratosis: thickening of the keratin layer; scale: fragment of dry skin; plaque: raised flat-topped lesion, usually over 2cm in diameter. Initial investigations (other tests in **bold** below): digital photography of lesion.

Main differential diagnoses and typical outline evidence, etc.	
Psoriasis	*Suggested by:* scaly, silvery scales on extensor surfaces and sites of minor trauma (Koebner's phenomenon); lesions usually clear after exposure to sun. *Confirmed by:* typical presence of plaques of scaly lesions covering extensor areas of trunk and limbs. *Finalized by the predictable outcome of management,* e.g. tar preparation, Dovobet®, short contact dithranol, or UVB. Immunosuppressants for extensive lesions.
Chronic eczema: atopic, contact	*Suggested by:* contact with certain objects or history of atopy. *Confirmed by:* improvement of condition after eliminating the offending subject. *Finalized by the predictable outcome of management,* e.g. removal of the cause; moisturizers, creams, and topical steroids. Antibiotics if there is infection.
Fungal infections	*Suggested by:* typical ring-like lesions (clearer centres) on the trunk and limbs in tinea corporis (ringworm) or lesions in the inner upper thigh, not involving the scrotum with an advancing scaly and pustular edge in tinea cruris. *Confirmed by:* **microscopy and culture of skin scrapings. Wood's UV light examination** for tinea capitis. *Finalized by the predictable outcome of management,* e.g. local or systemic antifungal agents.
Seborrhoeic dermatitis	*Suggested by:* scalp and facial involvement, excessive dandruff with an itchy and scaly eruption, affecting sides of nose, scalp margin, eyebrows, and ear. *Confirmed by:* typical skin lesions and distribution. *Finalized by the predictable outcome of management,* e.g. medicated shampoo alone or following the application of 2% sulphur ± preceding 2% salicylic acid for scalp lesions. Facial lesions treated with combined antimicrobial and steroid creams.
Lichen simplex chronicus	*Suggested by:* history of repeated rubbing or scratching of an area as a habit or caused by stress; typically Asian or Chinese patient. *Confirmed by:* presence of a single plaque on the back of the neck or in the perineum. *Finalized by the predictable outcome of management,* e.g. emollients and topical steroids.
Lichen planus	*Suggested by:* no FH, related to stress; presence of Koebner's phenomenon. *Confirmed by:* itchy, well-defined, raised, shiny-surfaced lesions with a violaceous colour divided by white streaks (Wickman's striae). *Finalized by the predictable outcome of management,* e.g. topical steroids, systemic steroids for very extensive lesions.

Solar keratosis	*Suggested by:* lesions on sites exposed to sun, patients work out of doors or history of excessive sunbathing, pipe smokers.
	Confirmed by: raised keratotic lesion <1cm in diameter with an irregular edge on face, back of the hands, arms and legs, and scalp in bald men. Lesions are pre-malignant.
	Finalized by the predictable outcome of management, e.g. cryotherapy for large and multiple lesions; trial of fluorouracil cream bd for 2wk.
Pityriasis versicolor	*Suggested by:* chronic brown or pinkish oval or round scaly patches on trunk and limbs; hypopigmented spots in tanned or racially dark skin.
	Confirmed by: typical appearance on **microscopy of skin scrapings**.
	Finalized by the predictable outcome of management, e.g. clotrimazole or miconazole creams, or the use of topical selenium sulphide or ketoconazole shampoos applied for 30min, and then washed off tds for 2wk. If resistant, itraconazole PO for 1wk.
Pityriasis rosea	*Suggested by:* acute onset of scaly oval papules, mainly on trunk, preceded by a 2–8cm in diameter single lesion called the 'herald patch'.
	Confirmed by: typical appearance of the rash and the herald patch.
	Finalized by the predictable outcome of management, e.g. symptomatic treatment.
Juvenile plantar dermatosis	*Suggested by:* child <10y, wearing socks and shoes made of synthetic material.
	Confirmed by: presence of red, dry, fissured, and shiny skin, usually on the forefoot ± the whole sole.
	Finalized by the predictable outcome of management, e.g. use of emollients.
Guttate psoriasis	*Suggested by:* acute, symmetrical appearance of drop-like, scaly skin lesions, on trunk and limbs in an adolescent or young adult typically with sore throat.
	Confirmed by: typical appearance of the rash.
	Finalized by the predictable outcome of management, e.g. topical steroids, coal tar, or narrow band UV.
Bowen's disease	*Suggested by:* indurated, crusted, well-defined, erythematous macule trunk or limbs ± exposure to sheep dip or weed-killers.
	Confirmed by: **biopsy**: carcinoma *in situ*.
	Finalized by the predictable outcome of management, e.g. cryotherapy, topical fluorouracil cream, photodynamic therapy.
Mycosis fungoides (cutaneous T-cell lymphoma)	*Suggested by:* scaly, erythematous patches progressing over months to years to fixed infiltrated plaques, then cancerous nodules.
	Confirmed by: **biopsy**.
	Finalized by the predictable outcome of management, e.g. topical steroids PUVA, or electron beam therapy depending on severity.

Main differential diagnoses and typical outline evidence, etc.

Drug-induced (e.g. β-blockers, carbamazepine)	*Suggested by:* history of taking suspected drug in the preceding 2–3wk. *Confirmed by:* accurate prescribing records. **Patch test**. *Finalized by the predictable outcome of management,* e.g. withdrawal of causative drug. Emollients and/or topical steroids.
Ichthyosis	*Suggested by:* mild to severe dry, scaly skin, seen mainly on the extensor surfaces with the flexures often spared ± FH. *Confirmed by:* typical appearance of skin and **biopsy**. *Finalized by the predictable outcome of management,* e.g. emollients and bath oils for mild cases.
Keratoderma	*Suggested by:* gradual onset in middle age, typically in post-menopausal female. *Confirmed by:* hyperkeratosis of palms and soles. *Finalized by the predictable outcome of management,* e.g. 5–10% salicylic acid ointment or 10% urea cream.
Erythroderma due to eczema, psoriasis, and lymphoma	*Suggested by:* severe systemic symptoms with patchy, then generalized erythema followed by scaling days later ± features of an underlying cause. *Confirmed by:* **skin biopsy.** *Finalized by the predictable outcome of management,* e.g. hospital admission for IV. fluids and steroids.
2° syphilis	*Suggested by:* history of previous chancre + presence of a non-itchy, pink-coloured, papular eruption, becoming scaly, on the trunk, limbs, palms, and soles. *Confirmed by:* +ve **serology for syphilis.** *Finalized by the predictable outcome of management,* e.g. benzyl-penicillin IM or Penicillin V orally for 14d (or doxycycline, erythromycin).

Itchy scalp

Initial investigations (other tests in **bold** below): digital photography of lesion.

Main differential diagnoses and typical outline evidence, etc.	
Head lice	*Suggested by:* intense itching of scalp, typically in a school child ± poor social and hygienic conditions. *Confirmed by:* seeing nits or lice on hair shafts. *Finalized by the predictable outcome of management*, e.g. malathion applied to scalp and left for 12h before being washed out, to be repeated in a week's time. Nits can be removed with a comb.
Seborrhoeic eczema	*Suggested by:* scalp and facial involvement, excessive dandruff with an itchy and scaly eruption, affecting sides of nose, scalp margin, eyebrows, and ear. *Confirmed by:* the above typical skin lesions and distribution. *Finalized by the predictable outcome of management*, e.g. medicated shampoo alone or 2% sulphur or 2% salicylic acid for scalp lesions. Facial lesions: combined antimicrobial and steroid creams.
Psoriasis	*Suggested by:* onset after period of stress, lesions at sites of minor trauma (Koebner's phenomenon) clearing after exposure to sun. *Confirmed by:* well-defined, raised, scaly, disc-shaped plaques on scalp hair margin. *Finalized by the predictable outcome of management*, e.g. 3% salicylic acid in a cream base applied daily in combination with a tar-containing shampoo. Trial of coconut oil compound.
Lichen simplex chronicus	*Suggested by:* history of repeated rubbing or scratching of an area habitually or during stress; typically Asian or Chinese. *Confirmed by:* single plaque on the back of the neck or in the perineum. *Finalized by the predictable outcome of management*, e.g. emollients and topical steroids.
Allergic contact dermatitis	*Suggested by:* exposure to suspect precipitant, e.g. hair dye. *Confirmed by:* improvement on removal of the offending agent. *Finalized by the predictable outcome of management*, e.g. avoid causative agent. Local steroid lotions.
Fungal infection (complicated by possible irreversible hair loss, if untreated)	*Suggested by:* mild, scaly, inflammatory areas with alopecia and broken hair shafts or an inflamed boggy pustular swelling called kerion. *Confirmed by:* **microscopy and culture of skin scrapings**. *Finalized by the predictable outcome of management*, e.g. griseofulvin for 1–2mo.

Herpes zoster	*Suggested by:* pain, tenderness, and paraesthesia in the affected area before the appearance of rash.
	Confirmed by: presence of typical unilateral lesions.
	Finalized by the predictable outcome of management, e.g. mild—analgesics, rest; local calamine lotion; if severe and seen within 72h of rash appearing: aciclovir, e.g. 800mg five times daily for 1wk.
Anxiety and depression	*Suggested by:* history of low mood, anxiety.
	Confirmed by: normal appearance of scalp initially and on follow-up.
	Finalized by the predictable outcome of management, e.g. explanation, psychotherapy.

Itchy skin with lesions but no wheals

Skin scratched or rubbed ± a number of secondary skin signs: excoriations (scratch marks), lichenification (skin thickening), papules (localized skin thickening), or nodules. Initial investigations (other tests in **bold** below): digital photography of lesion.

Main differential diagnoses and typical outline evidence, etc.	
Allergic contact dermatitis	*Suggested by:* exposure to a potential allergen, e.g. hair dye. *Confirmed by:* improvement on removal of the offending agent. *Finalized by the predictable outcome of management,* e.g. avoid causative agent. Local steroid lotions.
Candidiasis e.g. due to diabetes mellitus, AIDS, or Cushing's syndrome	*Suggested by:* itchy, symmetrical with 'satellite' pustules outside the outer edge of the skin rash. Symptoms and signs of underlying condition. *Confirmed by:* +ve swabs and **skin scrapings for yeasts**. *Finalized by the predictable outcome of management,* e.g. local clotrimazole or miconazole for 2–4wk. Systemic treatment for non-responding cases.
Discoid eczema	*Suggested by:* recurring itchy lesion in a middle-aged or an elderly man. *Confirmed by:* presence of coin-shaped lesions on the limbs with a symmetrical distribution. *Finalized by the predictable outcome of management,* e.g. potent steroid cream combined with an antibiotic.
Drug-induced eczema	*Suggested by:* itchy skin with a history of recent drug ingestion. *Confirmed by:* improvement on withdrawal of offending agent. *Finalized by the predictable outcome of management,* e.g. removal of the offending agent. Topical emollients and steroids.
Varicose eczema	*Suggested by:* associated varicose veins and swollen oedematous leg. *Confirmed by:* presence of an eczematous patch on the medial aspect of leg. *Finalized by the predictable outcome of management,* e.g. diuretics, leg elevation, compression bandage, emollient, and steroid creams.
Scabies	*Suggested by:* severe itching, especially at night; other member of family affected. *Confirmed by:* presence of burrows on sides of fingers, wrists, ankles, and nipples. **Microscopic examination** showing the mites. *Finalized by the predictable outcome of management,* e.g. malathion lotion applied on whole body for 24h ± reapplication after 2wk. Treat all close contacts. Wash all clothes and bedding.

Seborrhoeic dermatitis	*Suggested by:* scalp and facial involvement, excessive dandruff with an itchy and scaly eruption affecting sides of nose, scalp margin, eyebrows, and ear. *Confirmed by:* typical skin lesions and distribution. *Finalized by the predictable outcome of management,* e.g. medicated shampoo alone ± preceding 2% sulphur or 2% salicylic acid. Facial lesions treated with combined antimicrobial and steroid creams.
Asteatotic eczema	*Suggested by:* history of dryness and itching in elderly patient, excessive use of central heating, and washing. *Confirmed by:* presence of a scaly, red rash; in severe forms, fissuring and inflammation on leg. *Finalized by the predictable outcome of management,* e.g. emollients with or without topical steroids.
Dermatitis herpetiformis associated with gluten enteropathy	*Suggested by:* a young adult male with gluten sensitivity, with small symmetrical, very itchy blisters in the extensor surfaces. *Confirmed by:* **direct immunofluorescence studies** showing depositions and IgA antibodies in the dermis. *Finalized by the predictable outcome of management,* e.g. local and systemic antibiotics.
Lichen planus	*Suggested by:* related to stress and the presence of Koebner's phenomenon. *Confirmed by:* presence of itchy, well-defined, and raised, shiny-surfaced lesions with a violaceous colour interpreted by white streaks (Wickman's striae). *Finalized by the predictable outcome of management,* e.g. topical steroids; systemic steroids for very extensive lesions.
Psoriasis	*Suggested by:* scaly, silvery scales on extensor surfaces and sites of minor trauma (Koebner's phenomenon); lesions usually clear after exposure to sun. *Confirmed by:* typical presence of plaques of scaly lesions covering extensor areas of trunk and limbs. *Finalized by the predictable outcome of management,* e.g. tar preparation, Dovobet®, short contact dithranol or UVB. Immunosuppressants for extensive lesions.
Eczema herpeticum	*Suggested by:* previous history of atopic eczema in a child who is generally unwell. *Confirmed by:* presence of herpetic lesions on a background of eczematous skin. *Finalized by the predictable outcome of management,* e.g. admission to hospital for fluids IV + aciclovir.
Lichen sclerosus	*Suggested by:* presence of lesion on the genitals and perineum in a female. History of autoimmune conditions, e.g. vitiligo and pernicious anaemia. *Confirmed by:* itchy, atrophic patches of skin in the genital area. *Finalized by the predictable outcome of management,* e.g. moderate to potent local skin steroid cream.

Main differential diagnoses and typical outline evidence, etc.

Lichen simplex chronicus	*Suggested by:* history of habitual rubbing or scratching associated with stress and typically in Asian or Chinese patient. *Confirmed by:* presence of a single plaque on the back of the neck or in the perineum. *Finalized by the predictable outcome of management,* e.g. emollients and topical steroids.
Pellagra associated with carcinoid syndrome or anti-TB drugs.	*Suggested by:* diarrhoea, dementia, and dermatitis. May be history of associated condition. *Confirmed by:* response to nicotinic acid treatment. *Finalized by the predictable outcome of management,* e.g. correction of fluid and electrolyte imbalance + nicotinamide.
Polymorphic light eruption	*Suggested by:* recurrent lesions on exposure typically in a female. *Confirmed by:* presence of an eruption, which may range from a few inflamed papules to severely inflamed and oedematous skin. *Finalized by the predictable outcome of management,* e.g. avoid exposure to sun, use of sunscreens, topical and/or systemic steroids for the acute rash.
Pompholyx	*Suggested by:* history of atopy, stress, allergic reactions to fungal infections elsewhere. *Confirmed by:* presence of persistent, itchy, clear blisters on fingers and sometimes palms. *Finalized by the predictable outcome of management,* e.g. symptomatic with antihistamines, antibiotics, and local creams.

Itch with wheals

Initial investigations (other tests in **bold** below): digital photography of lesion.

Main differential diagnoses and typical outline evidence, etc.	
Chronic idiopathic urticaria	*Suggested by:* recurrent nature and by the appearance of wheals variable in size, shape, and number anywhere on skin with no obvious triggering factors. *Confirmed by:* disappearance of wheals in <24h and possible spontaneous resolution after 6mo. *Finalized by the predictable outcome of management,* e.g. cetirizine and systemic steroids for severe cases, anaphylactic shock treated with adrenaline and as per protocol in BNF.
Acute urticaria	*Suggested by:* sudden urticarial rash after the introduction of the known offending agent, e.g. eggs, fish, peanuts, antibiotics, or latex. *Confirmed by:* improvement after eliminating the offending agent. *Finalized by the predictable outcome of management,* e.g. avoiding the offending agent, cetirizine and systemic steroids for severe cases, anaphylactic shock treated with adrenaline and as per protocol in BNF.
Physical urticaria	*Suggested by:* appearance of wheals after exposure to cold, sun, pressure water, and stress. *Confirmed by:* dermographism and improvement when excluding the offending agent. *Finalized by the predictable outcome of management,* e.g. avoiding the offending agents for the acute condition; cetirizine or fexofenadine, and systemic steroid for more severe reaction. Adrenaline for anaphylaxis and as per BNF protocol.
Hereditary angioedema	*Suggested by:* +ve FH and an onset from childhood of episodes of angioedema affecting the larynx, impairing respiration and GI system, causing abdominal pain, and vomiting. *Confirmed by:* low levels of **C1-esterase inhibitor** and **complement studies** during the acute episode. *Finalized by the predictable outcome of management,* e.g. as for urticaria plus IV infusion of C1-esterase inhibitor.
Linear IgA disease	*Suggested by:* blisters and urticarial rash on back and extensor surfaces. *Confirmed by:* **direct immunofluorescence studies** revealing linear IgA at basement membrane. *Finalized by the predictable outcome of management,* e.g. symptomatic treatment

Itch with no skin lesion

Initial investigations (other tests in **bold** below): digital photography of lesion. FBC, U&E, LFT.

Main differential diagnoses and typical outline evidence, etc.	
Chronic liver disease	*Suggested by:* jaundice, spider naevi, enlarged liver. *Confirmed by:* **LFT**: ↑bilirubin and ↑alkaline phosphatase, prolonged prothrombin time, and low albumin. *Finalized by the predictable outcome of management,* e.g. colestyramine.
Chronic renal failure	*Suggested by:* dry, sallow skin itching. *Confirmed by:* ↑**urea and creatinine,** and ↓**Hb.** *Finalized by the predictable outcome of management:* dietary advice; salt and water management. Regular follow-up. When advanced, plan dialysis or renal transplant.
Iron deficiency	*Suggested by:* pale complexion and skin, koilonychias, angular stomatitis. *Confirmed by:* ↓**Hb,** ↓**MCV,** and ↓**ferritin.** *Finalized by the predictable outcome of management* iron replacement, e.g. ferrous sulfate; improvement after treating underlying causes.
Hyperhidrosis	*Suggested by:* excessive sweating, itching, obesity. *Confirmed by:* typical features and no other features on follow-up. *Finalized by the predictable outcome of management,* e.g. topical aluminium chloride; if intractable, sympathectomy.
1° hypothyroidism	*Suggested by:* dry skin, fatigue, slow-relaxing ankle jerk. *Confirmed by:* ↑**TSH,** ↓**T4.** *Finalized by the predictable outcome of management,* e.g. thyroxine replacement.
Lymphoma (Hodgkin's or non-Hodgkin's)	*Suggested by:* loss of weight, night sweats, lymphadenopathy, hepatosplenomegaly. *Confirmed by:* **biopsy**: Reed–Sternberg cells in Hodgkin's, not in non-Hodgkin's lymphoma, etc. *Finalized by the predictable outcome of management,* e.g. specialist confirmation of diagnosis and staging.
Malignancy	*Suggested by:* general ill health, loss of weight, hepatomegaly, clubbing of fingers, shadow in a **CXR**. *Confirmed by:* **CT scan** of suspect organ(s). *Finalized by the predictable outcome of management,* e.g. specialists confirmation of diagnosis, staging, and selection for potentially curative or palliative care.
1° biliary cirrhosis	*Suggested by:* non-tender hepatomegaly and splenomegaly, xanthoma, arthralgia, abnormal LFT. *Confirmed by:* +ve **anti-mitochondrial, US examination and liver biopsy**. *Finalized by the predictable outcome of management,* e.g. colestyramine; ursodeoxycholic acid (may increase life expectancy and avoid transplant).

Skin ulceration

Initial investigations (other tests in **bold** below): digital photography of lesion.

Main differential diagnoses and typical outline evidence, etc.	
Staphylococcal infection	*Suggested by:* thin-walled blisters, rupturing easily to leave a yellow, crusted area spreading rapidly, usually on face. *Confirmed by:* above typical appearance and site. *Finalized by the predictable outcome of management,* e.g. systemic antibiotic, avoiding local antibiotic due to risk of bacterial resistance.
Basal cell carcinoma	*Suggested by:* small, pearly nodule progressing to central necrosis, producing a crusted ulcer with a rolled edge or a large plaque with a central depression. *Confirmed by:* **histology.** *Finalized by the predictable outcome of management,* e.g. excision.
Squamous cell carcinoma	*Suggested by:* persistently ulcerated or crusted, firm, irregular lesion, usually on sun-exposed areas, e.g. ears, back of hands, bald scalp; in pipe smokers, and patients with leg ulcers. *Confirmed by:* **biopsy.** *Finalized by the predictable outcome of management,* e.g. excision.
Dermatomyositis	*Suggested by:* purple (heliotrope) rash on eyelid/face, Gottron's papules, muscle weakness. *Confirmed by:* +ve **auto-antibodies, skin and muscle biopsy.** *Finalized by the predictable outcome of management,* e.g. systemic steroids.
Pyoderma gangrenosum	*Suggested by:* recurring nodule, pustular ulcers, about 10cm wide, with a tender, red, necrotic edge, healing with pitted scars on legs, abdomen, and face. *Confirmed by:* dramatic response to dapsone. *Finalized by the predictable outcome of management,* e.g. saline cleansing and dapsone.
Rheumatoid arthritis with vasculitis	*Suggested by:* vasculitic ulcer ± purpura, swollen and deformed phalyngeal joints with ulnar deviation. Rheumatoid nodules. *Confirmed by:* +ve **rheumatoid factor**, erosive appearance on **joint X-ray**. *Finalized by the predictable outcome of management,* e.g. NSAIDs, steroids, disease-modifying drugs, skin grafting.

Syphilis	*Suggested by:* an isolated, painless genital ulcer (primary chancre).
	Confirmed by: **serology, histology** and typical appearance.
	Finalized by the predictable outcome of management, e.g. benzylpenicillin.
SLE	*Suggested by:* associated facial butterfly rash, photosensitivity (face, dorsum of hands, neck), red scaly rashes.
	Confirmed by: +ve and high titre **antinuclear auto-antibodies, immunofluorescence studies.**
	Finalized by the predictable outcome of management, e.g. symptomatic treatment, systemic steroids.
Wegener's granuloma	*Suggested by:* skin and mouth ulcers, nasal ulceration with epistaxis, cranial nerve lesions, haemoptysis.
	Confirmed by: **cANCA** +ve. **Biopsy** showing granulomatous vasculitis.
	Finalized by the predictable outcome of management, e.g. high-dose systemic steroids.

Photosensitive rash

The initial management of all these conditions will clearly involve avoidance of exposure to sunlight and use of sunblock creams. Initial investigations (other tests in **bold** below): digital photography of lesion.

Main differential diagnoses and typical outline evidence, etc.	
Polymorphic light eruptions	*Suggested by:* recurrent rash on exposure to sun, typically in a female patient. *Confirmed by:* presence of an eruption, which may range from a few inflamed papules to severely inflamed and oedematous skin. *Finalized by the predictable outcome of management*, e.g. improvement by avoiding the exposure to sun, use of sunscreen. Topical and/or systemic steroids for the acute rash.
Plant chemical hyperphotosensitivity	*Suggested by:* red-brown macules on arms, hands, and face (blistering first) after exposure to sunlight. *Confirmed by:* history of cutting plants (e.g. giant hogweed) without skin covering. *Finalized by the predictable outcome of management*, e.g. sunblock and avoidance of exposure to sun. Cosmetics to conceal pigmentation.
Actinic prurigo	*Suggested by:* presence since childhood with papules appearing on sun-exposed sites. *Confirmed by:* improvement after protecting the exposed site. *Finalized by the predictable outcome of management*, e.g. sunblock and avoidance of exposure to sun. Cosmetics to conceal pigmentation.
Drug-induced photosensitivity	*Suggested by:* intake of a drug or the application of a cream that are known to cause photosensitivity, e.g. amiodarone, furosemide, tetracycline, and sunscreen agents. *Confirmed by:* improvement after eliminating the offending agent. *Finalized by the predictable outcome of management*, e.g. emollients and steroid creams, and avoidance of exposure to sun.
Pellagra associated with carcinoid syndrome or anti-TB drugs	*Suggested by:* diarrhoea, dementia, and dermatitis. History of predisposing condition. *Confirmed by:* response to treatment with nicotinic acid. *Finalized by the predictable outcome of management*, e.g. correction of fluid and electrolyte imbalance + nicotinamide.

Solar urticaria **Idiopathic or drug-induced, e.g. aspirin or opiates**	*Suggested by:* urticarial rash appearing after exposure to sun. *Confirmed by:* no other features on follow-up. *Finalized by the predictable outcome of management,* e.g. avoidance of sun exposure, and use of cetirizine and local emollients.
SLE	*Suggested by:* facial butterfly rash, photosensitivity (face, dorsum of hands, neck), red scaly rashes. *Confirmed by:* +ve and high titre **antinuclear auto-antibodies. Direct skin immunoflorescence studies.** *Finalized by the predictable outcome of management,* e.g. improvement by avoiding exposure to sun, systemic steroids.
Subacute cutaneous lupus erythematosus	*Suggested by:* symmetrical, scaly plaques on sun-exposed areas of face and forearm. *Confirmed by:* presence of **anti-Ro antibodies. Biopsy.** *Finalized by the predictable outcome of management,* e.g. avoid exposure to sun and use sunscreen. Local steroid creams.
Pemphigus associated with autoimmune thyroiditis, hypothyroidism or myasthenia gravis	*Suggested by:* presence of superficial blisters on the scalp, face, back, chest, and flexures ± preceding mouth erosions. History of other autoimmune disease. *Confirmed by:* **IgG autoantibodies** to epidermal components. **Direct immunofluoresence studies** showing deposition of IgG antibodies. *Finalized by the predictable outcome of management,* e.g. avoid exposure to sun. High dose of prednisolone orally with or without azathioprine or cyclophosphamide.

Pigmented moles

A flat or raised pigmented spot in the skin. Initial investigations (other tests in **bold** below): digital photography of lesion.

Main differential diagnoses and typical outline evidence, etc.	
Blue melanocytic naevus	*Suggested by:* solitary with colour commonly on hands and feet. *Confirmed by:* above appearance with no change on follow-up over weeks to months. Biopsy, if in doubt. *Finalized by the predictable outcome of management,* e.g. no changes over time.
Spitz melanocytic naevus	*Suggested by:* fleshy, firm, reddish-brown, round papule or nodule, usually on face or leg of a child. *Confirmed by:* above appearance with no change on follow-up over weeks to months. *Finalized by the predictable outcome of management,* e.g. no changes over time.
Halo melanocytic naevus	*Suggested by:* presence of a white halo of depigmentation surrounding the original naevus, usually on trunk of a child or an adolescent. May be history of vitiligo. *Confirmed by:* above appearance with no change on follow-up over weeks to months. *Finalized by the predictable outcome of management,* e.g. no changes over time.
Becker's melanocytic naevus	*Suggested by:* large, hairy, pigmented area. Present unilaterally in an adolescent male on the upper back, shoulders, or chest. *Confirmed by:* above appearance with no change on follow-up over weeks to months. *Finalized by the predictable outcome of management,* e.g. same appearance over time.
Freckles	*Suggested by:* presence of small, pigmented macules <5mm in diameter on sun-exposed area of a fair-skinned person. *Confirmed by:* above appearance with no change on follow-up over weeks to months. *Finalized by the predictable outcome of management,* e.g. no changes over time.
Seborrhoeic wart	*Suggested by:* presence of round or oval pigmented spot on the trunk or face in an elderly or middle-aged person. Progression from small papule into a pigmented warty nodule. *Confirmed by:* 'stuck-on' appearance and multiplicity of lesions. *Finalized by the predictable outcome of management,* e.g. cryotherapy, curettage, or shave biopsy.

Chloasma	*Suggested by:* appearance of large (<5mm) areas of pigmentation during pregnancy.
	Confirmed by: resolution in months following delivery.
	Finalized by the predictable outcome of management, e.g. sunscreens and camouflage cosmetics.
Peutz–Jegher's syndrome (with risk of colonic and other neoplasms)	*Suggested by:* small (<5mm) macules on the lips, in the mouth, and around the eyes and nose; also around the anus, hands, and feet. Present since infancy or childhood and fade with age.
	Confirmed by: presence of *polyposis coli* on **colonoscopy**.
	No treatment but refer for regular colonoscopy to remove suspicious polyps.
Dysplastic naevi	*Suggested by:* irregular outline and deep pigmentation.
	Confirmed by: **biopsy.**
	Finalized by the predictable outcome of management, e.g. surgical excision.
Malignant melanoma 'superficial spreading', 'lentigo', 'acral lentiginous', 'nodular'	*Suggested by:* recent increase in the size of a naevus, irregular outline, variation of colour, itchiness, and oozing or bleeding. 'Superficial spreading' (up to 50%, typically on leg, female), 'lentigo' (up to 50%); acral lentiginous (10%) on palms, soles, and nailbed of dark-skin); 'nodular' (25%, typically on trunk).
	Confirmed by: **biopsy.**
	Finalized by the predictable outcome of management, e.g. dermatologists confirmation of diagnosis and surgical intervention. Prognosis is related to tumour thickness: 5-y survival rate: <1mm=95%; 1–2mm=90%; 2.1–4mm=77%; >4mm=65%.

A tumour on the skin

Initial investigations (other tests in **bold** below): digital photography of lesion.

Main differential diagnoses and typical outline evidence, etc.	
Seborrhoeic wart	*Suggested by:* a round or oval pigmented spot on the trunk or face in an elderly or middle-aged person, starting as a small papule, progressing to a pigmented warty nodule. *Confirmed by:* 'stuck-on' appearance and multiplicity of lesions. *Finalized by the predictable outcome of management,* e.g. cryotherapy, curettage, or shave biopsy.
Epidermal cyst	*Suggested by:* a cystic swelling on scalp, face, or trunk, with a firm consistency and skin-coloured. *Confirmed by:* typical appearance and little progression over weeks to months. *Finalized by the predictable outcome of management,* e.g. excision.
Milium	*Suggested by:* small, white cysts around the eyelids and on the cheeks, usually seen in children. *Confirmed by:* typical appearance. *Finalized by the predictable outcome of management,* e.g. extraction by a sterile needle.
Dermatofibroma	*Suggested by:* a nodular lesion in a young adult, typically on the lower leg of a female. *Confirmed by:* **biopsy.** *Finalized by the predictable outcome of management,* e.g. excision.
Pyogenic granuloma	*Suggested by:* a rapidly growing, easily bleeding, bright red, and may be pedunculated nodule, usually on a finger. *Confirmed by:* **excisional biopsy.** *Finalized by the predictable outcome of management,* e.g. excision.
Keloid	*Suggested by:* irregular and excessive skin growth at the site of a trauma, producing nodules or plaques on the upper back, neck, chest, and ear lobes. *Confirmed by:* typical appearance with failure to resolve. *Finalized by the predictable outcome of management,* e.g. steroid injections.
Campbell-de-Morgan spot	*Suggested by:* presence of small red papules on the trunk in elderly. *Confirmed by:* typical appearance with little change over months. *Finalized by the predictable outcome of management,* e.g. acceptance or cauterization.

Lipoma	*Suggested by:* soft, subcutaneous, fatty mass, usually multiple, and commonly found on trunk of neck.
	Confirmed by: above appearance, and slow or no progression over months to years.
	Finalized by the predictable outcome of management, e.g. excision, if unsightly.
Chondrodermatitis nodularis	*Suggested by:* a painful nodule on the sun-exposed helix of the pinna in elderly.
	Confirmed by: typical appearance and site.
	Finalized by the predictable outcome of management, e.g. excision.
Keratoacanthoma	*Suggested by:* a rapidly forming nodule on a sun exposed area. The centre falls leaving a crater.
	Confirmed by: **biopsy.**
	Finalized by the predictable outcome of management, e.g. excision.
Basal cell carcinoma	*Suggested by:* presence of a nodule, usually started as a papule, developing central necrosis and producing an ulcer with rolled edges, usually on sun-exposed sites, e.g. by the nose and on the temple.
	Confirmed by: **excisional biopsy.**
	Finalized by the predictable outcome of management, e.g. excision.
Squamous cell carcinoma	*Suggested by:* history of chronic sun exposure, pipe smoking, chronic ulceration, e.g. a burn or renal transplant.
	Confirmed by: **biopsy.**
	Finalized by the predictable outcome of management, e.g. surgical excision.
Malignant melanoma	*Suggested by:* recent increase in the size of itchiness, and oozing or bleeding naevus, irregular outline, variation of colour.
	Confirmed by: **biopsy**.
	Finalized by the predictable outcome of management, e.g. dermatologists confirmation of diagnosis and surgical intervention.

Hyperpigmented skin

Initial investigations (other tests in **bold** below): digital photography of lesion.

Main differential diagnoses and typical outline evidence, etc.	
Freckles	*Suggested by:* brown macules, usually on the face, and become darker on sun exposure. *Confirmed by:* above appearance and no progression over months to years. *Finalized by the predictable outcome of management,* e.g. no progression over time.
Lentigines	*Suggested by:* brown macules, not affected by exposure to sun, usually seen in elderly. *Confirmed by:* above appearance and no progression over months to years. *Finalized by the predictable outcome of management,* e.g. no changes over time.
Drug-induced	*Suggested by:* intake of a drug, e.g. amiodarone, phenothiazine, minocycline, and oestrogen. *Confirmed by:* improvement on removing the drug. *Finalized by the predictable outcome of management,* e.g. eliminate offending agent.
Addison's disease	*Suggested by:* pigmentation in palmar creases and buccal mucosa. Nausea, weight loss, ↓BP, etc. *Confirmed by:* ↑**ACTH** with ↓**cortisol,** and poor response to **Synacthen® stimulation test**. *Finalized by the predictable outcome of management,* e.g. replacement hydrocortisone and fludrocortisone.
Cushing's disease	*Suggested by:* pigmentation in palmar creases and buccal mucosa. *Confirmed by:* ↑**ACTH** with ↑**cortisol** with failure to suppress normally in **dexamethasone test**. *Finalized by the predictable outcome of management,* e.g. metyrapone initially, then plan for pituitary adenectomy.
Biliary cirrhosis	*Suggested by:* non-tender hepatomegaly, splenomegaly, xanthelasmatosis, xanthoma, arthralgia. *Confirmed by:* +ve **anti-mitochondrial antibodies and liver biopsy**. *Finalized by the predictable outcome of management,* e.g. colestyramine.
Pemphigoid	*Suggested by:* presence of tense, large blisters arising on a red or a normal-looking skin, usually in an elderly patient, on the limbs, trunk, and flexures, or mouth. *Confirmed by:* specific **IgG antibodies to the antigens BP230 and BP180, and direct immunofluorescence studies** show IgG and C3 antibodies in the subepidermis. *Finalized by the predictable outcome of management,* e.g. low dose of prednisolone orally ± azathioprine.

Pellagra	*Suggested by:* presence of diarrhoea, dementia, and dermatitis. History of carcinoid syndrome or anti-TB drugs.
	Confirmed by: response to nicotinic acid.
	Finalized by the predictable outcome of management, e.g. correction of fluid and electrolyte imbalance + nicotinamide.
Carotenaemia	*Suggested by:* eating many carrots or dye-containing foods.
	Confirmed by: dietary history and response to advice.
	Finalized by the predictable outcome of management, e.g. improvement after following a dietary advice.
Lichen planus	*Suggested by:* associated Koebner's phenomenon.
	Confirmed by: presence of itchy, well-defined, and raised, shiny-surfaced lesions with a violaceous colour interpreted by white streaks (Wickman's striae).
	Finalized by the predictable outcome of management, e.g. topical steroids; systemic steroids for extensive lesions.
Acanthosis nigricans	*Suggested by:* skin thickening and pigmentation.
	Confirmed by: presence of pigmented, velvety, and papillomatous skin lesion of flexures, neck, nipples, and umbilicus.
	Finalized by the predictable outcome of management, e.g. treatment of underlying problem, e.g. diabetes mellitus.

Hypopigmented skin

Initial investigations (other tests in **bold** below): digital photography of lesion.

Main differential diagnoses and typical outline evidence, etc.	
Vitiligo	*Suggested by:* presence of symmetrical, non-scaly, white macules ± history of injury or sun exposure, usually on hand, neck, and around mouth.
	Confirmed by: above appearance and little or no change over months or years.
	Finalized by the predictable outcome of management, e.g. camouflage cosmetics, sunscreens, PUVA.
Albinism	*Suggested by:* FH, white or pink skin, white hair, poor sight.
	Confirmed by: above appearance and little or no change over months or years.
	No treatment but advise to avoid sun exposure (risk of cancer).
Phenylketonuria	*Suggested by:* fair skin, learning difficulties.
	Confirmed by: ↑**phenylalanine in blood.**
	Finalized by the predictable outcome of management, e.g. low phenylalanine diet.

Cardiovascular symptoms and physical signs

Chest pain—alarming and increasing over minutes to hours 174
Severe lower chest or upper abdominal pain 176
Sudden breathlessness, onset over seconds 178
Breathlessness on minimal exertion or orthopnoea or
    paroxysmal nocturnal dyspnoea (PND) 180
Palpitations 182
Acute breathlessness, wheeze ± cough 184
Cough and pink frothy sputum 186
Syncope 188
Leg pain on walking—intermittent claudication 190
Leg pain on standing—relieved by lying down 191
Unilateral calf swelling 192
Bilateral ankle swelling 194
Thoughts on interpreting cardiovascular signs 196
Peripheral cyanosis 197
Central cyanosis 198
Tachycardia (e.g. pulse rate >120bpm) 200
Bradycardia (<60bpm) 202
Pulse irregular 204
Pulse volume high 205
Pulse volume low 206
Blood pressure high—hypertension 208
Blood pressure very low 210
Postural fall in blood pressure 212
BP/pulse difference between arms 214
BP/pulse difference between arm and legs 215
Prominent leg veins ± unilateral leg swelling 216
Unilateral leg and ankle swelling 218
Bilateral leg and ankle swelling 220
Raised jugular venous pressure 222
Abnormal apex impulse 224
Extra heart sounds 226
Diastolic murmur 228
Mid-systolic murmur 230
Pansystolic murmur 232
Murmurs not entirely in systole or diastole 233

Chest pain—alarming and increasing over minutes to hours

Ideally, the assessment should take place where resuscitation facilities are available. Serial ECG or blood changes (especially troponin) are needed to differentiate between the possible diagnoses.

- Normal troponin 12h after pain: probability of MI <0.3%.
- Troponin rise indicates episode of muscle necrosis ≤ 2wk before.
- Initial investigations (other tests in bold below): FBC, U&E, ECG, troponin from 6–12h after onset of the pain.

Main differential diagnoses and typical outline evidence, etc.	
Angina (new or unstable) or acute coronary syndrome (ACS) that also includes early stages of myocardial infarction	*Suggested by:* central pain ± radiating to jaw and either arm (left typically). Intermittent, relieved by rest or nitrates, and lasting <30min. *Confirmed by:* no ↑troponins after 12h ideally from earlier baseline, and no T wave or ST segment changes on **serial ECG**, positive exercise test or inducible ischaemia/angiogram. *Finalized by the predictable outcome of management,* e.g. O₂, high dose aspirin, clopidogrel, sublingual GTN, IV or oral β-blockers, statins, LMW heparin.
ST elevated myocardial infarction (STEMI)	*Suggested by:* central chest pain ± radiating to jaw and either arm (left typically). Continuous, typically over 30min, not relieved by rest or nitrates. *Confirmed by:* ↑ST 1mm in limb leads or 2mm in chest leads on **serial ECG**, focal akinesia on echocardiogram. *Finalized by the predictable outcome of management,* e.g. O₂, high dose aspirin, nitrates IV and/or oral, β-blockers, statins, and ACE inhibitor. Primary angioplasty (or if not possible, thrombolysis).
Non-ST elevation myocardial infarction (NSTEMI)	*Suggested by:* central chest pain ± radiating to jaw and either arm (left typically). Continuous, typically over 30min, not relieved by rest or nitrates. *Confirmed by:* ↑**troponin** after 6 or 12h. Ideally from earlier baseline. T wave or ST segment depression but no ↑ST on **serial ECG**. *Finalized by the predictable outcome of management,* e.g. O₂, high dose aspirin, nitrates, IV and/or oral, β-blockers, statins, and ACE inhibitor. LMW heparin, early angiogram ± primary angioplasty followed by low dose aspirin 75mg od ±clopidogrel 75mg od after considering GI bleeding risk.

Oesophagitis and oesophageal spasm	*Suggested by:* past episodes of pain when supine, after food, alcohol, NSAIDs. Relieved by antacids. *Confirmed by:* no ↑**troponin** after 12h and no serial changes on **ECG**. Oesophagitis on **endoscopy**. *Finalized by the predictable outcome of management,* e.g. PPI and lifestyle modification. Calcium antagonist, e.g. nifedipine, if spasm.
Pulmonary embolus/ infarction **(arising from deep veins or in fibrillating right atrium)**	*Suggested by:* sudden breathlessness, pleural rub, cyanosis/hypoxia, tachycardia, loud P2, signs of DVT, risk factors e.g. recent surgery, immobility, previous emboli, malignancy, etc. *Confirmed by:* **CT pulmonary angiogram** showing clot in pulmonary artery. *Finalized by the predictable outcome of management,* e.g. O_2 to maintain saturations 94%, LMW heparin (treatment dose), then warfarin. Thrombolysis if ↓BP, or acutely dilated right ventricle on **echocardiogram**.
Pneumothorax **('tension', moderate, or mild)**	*Suggested by:* pain in centre or side of chest with abrupt breathlessness, diminished breath sounds, and hyper-resonance to percussion. *Confirmed by:* above with tracheal deviation and distress, ↓BP, suggesting tension pneumothorax or **expiration CXR** showing loss of lung markings outside sharp line ('moderate' if >5cm gap from lung edge to chest wall; 'mild' if <5cm). *Finalized by the predictable outcome of management,* e.g. if tension pneumothorax, large Venflon inserted into 2nd intercostal (IC) space, mid-clavicular line, O_2 if hypoxic aiming for target sats 94–96% or 88–92% if COPD. Analgesia. Aspiration if 'moderate'; if not satisfactory or prior lung disease, IC drain inserted into 'triangle of safety'. If 'mild' (<5cm gap) and not breathless, observation. If recurrent or bilateral— surgical intervention.
Dissecting thoracic aortic aneurysm	*Suggested by:* 'tearing' pain, often radiating to back, abnormal or absent peripheral pulses, early diastolic murmur, low BP, and widened mediastinum on **CXR**. *Confirmed by:* loss of single, clear lumen on **CT scan** or **MRI**. *Finalized by the predictable outcome of management,* e.g. O_2, analgesia, large-bore IV access, blood transfusion (crossmatching 6 units), and urgent surgical intervention.
Chest wall pain **(e.g. Tietze's syndrome.)**	*Suggested by:* chest pain and tenderness of chest wall on twisting of neck or thoracic cage. *Confirmed by:* normal (or no changes in) **troponin, ECG**, and **CXR**. *Finalized by the predictable outcome of management,* e.g. simple analgesia (e.g. NSAIDs) and avoidance of strenuous activity until ↓pain.

Severe lower chest or upper abdominal pain

Upper abdominal pain may also be difficult for the patient to separate from lower chest pain, so the causes of chest pain also have to be borne in mind. Initial investigations (other tests in **bold** below): FBC, U&E, LFT, CRP, D-dimer, troponin, ECG, CXR.

Main differential diagnoses and typical outline evidence, etc.	
Gastro-oesophageal reflux/gastritis	*Suggested by:* central or epigastric burning pain, onset over hours, dyspepsia, worse on lying flat, worsened by food, alcohol, NSAIDs. *Confirmed by:* **troponin** normal after 12h and no ↑ST segments on **ECG**. Oesophagitis on **endoscopy**. *Finalized by the predictable outcome of management,* e.g. improvement with antacids, e.g. PPI. Calcium antagonist, e.g. nifedipine, if spasm.
Biliary colic	*Suggested by:* post-prandial chest or upper abdominal pain over hours (after fatty foods), severe, colicky, central, right upper quadrant, with radiation to right scapula ± fever. *Confirmed by:* **US scan** showing gallstones and biliary dilatation and also on **ERCP**. *Finalized by the predictable outcome of management,* e.g. analgesia (e.g. pethidine IM). Nil by mouth. Fluids IV. Antibiotics, e.g. IV cefuroxime/metronidazole if fever or ↑WCC. Avoiding fatty foods. If recurrent, surgical drainage of stones or gall bladder removal.
Pancreatitis (often due to gallstone impacted in common bile duct; often complicated by chronic pancreatitis.)	*Suggested by:* mid-epigastric pain radiating to back, associated with nausea and vomiting, gallstones. Onset over hours. Presence of risk factors (e.g. alcohol, gallstones, etc.). *Confirmed by:* ↑↑**serum amylase** (normal if gland destruction), pancreatic pseudocyst on **CT abdomen**. *Finalized by the predictable outcome of management,* e.g. opiate analgesia, e.g. pethidine IM, nil by mouth. Fluids IV, monitoring ± correcting glucose and Ca^{2+}, if ileus NG tube ± colloid and blood. Antibiotics, e.g. IV cefuroxime + metronidazole. If chronic: analgesics, pancreatic supplements, monitoring blood glucose.

Myocardial infarction (often inferior MI)	*Suggested by:* central chest pain ± radiating to jaw and either arm (left typically). Continuous, typically over 30min, not relieved by rest or nitrates.
	Confirmed by: ↑ST 1mm in limb leads or 2mm in chest leads on **serial ECG**. ↑**Troponin** 6–12h after chest pain onset, ideally from earlier baseline.
	Finalized by the predictable outcome of management, e.g. O$_2$, high dose aspirin, nitrates IV and/or oral, β-blockers, statins, and ACE inhibitor. Primary angioplasty or occasionally thrombolysis then followed by low dose aspirin 75mg od ±clopidogrel 75mg od after considering GI bleeding risk.

Sudden breathlessness, onset over seconds

This situation may be life-threatening; the severity of the underlying condition often creates helpful diagnostic information. Initial investigations (other tests in bold below): FBC, U&E, ABG, ECG, CXR.

Main differential diagnoses and typical outline evidence, etc.

Pulmonary embolus/ infarction (arising within the lung or from deep veins or right atrium) fibrillating	*Suggested by:* sudden breathlessness, pleural rub, cyanosis/hypoxia, tachycardia, loud P2, signs of DVT, risk factors, e.g. recent surgery, immobility, previous emboli, malignancy, etc. *Confirmed by:* **CT pulmonary angiogram** showing clot in pulmonary artery. *Finalized by the predictable outcome of management*, e.g. O2 to maintain saturations 94–96%, LMW heparin, then warfarin. Thrombolysis if ↓BP, or acutely dilated right ventricle on **echocardiogram**.
Pneumothorax ('tension', moderate, or mild)	*Suggested by:* pain in centre or side of chest with abrupt breathlessness, diminished breath sounds, and hyper-resonance to percussion. *Confirmed by:* above with tracheal deviation and distress, ↓ BP, suggesting tension pneumothorax or **expiration CXR** showing loss of lung markings outside sharp line ('moderate' if >5cm gap from lung edge to chest wall; 'mild' if <5cm). *Finalized by the predictable outcome of management*, e.g. if tension pneumothorax, large Venflon inserted into 2nd intercostal (IC) space, mid-clavicular line, O₂ if hypoxic aiming for target sats 94–96% or 88–92% if COPD. Analgesia. Aspiration if 'moderate'; if not satisfactory or prior lung disease, IC drain inserted into 'triangle of safety'. If 'mild' (<5cm gap) and not breathless, observation. If recurrent or bilateral— surgical intervention.
Anaphylaxis ?precipitant	*Suggested by:* dramatic onset over minutes, recent allergen exposure. Flushing, sweating facial oedema, urticaria, warm but clammy extremities, tachypnoea, bronchospasm, and wheeze. Tachycardia and hypotension. *Confirmed by:* precipitant identification. *Finalized by the predictable outcome of management*, e.g. removal of antigen (e.g. bee sting, medication). Adrenaline IM 1 in 1,000. High flow O₂, fast fluids IV, steroids IV, and antihistamines IV. If stridor, securing of airway in case of laryngeal oedema, and transfer to HDU/ITU.

Inhalation of foreign body	*Suggested by:* history of putting an object in mouth, e.g. peanut. Sudden stridor, severe cough, low-pitched, monophonic wheeze, and reduced breath sounds, more typically on the right.
	Confirmed by: if not in extremis, **CXR/CT thorax** or **bronchoscopy** to see foreign body.
	Finalized by the predictable outcome of management, e.g. slap back between the shoulder blades with patient leaning forward, or Heimlich manoeuvre.

Breathlessness on minimal exertion or orthopnoea or paroxysmal nocturnal dyspnoea (PND)

Orthopnoea is shortness of breath when lying flat. (Try to confirm by observing what happens when patient lies flat.) This can be explained by oedema gathering along the posterior length of the lungs or less efficient lung movement when the abdominal contents press against the diaphragm. PND can happen when the patient slides down in bed at night or by bronchospasm due to night-time asthma. Initial investigations (other tests in **bold** below): FBC, U&E, ECG, and CXR.

Main differential diagnoses and typical outline evidence, etc.

Pulmonary oedema (due to congestive (chronic) heart failure or left ventricular failure— due to ischaemic heart disease, mitral stenosis, etc.)	*Suggested by:* background fatigue and exertional breathlessness, cardiac risk factors. Displaced apex beat, 3rd heart sound, bilateral basal fine crackles. Raised JVP and leg swelling. *Confirmed by:* **CXR** showing fluffy opacification, especially near hila. Loss of costophrenic angle. Impaired left ventricular function on **echocardiogram.** *Finalized by the predictable outcome of management,* e.g. sitting patient up, if hypoxic, controlled O$_2$ aiming for saturations 94–96%, diuretics IV. Nitrates IV and diamorphine if very breathless and systolic BP >90. Chronic: thiazide or loop diuretic, ACE inhibitor (or angiotensin receptor blocker). β-blocker and spironolactone (monitoring potassium).
COPD	*Suggested by:* long history of cough ± sputum, >10-pack years smoking, recurrent 'exacerbations'. **CXR** radiolucent lungs. *Confirmed by:* **spirometry:** FEV$_1$ <80% predicted and FEV/FVC ratio <0.7. Emphysema on **CT chest.** *Finalized by the predictable outcome of management,* e.g. no more smoking. Bronchodilators prn, then regular long-acting bronchodilators. Regular inhaled steroids if FEV<60% predicted and three exacerbations in past year. Pulmonary rehabilitation and specialist testing, e.g. alpha-1 antitrypsin, etc. Controlled O$_2$ if hypoxic, aiming for sats of 88–92%, prednisolone 7–10d, and nebulized bronchodilators. If worsening breathlessness, cough and mucopurulent sputum, antibiotics. Check ABGs and NIV if respiratory acidosis or invasive ventilation.

Asthma	*Suggested by:* wheeze, chronic cough worse at night/early morning, specific triggers. Family history or childhood history of asthma or atopy.
	Confirmed by: ↓**peak flow** and ↓**FEV1** that improves by >15% with inhaled beta agonist, e.g. salbutamol.
	Finalized by the predictable outcome of management, e.g. identification of precipitants, smoking cessation, trial of bronchodilator prn, and inhaled steroids, long-acting β-agonist/steroid combinations, leukotriene inhibitors/antihistamines. Acute attacks: high flow O_2, prednisolone PO or hydrocortisone IV. Nebulized salbutamol and ipratropium ± magnesium IV + aminophylline IV.
Cardiac arrhythmia	*Suggested by:* palpitations, chest pain, dizziness, cardiac risk factors, pallor, hypotension, tachycardia (occasionally bradycardia), ±↓BP. No wheeze, ± bibasal crackles from associated left ventricular failure.
	Confirmed by: **ECG** (pulse typically >140 or <40) and improvement in symptoms/signs as pulse rate improves.
	Finalized by the predictable outcome of management, e.g. controlled O_2; if pulse> 140, vasovagal manoeuvres and rate-lowering medications, electric cardioversion if confusion, hypotension, chest pain); if bradycardia (e.g. pulse <40), O_2, atropine IV, pacing internal in a CCU.
Respiratory muscle (diaphragm) weakness	*Suggested by:* muscle weakness, orthopnoea, daytime sleepiness and/or early morning headaches (due to nocturnal hypoventilation). Muscle wasting, fasciculation, calf hypertrophy, etc. Abnormal ABG.
	Confirmed by: clinical presentation and muscle biopsy. Restrictive defect on **spirometry +** FVC, and fall in FVC by ≥20% on lying flat. Small volume lungs on CXR.
	Finalized by the predictable outcome of management, e.g. controlled oxygen if hypoxic aiming for target saturations 88–92%, NIV if ABGs show type 2 respiratory failure or sleep disturbed breathing.
Acute retention of urine with reactive pulmonary oedema	*Suggested by:* onset of breathlessness over minutes to hours, not passed urine for hours, history of poor stream, frequency, nocturia. Palpably distended bladder. CXR: fluffy opacification, especially near hila.
	Confirmed by: large volume of urine drained after catheterization with rapid resolution of breathlessness and CXR appearances.
	Finalized by the predictable outcome of management, e.g. symptom free after management of prostatism e.g with α-blockers ± bladder catheter ± TURP.

Palpitations

Very subjective and a poor lead (with many self-limiting undiagnosable causes) unless forceful, fast, prolonged, and associated with chest pain, dizziness, or loss of consciousness. Often no cause is found after multiple tests. Initial investigations (other tests in **bold** below): FBC, U&E, glucose, ECG, CXR.

Main differential diagnoses and typical outline evidence, etc.

Runs of SVT **?exercise-induced due to IHD** **?due to electrolyte abnormalities**	*Suggested by:* abrupt onset, sweats, and dizziness. *Confirmed by:* baseline **ECG** or **24h ECG** normal QRS complexes with absent or abnormal P waves >140/min. **Exercise ECG** showing precipitation by exercise. *Finalized by the predictable outcome of management,* e.g. O₂, vasovagal manoeuvres, trial of adenosine IV, verapamil, or amiodarone. If ↓BP, LVF, ↓consciousness, chest pain, DC cardioversion.
Episodic heart block	*Suggested by:* onset over minutes or hours, slow and forceful beats. Pallor or loss of consciousness. *Confirmed by:* fixed or progressive prolonged PR interval, A–V dissociation, and slow QRS rate on baseline or **24h ECG.** *Finalized by the predictable outcome of management,* e.g. O₂ if hypoxic, correction of electrolyte abnormalities, stopping β-blockers/verapamil/ digoxin. Temporary pacing wire if compromised, otherwise permanent pacemaker.
Sinus tachycardia **(multitude of causes, anxiety, caffeine, febrile illness, hypovolaemia, pulmonary embolism, hyperventilation, nebulizers, etc.)**	*Suggested by:* gradual onset over minutes of regular palpitations, clear history of precipitating cause and pulse <150/min. *Confirmed by:* basal **ECG.** Resolution by stopping precipitating factors. *Finalized by the predictable outcome of management,* e.g. O₂ if hypoxic aiming for saturations 94–96%, and address underlying cause. Unlikely cardiac cause if pulse <140.
AF **(acute (<24h) may have precipitating cause, e.g. MI, infection, electrolyte imbalance, thyrotoxicois)**	*Suggested by:* irregularly irregular pulse. *Confirmed by:* **ECG** showing no P waves and irregularly irregular normal QRS complexes. *Finalized by the predictable outcome of management,* e.g. treating cause (low K+, sepsis, etc.), anticoagulation. For onset <24h and/or HR >130, chemical cardioversion (β-blocker/digoxin/ verapamil/amiodarone) and **cardiac monitor.** DC shock for adverse signs (↓BP, chest pain, ↓consciousness). For rate <50, anticoagulation and treatment for bradycardia. For rate 50–100 and duration unknown, rate control and anticoagulation, outpatient cardioversion.

Ventricular ectopics unifocal (benign) or multifocal (may have underlying pathology)	*Suggested by:* palpitations, noted over hours or days, associated anxiety. *Confirmed by:* premature wide QRS complexes on **baseline ECG or 24h ECG.** *Finalized by the predictable outcome of management,* e.g. verapamil, and ACE inhibitors (if left ventricular dysfunction on echocardiogram).
Menopause	*Suggested by:* irregular episodes, amenorrhoea, worse over weeks or months. *Confirmed by:* ↓**serum oestrogen,** ↑**FSH/LH.** *Finalized by the predictable outcome of management,* e.g. combined oestrogen/progesterone HRT.
Thyrotoxicosis	*Suggested by:* onset over weeks or months. Irritability, weight loss, loose frequent stools, goitre, lid retraction and lag, brisk reflexes. *Confirmed by:* ↑**FT4** and/or ↑**FT3** and ↓**TSH.** *Finalized by the predictable outcome of management,* e.g. propranolol tds prn for symptom control. Carbimazole/propylthiouracil and thyroid anitbodies, US scan or Isotope scan to determine cause.
Phaeochromocytoma (rare)	*Suggested by:* abrupt episodes of anxiety, fear, chest tightness, sweating, headaches, and marked rises in BP. *Confirmed by:* catecholamines (**VMA, HMMA**) or ↑**free metadrenaline** in urine and blood soon after episode. *Finalized by the predictable outcome of management,* e.g. α- and β-blockers IV, then orally until vascular volume restored (monitor Hb/haematocrit for fall). Surgery for excision.

Acute breathlessness, wheeze ± cough

This symptom suggests airway narrowing. The commonest cause is bronchospasm (constriction of the smooth muscle in the distal bronchioles); less common causes are wheeze due to inhalation of a foreign body or hydrostatic pulmonary oedema, i.e. 'cardiac wheeze.' Initial investigations (other tests in **bold** below): FBC, U&E, CRP, ABG, ECG, and CXR.

Main differential diagnoses and typical outline evidence, etc.	
Exacerbation of asthma	*Suggested by:* widespread polyphonic wheeze with exacerbations over hours (silent chest if severe), anxiety, tachypnoea, tachycardia, and use of accessory muscles. *Confirmed by:* reduced peak flows. **FEV$_1$** that improves by >15% after inhaled beta agonist. *Finalized by the predictable outcome of management,* e.g. O$_2$ given if hypoxic aiming for saturations 94–96%, prednisolone PO or hydrocortisone IV. Nebulized salbutamol and ipratropium ± magnesium IV and aminophylline IV, hydration, and monitoring ABG and serum K$^+$. Antibiotics if infection. HDU if drowsy or ↑CO$_2$.
Exacerbation of COPD	*Suggested by:* long history of cough ± sputum daily, porgressive breathlessness and >10-pack years smoking, recurrent 'winter infections'. **CXR** radiolucent and hyperinflated lungs. *Confirmed by:* **spirometry:** FEV$_1$ <80% predicted and FEV/FVC ratio <0.7. Emphysema on **HRCT chest**. *Finalized by the predictable outcome of management,* e.g. controlled O$_2$, prednisolone for 7–10d, and nebulized bronchodilators, ± antibiotics for infection. ABGs and early NIV if respiratory acidosis. No more smoking. Trials of inhaled bronchodilators prn, then regular long-acting bronchodilators. Regular inhaled steroids if FEV<60% predicted and three exacerbations in last year. Home oxygen assesment and specialist testing e.g. alpha-1 antitrypsin, etc.
Acute viral or bacterial bronchitis	*Suggested by:* onset of wheeze over days, gradual progression. Fever, mucopurulent sputum, dyspnoea. *Confirmed by:* **sputum culture** and sensitivities. No consolidation on **CXR**, nor clinically. *Finalized by the predictable outcome of management,* e.g. simple analgesia and antibiotics, if continued purulent sputum.

Acute left ventricular failure due to ?cardiac event ?valvular disease ?electrolyte imbalance ?arrhythmia	*Suggested by:* onset over minutes to hours. Breathless, distressed, clammy; displaced tapping apex beat, 3rd heart sound, bilateral basal late fine inspiratory crackles. Often also signs of right ventricular failure (↑JVP, swollen legs).
	Confirmed by: **CXR:** fluffy opacification (greatest around the hila), horizontal linear opacities peripherally, bilateral effusions, large heart. Impaired left ventricular function on **echocardiogram.**
	Finalized by the predictable outcome of management, e.g. sitting patient up, controlled O_2, diuretics IV. Nitrates IV if severe and systolic BP >90. Chronic: thiazide or loop diuretic, ACE inhibitor (or angiotensin receptor blocker). β-blocker and spironolactone (monitor K^+).
Anaphylaxis ?precipitant	*Suggested by:* dramatic onset over minutes, recent allergen exposure, feeling of 'impending doom'. Flushing, sweating, facial oedema, urticaria, warm but clammy extremities, tachypnoea, bronchospasm, and wheeze. Tachycardia and hypotension.
	Confirmed by: precipitant identification and response to IM adrenaline (epinephrine).
	Finalized by the predictable outcome of management, e.g. remove antigen (e.g. bee sting, medication). Adrenaline IM 1 in 1,000. O_2 if hypoxic aiming for saturations 94–96%, fast fluids IV, steroids IV, and antihistamines IV. If stridor, secure airway early as laryngeal oedema may progress, and transfer to HDU/ITU.

Cough and pink frothy sputum

This is due to a combination of frothy sputum of pulmonary oedema mixed with blood from haemoptysis from pulmonary hypertension, causing distension and congestion of the pulmonary vasculature bed. Initial investigations (other tests in **bold** below): FBC, U&E, CRP, D-dimer, troponin, ECG, CXR.

Main differential diagnoses and typical outline evidence, etc.	
Acute pulmonary oedema due to left ventricular failure (due to ischaemic heart disease, mitral stenosis)	*Suggested by:* background fatigue and exertional breathlessness, cardiac risk factors. Displaced apex beat, 3rd heart sound, bilateral basal fine crackles. Raised JVP and leg swelling.
	Confirmed by: **CXR** fluffy opacification, especially near hila. Loss of costophrenic angle. Impaired left ventricular function on **echocardiogram.**
	Finalized by the predictable outcome of management, e.g. sitting patient up, controlled O$_2$ aiming for sats 94–96%, diuretics IV. Nitrates IV and diamorphine if BP >90. Chronic: thiazide or loop diuretic, ACE inhibitor (or angiotensin receptor blocker). β-blocker and spironolactone (monitor potassium).
Mitral stenosis (± dilated left atrium ± atrial fibrillation)	*Suggested by:* months to years of orthopnoea, mitral facies, tapping, displaced apex, loud 1st heart sound, diastolic murmur, fine bibasal crackles. AF on **ECG**. Enlarged left atrial shadow (behind heart) and splayed carina on **CXR**.
	Confirmed by: large left atrium and mitral stenosis on **echocardiogram.**
	Finalized by the predictable outcome of management, e.g. aspirin and or warfarin if AF. Valvotomy/ valve replacement, e.g. for high pressure gradient (>30mmHg) or very small valve area (<1.5cm^2).

Syncope

This is sudden loss of consciousness over seconds. Think of abnormal 'electrical' activity in the central nervous system or a temporary drop in cardiac output and BP that improves as soon as the patient is in a prone position. Fits can occur due to a profound fall in BP so they are not specific of epilepsy. Initial investigations (other tests in **bold** below): FBC, U&E, CRP, glucose, ECG, and CXR.

Main differential diagnoses and typical outline evidence, etc.	
Vasovagal attack— simple faint **? precipated by emotion, pain, fear, prolonged standing, etc.**	*Suggested by:* syncope within seconds or minutes of preceding precipitant. Nausea, sweating, and darkening of vision. Recovery within minutes. No incontinence. *Confirmed by:* history. No abnormal physical signs. *Finalized by the predictable outcome of management*, e.g. reassurance and advice regarding avoidance of precipating causes.
Postural hypotension (often due to BP-lowering drugs, hypovolaemia)	*Suggested by:* sudden loss of consciousness after getting up from sitting or lying position. *Confirmed by:* fall in BP from, e.g. >20mmHg reclining to standing. *Finalized by the predictable outcome of management*, e.g. minimize/ avoid precipitants (including drugs). Advice on posture and prolonged standing. Support stockings. Fludrocortisone PO or midodrine, if symptoms persist and disabling.
Stokes– Adams attack— arrhythmia	*Suggested by:* sudden loss of consciousness with no warning, pallor, then recovery within seconds or minutes, often with flushing. Q waves or other abnormalities. *Confirmed by:* **24h ECG** showing episodes of asystole or heart block, SVT or VT. *Finalized by the predictable outcome of management*, e.g. correct electrolyte disturbances, temporary/permanent pacemaker.
Aortic stenosis	*Suggested by:* syncope on exercise. Slow rising pulse, low BP and pulse pressure, and heaving apex. Mid-systolic crescendo murmur, soft S2. **ECG**: tall R waves, left ventricular hypertrophy, left axis deviation, ST/T wave changes of 'strain'. *Confirmed by:* **echocardiogram** and **cardiac catheter**: stenosed valve. *Finalized by the predictable outcome of management*, e.g. aspirin; keep on cardiac monitor if syncope due to VT/VF. Valve replacement.
Hypertrophic cardiomyopathy (HOCM)	*Suggested by:* syncope. Family history of sudden death or HOCM. Angina, breathless, jerky pulse, high JVP with 'a' wave, double apex beat, thrill and murmur best at left sternal edge. *Confirmed by:* **echocardiogram** showing hypertrophied septum and ventricular walls with small ventricular cavities, especially on left. *Finalized by the predictable outcome of management*, e.g. β-blockers, aspirin. Cardiac monitor. Referral to specialist centre.

Micturition syncope	*Suggested by:* sudden loss of consciousness after micturating. Often nocturnal and associated prostatism. *Confirmed by:* history. Normal examination. *Finalized by the predictable outcome of management,* e.g. advice om avoidance, treatment of prostatism, e.g. α–blocker.
Cough syncope	*Suggested by:* sudden loss of consciousness after severe bout of coughing. *Confirmed by:* history. Normal examination. *Finalized by the predictable outcome of management,* e.g. treating cause of cough.
Carotid sinus syncope	*Suggested by:* sudden syncope on turning head (e.g. while shaving). *Confirmed by:* history and reproducible symptoms on movement. *Finalized by the predictable outcome of management,* e.g. aspirin, carotid Doppler scans, surgery if >70% stenosis.
Hypoglycaemia ?insulin intake mismatch (e.g. meals, alcohol, etc.)	*Suggested by:* prior seconds or minutes of hunger, sweating, and darkening of vision esp. in known diabetic. *Confirmed by:* **blood sugar** <2mmol/L and exclusion of associated cardiac condition. *Finalized by the predictable outcome of management,* e.g. giving glucose (IV or oral glucose gel/glucagon. Reassessment of insulin requirements and lifestyle.
Epilepsy ?precipitant (e.g. alcohol, infection, electrolyte abnormalities, BP drop)	*Suggested by:* preceding aura for few minutes, then tonic phase with cyanosis, clonic jerks of limbs, incontinence of urine and/ or faeces. *Confirmed by:* history from witness. **EEG** changes, e.g. 'spike and wave'. *Finalized by the predictable outcome of management,* e.g. BLS algorithm, rectal or diazepam IV, phenytoin IV. Addressing of ting causes.
Cerebrovascular accident	*Suggested by:* residual sensorimotor deficit, may have pre-aura. *Confirmed by:* **CT head** showing infarct or bleed. *Finalized by the predictable outcome of management,* e.g. if infarct: high dose aspirin initially and (daily regular dose) aspirin ± thrombolysis within hours. Dipyridamole if stroke occurred whilst on aspirin. Control BP. Also nil by mouth and fluids IV, SALT assessment if ↓consciousness/dysphagia. DVT prophylaxis: stockings/LMW heparin (if no bleed). If haemorrhage: treatment of severe hypertension (systolic >200mmHg), neurosurgery.
Pulmonary embolism/ infarction (arising within the lung or from deep veins or right atrium) fibrillating	*Suggested by:* sudden breathlessness, pleural rub, cyanosis/ hypoxia tachycardia, loud P2, signs of DVT, risk factors such as recent surgery, immobility, previous emboli, malignancy, etc. *Confirmed by:* **CT pulmonary angiogram** showing clot in pulmonary artery. *Finalized by the predictable outcome of management,* e.g. O_2, to maintain saturations 94–96%, LMW heparin (treatment dose), then warfarin. Thrombolysis if ↓BP, or acutely dilated right ventricle on **echocardiogram**.

Leg pain on walking—intermittent claudication

This is analogous to angina, but pain comes on in the legs, instead of the chest, on exercise. Quantify the effect on daily activity (especially distance walked) and ability to cope at home, work, recreation, and rest. Initial investigations (other tests in bold below): FBC, U&E, D-dimer, CRP.

Main differential diagnoses and typical outline evidence, etc.	
Arterial disease in legs (if associated impotence=Leriche's syndrome) **Risk factors (e.g. smoking, poor diabetes control)**	*Suggested by:* predictable claudication distance. Worse on exertion, relieved with rest. Worse uphill, better downhill. Pain at rest (implies riask of gangrene). Sleeping with leg hanging over edge of bed or in chair. Poor peripheral pulses and perfusion of skin and toes. *Confirmed by:* **Doppler ultrasound** or **arteriogram** showing stenosis and poor flow. *Finalized by the predictable outcome of management,* e.g. regular aspirin 150mg od, addressing risk factors especially smoking, addressing skin and feet viability. Vascular surgery.
Spinal claudication	*Suggested by:* weakness associated with pain. Improves slowly with rest but variable. Worse downhill. Brisk/reduced reflexes. Sensory deficits according to level of compression. *Confirmed by:* **MRI spine** showing canal stenosis or disc compression of cord or cauda equina. *Finalized by the predictable outcome of management,* e.g. analgesia, e.g. NSAIDs, carbamazepine. Neurosurgery.

Leg pain on standing—relieved by lying down

Think of something relieved by reducing 'pressure' on lying down. Two possibilities are relief of the pressure transmitted down to leg tissues by incompetent venous valves or relief of pressure by the spinal column on to a damaged disc, aggravating its protrusion and pressure on adjacent nerve roots. Initial investigations (other tests in **bold** below): FBC, CRP, thoracic/lumbar spine X-rays.

Main differential diagnoses and typical outline evidence, etc.	
Peripheral venous disease and varicose veins	*Suggested by:* generalized ache, itching, varicose veins and venous eczema ± ulcers. Cough impulse. **Trendelenberg test** showing filling down along extent of communicating valve leaks.
	Confirmed by: clinical findings or **Doppler ultrasound** to confirm any incompetence in sapheno-femoral junction or short saphenous vein.
	Finalized by the predictable outcome of management, e.g. advice to avoid prolonged standing and keep leg(s) elevated when sitting. Compression bandages and support stockings. Surgery.
Disc protrusion ('slipped disc')	*Suggested by:* severe referred ache or shooting pains, affected by position. Neurological deficit in root distribution.
	Confirmed by: **MRI spine** showing disc impinging on nerve roots
	Finalized by the predictable outcome of management, e.g. analgesia, bed rest, surgery.

Unilateral calf swelling

Unilateral swelling implies local inflammation, damage or obstruction to a vein or lymphatic duct. Bilateral swelling implies a more systemic cause, proximal obstruction or bilateral local causes. The speed of onset allows one to imagine what process might be taking place—traumatic, thrombotic, or infective. Initial investigations (other tests in **bold** below): FBC, CRP, D-dimer, doppler ultrasound.

Main differential diagnoses and typical outline evidence, etc.	
Deep venous thrombosis	*Suggested by:* onset over hours. Legs tense, tender, and warm. Risk factors.
predisposed to by obesity, immobility, malignancy, contraceptive, smoking, previous clots	*Confirmed by:* poor flow on **Doppler ultrasound scan**, filling defect on **venogram**.
	Finalized by the predictable outcome of management, e.g. analgesia, treatment dose heparin then warfarin for at least 3mo. Address risk factors. Compression stockings to reduce risk of post-thrombotic syndrome.
Ruptured Baker's cyst	*Suggested by:* onset sudden over seconds, e.g. when walking up a step. Typically arthritic knee.
(leaking synovial fluid, sometimes no cyst)	*Confirmed by:* normal flow on **Doppler ultrasound** and extravascular collection of fluid. No filling defect on **venogram**. Leakage of contrast from joint capsule if **arthrogram** done soon after the event.
	Finalized by the predictable outcome of management, e.g. analgesia, rest, and leg elevation. Occasionally needs surgical excision.
Cellulitis	*Suggested by:* onset over days. Warm, tender erythema, tracking (red lines), fever, ↑**WBC**. Often break in skin e.g. ulcer or insect bite.
	Confirmed by: **skin swabs** if discharge from skin, **blood cultures**.
	Finalized by the predictable outcome of management, e.g. analgesia. Leg elevation. Response to high dose benzylpenicillin IV + flucloxacillin for 10–14d. Fusidic acid + vancomycin if penicillin allergy. Prophylactic heparin.
Abnormal lymphatic drainage	*Suggested by:* onset over years, firm, non-tender, non-pitting oedema.
often cryptogenic but causes include lymphoma or malignant infiltration (or trypanosomiasis in tropics). Rarely, hereditary in young women.	*Confirmed by:* obstruction to flow on **lymphangiogram**.
	Finalized by the predictable outcome of management, e.g. compression stockings and leg elevation, specialist nursing input.

Bilateral ankle swelling

This is caused by leakage of fluid from the intravascular compartment into the the tissues (3rd space). Think of imbalance in Starling's laws, i.e. increased pressure within the veins or lymphatic vessels or low albumin in the vascular space, bilateral damage to vein walls, lymphatics, or capillaries due to local inflammation. Initial investigations (other tests in **bold** below): FBC, U&E, LFT, CRP.

Main differential diagnoses and typical outline evidence, etc.	
Right ventricular failure due to pulmonary hypertension or congestive cardiac failure	*Suggested by:* ↑JVP, liver enlargement and pulsation, right ventricular heave, loud S2 and often presence of chronic lung disease. Onset over months typically. *Confirmed by:* dilated right ventricle on **echocardiogram**. *Finalized by the predictable outcome of management,* e.g. thiazide or loop diuretics, correcting hypoxia/ CO_2 retention. Loop diuretic and metolazone and fluid restriction in resistant cases.
Poor venous return due to abdominal or pelvic masses, post-phlebitic or thrombotic venous damage at inferior vena cava level or bilateral deep veins	*Suggested by:* onset over months. Worse on prolonged standing or sitting, varicosities, venous eczema, pigmentation, or ulceration. *Confirmed by:* clinical findings or **Doppler ultrasound** to determine incompetence in sapheno-femoral junction or short saphenous vein, **CT abdomen** and **pelvis**. *Finalized by the predictable outcome of management,* e.g. avoid prolonged standing and keep leg(s) elevated when sitting. Compression bandages/stockings. Long-term warfarin if clot. Surgical removal of pelvic obstruction. Vascular surgery if symptoms worsen.
Low albumin states due to liver failure, nephrotic syndrome, malnutrition or GI losses.	*Suggested by:* onset over months. Generalized oedema, often including face after lying down. *Confirmed by:* ↓**serum albumin**. *Finalized by the predictable outcome of management,* e.g. diuretics if gross oedema and BP stable. Correct cause, e.g. with quality diet/treatment of nephrotic syndrome/GI malabsorption.
Bilateral cellulitis often associated with diabetes mellitus	*Suggested by:* onset over days. Warm, red, and tender legs, thrombophlebitis and tracking, ulcers, etc. *Confirmed by:* ↑**WBC** positive **blood cultures/ skin swabs** (typically streptococcal or staphylococcal). ↑**blood sugar** in diabetes. *Finalized by the predictable outcome of management,* e.g. analgesia, leg elevation, high dose benzylpenicillin IV + flucloxacillin for 10–14d, fusidic acid + vancomycin if penicillin allergy. Prophylactic heparin.

Inferior vena cava (IVC) obstruction due to clot especially if prolonged immobility, carcinoma, and oral combined contraceptive use. Can also be caused by extrinsic compression of IVC	*Suggested by:* bilateral leg swelling, onset over hours, associated risk factors. May have symptoms/signs of pulmonary embolism (PE). *Confirmed by:* **CT abdomen**, low flow on **Doppler ultrasound**, or filling defect on **venogram**. *Finalized by the predictable outcome of management,* e.g. analgesia, treatment dose heparin until warfarin dose is therapeutic. Anticoagulation for at least 3mo and address underlying risk factors. IVC filter if large thrombus or recurrent PE despite anticoagulation.
Drugs e.g. calcium channel or α-blocker	*Suggested by:* onset over days to weeks since starting e.g. calcium channel blocker, gabapentin or steroids. *Confirmed by:* symptom improves when offending drug stopped. *Finalized by the predictable outcome of management,* e.g. stopping or substitute drug, e.g. calcium channel or α-blocker.
Bilateral thromboses	*Suggested by:* onset over hours. Legs firm, warm, tender. Presence of risk factors. *Confirmed by:* poor flow on **Doppler ultrasound scan**, filling defect on **venogram**. *Finalized by the predictable outcome of management,* e.g. analgesia, treatment dose heparin until warfarin provides therapeutic INR. Anticoagulation for at least 3mo and addressing underlying risk factors. Compression stockings to reduce the risk of post-thrombotic syndrome.
Impaired lymphatic drainage	*Suggested by:* firm, non-tender, non-pitting oedema of gradual onset over months to years. *Confirmed by:* obstruction to flow on **lymphangiogram**. *Finalized by the predictable outcome of management,* e.g. compression stockings, elevation, specialist nursing input.

Thoughts on interpreting cardiovascular signs

The findings are described in a sequence of the cardiovascular examination, thinking of cardiac output, beginning with general inspection (pallor, sweaty, cachexia) then hand warmth, checking the radial pulse, measuring the BP. Continuing to think of cardiac output, examine the carotids. Next, think of venous return by inspecting the JVP. Finally, inspect, palpate, percuss, and auscultate the heart. Examine the legs and again think of cardiac output (e.g. temperature of skin and peripheral pulses), venous return (e.g. pitting oedema, leg veins, and liver enlargement).

Peripheral cyanosis

Cyanosis of hands but not tongue. Initial investigations (other tests in **bold** below): FBC, CRP, blood cultures, ESR, ABG, CXR.

Main differential diagnoses and typical outline evidence, etc.

Raynaud's phenomenon due to exposure of hands to cold or vibration	*Suggested by:* blue hands after exposure to cold, vibrating tools, connective tissue disease, vasopressor drugs. *Confirmed by:* symptoms improving with warmth. *Finalized by the predictable outcome of management,* e.g. avoiding precipitating factors. Calcium channel blockers. Ilioprost infusions in a specialist setting if connective tissue disease.
Arterial obstruction due to atheroma or small vessel disease in diabetics	*Suggested by:* absent or poor pulsation of radial or dorsalis pedis. Cool skin, absent hair and skin atrophy (if chronic). *Confirmed by:* Doppler ultrasound (reduced blood flow) and angiography. *Finalized by the predictable outcome of management,* e.g. stop smoking. Aspirin. Optimize lipids, glucose control in diabetic, etc. Vascular surgery.
Haemorrhage due to external or internal bleeding	*Suggested by:* low BP, high pulse rate, poor peripheral perfusion and urine output. *Confirmed by:* **falling Hb.** *Finalized by the predictable outcome of management,* e.g. volume replacement by blood transfusion or plasma expander, correction of coagulopathy and controlling source of bleeding. OGD/colonoscopy/**CT abdomen.**
Low cardiac output due to pump failure, e.g. large myocardial infarction, severe valvular stenosis or incompetence, arrhythmia or electrolyte imbalance	*Suggested by:* onset over minutes or hours of breathlessness, distressed and clammy, displaced tapping apex beat, 3rd heart sound, bilateral basal late fine inspiratory crackles. Poor urine output. Often also signs of right ventricular failure (↑JVP, swollen legs). *Confirmed by:* **CXR:** fluffy opacification (greatest around the hila), horizontal linear opacities peripherally, bilateral effusions, large heart. Impaired left ventricular function on **echocardiogram.** *Finalized by the predictable outcome of management,* e.g. sitting patient up, O$_2$ aiming for saturations 94–96%, diuretics (usually IV) and nitrates IV (if systolic BP>80mmHg). Identify and treatment of cause.
Septicaemia due to Gram − ve organisms commonly	*Suggested by:* warm, well-perfused peripheries, bounding pulse, low BP, tachycardia. Poor urine output. *Confirmed by:* +ve **blood cultures,** and response to plasma expanders and control of infection. *Finalized by the predictable outcome of management,* e.g. fast fluids IV, e.g. normal saline stat and 2–4 hourly. Cefuroxime + metronidazole IV or co-amoxiclav/ piperacillin with tazobactam according to likely source.

Central cyanosis

Cyanosis of tongue and hands. Significant hypoxia is present to cause this sign, so higher flow O_2 and close monitoring of saturations with ABG is needed. Initial investigations (confirmatory tests in **bold** below): pulse oximetry, FBC, blood cultures, ABG, ECG, CXR.

Main differential diagnoses and typical outline evidence, etc.	
Right-to-left cardiac shunt due to congenital heart disease, e.g. Tetralogy of Fallot, Eisenmenger's syndrome, tricuspid atresia, Ebstein's anomaly, pulmonary AV fistula, transposition of the great vessels	*Suggested by:* breathlessness, clubbing, systolic or continuous murmur, right ventricular heave. *Confirmed by:* **echocardiogram** and **cardiac catheterization**. *Finalized by the predictable outcome of management,* e.g. antibiotic prophylaxis for procedures and supervision by paediatric cardiologist.
Right-to-left pulmonary shunt due to no perfusion of lung tissue from extensive collapse or consolidation due to alveolar infection or bronchial obstruction	*Suggested by:* breathlessness, poor chest movement, dullness to percussion, and absent breath sounds over a large area of the chest. *Confirmed by:* **CXR** and **bronchoscopy**. *Finalized by the predictable outcome of management,* e.g. high flow O_2 and also management of associated: Inhaled foreign body, see ➲ Reduced breath sounds, p.274. Extensive consolidation, see ➲ Unilateral poor chest expansion, p.262. Large/bilateral pulmonary embolus, see ➲ Pleural rub, p.281. Pneumothorax, see ➲ Trachea displaced, p.264. Severe COPD (cor pulmonale), see ➲ Chronic breathlessness, p.242.
Haemoglobin abnormalities due to congenital NADH diaphorase, Hb M disease, or acquired methaemoglobinaemia or sulfhaemoglobinaemia	*Suggested by:* no clubbing, no murmurs, normal chest movement, no chest signs. History from childhood or exposure to toxic drugs, e.g. aniline dyes, phenacatin, etc. *Confirmed by:* **Hb electrophoresis**. *Finalized by the predictable outcome of management,* e.g. high flow O_2. Long-term management by haematologist.

Exacerbation of severe asthma, see ➲ **Reduced breath sounds**, p.274.
Severe pulmonary fibrosis, see ➲ **Chronic breathlessness**, p.242.
Neuromuscular disease, see ➲ **Chronic breathlessness**, p.242.
Pulmonary hypertension, see ➲ **Chronic breathlessness**, p.242.
Pulmonary embolus, see ➲ **Sudden breathlessness, onset over seconds**, p.238.

Tachycardia (e.g. pulse rate >120bpm)

Initial investigations (other tests in **bold** below): FBC, U&E, CRP, D-dimer, troponin, ABG, ECG, CXR.

Main differential diagnoses and typical outline evidence, etc.

Fever	*Suggested by:* warm skin, erythema, sweats, temperature >38°C. *Confirmed by:* temperature chart, fever pattern. **Blood/sputum/urine/skin swab cultures**. *Finalized by the predictable outcome of management,* e.g. antipyretics. Provisional antibiotics: amoxicillin (for urine/chest/skin source), cefuroxime/ metronidazole/trimethoprim (bowel/urinary source). Antibiotics IV if severe infection. Fluids IV/ plasma expanders for ↓BP, poor urine output.
Haemorrhage	*Suggested by:* pallor, sweats, ↓BP, poor urine output, and peripheral perfusion. *Confirmed by:* **↓Hb** (can be normal initially), low central venous pressure. *Finalized by the predictable outcome of management,* e.g. control of bleeding source. Multiple large bore IV access, fluids IV resuscitation until blood available.
Hypoxia	*Suggested by:* cyanosis, distress. *Confirmed by:* **↓P_aO_2**. *Finalized by the predictable outcome of management,* e.g. controlled O_2 aiming to keep saturations above 88–92% or 94–96%, depending on underlying illness. Address underlying cause (see ➲ Peripheral cyanosis, p.197).
Thyrotoxicosis	*Suggested by:* sweating, fine tremor, weight loss, lid lag, frequent bowel movements. *Confirmed by:* **↑FT4 ± ↑FT3 and ↓TSH**. *Finalized by the predictable outcome of management,* e.g. propranolol for symptoms. Carbimazole/ propylthiouracil for thyrotoxicosis.
Severe anaemia ?due to acute blood loss or chronic pathology/ deficiencies (e.g. folate/iron/B_{12})	*Suggested by:* subconjunctival and nail-bed pallor. *Confirmed by:* **↓Hb**. *Finalized by the predictable outcome of management,* e.g. fluids/blood. Identifying and treating cause, e.g. control of bleeding, supplements for deficiencies or treatment of chronic pathology.

Heart failure (left ventricular, right ventricular, congestive) **associated with ischaemic heart disease, myocarditis, valvular disease, arrhythmias**	*Suggested by:* breathlessness, displaced apex beat, 3rd heart sound, bilateral basal crackles. ↑JVP, swollen legs. *Confirmed by:* **CXR:** fluffy opacification (esp. peri-hilar), horizontal linear opacities peripherally, bilateral effusions, large heart, poor R wave progression on ECG. Impaired left ventricular function on **echocardiogram**. *Finalized by the predictable outcome of management,* e.g. sitting patient up, controlled O₂, aiming for saturation 94–96%, diuretics IV. Nitrates IV if very breathless and systolic BP >90. Treating causes (e.g. see diagnosis column). Controlled with thiazide or loop diuretic, ACE inhibitor (or angiotensin receptor blocker). β-blocker and spironolactone (monitor K⁺). Biventricular pacing if intractible in selected patients.
Pulmonary embolus/ infarction **arising within the lung or from deep veins or left atrium**	*Suggested by:* sudden breathlessness, pleural rub, cyanosis/hypoxia, tachycardia, loud P2, signs of DVT, risk factors such as recent surgery, immobility, previous emboli, malignancy, etc. *Confirmed by:* **CT pulmonary angiogram** showing clot in pulmonary artery. *Finalized by the predictable outcome of management,* e.g. O₂, to maintain saturations 94–96%, LMW heparin (treatment dose), then warfarin. Thrombolysis if ↓BP, or acutely dilated right ventricle on **echocardiogram**.
Drugs **e.g. amphetamines, beta-agonists**	*Suggested by:* drug history. *Confirmed by:* normal heart rate when drug stopped.
Cardiac tachyarrhythmia **Supra-ventricular tachycardia, atrial flutter or fibrillation, ventricular tachycardia** **?associated with electrolyte imbalance especially hypokalaemia**	*Suggested by:* ECG appearance. *Confirmed by:* ECG: regular normal QRS complexes in SVT, irregularly irregular QRS complexes in AF, wide regular QRS complexes in VT, ↑K⁺ or ↓K⁺. *Finalized by the predictable outcome of management,* e.g. normal heart rate after beta-blocker for SVT or AF, amiodarone and correction of any electrolyte imbalance, e.g. ↑K⁺: calcium gluconate IV, glucose-insulin IV, Calcium Resonium® PO/PR. ↓K⁺: potassium chloride orally or slowly IV and reducing K⁺ loss (e.g. stopping diuretics).

Bradycardia (<60bpm)

Initial investigations (other tests in **bold** below): FBC, U&E, TFT, CRP.

Main differential diagnoses and typical outline evidence, etc.	
Athletic heart	*Suggested by:* young/fit, asymptomatic. *Confirmed by:* normal history/examination. *Finalized by the predictable outcome of management,* e.g. reassurance and happy outcome.
Drug effect	*Suggested by:* history, e.g. β-blockers, digoxin. *Confirmed by:* 'reverse tick' sign on **ECG** and serum levels in digoxin toxicity. *Finalized by the predictable outcome of management,* e.g. normal heart rate when drug stopped or antidote.
Sinoatrial disease ?myocardial ischaemia	*Suggested by:* elderly, known ischaemic heart disease. *Confirmed by:* **ECG**—abnormal P wave or P–R interval or pauses >25. *Finalized by the predictable outcome of management,* e.g. correction of abnormal electrolytes or atropine or temporary pacing when unstable or permanent pacemaker. **Echocardiogram** for left ventricular function if history of syncope.
Ventricular or supraventricular bigemini ?myocardial ischaemia	*Suggested by:* known associated ischaemic heart disease. *Confirmed by:* **ECG** and **24h ECG** premature ectopics with and compensatory pause. *Finalized by the predictable outcome of management,* e.g. correction of abnormal lectrolytes. Cardiac monitoring. Atropine or temporary pacing when unstable or permanent pacemaker/cardiac resynchromisation therapy. **Echocardiogram** for left ventricular function if history of syncope.
Myocardial infarction	*Suggested by:* central chest pain ± radiating to jaw and either arm (left typically). Continuous, typically over 30min, not relieved by rest or nitrates. *Confirmed by:* ↑ST of 1mm in limb leads or 2mm in chest leads on **serial ECG**. Troponin↑. *Finalized by the predictable outcome of management,* e.g. O_2, high dose aspirin, nitrates IV and/or oral, withhold β-blockers if pulse <60, statins, and ACE inhibitor. Primary angioplasty/or urgent thrombolysis.
Hypothyroid	*Suggested by:* constipation, weight gain, dry skin, dry hair, reduced reflexes/energy. *Confirmed by:* ↑**TSH**, ↓**T4**. *Finalized by the predictable outcome of management,* e.g. thyroxine replacement.

Hypothermia	*Suggested by:* history of exposure to cold temperature and/or prolonged immobility.
	Confirmed by: core temperature <35°C.
	Finalized by the predictable outcome of management, e.g. gentle rewarming (space blanket, warmed fluids IV, bladder irrigation).
Severe electrolyte disturbances esp.⇈K+ or ⇊K+	*Suggested by:* drug history, renal failure.
	Confirmed by: normal heart rate when electrolyte corrected. **ECG**: T wave changes.
	Initial management: fluids IV and correct electrolyte imbalance, e.g. ↑K^+: calcium gluconate IV, glucose-insulin IV, Calcium Resonium® PO/PR. ↓K^+: potassium chloride IV and stop K^+ loss (e.g. from diuretics).

Pulse irregular

Initial investigations (other tests in **bold** below): FBC, U&E, CRP, ECG, CXR.

Main differential diagnoses and typical outline evidence, etc.	
AF acute (<24h) may have precipitating cause (e.g. myocardial infarction, infection, electrolyte imbalance, thyrotoxicosis)	*Suggested by:* irregularly irregular pulse. *Confirmed by:* **ECG** showing no P waves, and irregularly irregular normal QRS complexes. *Finalized by the predictable outcome of management,* e.g. if (<24h) and/or rate >130: treatment of cause, anticoagulation, and chemical cardioversion (digoxin/verapamil/ amiodarone). **Cardiac monitor**. DC shock if unstable. If rate <50, anticoagulation and treatment of as bradycardia. If rate 50–100 and duration unknown, anticoagulation. If rate >100 and duration unknown or multiple morbidities, β-blockers and digoxin long-term with anticoagulation. Echocardiogram and outpatient DC cardioversion if no severe valvular disease.
Atrial flutter with variable heart block caused by ischaemic heart disease, etc.	*Suggested by:* irregularly irregular pulse. *Confirmed by:* **ECG** showing 'saw tooth' F waves, and irregularly irregular normal QRS complexes. *Finalized by the predictable outcome of management,* e.g. as AF above.
Atrial or ventricular ectopics caused by ischaemic heart disease, etc.	*Suggested by:* regular rate with irregular dropped beat. *Confirmed by:* **ECG** showing normal sinus rhythm with irregular QRS complexes not preceded by P wave, and compensatory absence of subsequent QRS. *Finalized by the predictable outcome of management,* e.g. **cardiac monitor.** Treatment of cause (e.g. MI, ↑K$^+$, etc.). If prolonged PR interval (>200ms) and/or syncope, pacemaker. β-blockers if multiple ectopics and ACE inhibitors if LV dysfunction.
Wenkenbach heart block caused by ischaemic heart disease, etc.	*Suggested by:* regular rate with regular dropped beat. *Confirmed by:* **ECG** showing progressive prolongation of PR interval with normal QRS complex, followed by an eventually 'dropped' absent QRS complex. *Finalized by the predictable outcome of management,* e.g. **cardiac monitor.** Treatment of cause (e.g. MI, ↑K$^+$, etc.). If prolonged PR and/or syncope, pacemaker. ACE inhibitors if LV dysfunction.

Pulse volume high

This is an indication of the width of the pulse pressure. It can be confirmed by a large difference between the systolic and diastolic blood pressure. Initial investigations (other tests in **bold** below): FBC, U&E, CRP, ECG, CXR.

Main differential diagnoses and typical outline evidence, etc.	
Aortic incompetence	*Suggested by:* 'water hammer' radial pulse. Systolic BP high (e.g. >160mmHg) and diastolic BP very low (e.g. <50mmHg), early diastolic murmur. *Confirmed by:* **echocardiogram** and **cardiac catheterization** showing aortic regurgitation. *Finalized by the predictable outcome of management,* e.g. if acute/signs of sepsis or vegetations on the valve, treatment for bacterial endocarditis with high dose antibiotics. If acute and severe chest/back/abdominal pain and low BP, treatment of for aortic dissection. If stable, start aspirin and cardiology follow-up ± valve replacement.
Arteriosclerosis	*Suggested by:* history of thrombi/emboli. Systolic hypertension (>160mmHg) without diastolic hypotension (>80mmHg). *Confirmed by:* palpable thickening of small arteries, e.g. radial and/or absence of some peripheral pulses, absence of features of differential diagnoses of high pulse pressure, **echocardiogram** also to exclude aortic incompetence. *Finalized by the predictable outcome of management,* e.g. aspirin, treatment of risk factors (smoking, cholesterol, BP, diabetes).
Severe anaemia ?due to acute blood loss or chronic pathology/ deficiencies (e.g. folate/iron/B$_{12}$)	*Suggested by:* subconjunctival and nail bed pallor. *Confirmed by:* **Hb↓**. *Finalized by the predictable outcome of management,* e.g. identification and treatment of cause, e.g. supplements for deficiencies or chronic disease. Fluids IV/transfusion if unstable.
Bradycardia of any cause with normal myocardium	*Suggested by:* slow heart rate (e.g. <50bpm). *Confirmed by:* **ECG** showing slow rate and type of rhythm. *Finalized by the predictable outcome of management,* e.g. see differential diagnosis of bradycardia in ➔ Bradycardia (<60bpm), p.202.
Hyperkinetic circulation e.g. due to hypercapnia, thyrotoxicosis, fever, Paget's disease, AV fistula	*Suggested by:* warm peripheries and features of cause, e.g. central cyanosis, tremor, lid lag, fever, skull deformity, etc. *Confirmed by:* **ABG**—↑P_aCO_2 (if hypercapnia) or TFT—↑FT4 ± ↑FT3 and ↓TSH (if thyrotoxic), or **septic screen** positive or ↑**hydroxyproline** (Paget's). *Finalized by the predictable outcome of management,* e.g. controlled O_2 and treatment of cause.

Pulse volume low

This is an indication of the width of the pulse pressure. It can be confirmed by a small difference between the systolic and diastolic blood pressure. Initial investigations (other tests in **bold** below): FBC, U&E, CRP, ECG, CXR.

Main differential diagnoses and typical outline evidence, etc.	
Poor cardiac contractility due to ischaemic heart disease, cardiomyopathy, cardiac tamponade, constrictive pericarditis	*Suggested by:* quiet heart sounds, ↑JVP, peripheral oedema, basal lung crackles. Poor R wave progression, low amplitude complexes on **ECG**. *Confirmed by:* **echocardiogram** showing poor left ventricular contractility, pericardial effusion, etc. *Finalized by the predictable outcome of management*, e.g. sitting patient up, controlled O_2 aiming for saturations 94–96%, diuretics IV. Nitrates IV and diamorphine if very breathless and systolic BP >90. Treatment of reversible causes. ACE inhibitor/angiotensin receptor blocker, β-blocker, and spironolactone (monitor K^+).
Hypovolaemia due to blood loss, dehydration	*Suggested by:* cold peripheries, thirst, dry skin, low urine output. ↑**urea**, ↑**creatinine**. *Confirmed by:* ↓**Hb** (in blood loss) or ↑ (if haemo-concentrated). *Finalized by the predictable outcome of management*, e.g. oral fluids. Large-bore IV access, fast IV resuscitation with fluids/blood transfusion if anaemic. Catheterization and hourly urine output. Identification and treatment of any blood loss.
Relative hypovolaemia due to poor vascular tone (vasodilation) typically due to septicaemic shock	*Suggested by:* warm peripheries, thirst, dry skin, ↑urine output. Symptoms/signs of infection. ↑**urea**, ↑**WCC**. *Confirmed by:* **positive blood cultures**. *Finalized by the predictable outcome of management*, e.g. fluids IV and response to antibiotics IV, e.g. cefuroxime and metronidazole (for urinary/gastrointestinal tract infections), benzylpenicillin and flucloxacillin (for skin infections), co-amoxiclav or cefuroxime (for chest infections).
Aortic stenosis	*Suggested by:* slow rising pulse, narrow pulse pressure, soft S2, systolic murmur. *Confirmed by:* **echocardiogram** and **cardiac catheterization**. *Finalized by the predictable outcome of management*, e.g. aspirin, and cardiology follow-up ± surgery.

Blood pressure high—hypertension

(Systolic >150mmHg and diastolic >90mmHg.)
The level treated depends on the presence of risk factors. Generally, any sustained systolic BP >150 is treated, but in diabetics, >140 systolic or >80 diastolic. Initial investigations (other tests in **bold** below): FBC, U&E, CRP, ECG.

Main differential diagnoses and typical outline evidence, etc.	
Temporary hypertension with no risk factors	*Suggested by:* normal BP <150mmHg systolic and <90mmHg diastolic, when repeated. *Confirmed by:* **24h ambulatory blood pressure** monitoring result in low risk range. *Finalized by the predictable outcome of management,* e.g. reassure and repeat BP check in 2–3mo.
Essential hypertension 95% cases	*Suggested by:* sustained hypertension. If well established, then end-organ damage, e.g. retinopathy, nephropathy, LV hypertrophy will be present. *Confirmed by:* **24h ambulatory blood pressure** monitoring. No symptoms or signs of cause, normal urea and electrolytes, and prompt control on treatment. *Finalized by the predictable outcome of management,* e.g. thiazide diuretic or calcium channel blocker or ACE inhibitor or β-blocker or α-blocker.
Hypertension of pregnancy (pre-eclampsia sometimes progressing to eclampsia)	*Suggested by:* only occurring during pregnancy, oedema, and proteinuria. Fits in eclampsia. Additionally, Haemolysis, Elevated Liver enzymes and Low Platelets in HELLP syndrome. *Confirmed by:* resolution or improvement when pregnancy over or brought to an early end. *Finalized by the predictable outcome of management,* e.g. β-blockers IV, hydralazine, methyldopa to bring diastolic BP <100mmHg. Specialist supervsion, delivery if >30–34wk gestation.
Obstructive sleep apnoea	*Suggested by:* daytime somnolence, witnessed apnoeas whilst asleep. Collar size >17in. *Confirmed by:* **apnoea-hypopnoea index >15 events per h** on sleep study. *Finalized by the predictable outcome of management,* e.g. weight reduction and continuous positive airways pressure (CPAP) whilst asleep.
Renal hypertension due to renovascular stenosis or 1° renal disease	*Suggested by:* persistently ↑**urea** and ↑**creatinine**, ↓**Hb**. *Confirmed by:* **renal ultrasound** and **renogram** of renal vasculature. *Finalized by the predictable outcome of management,* e.g. treatment of ment of cause (e.g. diabetes, autoimmune disease). Calcium channel blockers and β-blockers before ACE inhibitors (which precipitate renal failure if renovascular) and avoidance of diuretics if severe impairment.

Vascular hypertension due to coarctation of the aorta, subclavian artery stenosis	*Suggested by:* upper body hypertension (right arm) and diminished pulses in legs (and left arm in subclavian artery stenosis). Radio-radial/femoral delay. *Confirmed by:* **echocardiography** (also measure pressure gradients), **MR angiogram/angiography**. *Finalized by the predictable outcome of management, e.g.* aspirin, surgery.
Primary hyperaldosteronism (Conn's syndrome if tumour)	*Suggested by:* proximal muscle weakness, ↓K⁺. *Confirmed by:* **↑aldosterone** and **↓renin**. *Finalized by the predictable outcome of management, e.g.* spironolactone or tumour removal.
Cushing's syndrome	*Suggested by:* proximal muscle weakness, facial and truncal obesity, wasting of arms and legs, purple abdominal striae. *Confirmed by:* **↑24h urinary free cortisol**, etc. *Finalized by the predictable outcome of management, e.g.* metyrapone intially and then surgery.
Acromegaly	*Suggested by:* proximal muscle weakness. *Finalized by the predictable outcome of management,* e.g. ±medical treatment initially, e.g. octreotide or bromocriptine or pegvisomant then surgery.
Phaeochromo-cytoma	*Suggested by:* paroxysms of vascular symptoms. *Confirmed by:* **↑VMA** and **↑metadrenaline** in phaeochromocytoma. *Finalized by the predictable outcome of management, e.g.* β-blockers and α-blockers prior to surgery.
Drug-induced due to NSAIDs, oestrogen pill, steroids, erythropoeitin	*Suggested by:* drug history. *Confirmed by:* improvement or resolution when offending drug stopped.

Blood pressure very low

Initial investigations (other tests in **bold** below): FBC, U&E, CRP, ECG, glucose.

Main differential diagnoses and typical outline evidence, etc.	
Cardiogenic— low output due to poor myocardium, stenosis or regurgitation, etc.	*Suggested by:* very low BP, fast or slow heart rate, peripheral and central cyanosis, displaced apex beat, quiet heart sounds ± abnormal murmur. ↑JVP, crepitations at lung bases. *Confirmed by:* ↑central venous pressure, ECG abnormal ± rhythm abnormalities, cardiomegaly ± 'pulmonary oedema' on CXR. Abnormal myocardium ± valvular lesions on **echocardiogram**. *Finalized by the predictable outcome of management,* e.g. sitting patient up, controlled O_2, diuretics IV and nitrates IV (if systolic BP >80mmHg). Treatment of any identified causes.
Drug-induced due to excessive dose of any hypotensive agent	*Suggested by:* drug history (e.g. antihypertensives, L-dopa, carbidopa, phenothiazines, tricyclic antidepressants). *Confirmed by:* resolution or improvement after stopping or reducing drug.
Low circulating blood volume due to haemorrhage (GI, etc.), dehydration, etc.	*Suggested by:* very low BP, fast heart rate, cold peripheries often with peripheral cyanosis, ↓JVP, thirst, dry skin, low urine output. ↑**urea**, ↑creatinine. Background evidence of cause. *Confirmed by:* ↓**Hb** (in loss) or ↑ (if haemo-concentrated), ↓central venous pressure, improvement with fluid resuscitation. *Finalized by the predictable outcome of management,* e.g. resuscitation with fluids/transfusions monitored by catheterization and measuring urine output. Treatment of bleeding source.
Loss of vascular tone due to septicaemia, anaphylaxis, adrenal failure, etc.	*Suggested by:* fever, warm peripheries, shock, ↓JVP, ↓urine output, signs of anaphylaxis. *Confirmed by:* +ve **blood cultures**, response to plasma expanders/fluids and antibiotics, identified allergen. *Finalized by the predictable outcome of management,* e.g. fluids IV with central venous pressure monitoring and hourly urine output. Adrenaline IM/steroids IV if anaphylaxis. Antibiotics IV for infection.
Addison's disease Adrenal failure 2° to ACTH deficiency	*Suggested by:* ↑K^+, ↓Na^+ (in Addison's), ↓glucose, pallor (in ACTH deficiency) with hyperpigmentation skin/palmar creases (↓ in Addison's not in ACTH deficiency). *Confirmed by:* ↓**serum cortisol,** poor cortisol response to **Synacthen® test.** *Finalized by the predictable outcome of management,* e.g. hydrocortisone IV or prednisolone (for Addison's and ACTH deficiency) and fludrocortisone (if Addison's).

Spinal cord injuries/disease	*Suggested by:* sensorimotor deficits.
	Confirmed by: **MRI spine**.
	Finalized by the predictable outcome of management, e.g. dexamethasone or hydrocortisone IV, fluids IV, immobilization, analgesia and transfer to specialist unit.

Postural fall in blood pressure

To be a strong diagnostic lead, the systolic blood pressure must fall >20mmHg (or 15%) and stay down for at least 1min and be accompanied by dizziness/syncope; otherwise many of the 'causes' will be self-limiting, and no diagnosis will be confirmed. Initial investigations (other tests in **bold** below): FBC, U&E, CRP, ECG, CXR.

Main differential diagnoses and typical outline evidence, etc.	
Drug-induced due to excessive dose of any hypotensive agent	*Suggested by:* drug history (e.g. antihypertensives, L-dopa, carbidopa, phenothiazines, tricyclic antidepressants). *Confirmed by:* by resolution or improvement after stopping or reducing drug.
Autonomic neuropathy typically secondary to other diseases	*Suggested by:* long-standing diabetes, alcoholism, hypovolaemia (e.g. diarrhoea, vomiting, over diuresis). *Confirmed by:* **ECG monitor of beat-to-beat variation:** <10 beats per min change in heart rate on deep breathing at 6 breaths per min or getting up from lying. *Finalized by the predictable outcome of management,* e.g. Treating cause and stopping any contributing drugs. Advice on posture, e.g. getting up slowly. TED stockings, and in severe cases, fludrocortisone or sympathomimetics, e.g. midodrine.
Idiopathic orthostatic hypotension (due to blunting of autonomic tone, sino-atrial node, and vascular responses)	*Suggested by:* normal history. Typically elderly. Blunting of sino-atrial node and vascular responses. *Confirmed by:* postural hypotension with no other associated features. *Finalized by the predictable outcome of management,* e.g. treating cause and stopping any contributing drugs. Advice on posture, e.g. getting up slowly. TED stockings, and in severe cases, fludrocortisone or sympathomimetics, e.g. midodrine.
Cardiogenic—low output due to poor myocardium, stenosis or regurgitation, etc.	*Suggested by:* very low BP, fast or slow heart rate, peripheral and central cyanosis, S3, displaced apex beat, quiet heart sounds ± abnormal murmur. ↑JVP, crepitations at lung bases. *Confirmed by:* ↑central venous pressure, ECG abnormal ± rhythm abnormalities, cardiomegaly ± 'pulmonary oedema' on CXR. Abnormal myocardium ± valvular lesions on **echocardiogram**. *Finalized by the predictable outcome of management,* e.g. sitting patient up, controlled O_2, diuretics IV and nitrates IV (if systolic BP >80mmHg). Treatment of any identified causes.

Low circulating blood volume due to haemorrhage (GI, etc.) dehydration, etc.	*Suggested by:* very low BP, fast heart rate, cold peripheries, peripheral cyanosis, ↓JVP. Thirst, dry skin, low urine output. ↑**urea** and **creatinine**. Background evidence of cause. *Confirmed by:* ↓Hb (in loss) or ↑ (if haemo-concentrated), ↓central venous pressure, improvement with fluid resuscitation. *Finalized by the predictable outcome of management,* e.g. resuscitatation with fluids/transfusions. Catheterize and hourly urine output. Identify and treatment of any bleeding or negative fluid balance.
Loss of vascular tone due to septicaemia, adrenal failure, etc.	*Suggested by:* fever, warm peripheries, shock, ↓JVP, ↓urine output, signs of anaphylaxis. *Confirmed by:* +ve **blood cultures**, response to plasma expanders/fluids and antibiotics, identified allergen. *Finalized by the predictable outcome of management,* e.g. fast fluids IV with central venous pressure monitoring and hourly urine output. Adrenaline IM/ steroids IV if anaphylaxis. Antibiotics IV for infection.
Central nervous system diseases, e.g. multiple sclerosis, Parkinson's disease	*Suggested by:* history. *Confirmed by:* **abnormal neurological signs consistent with disease.** *Finalized by the predictable outcome of management,* e.g. advice on posture, e.g. stand slowly. TED stockings, and in severe cases, fludrocortisone or sympathomimetics, e.g. midodrine.
Also	Primary autonomic neuropathies (e.g. Shy–Drager syndrome), B_{12} deficiency and subacute combined degeneration of the spinal cord, amyloidosis, porphyria, Guillain–Barré, phaeochromocytoma, myelopathies.

BP/pulse difference between arms

Right different from left by 15mmHg. Initial investigations (other tests in **bold** below): FBC, U&E, ECG, CXR.

Main differential diagnoses and typical outline evidence, etc.	
Old or acute thrombosis in atheromatous artery or aneurysm or dissection of ascending aorta	*Suggested by:* associated peripheral vascular disease. *Confirmed by:* **CT chest** and arms with contrast in arterial phase, **MRA/angiography**. *Finalized by the predictable outcome of management,* e.g. resuscitatation with fluids IV/transfusions. Surgical correction.
Supravalvular aortic stenosis (congenital)	*Suggested by:* 'elfin-like' facies, ejection systolic murmur, angina, and syncope. *Confirmed by:* **echocardiography, MRI** and **angiography**. *Finalized by the predictable outcome of management,* e.g. monitor BP in specialist clinic, surgery.
Subclavian steal syndrome	*Suggested by:* associated neurological symptoms. Exercising right arm inducing cerebral ischaemia. *Confirmed by:* **Doppler scans** and **angiography** showing abnormal subclavian artery. *Finalized by the predictable outcome of management,* e.g. antiplatelets or anticoagulation, surgery.
Thoracic inlet syndrome	*Suggested by:* bracing shoulder aggravates BP difference. *Confirmed by:* **MR angiogram/angiography** showing abnormal subclavian artery. **CT thoracic inlet** also needed to view external occluding structure. *Finalized by the predictable outcome of management,* e.g. surgery: vein bypass graft and offending structure (e.g. aneurysm, congenital band, accessory rib) removed at the same time.
Aortic arch syndrome, Takayasu's syndrome	*Suggested by:* typically young Asian female with cerebral and peripheral ischaemic symptoms. Fever, weight loss, fatigue, and arthralgia. Vascular bruits and pulseless extremities. ⇈ESR. *Confirmed by:* **angiography** showing abnormal subclavian artery. *Finalized by the predictable outcome of management,* e.g. corticosteroids and cyclophosphamide.

BP/pulse difference between arm and legs

Difference of 15mmHg. Need wide cuff for thigh. NB Patient's arms and legs must be level. Initial investigations (other tests in **bold** below): FBC, U&E, ECG, CXR.

Main differential diagnoses and typical outline evidence, etc.	
Old or acute thrombosis in atheromatous artery	*Suggested by:* associated peripheral vascular disease. Atrophic skin and hair loss on lower legs. *Confirmed by:* **Doppler ultrasound** of legs to try to find remediable flow reduction. **Angiography** to try to identify surgically remediable arterial stenosis. *Finalized by the predictable outcome of management,* e.g. aspirin and heparin. Urgent surgery if acute thrombosis and signs of ischaemic leg.
Aneurysm or dissection of descending thoracic or abdominal aorta or iliac arteries, especially in diabetics	*Suggested by:* associated peripheral vascular disease, severe abdominal/back/groin pain. Signs of shock. *Confirmed by:* **CT abdomen and pelvis**. *Finalized by the predictable outcome of management,* e.g. large-bore IV access. Resuscitatation with fluids IV/transfusions. Surgery.
Coarctation of aorta	*Suggested by:* ejection systolic murmur, presenting in childhood or early adult life. *Confirmed by:* rib notching on **CXR** and a narrowing in the aorta at site of coarctation on **CT angiography**. *Finalized by the predictable outcome of management,* e.g. surgery.

Prominent leg veins ± unilateral leg swelling

Initial investigations (other tests in **bold** below): FBC, U&E, CRP, D-dimer.

Main differential diagnoses and typical outline evidence, etc.	
Varicose veins ± competent communicating valves	*Suggested by:* generalized ache, itching, varicose veins, and venous eczema ± ulcers. Cough impulse. **Trendelenberg test** showing filling down along extent of communicating valve leaks. *Confirmed by:* clinical findings or **Doppler ultrasound** to confirm any incompetence in sapheno-femoral junction or short saphenous vein. *Finalized by the predictable outcome of management,* e.g. advice to avoid prolonged standing and keep leg(s) elevated when sitting. Compression bandages and support stockings. Vascular surgery if symptoms debilitating.
Thrombophlebitis	*Suggested by:* tender, hot veins with redness of surrounding skin. *Confirmed by:* history. Resolution on antibiotics. *Finalized by the predictable outcome of management,* e.g. NSAIDs and amoxicillin.
Deep vein thrombosis	*Suggested by:* immobility, prominent dilated veins, warm and tender swollen calf. *Confirmed by:* reduced flow on compression **Doppler**, filling defect seen on **venography.** *Finalized by the predictable outcome of management,* e.g. analgesia, treatment dose heparin until therapeutic warfarin. Anticoagulaion for at least 3mo. Treatment of underlying cause.

Unilateral leg and ankle swelling

Initial investigations (other tests in **bold** below): FBC, U&E, CRP, D-dimer.

Main differential diagnoses and typical outline evidence, etc.	
Deep vein thrombosis	*Suggested by:* immobility, prominent dilated veins, warm and tender swollen calf.
	Confirmed by: reduced flow on compression **Doppler**, filling defect seen on **venography.**
	Finalized by the predictable outcome of management, e.g. analgesia, treatment dose heparin until therapeutic anticoagulation on warfarin acheived. Anticoagulation for at least 3mo.
Ruptured Baker's cyst	*Suggested by:* onset sudden over seconds, e.g. when walking up a step. Typically arthritic knee.
	Confirmed by: normal flow on **Doppler ultrasound** and extravascular collection of fluid. No filling defect on **venogram**. Leakage of contrast from joint capsule if **arthrogram** done soon after the event.
	Finalized by the predictable outcome of management, e.g. analgesia, rest, and leg elevation.
Cellulitis from infection due to breaks in skin	*Suggested by:* onset over days. Warm and tender erythema, tracking (red lines), fever, ↑**WBC**.
	Confirmed by: **skin swabs** if discharge from skin, **blood cultures**, response to antibiotics.
	Finalized by the predictable outcome of management, e.g. analgesia. Leg elevation. High dose benzylpenicillin IV + flucloxacillin for 10–14d. Fusidic acid and vancomycin if penicillin allergy. Prophylactic heparin.
Unilateral varicose veins	*Suggested by:* distended and tortuous veins made worse when standing.
	Confirmed by: **Doppler ultrasound** probe to confirm where incompetence is present.
	Finalized by the predictable outcome of management, e.g. advice not to do prolonged standing and keep leg(s) elevated when sitting. Compression bandages and support stockings. Vascular surgery if symptoms worsen.
Chronic venous insufficiency from old deep vein thromboses (e.g. post-thrombotic syndrome)	*Suggested by:* past history, veins distended and made worse on standing.
	Confirmed by: **Doppler ultrasound** probe to where incompetence is present.
	Finalized by the predictable outcome of management, e.g. advice not to do prolonged standing and keep leg(s) elevated when sitting. Compression bandages and support stockings.

Venous insufficiency from obstruction by tumour or lymph node	*Suggested by:* onset over weeks, veins distended.
	Confirmed by: **Doppler ultrasound. CT abdomen/pelvis** and **venography** to explore where obstruction is present.
	Finalized by the predictable outcome of management, e.g. relief of obstruction.
Immobility (e.g. disabling cerebrovascular accident, hemiplegia, trauma)	*Suggested by:* history of immobility.
	Confirmed by: response to elevation legs and mobilization.
	Finalized by the predictable outcome of management, e.g. TED stockings, physiotherapy.
Abnormal lymphatic drainage caused by lymphoma or malignant infiltration (or trypanosomiasis in tropics).	*Suggested by:* onset over years, firm, non-tender, non-pitting oedema.
	Confirmed by: obstruction to flow on **lymphangiogram**.
	Finalized by the predictable outcome of management, e.g. compression stockings and leg elevation, specialist nursing input.
Congenital oedema (Milroy's syndrome)	*Suggested by:* presence since childhood. Worse pre-menstrually, in warm weather.
	Confirmed by: history and **lymphangiogram** showing primary lymphatic hypoplasia.
	Finalized by the predictable outcome of management, e.g. compression stockings and leg elevation, specialist nursing input.
Acute lymphatic obstruction due to streptococcal lymphangitis	*Suggested by:* sudden, unilateral swelling developing over hours. No venous dilatation but lymphangitic streaks.
	Confirmed by: clinical features and response to penicillin. **Doppler ultrasound** to show normal venous flow.
	Finalized by the predictable outcome of management, e.g. penicillin and leg elevation. Prophylactic heparin to cover immobility.

Bilateral leg and ankle swelling

Initial investigations (other tests in **bold** below): FBC, U&E, LFT, CRP, ECG, CXR.

Main differential diagnoses and typical outline evidence, etc.	
Bilateral varicose veins or old deep vein thromboses	*Suggested by:* veins distended and tortuous made worse when standing. *Confirmed by:* **Doppler ultrasound** probe to confirm where incompetence is present. *Finalized by the predictable outcome of management,* e.g. mobilization. Avoiding prolonged standing. Compression stockings, anticoagulation if clots.
Low albumin **due to poor nutrition, malabsorption, liver failure, nephrotic syndrome, protein-losing enteropathy**	*Suggested by:* history of facial puffiness in morning *Confirmed by:* ↓**serum albumin** (<30g/L). *Finalized by the predictable outcome of management,* e.g. treatment of cause, oral dietary supplements, NG/PEG feeding.
Congestive cardiac failure **due to ischaemic heart disease, mitral stenosis, cardiomyopathy, etc.**	*Suggested by:* very low BP, fast or slow heart rate, peripheral and central cyanosis, S3, displaced apex beat, quiet heart sounds ± abnormal murmur. ↑JVP, crepitations at lung bases. *Confirmed by:* ↑central venous pressure, ECG abnormal ± rhythm abnormalities, cardiomegaly ± 'pulmonary oedema' on CXR. Abnormal myocardium ± valvular lesions on **echocardiogram**. *Finalized by the predictable outcome of management,* e.g. sitting patient up, controlled O_2, diuretics IV and nitrates IV (if systolic BP >80mmHg). Treatment of any identified causes.
Cor pulmonale (right heart failure due to pulmonary hypertension) **due to long-standing lung disease, old pulmonary emboli, etc.)**	*Suggested by:* chronic hypoxia, ↑JVP, hepatomegaly, loud pulmonary 2nd sound, and right ventricular heave. Signs of chronic lung disease. *Confirmed by:* **CXR** showing pulmonary disease, **ECG** showing right axis deviation. **Echocardiogram:** high estimated pulmonary artery pressures, right ventricular dysfunction. *Finalized by the predictable outcome of management,* e.g. treatment of hypoxia. Diuretics.
Immobility	*Suggested by:* history of immobility. *Confirmed by:* response to elevation legs and mobilization. *Finalized by the predictable outcome of management,* e.g. TED stockings, physiotherapy.

Abnormal lymphatic drainage **caused by lymphoma or malignant infiltration (or trypanosomiasis in tropics).**	*Suggested by:* onset over years, firm, non-tender, non-pitting oedema. *Confirmed by:* obstruction to flow on **lymphangiogram** *Finalized by the predictable outcome of management,* e.g. compression stockings and leg elevation, specialist nursing.
Congenital oedema (Milroy's syndrome)	*Suggested by:* presence since childhood. worse pre-menstrually, in warm weather. *Confirmed by:* history and **lymphangiogram** showing primary lymphatic hypoplasia *Finalized by the predictable outcome of management,* e.g. compression stockings and leg elevation, specialist nursing.
Acute lymphatic obstruction due to streptococcal lymphangitis	*Suggested by:* sudden, unilateral swelling developing over hours. No venous dilatation but lymphangitic streaks. *Confirmed by:* clinical features and response to penicillin. **Doppler ultrasound** to show normal venous flow. *Finalized by the predictable outcome of management,* e.g. penicillin and leg elevation. Prophylactic heparin to cover immobility.

Raised jugular venous pressure

Measured with patient lying at 45°. Undetectably low if external jugular empties when compressing finger released. Initial investigations (other tests in **bold** below): FBC, U&E, ECG, CXR.

Main differential diagnoses and typical outline evidence, etc.	
Fluid volume overload	*Suggested by:* history of high input of fluids IV. Pulsatile. JVP with 'a' waves. Normal left ventricular function in echocardiogram. *Confirmed by:* drop in JVP with fluid management. *Finalized by the predictable outcome of management,* e.g. fluid restriction/diuretics.
Congestive cardiac failure	*Suggested by:* breathlessness, fatigue, orthopnoea. ↑JVP, liver large, fine bibasal crackles at bases, 3rd heart sound. *Confirmed by:* **CXR**: cardiomegaly, upper lobe vascular prominence, pleural effusions. **Echocardiogram**: ventricular dysfunction. *Finalized by the predictable outcome of management,* e.g. sitting patient up, controlled O_2, diuretics IV. Nitrates IV if very breathless and systolic BP >90. Treatment of reversible causes. ACE inhibitor/angiotensin receptor blocker, β-blocker and spironolactone (monitor K^+).
Cor pulmonale due to high right atrial pressure	*Suggested by:* large 'a' waves present in JVP. *Confirmed by:* **ECG** showing tall P wave, right axis deviation, right heart strain pattern. *Finalized by the predictable outcome of management,* e.g. treatment of hypoxia. Diuretics.
AF acute (<24h) may have precipitating cause (e.g. myocardial infarction, infection, electrolyte imbalance, thyrotoxicosis)	*Suggested by:* irregularly irregular pulse. *Confirmed by:* **ECG** showing no P waves, and irregularly irregular normal QRS complexes. *Finalized by the predictable outcome of management,* e.g. If new onset (<24h) and/or heart rate >130: treatment of cause, anticoagulation, and chemicalcardioversion (digoxin/verapamil/amiodarone). **Cardiac monitor**. DC shock if unstable. If rate <50, anticoagulation and treatment as bradycardia. If rate 50–100 and duration unknown, anticoagulate. If rate >100 and duration unknown or multiple morbidities, β-blockers and digoxin long-term with anticoagulation. Echocardiogram and outpatient DC cardioversion if no severe valvular disease.
Complete heart block	*Suggested by:* intermittent giant 'v' waves. Bradycardia. *Confirmed by:* **ECG** showing no association between P waves and QRS complex. *Finalized by the predictable outcome of management,* e.g. cardiac monitor. Temporary pacing if symptomatic. Treatment of identifiable cause. Assess for permanent pacemaker.

Tricuspid regurgitation ?right ventricular dilatation due to pulmonary embolus, endocarditis, cor pulmonale	*Suggested by: large 'v' waves.* Pansystolic murmur present. *Confirmed by:* **echocardiogram** showing large right atrium and tricuspid incompetence. *Finalized by the predictable outcome of management,* e.g. diuretics. Treatment of identifiable cause (oxygenation, anticoagulation, etc).
Pericardial effusion ?due to myocardial infarction, haemorrhagic, infective, inflammation, malignant, autoimmune	*Suggested by:* pulsatile JVP with 'a' wave and rapid descent. Very breathless. Quiet heart sounds. Globular heart shadow on **CXR**. Low voltage QRS complexes on **ECG**. *Confirmed by:* significant effusion on **echocardiogram**. *Finalized by the predictable outcome of management,* e.g. diagnostic/therapeutic pericardiocentesis. Treatment of identifiable cause.
Constrictive pericarditis ?due infection, uraemia, hypothyroidism, trauma, autoimmune	*Suggested by:* rapid descent of 'a' waves. Quiet heart sounds. Pericardial rub. Chest pain relieved on sitting forward. **ECG** showing widespread concave 'saddle-shaped' ↑ST except in AVR and V1–2, which have ↓ST. *Confirmed by:* **echocardiogram** showing small cavity and little contraction. *Finalized by the predictable outcome of management,* e.g. analgesia (NSAIDs), steroids, pericardiocentesis if significant effusion or signs of tamponade. Treatment of identifiable cause.
Jugular vein obstruction ?luminal (e.g. thrombus) or extraluminal (e.g. tumour)	*Suggested by:* no JVP pulsation, external jugular vein also distended (often plethoric face with oedema.) *Confirmed by:* **US** or **CT scan** to explore site of obstruction. *Finalized by the predictable outcome of management,* e.g. steroids, anticoagulation, treatment of obstruction e.g. urgent radiotherapy for compressing tumour.

Abnormal apex impulse

Look for displacement from normal site in mid-clavicular line, heave, and character of impulse (tapping, double). Initial investigations (other tests in **bold** below): FBC, ECG, CXR.

Main differential diagnoses and typical outline evidence, etc.	
Fat, fluid, or air between the apex and palpating hand	*Suggested by:* impalpable apex. *Confirmed by:* evidence of obesity, emphysema, pneumothorax, pleural effusion, pericardial effusion. *Finalized by the predictable outcome of management,* e.g. pneumothorax (see ⊃ Hyper-resonant percussion, p.272), pericardial effusion (see ⊃ Raised jugular venous pressure, p.222), emphysema (see ⊃ Bilateral poor chest expansion, p.260; ⊃ Hyper-resonant percussion, p.272).
Dextrocardia	*Suggested by:* apex on the right side of chest. *Confirmed by:* **CXR**. *Finalized by the predictable outcome of management,* e.g. congenital cardiac abnormalities, bronchiectasis (Kartagener's syndrome and situs inversus).
Large left ventricle due to ischaemic cardiomyopathy, mitral incompetence, aortic incompetence, right-to-left ventral septal defect shunt	*Suggested by:* apex heaving and displaced. *Confirmed by:* **echocardiogram** showing left ventricular dysfunction. *Finalized by the predictable outcome of management,* e.g. O_2 and diuretics ± ACE inhibitors and β-blockers for heart failure. Surgery for ventriculoseptal defect (VSD). Investigation of underlying cause e.g. ischaemia, valvular regurgitation, alcohol, etc. versus idiopathic.
Hypertrophied left ventricle due to hypertension, aortic stenosis	*Suggested by:* apex heaving but not displaced. *Confirmed by:* **echocardiogram** showing left ventricular dysfunction. *Finalized by the predictable outcome of management,* e.g. treatment of BP (aim for <140/80mmHg). Aspirin and ACE inhibitors.
Hypertrophic cardiomyopathy (HOCM)	*Suggested by:* double apex beat, angina, jerky pulse, ↑JVP with 'a' wave, thrill and murmur at left sternal edge. *Confirmed by:* **echocardiogram** showing hypertrophied septum and ventricular walls with small ventricular cavities, more on left side. *Finalized by the predictable outcome of management,* e.g. β-blockers (main risk is ventricular fibrillation) and aspirin. Cardiac investigation and genetic counselling.

Ventricular aneurysm	*Suggested by:* double impulse. Persistently raised ST segments on **ECG**.
	Confirmed by: paradoxical movement of ventricular wall on **echocardiogram**.
	Finalized by the predictable outcome of management, e.g. aspirin/anticoagulation for at least 3mo, if associated thrombus. ACE inhibitor. Cardiology supervision ±surgery.
Mitral stenosis	*Suggested by:* tapping left ventricular impulse (palpable 1st heart sound) and rumbling diastolic murmur.
	Confirmed by: **ECG** findings, **echocardiogram** and **cardiac catheterization**.
	Finalized by the predictable outcome of management, e.g. aspirin, anticoagulation if AF. Cardiology supervision ±surgery.
Right ventricular hypertrophy due to pulmonary hypertension or pulmonary stenosis	*Suggested by:* left parasternal heave.
	Confirmed by: **ECG** findings and **echocardiogram**.
	Finalized by the predictable outcome of management, e.g. correction of hypoxia, anticoagulation if clot/pulmonary hypertension. Diuretics. Specialist supervision.

Extra heart sounds

Initial investigations (other tests in **bold** below): FBC, ECG, CXR, echocardiogram.

Main differential diagnoses and typical outline evidence, etc.	
Normal young heart	*Suggested by:* 4th heart sound. *Confirmed by:* normal **CXR** and **echocardiogram**. *Finalized by the predictable outcome of management,* e.g. reassurance and normal healthy life.
Heart failure	*Suggested by:* breathlessness, ankle oedema, ↑JVP, displaced apex, 3rd heart sound, crackles at both bases. *Confirmed by:* normal **CXR** and **echocardiogram**. *Finalized by the predictable outcome of management,* e.g. sitting patient up, if hypoxic, controlled O_2 aiming for saturations 94–96%, diuretics IV. Nitrates IV and diamorphine if very breathless and systolic BP >90. Chronic: thiazide or loop diuretic, ACE inhibitor (or angiotensin receptor blocker). β-blocker and spironolactone (monitoring potassium)
Cardiomyopathy	*Suggested by:* fatigue, shortness of breath, 3rd heart sound, quiet 1st heart sound impalpable apex beat, ± pansystolic murmur (if tricuspid incompetence) *Confirmed by:* large heart with sharp (slow moving) outline on **CXR** and **echocardiogram** appearance. *Finalized by the predictable outcome of management,* e.g. thiazide or loop diuretic, ACE inhibitor (or angiotensin receptor blocker). β-blocker and spironolactone (monitoring potassium).
Constrictive pericarditis due to radiation, cardiac surgery, past TB, mesothelioma	*Suggested by:* fatigue, breathlessness, low BP, raised JVP with rapid descent of 'a' waves. Quiet heart 1st and 2nd sounds. Prominent 3rd heart sound. Peripheral oedema, ascities. **ECG** showing widespread concave 'saddle-shaped' ↑ST except in AVR and V1–2, which have ↓ST. *Confirmed by:* **echocardiogram** showing small cavity and little contraction, CXR, CT scan or MRI appearance. *Finalized by the predictable outcome of management,* e.g. diuretics, cardiac surgery.

Severe heart failure	*Suggested by:* breathlessness, ankle oedema, ↑JVP, displaced apex, 3rd and 4th heart sound (gallop rhythm), dullness to percussion and crackles at both bases.
	Confirmed by: **CXR** showing large heart, fluffy opacification at hila and both bases and **echocardiogram** showing dilated heart and poor contractility.
	Finalized by the predictable outcome of management, e.g. sitting patient up, if hypoxic, controlled O_2 aiming for saturations 94–96%, diuretics IV. Nitrates IV and diamorphine if very breathless and systolic BP >90. Chronic: thiazide or loop diuretic, ACE inhibitor (or angiotensin receptor blocker). β-blocker and spironolactone (monitoring potassium).

Diastolic murmur

Find where it is heard best (e.g. apex or left sternal edge). For any significant valvular heart disease, antibiotic prophylaxis should be considered for procedures that carry a risk of bacteraemia. Monitor for resulting ventricular compromise. Initial investigations (other tests in **bold** below): FBC, ECG, CXR, echocardiogram.

Main differential diagnoses and typical outline evidence, etc.	
Mitral stenosis	*Suggested by:* tapping left ventricular impulse (palpable 1st heart sound) and rumbling diastolic murmur.
	Confirmed by: ECG findings, **echocardiogram**, and **cardiac catheterization**.
	Finalized by the predictable outcome of management, e.g. aspirin, anticoagulation if AF. Prophylactic antibiotics for surgical procedures. Cardiology supervison ± surgery.
Mitral stenosis with pliable valve	*Suggested by:* opening snap.
	Confirmed by: **echocardiogram**.
	Finalized by the predictable outcome of management, e.g. aspirin, anticoagulation if AF. Prophylactic antibiotics for surgical procedures. Cardiology supervison ± surgery.
Aortic incompetence ?due to aortic dissection, endocarditis, Marfan's, connective tissue disease.	*Suggested by:* ↑BP, collapsing pulse, displaced apex beat, early diastolic murmur best heard at left sternal edge.
	Confirmed by: **echocardiogram** and **cardiac catheter** displaying valve lesion.
	Finalized by the predictable outcome of management, e.g. if acute onset and unstable—O$_2$, diuretics, blood cultures x3, and immediate IV (broad spectrum) antibiotics, monitor ABG and serial ECG. Prophylactic antibiotics for surgical procedures. Aortic valve replacement.

Mid-systolic murmur

Mid-systolic murmur means that the 1st and 2nd heart sounds can be heard clearly. Monitor for any resulting ventricular compromise. Initial investigations (other tests in **bold** below): FBC, CRP, ECG, CXR, echocardiogram.

Main differential diagnoses and typical outline evidence, etc.	
Aortic stenosis	*Suggested by:* cool extremities, slow rising pulse, low BP and pulse pressure, heaving apex, and soft or absent aortic component of 2nd heart sound (A_2). **ECG:** tall R waves and left axis deviation.
	Confirmed by: **echocardiogram** and **cardiac catheter** stenosed valve.
	Finalized by the predictable outcome of management, e.g. aspirin. Treatment of any ischaemic heart disease. Prophylactic antibiotics for surgical procedures. Surgery.
Hypertrophic cardiomyopathy (HOCM)	*Suggested by:* double apex beat, angina, jerky pulse, ↑JVP with 'a' wave, thrill and murmur at left sternal edge.
	Confirmed by: **echocardiogram** showing hypertrophied septum and ventricular walls with small ventricular cavities, more on left side.
	Finalized by the predictable outcome of management, e.g. β-blockers (main risk is ventricular fibrillation) and aspirin. Surgery. Genetic counselling.
Aortic sclerosis	*Suggested by:* normal pulse and BP ± no heaving apex. Typically elderly and evidence of atherosclerosis, e.g. palpably thickened arteries or absent pulses. Aortic calcification on CXR.
	Confirmed by: normal **ECG** and sclerotic valve on **echocardiogram**.
	Finalized by the predictable outcome of management, e.g. aspirin, keep BP <140/80mmHg and treatment of associated risk factors/ischaemia. Echocardiogram every 12mo.
Pulmonary high flow	*Suggested by:* normal pulse and BP, normal JVP, and no left parasternal heave. Typically in young women.
	Confirmed by: normal **ECG** and **echocardiogram**, showing no pulmonary hypertension or other lesion.
	Finalized by the predictable outcome of management, e.g. normal active life.
Atrial septal defect (rare) causing high pulmonary flow	*Suggested by:* normal pulse and BP, normal JVP, and left parasternal heave present. **ECG:** peaked P waves, right axis deviation in secundum defect, left axis deviation in primum defect.
	Confirmed by: **echocardiogram** and **cardiac catheter**.
	Finalized by the predictable outcome of management, e.g. cardiology supervision/surgery.

Pulmonary stenosis	*Suggested by:* low pulse, ↑JVP, and left parasternal heave. Right bundle branch block and right axis deviation on **ECG**. *Confirmed by:* **echocardiogram** and **cardiac catheter**. *Finalized by the predictable outcome of management,* e.g. aspirin, angioplasty/surgical repair.

Pansystolic murmur

Pansystolic murmurs mean that the 1st and 2nd heart sounds cannot be heard in all areas. Initial investigations (other tests in bold below): FBC, CRP, ECG, CXR, echocardiogram.

Main differential diagnoses and typical outline evidence, etc.	
Mitral incompetence due to rheumatic heart disease, valve dysfunction after myocardial infarction	*Suggested by:* pansystolic murmur at apex with radiation to axilla. No large JVP, 'V' waves. Displaced heaving apex beat. **CXR:** large round opacity 'behind heart' (big left atrium). **ECG:** 'M'-shaped P wave. *Confirmed by:* **echocardiogram** and **cardiac catheter**. *Finalized by the predictable outcome of management,* e.g. aspirin/anticoagulation if AF. Treatment of left ventricular dysfunction. Prophylactic antibiotics for surgical procedures. Referral to cardiology for assessment for possible surgery.
Tricuspid incompetence (rarely alone, e.g. severe cor pulmonale or after pulmonary embolus)	*Suggested by:* pansystolic murmur at left sternal edge. Large JVP 'V' waves. Left parasternal heave. **ECG:** tall peaked 'P' waves, right axis deviation and right bundle branch block. *Confirmed by:* **echocardiogram** and **cardiac catheter** show incompetence. *Finalized by the predictable outcome of management,* e.g. treatment of primary causes. O_2 and diuretics if associated cor pulmonale.
Ventricular septal defect typically congenital, sometimes rupture of septum after infarction	*Suggested by:* pansystolic murmur loud and rough. ↑JVP. Central cyanosis if right-to-left shunt. Displaced heaving apex beat. Right bundle branch block and right axis deviation in **ECG**. *Confirmed by:* **echocardiogram** and **cardiac catheter** show defect. *Finalized by the predictable outcome of management,* e.g. aspirin/anticoagulation if AF. Treatment of left ventricular dysfunction. Prophylactic antibiotics for surgical procedures. Referral to cardiology for assessment for possible surgery.

Murmurs not entirely in systole or diastole

Initial investigations (other tests in **bold** below): FBC, CRP, ECG, CXR, echocardiogram.

Main differential diagnoses and typical outline evidence, etc.	
Patent ductus arteriosus	*Suggested by:* newborn infant, high pulse volume, diastolic and systolic murmur to give continuous murmur. *Confirmed by:* **echocardiogram** and **cardiac catheter**. *Finalized by the predictable outcome of management,* e.g. aspirin/anticoagulation if AF. Cardiology supervision ± surgery.
Pericarditis with pericardial friction rub **?due to myocardial infarction, infection, uraemia, hypothyroidism, trauma, autoimmune**	*Suggested by:* rapid descent of 'a' waves. Quiet heart sounds. Pericardial rub. Chest pain relieved on sitting forward. **ECG** showing widespread concave 'saddle-shaped' ↑ST except in AVR and V1–2, which have ↓ST. *Confirmed by:* **echocardiogram** showing bright pericardium, if constrictive then small cavity and little contraction. *Finalized by the predictable outcome of management,* e.g. analgesia, steroids, pericardiocentesis if significant effusion or signs of tamponade. Treatment of identifiable causes.

Respiratory symptoms and physical signs

Chest pain—sharp and aggravated by breathing or
movement 236
Sudden breathlessness, onset over seconds 238
Acute breathlessness, wheeze ± cough 240
Chronic breathlessness 242
Frank haemoptysis (or sputum streaked with blood) 244
Cough with sputum 248
Persistent dry cough with no sputum 250
Hoarseness 252
Some thoughts when examining the respiratory system 254
Appearance suggestive of blood gas disturbance 255
Respiratory rate low (<10/min) 256
Chest wall abnormalities 258
Bilateral poor chest expansion 260
Unilateral poor chest expansion 262
Trachea displaced 264
Reduced tactile vocal fremitus 266
Increased tactile vocal fremitus 267
Stony dull percussion 268
Dull to percussion but not stony dull 270
Hyper-resonant percussion 272
Reduced breath sounds 274
Bronchial breathing 277
Fine inspiratory crackles 278
Coarse crackles 280
Pleural rub 281
Stridor ± inspiratory wheeze 282
Inspiratory monophonic wheeze 283
Expiratory monophonic wheeze 284
Expiratory polyphonic, high-pitched wheeze 286

Chest pain—sharp and aggravated by breathing or movement

This is a common symptom that is experienced in mild or transient forms by many in the population and resolves with no cause being discovered. It frightens a patient into seeking advice when it is severe or accompanied by other symptoms such as breathlessness. Initial investigations (other tests in **bold** below): FBC, U&E, ECG, troponin 12h after onset of the pain.

Main differential diagnoses and typical outline evidence, etc.	
Musculoskeletal injury or inflammation	*Suggested by:* associated focal tenderness ± history of trauma or lying awkwardly. *Confirmed by:* normal (or no changes in) troponins, ECG, and CXR. Good response to simple analgesia. *Finalized by the predictable outcome of management,* e.g. simple analgesia (e.g. NSAIDs) and avoidance of strenuous activity until pain improves.
Chest wall pain e.g. Tietze's syndrome	*Suggested by:* chest pain and tenderness of chest wall on twisting of neck or thoracic cage. *Confirmed by:* normal (or no changes in) troponins, ECG, and CXR. Good response to simple analgesia. *Finalized by the predictable outcome of management,* e.g. simple analgesia (e.g. NSAIDs) and avoidance of strenuous activity until pain improves.
Pneumonia with pleurisy	*Suggested by:* onset over hours or days, rusty brown sputum ± blood. Sharp pain worse on inspiration, fever, cough, crackles, dullness to percussion, bronchial breathing, **WCC:** ↑neutrophils, ↑**CRP**. *Confirmed by:* patchy shadowing on **CXR** and organisms grown in **sputum/blood culture**. *Finalized by the predictable outcome of management,* e.g. analgesia and provisional antibiotic, e.g. amoxicillin/clarithromycin PO for 5d. If >2 features of Confusion, Resp. rate >30/min, BP <90/60, age >65y), then antibiotic IV, e.g. amoxicillin/co-amoxiclav or cefuroxime + controlled O₂ and fluids. If suspected aspiration, then anti-anaerobics, e.g. cefuroxime/metronidazole IV. If hospital/nursing home acquired, cefuroxime or piperacillin with tazobactam IV.
Pulmonary embolus/ infarction arising from deep veins or in left atrium	*Suggested by:* sudden breathlessness, pleural rub, cyanosis, tachycardia, loud P2, associated DVT or risk factors such as recent surgery, immobility, previous emboli, malignancy, etc. *Confirmed by:* **CT pulmonary angiogram** showing clot in pulmonary artery. *Finalized by the predictable outcome of management,* e.g. LMW heparin (treatment dose), then warfarin. Thrombolysis if ↓BP, large bilateral clots, or acutely dilated right ventricular on echocardiogram.

Pneumothorax ('tension', moderate, or mild)	*Suggested by:* pain in centre or side of chest with abrupt breathlessness, diminished breath sounds, and hyper-resonance to percussion. *Confirmed by:* above findings, tracheal deviation, and distress suggesting tension pneumothorax, or **expiration CXR** showing loss of lung markings outside sharp line ('moderate' if >5cm gap from lung edge to chest wall; 'mild' if <5cm). *Finalized by the predictable outcome of management,* e.g. if tension pneumothorax, insertion of large Venflon into 2nd intercostal (IC) space, midclavicular line. Giving O_2 if breathless. Analgesia. Aspiration if moderate; if unsatisfactory or prior lung disease, insertion of IC drain into 'triangle of safety'. If 'mild' (<5cm gap) and not breathless, observation.
Pericarditis caused by myocardial infarction, infection (especially viral), malignancy, uraemia, connective tissue diseases	*Suggested by:* sharp pain worse lying flat, but relieved by leaning forward. Pericardial rub. *Confirmed by:* ECG: concave ↑ST, 'bright' pericardial signal on **echocardiogram**. **CXR** showing cardiomegaly and globular heart shadow if significant pericardial effusion. *Finalized by the predictable outcome of management,* e.g. close cardiac monitoring, NSAIDs and treating cause (e.g. viral—typically self-limiting; if uraemic, treating renal failure; steroids if autoimmune).
Referred cervical root pain	*Suggested by:* previous minor episodes of exacerbation of chest pain by neck movement (producing closure of nerve root foramina related to area of pain). *Confirmed by:* clinical features and **MRI scan.** *Finalized by the predictable outcome of management,* e.g. analgesia, trial of neck collar, and physiotherapy.
Shingles	*Suggested by:* pain (often burning in nature) in a dermatomal distribution, recent exposure to chicken pox, or previous shingles attacks. *Confirmed by:* vesicles appearing within days in the same dermatome. *Finalized by the predictable outcome of management,* e.g. NSAIDs ± co-analgesics, e.g. cabamazepine/gabapentin. Aciclovir if severe/immunosuppressed.

Sudden breathlessness, onset over seconds

This situation may be life-threatening. Initial investigations (other tests in bold below): FBC, U&E, CXR, ECG, D-dimer.

Main differential diagnoses and typical outline evidence, etc.	
Pulmonary embolus/ infarction arising from deep veins or in left atrium	*Suggested by:* sudden breathlessness, pleural rub, cyanosis, tachycardia, loud P2, associated DVT, or risk factors such as recent surgery, immobility, previous emboli, malignancy, etc. *Confirmed by:* **CT pulmonary angiogram** showing clot in pulmonary artery. *Finalized by the predictable outcome of management,* e.g. LMW heparin (treatment dose), then warfarin. Thrombolysis if ↓BP, large bilateral clots or acutely dilated right ventricular on echocardiogram.
Pneumothorax ('tension', moderate, or mild)	*Suggested by:* pain in centre or side of chest with abrupt breathlessness, diminished breath sounds and hyper-resonance to percussion. *Confirmed by:* tracheal deviation and distress suggesting tension pneumothorax, or **expiration CXR** showing loss of lung markings outside sharp line ('moderate' if >5cm gap from lung edge to chest wall; 'mild' if <5cm). *Finalized by the predictable outcome of management,* e.g. if tension pneumothorax, insertion of large Venflon into 2nd intercostal (IC) space, mid-clavicular line. Giving O₂ if breathless and analgesia. Aspiration if moderate; if this is unsatisfactory or prior lung disease, insertion of IC drain into 'triangle of safety'. If 'mild' (<5cm gap) and not breathless, observation.
Anaphylaxis	*Suggested by:* onset over minutes, history of recent allergen exposure, feeling of dread, flushing, sweating, facial oedema, urticaria, warm clammy extremities, dyspnoea and tachypnoea, wheeze. Tachycardia and ↓BP. *Confirmed by:* clinical presentation and response to adrenaline (epinephrine) IM. Results of controlled allergen exposure. *Finalized by the predictable outcome of management,* e.g. removal of antigen (e.g. bee sting, medication). Adrenaline IM 1 in 1,000. Securing of airway early if stridor. High flow O₂, fast fluids IV, steroids IV and antihistamines IV. Transferring to HDU/ITU.

Inhalation of foreign body	*Suggested by:* history of putting an object in mouth, e.g. peanut. Sudden stridor, severe cough, low-pitched, monophonic wheeze, and reduced breath sounds, typically on the right.
	Confirmed by: if not *in extremis*, **CXR/CT thorax** or **bronchoscopy** to show foreign body.
	Finalized by the predictable outcome of management, e.g. if *in extremis*, slap back between the shoulder blades with patient leaning forward. If fails, perform Heimlich manoeuvre.
Cardiac arrhythmia	*Suggested by:* palpitations, chest pain, dizziness, pallor, hypotension, tachycardia or ± ↓BP.
	Confirmed by: **ECG** (pulse typically >140 or <40) and improvement in symptoms/signs as pulse rate improves.
	Finalized by the predictable outcome of management, e.g. controlled O_2. If pulse >140, vasovagal manoeuvres or rate-lowering medication or electric cardioversion. If pulse <40, atropine IV or pacing (external, temporary internal), transferring to CCU.

Acute breathlessness, wheeze ± cough

This symptom suggests airway narrowing. The commonest cause is bronchospasm (constriction of the smooth muscle in the distal bronchioles); less common causes are wheeze due to inhalation of a foreign body or hydrostatic pulmonary oedema, i.e. 'cardiac wheeze.' Initial investigations (other tests in **bold** below): FBC, U&E, CRP, ABG, ECG, CXR.

Main differential diagnoses and typical outline evidence, etc.

Exacerbation of asthma	*Suggested by:* widespread polyphonic wheeze with exacerbations over hours. Silent chest if severe. Anxiety, tachypnoea, tachycardia, and use of accessory muscles.
	Confirmed by: reduced peak flows. **FEV$_1$** that improves by >15% with treatment.
	Finalized by the predictable outcome of management, e.g. high flow O$_2$, prednisolone PO or hydrocortisone IV. Nebulized salbutamol and ipratropium ± magnesium IV and aminophylline IV. NB. Keeping hydrated, and monitor ABG and serum K$^+$. HDU if drowsy, ↑CO$_2$.
Exacerbation of COPD	*Suggested by:* long history of cough ± sputum, many pack years of smoking, recurrent 'exacerbations'. **CXR**: radiolucent lungs.
	Confirmed by: **spirometry:** FEV$_1$ <80% predicted and FEV/FVC ratio <0.7. <15% reversibility. Emphysema on **CT chest** ± reduced α1-antitrypsin levels.
	Finalized by the predictable outcome of management, e.g. controlled O$_2$, prednisolone 7–10d, and nebulized bronchodilators. Antibiotics if worsening breathlessness, cough, and mucopurulent sputum. Stopping smoking. Trials of bronchodilators prn, then regular long-acting bronchodilators. Regular inhaled steroids if FEV<50% predicted and three COPD exacerbations per year.
Acute viral or bacterial bronchitis	*Suggested by:* onset of wheeze over days. No dramatic progression. Fever, mucopurulent sputum, dyspnoea.
	Confirmed by: **sputum culture** and sensitivities. No consolidation on **CXR.**
	Finalized by the predictable outcome of management, e.g. simple analgesia and antibiotics if continued purulent sputum.

Acute left ventricular failure due to ?cardiac event, valvular disease, electrolyte imbalance, arrhythmia	*Suggested by:* onset minutes to hours. Breathless, distressed and clammy, displaced tapping apex beat, 3rd heart sound, bilateral basal late fine inspiratory crackles. Often also signs of right ventricular failure (↑JVP, swollen legs).
	Confirmed by: **CXR**: fluffy opacification (greatest around the hila), horizontal linear opacities peripherally, bilateral effusions, large heart. Impaired left ventricular function on **echocardiogram.**
	Finalized by the predictable outcome of management, e.g. sitting patient up, controlled O_2, diuretics IV. Nitrates IV if very breathless and systolic BP >90. Identifying and treating potential causes. Chronic: thiazide or loop diuretic, ACE inhibitor (or angiotensin receptor blocker). β-blocker and spironolactone (monitor K^+).
Anaphylaxis ?precipitant	*Suggested by:* dramatic onset over minutes, recent allergen exposure. Flushing, sweating facial oedema, urticaria, and warm but clammy extremities, tachypnoea, bronchospasm, and wheeze. Tachycardia and hypotension.
	Confirmed by: precipitant identification and response to adrenaline (epinephrine) IM.
	Finalized by the predictable outcome of management, e.g. removal of antigen (e.g. bee sting, medication). Adrenaline IM 1 in 1,000. High flow O_2, fast fluids IV, steroids IV, and antihistamines IV. If stridor, securing of airway early as laryngeal oedema may progress, and HDU/ITU care.

Chronic breathlessness

Initial investigations (other tests in **bold** below): FBC, U&E, ECG, CXR, serial peak expiratory flow rates (PEFRs).

Main differential diagnoses and typical outline evidence, etc.

Obesity and muscle deconditioning	*Suggested by:* more breathlessness on exertion. No cough or other symptoms. High BMI, but no other abnormality on examination, and normal baseline tests. *Confirmed by:* normal or mild restrictive defect on **spirometry, CXR,** and **ECG.** Improvement with weight loss and graduated aerobic exercise programme. *Finalized by the predictable outcome of management,* e.g. weight loss and reconditioning.
Asthma precipitated by allergens, e.g. pollen, house mites, etc.	*Suggested by:* wheeze, chronic cough worse at night/early morning, specific triggers. Family history or childhood history of asthma or atopy. *Confirmed by:* **spirometry**: reduced peak flow. FEV$_1$ that improves by >15% with treatment. *Finalized by the predictable outcome of management,* e.g. high flow O$_2$, prednisolone PO or hydrocortisone IV. Nebulized salbutamol and ipratropium ± magnesium IV and aminophylline IV. Long-term care: identifying precipitants. Stopping smoking. Trial of bronchodilator prn and inhaled steroids, long-acting β-agonist/steroid combinations, leukotriene inhibitors/antihistamines.
COPD caused by smoking, smoke pollution, α1-antitrypsin deficiency	*Suggested by:* long history of cough ± sputum, many pack years of smoking, recurrent 'exacerbations'. **CXR:** radiolucent lungs. *Confirmed by:* **spirometry**: FEV$_1$<80% predicted and FEV/FVC ratio <0.7. <15% reversibility. Emphysema on **CT chest** ± ↓**α1-antitrypsin levels.** *Finalized by the predictable outcome of management,* e.g. stopping smoking. Trials of bronchodilators prn, then regular long-acting bronchodilators. Regular inhaled steroids if FEV <50% predicted and three COPD exacerbations per year. If cough and breathless persists, prednisolone PO. If respiratory failure, home O$_2$.
Left ventricular dysfunction caused or made worse by atrial fibrillation, ischaemic heart disease, mitral stenosis, or regurgitation, hypertension. Anaemia, thyrotoxicosis, chest infections	*Suggested by:* fatigue, orthopnoea, and reduced exercise capability. Resting tachycardia with S3 and displaced apex, bibasal crackles. Evidence of causes. *Confirmed by:* reduced left ventricular function on **echocardiogram. CXR**: large cardiac shadow, upper lobe vein dilatation, loss of costophrenic angle, hilar shadows. *Finalized by the predictable outcome of management,* e.g. thiazide or loop diuretics. ACE inhibitors (or angiotensin receptor blockers). β-blockers, spironolactone to improve prognosis. Treating causes.

Pulmonary fibrosis/ interstitial lung disease **NB majority of cases have no cause identified**	*Suggested by:* chronic dry cough, occupational exposure or evidence of underlying connective tissue disease. Clubbing, cyanosis, reduced chest expansion, coarse late inspiratory bibasal crackles. *Confirmed by:* ↓lung volumes and reticular nodular shadowing on **CXR**. Interstitial shadowing and/or subpleural fibrosis on **high resolution CT chest.** *Finalized by the predictable outcome of management,* e.g. home O₂ if saturations <93%. Specialist opinion for detailed lung function, lung biopsy, immunosupression, antifibrotics, palliation.
Neuromuscular disease complicated by respiratory failure	*Suggested by:* muscle weakness, orthopnoea, daytime sleepiness and/or early morning headaches (due to nocturnal hypoventilation). Muscle wasting, fasciculation, calf hypertrophy, etc. Abnormal ABG. *Confirmed by:* clinical presentation and muscle biopsy. Restrictive defect on **spirometry + FVC**, and fall in FVC by ≥20% on lying flat. Small volume lungs on CXR. *Finalized by the predictable outcome of management,* e.g. non-invasive ventilation if ABGs show respiratory failure. Follow-up by neurologist and multidisciplinary team.
Pulmonary hypertension (1° pulmonary hypertension in 20%; in 80%, 2° to previous pulmonary emboli, vasculitis, chronic lung disease)	*Suggested by:* features of underlying cause. Loud P2. Desaturation in pulse oximetry on walking and low transferring factor. *Confirmed by:* ↑pulmonary pressures and/or right ventricular dysfunction on **echocardiogram.** *Finalized by the predictable outcome of management,* e.g. treat underlying cause (anticoagulate with heparin and warfarin if severe pulmonary hypertension—even if no proven pulmonary emboli). O₂ to maintain saturations >93%. Managed in chest clinic.
Psychogenic	*Suggested by:* no other associated features of pulmonary or cardiac disease. Underlying anxiety (e.g. high Nijmegan score), triggered by stressful situations. *Confirmed by:* no appearance of organic cause over time *Finalized by the predictable outcome of management,* e.g. relaxation, control breathing exercises. Explanation and reassurance.
Chronic thrombo- emboli with or without pulmonary hypertension	*Suggested by:* underlying risk factors, borderline hypoxia (e.g. saturations of 92–95%), resting tachycardia. No loud P2. *Confirmed by:* **echocardiogram** showing no signs of pulmonary hypertension. **CT-PA** showing occluded vessels or **V/Q scans** (showing ventilation/perfusion mismatch (better at detecting peripheral smaller clots below 4th division of pulmonary arteries). *Finalized by the predictable outcome of management,* e.g. warfarin for at least 3mo, treating risk factors.

Frank haemoptysis (or sputum streaked with blood)

Haemoptysis rarely causes hypovolaemia from blood loss, but if there is hypotension or tachycardia, consider their causes (see ➲ Blood pressure very low, p.210; ➲ Tachycardia (e.g. pulse rate >120bpm), p.200). If tuberculosis (TB) is suspected, patient should be isolated whilst tests are carried out. Initial investigations (other tests in **bold** below): FBC, U&E, CXR.

Main differential diagnoses and typical outline evidence, etc.	
Acute viral or bacterial bronchitis	*Suggested by:* days of fever, mucopurulent sputum, dyspnoea. Typically only streaky haemoptysis and self-limiting.
	Confirmed by: **sputum culture** and sensitivities, response to appropriate antibiotics.
	Finalized by the predictable outcome of management, e.g. analgesia and antibiotics.
Pulmonary embolus/ infarction arising from deep veins	*Suggested by:* sudden breathlessness, pleural rub, cyanosis, tachycardia, loud P2, associated DVT, or predisposing risk factors such as recent surgery, immobility, malignancy, etc.
	Confirmed by: **CT pulmonary angiogram** showing clot in pulmonary artery.
	Finalized by the predictable outcome of management, e.g. LMW heparin (treatment dose), then warfarin. Thrombolysis if ↓BP, large bilateral clots, or acutely dilated right ventricle on echocardiogram.
Carcinoma of lung	*Suggested by:* weeks or months of weight loss, chest pain, typically smoking history, associated with new or worsening cough. Opacity on **CXR and/or CT**.
	Confirmed by: tumour cells on **sputum cytology** or on endobronchial/**CT guided biopsy.**
	Finalized by the predictable outcome of management, e.g. O₂ if dyspnoea or hypoxic. Analgesia, including diamorphine if distressed. Nebulized adrenaline and tranexamic acid PO before an urgent bronchoscopy.
Pulmonary TB	*Suggested by:* weeks or months of fever, malaise, weight loss, and a contact history/high-risk groups.
	Confirmed by: **CXR**: opacification, especially in apical segments but can be anywhere. Acid-fast bacilli (AFB) on **smear sputum**, **culture** and/or response to treatment (when cultures negative and no other explanation for symptoms).
	Finalized by the predictable outcome of management, e.g. isolating patient until smear test known and preferably at least 2 weeks treatment. Initially 4 drug regime of rifampicin, isoniazid, pyrazinamide, ethambutol, and if malnourished, adding pyridoxine. Specialist management and contact tracing.

Upper respiratory tract infection (URTI), abnormalities, and bleeding, e.g. nasal polyps, laryngeal carcinoma, pharyngeal tumours	*Suggested by:* days of purulent rhinorrhoea (blood from URTI swallowed or inhaled and coughed back up). *Confirmed by:* **nasendoscopy**, **CT/MRI**, **head and neck and surgery/biopsy.** *Finalized by the predictable outcome of management*, e.g. packing, cautery of (Little's) bleeding area, removal of lesion.
Lung abscess	*Suggested by:* days or weeks of copious and foul-smelling sputum, fevers, chest pain. Typically preceded by a prior significant respiratory infection (e.g. pneumonia). *Confirmed by:* **CXR**: circular opacity with fluid level, **sputum culture/culture of CT guided aspirate.** *Finalized by the predictable outcome of management*, e.g. analgesia, high dose broad-spectrum antibiotics IV for Gram +ve and Gram –ve bacteria, e.g. co-amoxiclav + flucloxacillin + metronidazole for 14d ± CT guided drainage (send for TB and fungal cultures) or surgical removal.
Bronchiectasis	*Suggested by:* progression over months or years. Cupful(s) of pus-like sputum per day. Clubbing, typically bilateral consolidation, and bilateral coarse late inspiratory crackles. Typically obstructive deficit on **spirometry**. *Confirmed by:* **CXR**: cystic shadowing; high resolution **CT chest**: honeycombing and thickened dilated bronchi. *Finalized by the predictable outcome of management*, e.g. chest physiotherapy (including postural drainage and cough clearance), sputum cultures. Mucolytics, bronchodilators, regular exercise, winter vaccinations. When unwell, treatment with 10–14d antibiotics IV according to last sputum cultures. NB. Anti-*pseudomonas* treatment (aminoglycoside cover). Monitoring for weight loss and managing secondary causes.
Wegener's granulomatosis	*Suggested by:* months of cough, breathless ± microscopic haematuria (i.e. triad of upper/lower respiratory tract and renal abnormalities). Arthritis, myalgia, skin rashes, and nasal bridge collapse. Renal impairment. *Confirmed by:* **CXR** showing cavitating shadows. **↑cANCA antibody titre**, and microscopic arteritis on **biopsy.** *Finalized by the predictable outcome of management*, e.g. immunosuppression with steroids, azathioprine, and cyclophosphamide jointly by renal, respiratory physicians, etc.

Pneumonia	*Suggested by:* onset over hours or days. Rusty brown sputum (i.e. purulent sputum tinged with blood). Sharp chest pains worse on inspiration, fever, cough, signs of consolidation, etc. *Confirmed by:* patchy shadowing on **CXR** and **sputum/blood culture.** *Finalized by the predictable outcome of management,* e.g. 5d course of oral amoxicillin/clarithromycin PO unless more features of CRB-65 (Confusion, Respiratory rate >30/min, Blood pressure <90/60 mmHg and age >65y). If so, amoxicillin/co-amoxiclav IV or cefuroxime with controlled O_2 and fluids. If reduced consciousness/aspiration, then cefuroxime/metronidazole IV. If hospital/nursing home acquired, cefuroxime or piperacillin with tazobactam IV.
Pulmonary arterio-venous malformation	*Suggested by:* haemoptysis alone. No other symptoms. CXR normal or showing coin-shaped lesion with feeding blood vessel. *Confirmed by:* vascular red-blue lesion on **bronchoscopy** (if endobronchial) or enhancing lesion on a **CT chest** with (delayed) contrast, **pulmonary arteriogram** shows feeding vessels. *Finalized by the predictable outcome of management,* e.g. embolization if bleeding is recurrent or a large quantity. Lobectomy if this fails.
Also	Opportunistic mycobacteria, Goodpasture's syndrome, aspergilloma, mitral valve stenosis (if on warfarin), other endobronchial tumours (including benign lesions), hereditary haemorrhagic telangiectasia, endobronchial amyloid, any cause of systemic clotting abnormality.

Cough with sputum

Initial investigations (other tests in **bold** below): FBC, U&E, CXR.

Main differential diagnoses and typical outline evidence, etc.	
COPD caused by smoking, smoke pollution, α-antitrypsin deficiency	*Suggested by:* long history of cough ± sputum, many pack years of smoking, recurrent 'exacerbations'. CXR: radiolucent lungs. *Confirmed by:* **spirometry:** FEV <80% predicted and FEV/ FVC ratio <0.7. <5% reversibility. Emphysema on CT chest ± ↓α-antitrypsin levels. *Finalized by the predictable outcome of management,* e.g. stopping smoking. Trials of bronchodilators prn, then regular long-acting bronchodilators. Inhaled steroids if FEV <50% predicted and three COPD exacerbations per year. If cough and breathlessness persists, prednisolone PO. If respiratory failure, home O_2.
Acute viral bronchitis	*Suggested by:* onset over hours or days. Fever, myalgia, fatigue, and white/yellow sputum. *Confirmed by:* no focal chest signs, no consolidation on **CXR**, resolution within 5d. *Finalized by the predictable outcome of management,* e.g. rest and simple analgesia such as paracetamol.
Acute bacterial bronchitis	*Suggested by:* onset over hours or days. Fever, mucopurulent sputum, dyspnoea. *Confirmed by:* no focal chest signs, **FBC**: ↑neutrophils, no consolidation on **CXR**, pathogens in sputum culture, and rapid response to appropriate antibiotics. *Finalized by the predictable outcome of management,* e.g. simple analgesia, amoxicillin/clarithromycin PO for 5–7d.
Pneumonia	*Suggested by:* onset over hours or days. Rusty brown sputum. Sharp chest pain (worse on inspiration), fever, cough, signs of consolidation. *Confirmed by:* patchy shadowing on **CXR** and sputum/blood culture. *Finalized by the predictable outcome of management,* e.g. 5d course of amoxicillin/clarithromycin PO unless 2 or more features of CRB-65 (Confusion, Respiratory rate >30min, Blood pressure <90/60mmHg and age >65y). If so, amoxicillin/co-amoxiclav IV or cefuroxime with controlled O_2 and fluids. If reduced consciousness/aspiration, then cefuroxime/metronidazole IV. If hospital/nursing home acquired, cefuroxime or piperacillin with tazobactam IV.

Lung abscess	*Suggested by:* days or weeks of copious and foul-smelling sputum, fever, chest pain. Typically preceded by a prior significant respiratory infection (e.g. pneumonia).
	Confirmed by: **CXR**: circular opacity with fluid level, **sputum culture/culture of CT guided aspirate.**
	Finalized by the predictable outcome of management, e.g. analgesia, high dose broad-spectrum antibiotics IV for Gram +ve and Gram –ve bacteria, e.g. co-amoxiclav + flucloxacillin + metronidazole for 14d ± CT guided drainage (send for TB and fungal cultures) or surgical removal.
Also	Broncho-alveolar cell carcinoma, pulmonary alveolar proteinosis, bronchiectasis associated with immunodeficiency states/primary ciliary dyskinesia, etc.

Persistent dry cough with no sputum

The duration of symptoms, severity, and progression will help determine the causes of a dry cough. No cause is found in up to 15% patients. As this symptom is non-life-threatening, initial management can be delayed until the exact cause is found. Initial investigations (other tests in **bold** below): FBC, U&E, CXR.

Main differential diagnoses and typical outline evidence, etc.	
Smoking	*Suggested by:* smoking history.
	Confirmed by: stopping smoking, cough often worsens initially as ciliary motility is restored, but improves within 3mo.
	Finalized by the predictable outcome of management, e.g. giving generic advice and adjunct pharmacotherapy. Referring to smoking cessation specialist, if available, and patient is keen to stop.
Chronic asthma	*Suggested by:* chronic cough, worse at night and early morning. Seasonal variation and other specific triggers (e.g. aerosol sprays, cold air, perfumes, smoke, infections exercise, etc.). Family history or childhood history of asthma or atopy.
	Confirmed by: reduced or variable peak flow (classical dipping early morning/late evening) and **FEV_1** that improve by >15% with treatment.
	Finalized by the predictable outcome of management, e.g. identifying precipitants, stopping smoking, trial of bronchodilator prn, regular inhaled steroids, long-acting β-agonist/steroid combinations, leukotriene inhibitors/antihistamines. Managed in chest clinic.
Gastro-oesophageal reflux	*Suggested by:* cough worse lying flat and after heavy meals. Heart burn/indigestion. Absent stomach bubble on **CXR** (of hiatus hernia).
	Confirmed by: **24h oseophageal pH monitoring** or improvement in cough on raising head of bed and with acid suppression (often need very high doses of more than one antacid, combined with promotility drugs).
	Finalized by the predictable outcome of management, e.g. proton pump inhibitor (PPI) bd combined with H_2 antagonist (e.g. ranitidine 150mg bd) and metoclopramide tds, domperidone 20mg tds, and even baclofen bd, in a stepwise fashion.
Post-nasal drip	*Suggested by:* feeling of catarrh and drip in back of throat, worse at night, nasal polyps.
	Confirmed by: improvement with nasal decongestion.
	Finalized by the predictable outcome of management, e.g. nasal steroids and or nasal ipratropium sprays. Antihistamines. ENT specialist if fails.
Viral infection with slow recovery	*Suggested by:* original onset over days, fever, sore throat, generalized aches.
	Confirmed by: spontaneous (slow) improvement.
	Finalized by the predictable outcome of management, e.g. observation.

ACE inhibitors	*Suggested by:* drug history. (NB Symptoms can start after taking ACE inhibitors for a long time.)
	Confirmed by: cough improves when ACE inhibitor stopped, may take several months.
	Finalized by the predictable outcome of management, e.g. substitute with angiotensin receptor blocker for ACE inhibitor.
COPD caused by smoking, smoke pollution, α1-antitrypsin deficiency	*Suggested by:* long history of cough ± sputum, many pack years of smoking, recurrent 'exacerbations'. **CXR**: radiolucent lungs.
	Confirmed by: **spirometry**: FEV_1 <80% predicted and FEV/FVC ratio <0.7. <15% reversibility. Emphysema on **CT chest** ± ↓α1-antitrypsin levels.
	Finalized by the predictable outcome of management, e.g. stopping smoking. Trials of bronchodilators prn, then regular long-acting bronchodilators. Inhaled steroids if FEV <50% predicted and three COPD exacerbations per year. If cough and breathless persists, prednisolone PO. If respiratory failure, home O_2.
Carcinoma of lung	*Suggested by:* weeks or months of weight loss, chest pain, typically smoking history, associated with new or worsening cough. Opacity on **CXR and/or CT**.
	Confirmed by: tumour cells on **sputum cytology** or on endobronchial/**CT guided biopsy.**
	Finalized by the predictable outcome of management, e.g. O_2 if dyspnoea or hypoxic. Surgery, chemoradiotherapy, and supportive care.
Pulmonary TB	*Suggested by:* weeks or months of fever, malaise, weight loss, and a contact history/high-risk groups.
	Confirmed by: **CXR**: opacification, especially in apical segments, but can be anywhere. AFB on **smear sputum, culture,** and/or response to treatment (when cultures negative and no other explanation for symptoms).
	Finalized by the predictable outcome of management, e.g. isolating patient until smear test known and preferably at least 2 weeks treatment. Initially 4 drug regime of rifampicin, isoniazid, pyrazinamide, ethambutol, and if malnourished, adding pyridoxine. Specialist management and contract tracing.
Interstitial lung disease	*Suggested by:* chronic dry cough, occupational exposure, or evidence of underlying connective tissue disease. NB Majority of cases have no cause identified. Clubbing, cyanosis, reduced chest expansion, coarse late inspiratory bibasal crackles.
	Confirmed by: reduced lung volumes and reticular nodular shadowing on **CXR**. Interstitial shadowing and/or subpleural fibrosis on **high resolution CT chest.**
	Finalized by the predictable outcome of management, e.g. O_2 if saturations <93%. Specialist opinion for detailed lung function, lung biopsy, immunosuppression, antifibrotics, palliation.
Also	Inhaled foreign body, benign endobronchial lesions (e.g. hamartomas), psychogenic.

Hoarseness

Hoarseness of some weeks' or months' duration may have some sinister causes that need urgent attention. Initial investigations (other tests in **bold** below): FBC, U&E, CXR.

Main differential diagnoses and typical outline evidence, etc.	
Inhaled steroids	*Suggested by:* drug history. *Confirmed by:* improvement on stopping steroids. *Finalized by the predictable outcome of management,* e.g. improve inhaler technique (especially using spacer) and rinsing mouth after inhalers.
Chronic laryngitis	*Suggested by:* onset over months or years. History of recurrent acute laryngitis. *Confirmed by:* inflamed cords at **laryngoscopy** and no other pathology. *Finalized by the predictable outcome of management,* e.g. stopping smoking and reduce alcohol.
Singer's nodes	*Suggested by:* onset over months. Long history, often occupational, in teachers or singers due to voice strain, singing, alcohol, fumes, etc. *Confirmed by:* nodules on cord at **laryngoscopy**. *Initial management:* speech therapy, surgical removal.
Laryngeal carcinoma (glottic, supra-glottic, or subglottic tumour)	*Suggested by:* progressive hoarseness over weeks to months. Smoker, including cannabis. Dysphagia, haemoptysis, ear pain. *Confirmed by:* **laryngoscopy**, biopsy, staging. *Finalized by the predictable outcome of management,* e.g. surgical removal.
Vocal cord paresis due to vagal nerve trauma, cancer (thyroid, oesophagus, pharynx, bronchus) **or tuberculosis, multiple sclerosis, polio, syringomyelia, (no cause identified in 15%)**	*Suggested by:* onset after surgery or otherwise over weeks and months. Bovine cough. Symptoms of cause. Abnormal **CXR, barium swallow, MRI**. *Confirmed by:* paresis or abnormal movement of cords on **laryngoscopy.** *Finalized by the predictable outcome of management,* e.g. urgent ENT referral. May be considered for vocal cord prosthesis/implant after treatment of cause.
Functional hoarseness	*Suggested by:* recurrence at times of stress. Variable symptoms, able to cough normally. *Confirmed by:* no abnormality **laryngoscopy.** *Finalized by the predictable outcome of management,* e.g. counselling and behavioural therapy.

Myxoedema	*Suggested by:* onset over months or years. Fatigue, puffy face, obesity, cold intolerance, bradycardia, slow relaxing reflexes.
	Confirmed by: swollen vocal cords at **laryngoscopy. ↑TSH, ↓FT4.**
	Finalized by the predictable outcome of management, e.g. thyroxine replacement.
Acromegaly	*Suggested by:* swollen vocal cords at **laryngoscopy.** Large, wide face, embossed forehead, jutting jaw (prognathism), widely spaced teeth, and large tongue.
	Confirmed by: **↑IGF**, failure to suppress growth hormone to <2mU/L with **oral GTT. Skull X-ray** confirming bony abnormalities. **Hand X-ray** showing typical tufts on terminal phalanges. **MRI** or **CT scan** showing enlarged pituitary fossa.
	Finalized by the predictable outcome of management, e.g. hormone replacement and pituitary surgery/ radiotherapy.
Sicca syndrome due to old age, Sjögren's syndrome, rheumatoid, sarcoid, etc.	*Suggested by:* onset over months to years. Dry mouth and eyes.
	Confirmed by: clinical presentation and inflamed cords at laryngoscopy and no other pathology.
	Finalized by the predictable outcome of management, e.g. lubricant lozenges ± artificial tears, address related conditions.
Granulomas due to syphilis, TB, sarcoid, Wegener's	*Suggested by:* onset over months with symptoms and signs in other systems. Abnormal CXR or other system involvement.
	Confirmed by: granulomata on cords at **laryngoscopy. Biopsy. Culture and sensitivity.**
	Finalized by the predictable outcome of management, e.g. if TB cultured, 6mo of triple/quadruple therapy. If Wegener's granulomatosis/sarcoid, immunosuppression with systemic steroids + azathioprine + cyclophosphamide. Surgical intervention for possible vocal cord prosthesis.

Some thoughts when examining the respiratory system

The findings are described here in the sequence of inspection, palpation, percussion, and then auscultation. While inspecting, think of blood gas status, and when palpating, think of the mechanisms of ventilation. When percussing, think of the pleural surfaces, contents of the pleural cavity, and lung tissue. When auscultating, think of the state of the lung and overlying tissue as well as the airways.

Appearance suggestive of blood gas disturbance

Look at hands for cyanosis, feel for warmth, ask patient to hold arms out and extended at the wrists to see if there is a coarse tremor and/or muscle twitching in the arms. Look at the fingers for peripheral cyanosis and more importantly here, the tongue and lips for central cyanosis. Initial investigations (other tests in **bold** below): FBC, U&E, CXR, ABG.

Main differential diagnoses and typical outline evidence, etc.	
Hypoxic	*Suggested by:* blue fingernails (peripheral) and tongue (central cyanosis), restless, confused, drowsy, or unconscious. *Confirmed by:* **P$_a$O$_2$** <8kPa on **blood gas analysis** (or **pulse oximetry** of <92% (mild) or <85% (severe). *Finalized by the predictable outcome of management,* e.g. controlled O$_2$ via Venturi and continuous clinical/physiological monitoring whilst addressing underlying cause.
CO$_2$ retention	*Suggested by:* warm hands, bounding pulse, dilated veins on hands and face, twitching of facial muscles, headaches, confusion, and drowsy. *Confirmed by:* **P$_a$CO$_2$** >6.5kPa on **blood gas analysis**. Typically >8.0 kPa to be symptomatic. *Finalized by the predictable outcome of management,* e.g. control O$_2$ delivery <28% (with Venturi mask to keeping O$_2$ saturation 88–92%). Address underlying cause of respiratory depression if respiratory rate <10 breaths per min.
Hypocapnia	*Suggested by:* dizzy, anxious, paraesthesiae around lips or fingers, tachypnoea. *Confirmed by:* P$_a$CO$_2$ <4.0kPa on **blood gas analysis.** *Finalized by the predictable outcome of management,* e.g. address underlying illness; giving supplemental O$_2$. If CO$_2$ low, then slow breathing by getting patient to relax; can try rebreathing with a paper bag.

Respiratory rate low (<10/min)

Count the number of respirations for a whole minute if rate appears low. Initial management is to check patient is conscious and securing of airway as per Basic Life Support. Removal of any obvious cause (e.g. high flow O_2 if saturations are >88%, needlesticks, etc). These patients typically have reduced consciousness and, therefore, are at risk of losing their airway patency (e.g. aspiration), so they must be treated in a high-dependency area. Initial investigations (other tests in **bold** below): FBC, U&E, CXR, ABGs.

Main differential diagnoses and typical outline evidence, etc.	
CO_2 narcosis (very high blood CO_2) due to excess O_2 administration	*Suggested by:* warm hands, bounding pulse, dilated veins on hands and face, twitching of facial muscles, drowsy. High flow O_2 being given. *Confirmed by:* P_aCO_2 >6.5kPa on **blood gas analysis.** *Finalized by the predictable outcome of management,* e.g. reduce inhaled O_2 to keeping saturation 88–92%. Address underlying cause of respiratory depression if respiratory rate is <10 breaths per min.
Drugs, e.g. opiates, alcohol, benzodiazepines, muscle relaxants	*Suggested by:* pinpoint pupils (needle track marks). History of ingestion, empty medication bottle. *Confirmed by:* response to drug withdrawal or antidotes, e.g. naloxone IV/IM, flumazenil IV. Drug levels on **toxicology screen.** *Finalized by the predictable outcome of management,* e.g. if saturations >90% and no other airway or cardiovascular compromise, observation only until the sedative wears off. Securing of airway and trial of antidote; needs high dependency setting with anaesthetist support.
Raised intracranial pressure	*Suggested by:* papilloedema, focal neurology, severe headaches, and vomiting. *Confirmed by:* **CT brain** (loss of normal sulci, cerebral oedema). *Finalized by the predictable outcome of management,* e.g. securing of airway, breathing, and circulation. Monitor neuro-observations. Nurse with head up at 45°. Dexamethasone IV, mannitol IV, and phenytoin IV if fits. Neurology referral.

Head injury (without raised intracranial pressure) or cervical cord trauma	*Suggested by:* history and signs of assault/trauma. Other abnormal neurology (upper or lower motor neurone signs).
	Confirmed by: **CT brain** (loss of normal sulci, cerebral oedema).
	Finalized by the predictable outcome of management, e.g. ATLS (Advanced Trauma Life Support) algorithm. NB Care stabilizing cervical spine.
Acute (-on-chronic) neuromuscular disease, e.g. Guillain-Barré syndrome	*Suggested by:* known neurological disease, recent viral illness, autonomic dysfunction, ascending weakness, etc. ± other lower motor neurone signs.
	Confirmed by: muscle weakness and $\downarrow P_aO_2$, $\uparrow P_aCO_2$ **on blood gas analysis.**
	Finalized by the predictable outcome of management, e.g. ventilatory support (if appropriate), supplemental O_2. Specific measures depending on cause.
Severe hypothermia	*Suggested by:* exposure, immobility, reduced **GCS**, bradycardia.
	Confirmed by: core temp <33°C.
	Finalized by the predictable outcome of management, e.g. gentle rewarming (space blankets, fluids IV, bladder irrigation, etc.)

Chest wall abnormalities

Inspect the chest shape and then its change on movement for asymmetry.
Initial investigations (other tests in **bold** below): FBC, U&E, CXR, ABGs.

Main differential diagnoses and typical outline evidence, etc.

Pectus carinatum (developmental or associated with emphysema)	*Suggested by:* prominent sternum, often associated with indrawing of the ribs (Harrison's sulci) above the costal margins. *Confirmed by:* **CXR.** *Finalized by the predictable outcome of management,* e.g. manage emphysema.
Pectus excavatum (developmental defect)	*Suggested by:* depression of the lower end or whole sternum. *Confirmed by:* **CXR.** *Finalized by the predictable outcome of management,* e.g. explanation.
Kyphosis (congenital or due to anterior collapse of spinal vertebrae, e.g. severe osteoporosis, spinal TB)	*Suggested by:* spine curved forward. *Confirmed by:* **CXR, spinal X-ray.** *Finalized by the predictable outcome of management,* e.g. assess partly using **blood gases**, need for (nocturnal) Non-Invasive Ventilatory support (NIV) if symptoms of ventilatory failure and/or P_aO_2 <8kPa with P_aCO_2 >6.5kPa.
Scoliosis (congenital, neuromuscular disease, surgery, spinal TB)	*Suggested by:* spine curved laterally. *Confirmed by:* CXR, spinal X-ray. *Finalized by the predictable outcome of management,* e.g. assess partly using blood gases, need for (nocturnal) Non-Invasive Ventilatory support (NIV) if symptoms of ventilatory failure and/or $\downarrow P_aO_2$ <8kPa with $\uparrow P_aCO_2$ >6.5kPa.
Absence of part of chest wall bone structure (congenital—Poland's syndrome—or post-surgery, e.g. thoracoplasty for TB, cancer)	*Suggested by:* absence of ribs, pectoralis muscle, clavicle, etc. *Confirmed by:* history, scars, **CXR, spinal X-ray.** *Finalized by the predictable outcome of management,* e.g. assess partly using **blood gases**, need for (nocturnal) NIV support if symptoms of ventilatory failure and/or P_aO_2 <8kPa with P_aCO_2 >6.5kPa.

Bilateral poor chest expansion

Consider all the causes of a low respiratory rate (see ➡ Respiratory rate low (<10/min), p.256) and also the following that typically do not cause a low respiratory rate. Initial investigations (other tests in **bold** below): FBC, U&E, CXR, ABG.

Main differential diagnoses and typical outline evidence, etc.

Obesity possibly causing obesity hypoventilation syndrome	*Suggested by:* insidious onset of breathlessness in obese individual. *Confirmed by:* examination (BMI often needs to be >40kg/m² to cause chest wall compromise). *Finalized by the predictable outcome of management,* e.g. weight loss, including dietitian referral and weight-lowering medications. Assess partly using **blood gases**, need for (nocturnal) NIV support if symptoms of ventilatory failure and P_aO_2 <8kPa with P_aCO_2 >6.5kPa (obesity hypoventilation syndrome).
Emphysema (overlaps with COPD) caused by smoking, smoke pollution, α1-antitrypsin deficiency	*Suggested by:* long history of cough ± sputum, many pack years of smoking, recurrent 'exacerbations', pursed lip, breathing (a chronic behavioural adaptation), hyperinflation, reduced chest expansion, reduced breath sounds and hyper-resonance. **CXR:** radiolucent lungs. *Confirmed by:* **spirometry:** FEV_1 <80% predicted and FEV/FVC ratio <0.7. <15% reversibility. Emphysema on **CT chest ±↓α1-antitrypsin levels.** *Finalized by the predictable outcome of management,* e.g. stopping smoking. Trials of bronchodilators prn, regular long-acting bronchodilators. Regular inhaled steroids if FEV <50% predicted and three COPD exacerbations per year. If cough and breathless persists, prednisolone PO. If respiratory failure, home O_2.
Pulmonary fibrosis/ interstitial lung disease NB Majority of cases have no cause identified	*Suggested by:* chronic dry cough, occupational exposure, or evidence of underlying connective tissue disease. Clubbing, cyanosis, reduced chest expansion, coarse late inspiratory bibasal crackles. *Confirmed by:* ↓lung volumes and reticular nodular shadowing on **CXR.** Interstitial shadowing and/or subpleural fibrosis on **high resolution CT chest.** *Finalized by the predictable outcome of management,* e.g. home O_2 if saturations <93%. Specialist opinion about detailed lung function, lung biopsy, immunosuppression, antifibrotics, palliation.

Muscular dystrophy (other rarer myopathies, e.g. limb-girdle dystrophy, acid maltase deficiency, etc.)	*Suggested by:* early age onset, family history, calf hypertrophy, lower motor neurone signs. *Confirmed by:* restrictive deficit on **spirometry** (especially when lying flat). Sparing of transferring factor, globally low volumes, especially reduced residual volumes and mouth (inspiratory) pressures on **detailed lung function; muscle biopsy.** *Finalized by the predictable outcome of management, e.g.* assess need for (nocturnal) NIV support if symptoms of ventilatory failure and/or **blood gases** show P_aO_2 <8kPa with P_aCO_2 >6.5kPa. Neurology clinic for long-term care.
Motor neurone disease	*Suggested by:* late-onset mixed upper and lower motor neurone signs, tongue fasciculation, bulbar palsy. *Confirmed by:* clinical and **electromyography** (EMG). Restrictive deficit (globally low volumes) on **spirometry** (especially when lying flat). Sparing of transferring factor, reduced residual volumes and mouth (inspiratory) pressures on **detailed lung function.** *Finalized by the predictable outcome of management, e.g.* medications to reduce upper airway secretions. Assess need for (nocturnal) NIV support if symptoms of ventilatory failure and/or **blood gases** show P_aO_2 <8kPa with P_aCO_2 >6.5kPa. Urgent referral to neurologist.
Multiple sclerosis	*Suggested by:* restrictive deficit (globally low volumes) on spirometry (especially when lying flat). *Confirmed by:* **MRI brain**, **visual evoked responses**. Sparing of transferring factor, reduced residual volumes and mouth (inspiratory) pressures on **detailed lung function.** *Finalized by the predictable outcome of management, e.g.* assess need for (nocturnal) NIV support if symptoms of ventilatory failure and/or **blood gases** show P_aO_2 <8kPa with P_aCO_2 >6.5kPa. Neurology clinic for long-term care.
Guillain–Barré syndrome	*Suggested by:* ascending weakness, autonomic disturbances, and recent infection. Restrictive deficit on **lung function** (especially when lying flat). *Confirmed by:* rapid deterioration on lung function (FVC). Sparing of corrected transferring factor. Progress of illness worsening over days to weeks, then improvement. *Finalized by the predictable outcome of management, e.g.* ventilatory support if P_aO_2 falling and/or P_aCO_2 rising, steroids, and plasmapheresis/immunoglobulin infusions.
Also	Myasthenia gravis, Eaton–Lambert syndrome, muscle relaxant drugs, e.g. suxamethonium, neurotoxins (including organophosphates), severe electrolyte abnormalities ($\downarrow\uparrow K^+$, $\downarrow Ca^{2+}$).

Unilateral poor chest expansion

If the patient has become ill rapidly, then this sign has a short differential diagnosis: tension pneumothorax (which needs to be treated without doing 'initial tests'), flail segment, or severe pneumonia, and needs rapid diagnosis and urgent treatment. Less urgent causes are more common; the more dangerous are giving in precedent here. Initial investigations (other tests in **bold** below): FBC, U&E, CXR, ABG.

Main differential diagnoses and typical outline evidence, etc.	
Pneumothorax ('tension', moderate, or mild)	*Suggested by:* pain in centre or side of chest with abrupt breathlessness, diminished breath sounds, and hyper-resonance to percussion. *Confirmed by:* tracheal deviation and distress suggesting tension pneumothorax, or **expiration CXR** showing loss of lung markings outside sharp line ('moderate' if >5cm gap from lung edge to chest wall, 'mild' if <5cm.) *Initial management:* if tension pneumothorax, insertion of large Venflon into 2nd intercostal (IC) space, mid-clavicular line. Giving O₂ if breathless. Analgesia. Aspiration if moderate; if this is unsatisfactory or prior lung disease, insertion of IC drain into 'triangle of safety'. If 'mild' (<5cm gap) and not breathless, observation.
Flail segment following trauma	*Suggested by:* paradoxical movement of part of chest wall. *Confirmed by:* **CXR.** *Finalized by the predictable outcome of management,* e.g. apply direct pressure and 'splint' the segment. Apply ATLS algorithm.
Extensive consolidation due to bacterial infection, but possibly autoimmune disease, malignancy, or drugs	*Suggested by:* reduced breath sounds, bronchial breathing, increased tactile vocal fremitus, reduced percussion note. *Confirmed by:* CXR. *Finalized by the predictable outcome of management,* e.g. if not very ill, but fever and ↑neutrophil count, analgesia, and an empiric 5d course of amoxicillin/clarithromycin PO. If ≥2 features of CRB-65, then amoxicillin/co-amoxiclav IV or cefuroxime with controlled O₂ and fluids. If history of reduced consciousness/aspiration, then cefuroxime/metronidazole IV. If hospital/nursing home acquired infection, cefuroxime or piperacillin with tazobactam IV. If no fever or WCC normal, investigate non-infective possibilities.
Fractured ribs possibly complicated by pneumothorax, haemothorax	*Suggested by:* history of trauma, focal tenderness. *Confirmed by:* **CXR.** *Finalized by the predictable outcome of management,* e.g. analgesia and rest. Admit to hospital for observation if breathless or worsening pain.

Pleural effusion	*Suggested by:* reduced breath sounds, reduced tactile vocal fremitus, stony dull percussion note.
	Confirmed by: homogeneous opacification with meniscus level on **CXR** and fluid on **US scan/CT chest.**
	Finalized by the predictable outcome of management, e.g. if breathless at rest, aspiration of 500mL (therapeutic) and send fluid for tests, not draining to dryness if cause unknown as thoracoscopy/pleural biopsy required. If known malignancy, also insertion of IC drain directly and pleurodesis.
Musculoskeletal e.g. previous thoracoplasty	*Suggested by:* history, scar.
	Confirmed by: **CXR.**
	Finalized by the predictable outcome of management, e.g. assess need for (nocturnal) NIV support if symptoms of ventilatory failure and/or **blood gases** show P_aO_2 <8kPa with P_aCO_2 >6.5kPa. Neurology clinic for long-term care.

Trachea displaced

First assess the patient—if clinically compromised, suspect tension pneumothorax. Although this is a rare cause of displaced trachea, it must be managed immediately both in primary and secondary care. Palpate with middle finger and with the index and ring finger on either side of trachea. Localize apex beat to see if lower mediastinum is also displaced. Initial investigations (after treating ing any tension pneumothorax based on clinical diagnosis—other tests in **bold** below): FBC, U&E, CXR, ABG.

Main differential diagnoses and typical outline evidence, etc.	
Pushed by contralateral tension pneumothorax	*Suggested by:* in extremis with high pulse rate and hypotension, reduced/absent breath sounds, reduced tactile vocal fremitus, hyper-resonant percussion note.
	Confirmed by: escape of air after insertion of a Venflon into 2nd IC space, opposite side of tracheal deviation.
	Finalized by the predictable outcome of management, e.g. insertion of a Venflon as above; expertly secured emergency IC drain insertion of ion. O_2 and analgesia.
Pulled by ipsilateral pneumothorax ('tension', moderate, or mild)	*Suggested by:* pain in centre or side of chest with abrupt breathlessness, diminished breath sounds, and hyper-resonance to percussion.
	Confirmed by: tracheal deviation and distress suggesting tension pneumothorax, or **expiration CXR** showing loss of lung markings outside sharp line ('moderate' if >5cm gap from lung edge to chest wall, 'mild' if <5cm).
	Initial management: O_2 if breathless. Analgesia. Aspiration if moderate; if this is unsatisfactory or prior lung disease, insertion of IC drain into 'triangle of safety'. If 'mild' (<5cm gap) and not breathless, observation.
Pulled by ipsilateral upper lobe fibrosis, collapse, or removal	*Suggested by:* TB (chronic), radiation fibrosis (skin changes, tattoo marks), surgery (scar), ankylosing spondylitis, chronic sarcoidosis. If smoker and focal lobar collapse, endobronchial tumour. Reduced upper chest wall expansion.
	Confirmed by: **CXR** showing diminished abnormal chest anatomy 'pulling' on mediastinum with trachea deviated towards the same side.
	Finalized by the predictable outcome of management, e.g. review old CXR; for **CT chest and bronchoscopy** if new upper lobe collapse. Assess need for (nocturnal) NIV support if symptoms of ventilatory failure and/or **blood gases** show P_aO_2 <8kPa with P_aCO_2 >6.5kPa.

Pushed by contralateral pleural effusion	*Suggested by:* reduced breath sounds, reduced tactile vocal fremitus, stony dull percussion note. *Confirmed by:* **CXR** showing large homogeneous white opacification 'pushing' on mediastinum. *Finalized by the predictable outcome of management,* e.g. if breathless at rest, aspiration of 500mL (therapeutic) and send fluid for tests. Do not drain to dryness if cause unknown, thoracoscopy/pleural biopsy is required. If known cause (e.g. malignancy), aspiration of 500mL or insertion of IC drain directly and pleurodesis.
Scoliosis	*Suggested by:* chest wall deformity and curved spine. *Confirmed by:* **spinal X-ray, CXR.** *Finalized by the predictable outcome of management,* e.g. analgesia, physiotherapy, calcium supplements. Assess need for (nocturnal) NIV support if symptoms of ventilatory failure and/or **blood gases** show P_aO_2 <8kPa with P_aCO_2 >6.5kPa.

Reduced tactile vocal fremitus

If *in extremis*, treat as tension pneumothorax. If not, Initial investigations (other tests in **bold** below): FBC, U&E, CXR.

Main differential diagnoses and typical outline evidence, etc.	
Pleural effusion	*Suggested by:* reduced breath sounds, reduced tactile vocal fremitus, stony dullness to percussion.
	Confirmed by: homogeneous opacification with meniscus level on **CXR** and fluid on **US scan/CT chest**.
	Initial management: if breathless at rest, aspiration of 500mL (therapeutic) and send fluid for tests. Do not drain to dryness if cause unknown, thoracoscopy/pleural biopsy is required. If known cause (e.g. malignancy), aspiration of 500mL or insertion of IC drain directly and pleurodesis.
Pneumothorax ('tension', moderate or mild)	*Suggested by:* pain in centre or side of chest with abrupt breathlessness, diminished breath sounds, and hyper-resonance to percussion.
	Confirmed by: above findings, tracheal deviation, and distress suggesting tension pneumothorax, or **expiration CXR** showing loss of lung markings outside sharp line ('moderate' if >5cm gap from lung edge to chest wall, 'mild' if <5cm.)
	Initial management: if tension pneumothorax, insertion of large Venflon into 2nd IC space, mid-clavicular line. Giving O_2 if breathless. Analgesia. Aspiration if moderate; if this unsatisfactory or prior lung disease, insert IC drain into 'triangle of safety'. If 'mild' (<5cm gap) + not breathless, observation.
Collapsed lobe with no consolidation	*Suggested by:* reduced breath sounds, reduced expansion, normal percussion note.
	Confirmed by: **CXR** (collapse of different lobes will have different patterns radiologically, e.g. showing fan-shaped shadow arising from mediastinum, mediastinal shift, raised hemidiaphragm, displaced horizontal fissure or 'sail sign'). **CT thorax** confirms lobar collapse.
	Finalized by the predictable outcome of management, e.g. bronchoscopy to removal of any foreign body or debris, or to biopsy obstructive growth.

Increased tactile vocal fremitus

Initial investigations (other tests in **bold** below): FBC, U&E, CXR.

Main differential diagnoses and typical outline evidence, etc.

Extensive consolidation due to bacterial infection, but possibly autoimmune disease, malignancy, or drugs	*Suggested by:* reduced breath sounds, bronchial breathing, increased tactile vocal fremitus, reduced percussion note. *Confirmed by:* **CXR**. *Finalized by the predictable outcome of management,* e.g. if not very ill, but fever and ↑neutrophil count on **FBC**, analgesia and an empiric 5d course of amoxicillin/clarithromycin PO. If ≥2 features of CRB-65, then amoxicillin/co-amoxiclav IV or cefuroxime with controlled O_2 and fluids. If history of reduced consciousness/aspiration, then cefuroxime/metronidazole IV. If hospital/nursing home acquired infection, cefuroxime or piperacillin with tazobactam IV. If no fever or WCC normal, investigate non-infective possibilities.

Stony dull percussion

This implies pleural effusion. The causes of pleural effusion are traditionally divided into transudates and exudates. Initial investigations (other tests in **bold** below): FBC, U&E, CXR, diagnostic pleural aspiration.

Main differential diagnoses and typical outline evidence, etc.	
Transudates	*Suggested by:* bilateral effusions, underlying clinical cause.
	Confirmed by: **protein in pleural effusion** <30g/L or <0.5 ratio to serum protein (except can be higher in treated heart failure).
Left heart failure (LVF), superior vena cava (SVC) obstruction, pericarditis, peritoneal dialysis	*Suggested by:* peripheral oedema, ↑JVP, basal crackles, 3rd heart sound, if LVF. Headache, swollen/plethoric face, and dilated superficial venules across anterior chest if SVC obstruction.
	Confirmed by: **CXR, echocardiogram, CT thorax** (if considering SVC obstruction).
	Initial treatment: diuretics and ACE inhibitors if LVF. Steroids and anticoagulation if SVC obstruction. NSAIDs and treating cause if pericardial effusion.
Low albumin states, e.g. liver cirrhosis, nephrotic syndrome	*Suggested by:* malnutrition, generalized oedema. Evidence of other disease.
	Confirmed by: ↓**serum albumin**.
	Initial treatment: try to correct serum albumin with appropriate diet.
Rare causes	Hypothyroidism, Meig's syndrome.
Exudates	*Suggested by:* typically unilateral effusion (but may be bilateral). Signs and symptoms of underlying disease.
	Confirmed by: **protein in effusion** >30g/dL or >0.5 ratio to serum protein.
Infective: bacterial/empyema, TB, viral, etc.	*Suggested by:* history, fever, ↓pH, ↓glucose in pleural fluid.
	Confirmed by: **pleural aspiration** of pus with organisms on **Gram stain or culture** in bacterial pneumonia. ↑lymphocytes suggest TB (confirmed by +ve cultures or **Ziehl–Neelsen (ZN)** stain on fluid or pleural biopsy or of caseating granuloma).
	Finalized by the predictable outcome of management, e.g. appropriate antibiotic treatment and IC drain to remove fluid or pus, or surgery.
Neoplastic: lung 1° or 2°, breast, ovarian, reticuloses, Kaposi's, local chest wall tumours, mesothelioma	*Suggested by:* history, especially weight loss. Signs of local or distal spread.
	Confirmed by: **pleural aspiration** (cytology), **pleural biopsy** or other tissue histology.
	Finalized by the predictable outcome of management, e.g. once cancer confirmed, typically needs IC drain, and drain to dryness followed by pleurodesis. Oncology opinion for active treatment or palliative care.

Rheumatoid, systemic lupus erythematosus, etc.	*Suggested by:* history, other organ specific involvement, e.g. joints, +ve rheumatoid factor in fluid, very low fluid glucose.
	Confirmed by: +ve **autoantibodies** and clinical criteria, response to immunosuppression.
	Finalized by the predictable outcome of management, e.g. steroids/azathioprine/cyclophosphamide.
Pulmonary infarction/ embolus	*Suggested by:* sudden/acute worsening of breathlessness, pleural rub, cyanosis, tachycardia, loud P2, associated DVT, or risk factors such as recent surgery, immobility, previous emboli, malignancy, etc. Other tests typically show raised D-dimers, tachycardia or right heart strain, and rarely S1Q3T3 on ECG.
	Confirmed by: **CT pulmonary angiogram** showing clot in pulmonary artery. Echocardiogram (right heart strain) is useful for risk stratification if pulmonary embolus confirmed.
	Finalized by the predictable outcome of management, e.g. LMW heparin (treatment dose not prophylactic dose) and 3mo anticoagulation with warfarin (longer if ongoing risk factors). Thrombolysis if ↓BP, large and bilateral clots, no response to anticoagulation or acutely dilated right ventricle on echocardiogram.

Dull to percussion but not stony dull

Initial investigations (other tests in **bold** below): FBC, U&E, CXR.

Main differential diagnoses and typical outline evidence, etc.

Consolidation due to bacterial infection, but possibly autoimmune disease, malignancy, or drugs.	*Suggested by:* reduced breath sounds, bronchial breathing, increased tactile vocal fremitus, reduced percussion note. *Confirmed by:* **CXR.** *Finalized by the predictable outcome of management,* e.g. if not very ill, but fever and ↑neutrophil count on **FBC**, analgesia and an empiric 5d course of amoxicillin/clarithromycin PO. If ≥2 features of CRB-65, then amoxicillin/co-amoxiclav IV or cefuroxime with controlled O_2 and fluids. If history of reduced consciousness/aspiration, then cefuroxime/metronidazole IV. If hospital/nursing home acquired infection, cefuroxime or piperacillin with tazobactam IV. If no fever or WCC normal, investigate non-infective possibilities.
Pulmonary oedema due to acute left ventricular failure or chronic (congestive) cardiac failure due to ischaemic heart disease, mitral stenosis	*Suggested by:* background fatigue and exertional breathless, cardiac risk factors. Displaced apex beat, 3rd heart sound, bilateral basal fine crackles. ↑JVP and leg swelling. *Confirmed by:* **CXR**: fluffy opacification, especially near hila. Loss of costophrenic angle. Impaired left ventricular function on **echocardiogram.** *Finalized by the predictable outcome of management,* e.g. sitting patient up, controlled O_2, diuretics IV. Nitrates IV if very breathless and systolic BP> 90. *In the long term:* thiazide or loop diuretic, ACE inhibitor (or angiotensin receptor blocker). β-blocker and spironolactone (monitor K^+).
Elevated hemidiaphragm	*Suggested by:* typically asymptomatic, reduced/absent breath sounds, no other abnormalities unless from underlying cause, e.g. pulmonary embolus, tumour, phrenic nerve scar, etc. (often no cause found). *Confirmed by:* **CXR.** *Finalized by the predictable outcome of management,* e.g. anticoagulate if pulmonary embolus, seek old CXR to see if longstanding.
Severe fibrosis/ collapse	*Suggested by:* clubbing and signs of underlying cause, reduced chest expansion, tracheal deviation. Reduced breath sounds, course crackles. *Confirmed by:* **CXR, high resolution CT thorax.** *Finalized by the predictable outcome of management,* e.g. bronchoscopy if new lobar collapse to remove foreign body.

Severe pleural thickening, e.g. due to pleural secondaries or mesothelioma	*Suggested by:* chest pain, weight loss, history of asbestos exposure, clubbing, reduced breath sounds.
	Confirmed by: **CT thorax and pleural biopsy.**
	Finalized by the predictable outcome of management, e.g. analgesia (e.g. opiates) and controlled O_2. Oncologist/ chest physician for specialist treatment.

Hyper-resonant percussion

If *in extremis*, the rare, but immediately life-threatening, cause of tension pneumothorax. Initial investigations (other tests in **bold** below): FBC, U&E, CXR, ABG.

Main differential diagnoses and typical outline evidence, etc.	
Emphysema (overlaps with COPD) caused by smoking, smoke pollution, α-1 antitrypsin deficiency	*Suggested by:* long history of cough ± sputum, many pack years of smoking, recurrent 'exacerbations', pursed lip, breathing (a chronic 'behavioural adaptation), hyperinflation, reduced chest expansion, reduced breath sounds, and hyper-resonance. CXR: radiolucent lungs.
	Confirmed by: **spirometry**: FEV_1 <80% predicted and FEV/FVC ratio <0.7, <15% reversibility. Emphysema on **CT chest** ± ↓α1-antitrypsin levels.
	Finalized by the predictable outcome of management, e.g. stopping smoking. Trials of bronchodilators prn, regular long-acting bronchodilators. Regular inhaled steroids if FEV <50% predicted and three COPD exacerbations per year. If cough and breathlessness persists, prednisolone PO. If respiratory failure, home O_2.
Large bullae	*Suggested by:* other signs of emphysema but can be isolated finding, and often congenital in otherwise normal lungs.
	Confirmed by: **CT thorax.**
	Finalized by the predictable outcome of management, e.g. observation. Can mimic partial pneumothorax (NO insertion of intercostal drain!). Cardiothoracic surgical referral for bullectomy or endobrachial valve if symptomatic and no widespread emphysema.
Pneumothorax ('tension', moderate, or mild)	*Suggested by:* pain in centre or side of chest with abrupt breathlessness, diminished breath sounds, and hyper-resonance to percussion.
	Confirmed by: above findings, tracheal deviation, and distress suggesting tension pneumothorax, or **expiration CXR** showing loss of lung markings outside sharp line ('moderate' if >5cm gap from lung edge to chest wall, 'mild' if <5cm).
	Initial management: if tension pneumothorax, insert large Venflon into 2nd IC space, mid-clavicular line. Give O_2 if breathless. Analgesia. Aspiration if moderate; if this is unsatisfactory or prior lung disease, insert IC drain into 'triangle of safety'. If 'mild' (<5cm gap) and not breathless, observation.

Reduced breath sounds

When auscultating the lungs, think of the underlying lung parenchyma and overlying tissues. Ensure patient breathes with mouth open, regularly and deeply, and does not vocalize (e.g. groaning). Reduced breath sounds may be because:

- air is not entering/leaving the lung(s);
- excess air, fat, or fluid between lung and your stethoscope;
- good air entry but abnormal lung parenchyma.

Initial investigations (other tests in **bold** below): FBC, U&E, CXR, ABG.

Air is not entering/leaving the lung(s): Main differential diagnoses and typical outline evidence, etc.	
Poor respiratory effort	*Suggested by:* reduced consciousness/cooperation, any cause of poor chest wall expansion (see ⊃ Bilateral poor chest expansion, p.260). *Confirmed by:* **ABG** (type 2 failure). *Finalized by the predictable outcome of management,* e.g. treating cause (e.g. removal of high flow O_2, respiratory sedative) and non-invasive ventilation.
Endobronchial obstruction, e.g. tumour, retained secretions, inhaled foreign body	*Suggested by:* cough, stridor, unilateral signs of dullness to percussion, crackles, and unilateral reduced breath sounds (unless pathology is above the carina). *Confirmed by:* **CT thorax, bronchoscopy.** *Finalized by the predictable outcome of management,* e.g. bronchoscopy and removal obstruction, if possible.
Severe asthma or anaphylaxis (bronchoconstriction)	*Suggested by:* history, sudden onset, often precipitating factor. Patient *in extremis,* reduced consciousness. *Confirmed by:* **peak flow rate** undetectable. **ABG** shows type 2 respiratory failure. *Finalized by the predictable outcome of management,* e.g. high flow O_2, high dose bronchodilators (β2-agonists and anticholinergics) via nebulizer. Hydrocortisone IV 200mg. magnesium IV, antihistamines IV, and aminophylline IV can be considered. NB Keeping hydrated and monitor ABG and serum K^+. HDU if drowsy, $\uparrow CO_2$ (as this is an ominous sign in asthma).

Excess air, fat, or fluid between lung and your stethoscope:
Main differential diagnoses and typical outline evidence, etc.

Obesity (leading to ventilatory failure = obesity hypoventilation syndrome)	*Suggested by:* insidious onset of breathlessness with rising weight. *Confirmed by:* examination (BMI typically >40kg/m² to cause chest wall compromise). *Finalized by the predictable outcome of management,* e.g. weight loss, including dietitian referral and weight-lowering medications. Assess need for (nocturnal) NIV support (i.e. if symptoms of ventilatory failure and P_aO_2 <8kPa with P_aCO_2 >6.5kPa).
Pneumothorax ('tension', moderate, or mild)	*Suggested by:* pain in centre or side of chest with abrupt breathlessness, diminished breath sounds, and hyper-resonance to percussion. *Confirmed by:* above findings, tracheal deviation, and distress suggesting tension pneumothorax, or **expiration CXR** showing loss of lung markings outside sharp line ('moderate' if >5cm gap from lung edge to chest wall, 'mild' if <5cm). *Initial management:* if tension pneumothorax, insertion of large Venflon into 2nd IC space, mid-clavicular line. O_2 if breathless. Analgesia. Aspiration if moderate; if this is unsatisfactory or prior lung disease, insertion of IC drain into 'triangle of safety'. If 'mild' (<5cm gap) and not breathless, observation.
Pleural effusion	*Suggested by:* reduced breath sounds, reduced tactile vocal fremitus, stony dull percussion note. *Confirmed by:* homogeneous opacification with meniscus level on **CXR** and fluid on **US scan/CT chest.** *Finalized by the predictable outcome of management,* e.g. if breathless at rest, aspiration of 500mL (therapeutic) and send fluid for tests, not draining to dryness if cause unknown, as thoracoscopy/pleural biopsy required. If known malignancy, also insertion of IC drain directly and pleurodesis.
Severe pleural thickening, e.g. due to pleural secondaries or mesothelioma	*Suggested by:* chest pain, weight loss, history of asbestos exposure, clubbing, reduced breath sounds. *Confirmed by:* **CT thorax and pleural biopsy**. *Finalized by the predictable outcome of management,* e.g. analgesia (e.g. opiates) and controlled O_2. Oncologist/chest physician for specialist treatment.

Good air entry but abnormal lung parenchyma:
Main differential diagnoses and typical outline evidence, etc.

Emphysema (overlaps with COPD) caused by smoking, smoke pollution, α1-antitrypsin deficiency	*Suggested by:* long history of cough ± sputum, many pack years of smoking, recurrent 'exacerbations', pursed lip, breathing (a chronic behavioural adaptation), hyperinflation, reduced chest expansion, reduced breath sounds, and hyper-resonance. CXR: radiolucent lungs.
	Confirmed by: **spirometry**: FEV_1 <80% predicted and FEV/FVC ratio <0.7. <15% reversibility. Emphysema on **CT chest ± ↓α1-antitrypsin levels.**
	Finalized by the predictable outcome of management, e.g. stopping smoking. Trials of bronchodilators prn, regular long-acting bronchodilators. Regular inhaled steroids if FEV <50% predicted and three COPD exacerbations per year. If cough and breathlessness persists, prednisolone PO. If respiratory failure, home O_2.
Large bullae	*Suggested by:* other signs of emphysema but can be isolated finding, and often congenital in otherwise normal lungs.
	Confirmed by: **CT thorax**.
	Initial treatment: observation. Can mimic partial pneumothorax, but do NOT insert IC drain. Refer to cardiothoracics for bullectomy or endobronchial valve if symptomatic and not widespread emphysema.
Consolidation due to bacterial infection, but possibly autoimmune disease, malignancy, or drugs	*Suggested by:* reduced breath sounds, bronchial breathing, increased tactile vocal fremitus, reduced percussion note.
	Confirmed by: **CXR.**
	Finalized by the predictable outcome of management, e.g. if not very ill, but fever and ↑neutrophil count, analgesia, an empiric 5d course of amoxicillin/clarithromycin PO. If ≥2 features of CRB-65, then amoxicillin/co-amoxiclav IV or cefuroxime with controlled O_2 and fluids. If history of reduced consciousness/aspiration, then cefuroxime/ metronidazole IV. If hospital/nursing home acquired infection, cefuroxime or piperacillin with tazobactam IV. If no fever or WCC normal, investigation for non-infective possibilities.

Bronchial breathing

Prolonged expiration phase with a definite silence between inspiration and expiration (same as sound heard with stethoscope bell over trachea). Initial investigations (other tests in **bold** below): FBC, U&E, CXR.

Main differential diagnoses and typical outline evidence, etc.

Consolidation due to bacterial infection, but possibly autoimmune disease, malignancy, or drugs	*Suggested by:* reduced breath sounds, bronchial breathing, increased tactile vocal fremitus, reduced percussion note. *Confirmed by:* **CXR**. *Finalized by the predictable outcome of management,* e.g. if not very ill, but fever and ↑neutrophil count on FBC, analgesia, and an empiric 5d course of amoxicillin/clarithromycin PO. If ≥2 features of CRB-65, then amoxicillin/co-amoxiclav IV or cefuroxime with controlled O₂ and fluids. If history of reduced consciousness/aspiration, then cefuroxime/metronidazole IV. If hospital/nursing home acquired infection, cefuroxime or piperacillin with tazobactam IV. If no fever or WCC normal, investigation for non-infective possibilities.
Lung cavity	*Suggested by:* localized bronchial breathing, otherwise normal examination. *Confirmed by:* **CXR**, **CT thorax** (should have greater than 2mm wall thickness to differentiate from a lung cyst). *Finalized by the predictable outcome of management,* e.g. compare with old CXR. Consider TB and lung cancer. Chest clinic follow-up.
Pulmonary fibrosis/interstitial lung disease NB Majority of cases have no cause identified	*Suggested by:* chronic dry cough, occupational exposure or evidence of underlying connective tissue disease. Clubbing, cyanosis, reduced chest expansion, coarse late inspiratory bibasal crackles. *Confirmed by:* ↓lung volumes and reticular nodular shadowing on **CXR**. Interstitial shadowing and/or subpleural fibrosis on **high resolution CT chest**. *Finalized by the predictable outcome of management,* e.g. home O₂ if saturations <93%. Specialist opinion about detailed lung function, lung biopsy, immunosuppression, antifibrotics, palliation.

Fine inspiratory crackles

Very fine crackles are like the sound made when hair next to the ear is rolled between finger and thumb, or opening a velcro pad! Initial investigations (other tests in **bold** below): FBC, U&E, CXR, ABG.

Main differential diagnoses and typical outline evidence, etc.	
Incidental due to normal secretions	*Suggested by:* late in inspiration, disappear on coughing. *Confirmed by:* **CXR** showing normal lung fields.
Pulmonary oedema due to acute left ventricular failure or chronic (congestive) cardiac failure due to ischaemic heart disease, mitral stenosis	*Suggested by:* background fatigue and exertional breathless, cardiac risk factors. Displaced apex beat, 3rd heart sound, bilateral basal fine crackles. ↑JVP and leg swelling. *Confirmed by:* **CXR**: fluffy opacification, especially near hila. Loss of costophrenic angle. Impaired left ventricular function on **echocardiogram.** *Finalized by the predictable outcome of management,* e.g. sitting patient up, controlled O_2, diuretics IV. Nitrates IV if very breathless and systolic BP >90. Chronic: thiazide or loop diuretic, ACE inhibitor (or angiotensin receptor blocker). β-blocker and spironolactone (monitor K^+).
Pulmonary oedema due to acute lung injury/acute respiratory distress syndrome (ARDS)	*Suggested by:* Acutely ill patient with severe hypoxia. History of precipitating cause (e.g. smoke inhalation, aspiration, drug exposure, fat/amniotic fluid emboli, viral infection, disseminated intravascular coagulation (DIC)), no clinical signs of left ventricular failure. CXR: symmetrical, diffuse, poorly defined opacities, which become confluent. Normal heart size. *Confirmed by:* (1) acute onset, (2) bilateral infiltrates, (3) pulmonary capillary wedge pressure <19mmHg or no congestive cardiac failure, (4) PaO_2:FiO_2<200 in the presence of good left ventricular function. *Finalized by the predictable outcome of management,* e.g. intubation; ventilation with small volumes and consider prone ventilation/steroids. Treatment of underlying cause.
Pulmonary fibrosis/ interstitial lung disease NB Majority of cases have no cause identified	*Suggested by:* chronic dry cough, occupational exposure or evidence of underlying connective tissue disease. Clubbing, cyanosis, reduced chest expansion, coarse late inspiratory bibasal crackles. *Confirmed by:* ↓lung volumes and reticular nodular shadowing on **CXR**. Interstitial shadowing and/or subpleural fibrosis on **high resolution CT chest.** *Finalized by the predictable outcome of management,* e.g. home O_2 if saturations <93%. Specialist opinion about detailed lung function, lung biopsy, immunosuppression, antifibrotics, palliation.

Chronic bronchitis (overlaps with COPD)	*Suggested by:* long history of cough (productive grey/ white sputum or dry). Typically >10-pack year smoking. Recurrent 'exacerbations' of cough lasting days, needing antibiotics. *Confirmed by:* spirometry shows FEV$_1$ <80% predicted and FEV/FVC ratio <0.7, little reversibility (FEV$_1$ improves <15% with treatment). *Finalized by the predictable outcome of management,* e.g. stopping smoking. Winter vaccinations. Improvement with inhalers.
Emphysema (overlaps with COPD) caused by smoking, smoke pollution, α1-antitrypsin deficiency	*Suggested by:* long history of cough ± sputum, many pack years of smoking, recurrent 'exacerbations', pursed lip, breathing (a chronic behavioural adaptation), hyperinflation, reduced chest expansion, reduced breath sounds, and hyper-resonance. **CXR**: radiolucent lungs. *Confirmed by:* **spirometry**: FEV$_1$ <80% predicted and FEV/FVC ratio <0.7. <15% reversibility. Emphysema on **CT chest ± ↓α1-antitrypsin levels.** *Finalized by the predictable outcome of management,* e.g. stopping smoking. Trials of bronchodilators prn, regular long-acting bronchodilators. Regular inhaled steroids if FEV <50% predicted and three COPD exacerbations per year. If cough and breathless persists, prednisolone PO. If respiratory failure, home O$_2$.
Consolidation due to bacterial infection, but possibly autoimmune disease, malignancy, or drugs.	*Suggested by:* reduced breath sounds, bronchial breathing, increased tactile vocal fremitus, reduced percussion note. *Confirmed by:* **CXR**. *Finalized by the predictable outcome of management,* e.g. if not very ill, but fever and ↑neutrophil count on **FBC**, analgesia, and an empiric 5d course of oral amoxicillin/clarithromycin. If ≥2 features of CRB-65, then amoxicillin/co-amoxiclav IV or cefuroxime with controlled O$_2$ and fluids. If history of reduced consciousness/aspiration, then cefuroxime/ metronidazole IV. If hospital/nursing home acquired infection, cefuroxime or piperacillin with tazobactam IV. If no fever or WCC normal, investigate non-infective possibilities.

Coarse crackles

Bubbly crackles, often heard in both inspiration and expiration. Initial investigations (other tests in **bold** below): FBC, U&E, CXR.

Main differential diagnoses and typical outline evidence, etc.	
Bronchiectasis	*Suggested by:* progression over months or years. Cupful(s) of pus-like sputum per day. Clubbing, typically bilateral consolidation, and bilateral coarse late inspiratory crackles. Typically obstructive deficit on **spirometry**. *Confirmed by:* **CXR**: cystic shadowing; high resolution **CT chest**: honeycombing and thickened dilated bronchi. *Finalized by the predictable outcome of management,* e.g. chest physiotherapy (including postural drainage and cough clearance), sputum cultures. Mucolytics, bronchodilators, regular exercise, winter vaccinations. When unwell, treatment with 10–14d antibiotics IV according to last sputum cultures. NB Anti-*pseudomonas* treatment (aminoglycoside cover). Monitor for weight loss.
Pulmonary fibrosis/ interstitial lung disease NB Majority of cases have no cause identified	*Suggested by:* chronic dry cough, occupational exposure or evidence of underlying connective tissue disease. Clubbing, cyanosis, reduced chest expansion, coarse late inspiratory bibasal crackles. *Confirmed by:* ↓lung volumes and reticular nodular shadowing on **CXR**. Interstitial shadowing and/or subpleural fibrosis on **high resolution CT chest.** *Finalized by the predictable outcome of management,* e.g. home O_2 if saturations <93%. Specialist opinion about detailed lung function, lung biopsy, immunosuppression, antifibrotics, palliation.

Pleural rub

This sound can be reproduced by placing one finger over your ear and scratching the nail bed with your opposite index finger (or crunching through snow). Pleural rub is caused by inflammation of the pleura. Initial investigations (other tests in **bold** below): FBC, U&E, CXR.

Main differential diagnoses and typical outline evidence, etc.	
Pneumonia with pleurisy	*Suggested by:* onset over hours or days, rusty brown sputum ± blood. Sharp pains worse on inspiration, fever, cough, crackles, dullness to percussion, bronchial breathing, **WCC**: ↑neutrophils, ↑**CRP**. *Confirmed by:* patchy shadowing on **CXR** and sputum/blood culture. *Initial management:* analgesia and provisional antibiotic e.g. amoxicillin/clarithromycin PO for 5d. If >2 features of <u>C</u>onfusion, <u>R</u>esp. rate >30/min, <u>B</u>P <90/60, age >65y), then antibiotic IV, e.g. amoxicillin/ co-amoxiclav or cefuroxime, and controlled O₂ and fluids. If suspected aspiration, then anti-anaerobics, e.g. cefuroxime/metronidazole IV. If hospital/nursing home acquired, cefuroxime or piperacillin with tazobactam IV.
Pulmonary embolus/infarction arising from deep veins or in left atrium	*Suggested by:* sudden breathlessness, pleural rub, cyanosis, tachycardia, loud P2, associated DVT, or risk factors such as recent surgery, immobility, previous emboli, malignancy, etc. *Confirmed by:* **CT pulmonary angiogram** showing clot in pulmonary artery. *Finalized by the predictable outcome of management,* e.g. LMW heparin (treatment dose), then warfarin. Thrombolysis if ↓BP, large bilateral clots or acutely dilated right ventricle on echocardiogram.
Severe pleural thickening, e.g. due to pleural secondaries or mesothelioma	*Suggested by:* chest pain, weight loss, history of asbestos exposure, clubbing, reduced breath sounds. *Confirmed by:* **CT thorax** and **pleural biopsy.** *Finalized by the predictable outcome of management,* e.g. analgesia (e.g. opiates) and controlled O₂. Oncologist/ chest physician for specialist treatment.

Stridor ± inspiratory wheeze

This suggests obstruction in or near the larynx. This represents a *medical emergency*. Attempts to examine the upper airway outside of a specialist setting may make matters worse. Initial investigations (other tests in **bold** below): FBC, U&E, CXR.

Main differential diagnoses and typical outline evidence, etc.	
Epiglottitis	*Suggested by:* fever, URTI coryzal symptoms (the 4 Ds = drooling, drawn facies, dysphonia, dysphagia). *Confirmed by:* **indirect laryngoscopy** under controlled (anaesthetic) conditions. *Finalized by the predictable outcome of management*, e.g. penicillin IV, and refer for emergency treatment with ENT and anaesthetic opinion.
Croup	*Suggested by:* high-pitched cough in infants. *Confirmed by:* above presentation and findings. *Finalized by the predictable outcome of management*, e.g. paediatric support if respiratory compromise.
Inhaled foreign body	*Suggested by:* history of inhaled peanut, bead, etc. typically right-sided chest signs. *Confirmed by:* **CXR, CT thorax, bronchoscopy.** *Finalized by the predictable outcome of management*, e.g. slap between shoulder blades/Heimlich manoeuvre if acutely ill. CT and bronchoscopy if not acutely ill.
Rapidly progressive laryngomalacia	*Suggested by:* change in voice over months to years. *Confirmed by:* **indirect laryngoscopy, CT thorax.** *Finalized by the predictable outcome of management*, e.g. ENT surgical intervention.
Laryngeal papillomas	*Suggested by:* change in voice over weeks to months. *Confirmed by:* **indirect laryngoscopy.** *Finalized by the predictable outcome of management*, e.g. ENT surgical intervention.
Anaphylaxis causing laryngeal oedema	*Suggested by:* onset over minutes, history of recent allergen exposure, feeling of dread, flushing, sweating, facial oedema, urticaria, warm clammy extremities, dyspnoea and tachypnoea, wheeze. Tachycardia and ↓BP. *Confirmed by:* clinical presentation and response to adrenaline (epinephrine) IM. Results of controlled allergen exposure. *Finalized by the predictable outcome of management*, e.g. removal of antigen (e.g. bee sting, medication). Adrenaline IM 1 in 1,000. Securing of airway early if stridor. High flow O_2, fast fluids IV, steroids IV, and antihistamines IV. HDU/ITU care.

Inspiratory monophonic wheeze

This suggests large airway obstruction, often very proximal. A lesion just above the carina can be immediately life-threatening as neither lung can be ventilated, and tracheostomy will also not get below the obstruction. Initial investigations (other tests in **bold** below): FBC, U&E, CXR.

Main differential diagnoses and typical outline evidence, etc.	
Acute bilateral vocal cord paralysis	*Suggested by:* change in voice, bilateral reduced breath sounds, and wheeze. *Confirmed by:* **laryngoscopy.** *Finalized by the predictable outcome of management,* e.g. ENT surgical intervention.
Inhalation of foreign body	*Suggested by:* history of putting an object in mouth, e.g. peanut. Sudden stridor, severe cough, low-pitched, monophonic wheeze, and reduced breath sounds, typically on the right. *Confirmed by:* if not *in extremis*, **CXR/CT thorax** or **bronchoscopy** to show foreign body. *Finalized by the predictable outcome of management,* e.g. if *in extremis*, slap back between the shoulder blades with patient leaning forward; if fails, perform Heimlich manoeuvre.
Tracheal tumours or stenosis after ventilation	*Suggested by:* stridor, over weeks to months, bilateral reduced breath sounds, and bilateral wheeze. *Confirmed by:* **CXR, CT thorax and neck, bronchoscopy**. *Initial treatment:* controlled O_2, and/or steroids IV.
Extrinsic compression of large airways by mediastinal masses	*Suggested by:* neck/chest discomfort ± swelling over weeks to months. Look for signs of SVC obstruction. Can be focal (unilateral) or bilateral wheeze, depending on site of obstruction. *Confirmed by:* **CT thorax and neck.** *Finalized by the predictable outcome of management,* e.g. steroids and palliative chemo-radiotherapy.
Extrinsic compression by oesophageal tumours	*Suggested by:* dysphagia, weight loss over weeks to months. *Confirmed by:* **CT thorax and neck.** *Finalized by the predictable outcome of management,* e.g. soft pureed diet. Barium swallow if high dysphagia or oesophagogastroduodenoscopy (OGD) if low dysphagia.
Tracheal blunt trauma	*Suggested by:* history, pain and swelling, change in voice over minutes or hours after trauma. *Confirmed by:* **laryngoscopy, bronchoscopy.** *Finalized by the predictable outcome of management,* e.g. early intubation and steroids.

Expiratory monophonic wheeze

This suggests obstruction of a large airway. Initial investigations (other tests in **bold** below): FBC, U&E, CXR.

Main differential diagnoses and typical outline evidence, etc.

Endobronchial carcinoma (benign lesions very rare)	*Suggested by:* smoker, weight loss, cough, chest pain, and haemoptysis, clubbed. Unilateral wheeze (typically occur below the carina) and unilateral reduced breath sounds. Often signs of consolidation distal to obstruction. CXR can be normal. *Confirmed by:* **sputum cytology, CT chest, bronchoscopy and biopsy.** *Finalized by the predictable outcome of management,* e.g. possible radiotherapy, tracheal stenting, cryotherapy, laser therapy, brachytherapy (radioactive source put close to tumour).
Acute bilateral vocal cord paralysis	*Suggested by:* change in voice, bilateral reduced breath sounds, and wheeze. *Confirmed by:* **laryngoscopy.** *Finalized by the predictable outcome of management,* e.g. ENT surgical intervention for possible intubation and tracheostomy.
Inhalation of foreign body	*Suggested by:* history of putting an object in mouth, e.g. peanut. Sudden stridor, severe cough, low-pitched, monophonic wheeze, and reduced breath sounds, typically on the right. *Confirmed by:* if not *in extremis,* **CXR/CT thorax or bronchoscopy** to show foreign body. *Finalized by the predictable outcome of management,* e.g. if *in extremis,* slap back between the shoulder blades with patient leaning forward; if fails, perform Heimlich manoeuvre. CT and bronchoscopy if not acutely ill.
Tracheal tumours	*Suggested by:* stridor over weeks to months, bilateral reduced breath sounds, and bilateral wheeze. *Confirmed by:* **CXR, CT thorax and neck, bronchoscopy.** *Initial treatment:* controlled O_2, and/or steroids IV.
Extrinsic compression by mediastinal masses	*Suggested by:* neck/chest discomfort ± swelling over weeks to months. Look for signs of SVC obstruction. Can be focal (unilateral) or bilateral wheeze, depending on site of obstruction. *Confirmed by:* **CT thorax and neck.** *Finalized by the predictable outcome of management,* e.g. steroids and palliative chemo-radiotherapy.

Extrinsic compression by oesophageal tumours	*Suggested by:* dysphagia, weight loss over weeks to months. *Confirmed by:* **CT thorax and neck.** *Finalized by the predictable outcome of management,* e.g. soft pureed diet. Barium swallow if high dysphagia or OGD if low dysphagia.
Tracheal blunt trauma	*Suggested by:* history, pain and swelling, change in voice over minutes or hours after trauma. *Confirmed by:* **laryngoscopy, bronchoscopy.** *Finalized by the predictable outcome of management,* e.g. steroids and ENT intervention for possible intubation and tracheostomy.

Expiratory polyphonic, high-pitched wheeze

This suggests small airways obstruction. Initial investigations (other tests in **bold** below): FBC, U&E, CXR.

Main differential diagnoses and typical outline evidence, etc.

Exacerbation of asthma	*Suggested by:* widespread polyphonic wheeze with exacerbations over hours. Silent chest if severe. Anxiety, tachypnoea, tachycardia, and use of accessory muscles. *Confirmed by:* reduced peak flows. **FEV₁** that improves by >15% with treatment. *Finalized by the predictable outcome of management,* e.g. high flow O_2, prednisolone PO or hydrocortisone IV. Nebulized salbutamol and ipratropium ± magnesium IV and aminophylline IV. NB. Keeping hydrated, and monitor ABG and serum K⁺. HDU care if drowsy, ↑CO_2 or silent chest.
'Wheezy bronchitis'	*Suggested by:* wheeze association with infective episodes of bronchitis alone. *Confirmed by:* **FEV₁** response to bronchodilators and antibiotics. *Finalized by the predictable outcome of management,* e.g. antibiotics if high fever, mucopurulent sputum.
Viral wheeze	*Suggested by:* wheeze associated URTI viral illness, poor response to bronchodilators. *Confirmed by:* resolving spontaneously. *Finalized by the predictable outcome of management,* e.g. analgesic and antipyretic, e.g. paracetamol.
Anaphylaxis	*Suggested by:* onset over minutes, history of recent allergen exposure, feeling of dread, flushing, sweating, facial oedema, urticaria, warm clammy extremities, dyspnoea and tachypnoea, wheeze. Tachycardia and ↓BP. *Confirmed by:* clinical presentation and response to adrenaline (epinephrine) IM. Results of controlled allergen exposure. *Finalized by the predictable outcome of management,* e.g. removal of antigen (e.g. bee sting, medication). Adrenaline IM 1 in 1,000. Securing of airway early if stridor. High flow O_2, fast fluids IV, steroids IV, and antihistamines IV. HDU/ITU care.
Pulmonary oedema due to acute left ventricular failure or chronic (congestive) cardiac failure due to ischaemic heart disease, mitral stenosis	*Suggested by:* background fatigue and exertional breathless, cardiac risk factors. Displaced apex beat, 3rd heart sound, bilateral basal fine crackles. ↑JVP and leg swelling. *Confirmed by:* **CXR**: fluffy opacification, especially near hila. Loss of costophrenic angle. Impaired left ventricular function on **echocardiogram.** *Finalized by the predictable outcome of management,* e.g. sitting patient up, controlled O_2, diuretics IV. Nitrates IV if very breathless and systolic BP >90. Chronic: thiazide or loop diuretic, ACE inhibitor (or angiotensin receptor blocker). β-blocker and spironolactone (monitor K⁺).

Gastrointestinal symptoms and physical signs

Unintentional weight loss over weeks or months   290
Weight gain   292
Vomiting   294
Vomiting with weight loss   295
Vomiting without weight loss   296
Vomiting shortly after food   298
Vomiting with abdominal pain and fever   300
Vomiting with abdominal pain alone (unrelated to food and no fever)—non-metabolic causes   302
Vomiting with abdominal pain alone (unrelated to food and no fever)—metabolic causes   304
Vomiting with headache alone (unrelated to food and no abdominal pain)   306
Vomiting alone (unrelated to food and without abdominal pain or headaches)   308
Jaundice   310
Pre-hepatic jaundice due to haemolysis   312
Hepatic jaundice due to congenital enzyme defect   313
Hepatocellular jaundice (due to hepatitis or very severe liver failure)   314
Obstructive jaundice   316
Dysphagia for solids that stick   318
Dysphagia for solids (that do not stick) > fluids   319
Sore throat   320
Dysphagia for fluids > solids   322
Acute pain in the upper abdomen   324
Acute central abdominal pain   326
Acute lateral abdominal pain   327
Acute lower central (hypogastric) abdominal pain   328
Acute abdominal pain in children   329
Recurrent abdominal pain in children   330
Sudden diarrhoea, fever, and vomiting   332
Recurrent diarrhoea with blood ± mucus—bloody flux   334
Acute bloody diarrhoea ± mucus—'dysentery'   335
Watery diarrhoea   336
Recurrent diarrhoea with no blood in the stools, no fever   338
Chronic diarrhoea in children   340
Constipation   342

Change in bowel habit *344*
Haematemesis ± melaena *346*
Passage of blood per rectum *348*
Tenesmus *350*
Anorectal pain *351*
Distended abdomen *352*
Distended abdominal veins *354*
Abdominal bruising *355*
Poor abdominal movement *356*
Localized tenderness in the hypogastrium (suprapubic area) *357*
Localized tenderness in the right upper quadrant *358*
Localized tenderness in the left upper quadrant *360*
Localized tenderness in the epigastrium or central abdomen *361*
Localized tenderness in the left or right loin *362*
Localized tenderness in left or right lower quadrant *363*
Hepatomegaly—smooth and tender *364*
Hepatomegaly—smooth but not tender *366*
Hepatomegaly—irregular, not tender *368*
Splenomegaly—slight (<3 fingers) *370*
Splenomegaly—moderate (3–5 fingers) *372*
Splenomegaly—massive (>5 fingers) *373*
Bilateral masses in upper abdomen *374*
Unilateral mass in right or left upper quadrant *375*
Mass in epigastrium (± umbilical area) *376*
Mass in right lower quadrant *377*
Mass in hypogastrium (suprapubic region) *378*
Mass in left lower quadrant *379*
Central dullness, resonance in flank *380*
Shifting dullness *381*
Silent abdomen with no bowel sounds *382*
High-pitched bowel sounds *383*
Abdominal/loin bruit *384*
Lump in the groin *386*
Scrotal swelling *388*
Anal swelling *390*
Enlargement of prostate *391*
Melaena on finger *392*
Fresh blood on finger on rectal examination *396*

Unintentional weight loss over weeks or months

Unintentional weight loss over weeks or months

The more rapid and severe the weight loss, the more probable it is to be due to a serious cause. Initial investigations (other tests in **bold** below): test urine for sugar and protein, FBC, ESR or CRP, fasting blood glucose, U&E, calcium and bone profile, LFT, PSA, TSH, and FT4, CXR, US scan abdomen.

Main differential diagnoses and typical outline evidence, etc.	
Any advanced malignancy (e.g. gastrointestinal (GI), lung, lymphoma)	*Suggested by:* progressive onset over weeks or months of specific symptoms, e.g. change of bowel habit, rectal bleeding, haemoptysis, neurological deficit, etc. *Confirmed by:* tumour on GI endoscopy or **bronchoscopy**, lymph node biopsy, metastases on CXR or CT thorax, metastases on **US scan of liver or CT abdomen**, or leukaemic changes on FBC, etc. *Finalized by the predictable outcome of management,* e.g. dietary advice, food supplements, counselling, analgesia if pain, planning treatment of any underlying diagnosis.
Psychiatric illness (mainly severe depression)	*Suggested by:* sleep disorder, poor concentration, social withdrawal, lack of interest in usual activities, etc. *Confirmed by:* history and mental state examination. *Finalized by the predictable outcome of management,* e.g. psychotherapy and anti-depressants, e.g. selective serotonin reuptake inhibitors (SSRI).
Non-malignant GI diseases (e.g. peptic ulcer disease, inflammatory bowel disease, malabsorption, etc.)	*Suggested by:* dysphagia, vomiting, diarrhoea, abdominal pain, melaena, alcohol intake. etc. *Confirmed by:* **GI endoscopy, US scan of abdomen,** anaemia on FBC, etc. *Finalized by the predictable outcome of management,* e.g. dietary intervention, e.g. food supplements, counselling, analgesia if pain, treatment of underlying condition.
Alcoholism (complicated by liver disease, gastritis, peptic ulceration, seizures, or delirium tremens on withdrawal)	*Suggested by:* depression, anxiety, visual hallucination, social withdrawal, lack of interest in non-drinking activities, anorexia, etc. *Confirmed by:* history of alcohol abuse, presence of signs of chronic liver disease, etc. *Finalized by the predictable outcome of management,* e.g. withdrawal of alcohol, short course of sedative to prevent withdrawal symptoms, benzodiazepine if seizure occurs.
Undiagnosed or uncontrolled diabetes mellitus	*Suggested by:* thirst, polydipsia, polyuria, pruritus. *Confirmed by:* **fasting blood glucose** ≥7.0 mmol/L (on two occasions) OR random or **GTT** glucose ≥11.1mmol/L once only in the presence of symptoms. *Finalized by the predictable outcome of management,* e.g. lifestyle modification—diet, exercise ± metformin. Insulin if type 1 diabetes or ketotic.

Thyrotoxicosis	*Suggested by:* heat intolerance, tremor, nervousness, palpitation, frequency of bowel movements, goitre, fine tremor, warm and moist palm.
	Confirmed by: ↓TSH, ↑FT4 ± ↑FT3. Anti-TSH receptor antibody if Graves' disease.
	Finalized by the predictable outcome of management, e.g. propranolol to control symptoms. Carbimazole or propylthiouracil to reduce T4.
Pulmonary tuberculosis (TB)	*Suggested by:* night sweats, fever, malaise, **chronic** cough.
	Confirmed by: CXR showing opacification of pneumonia and presence of **acid-fast bacilli (AFB) in sputum** on microscopy and culture.
	Finalized by the predictable outcome of management, e.g. initiation of antituberculous regimen, e.g. isoniazid, rifampicin, pyrazinamide, and ethambutol for 2mo, then isoniazid and rifampicin for 4mo with pyridoxine supplement.
Addison's disease	*Suggested by:* lethargy, weakness, dizziness, pigmentation (buccal, scar), hypotension.
	Confirmed by: ↓9a.m. plasma cortisol and impaired response to **short Synacthen® test**.
	Finalized by the predictable outcome of management, e.g. if ↓BP, fluids IV or colloids; if ↓glucose, 10% glucose IV. If ill, hydrocortisone IV, otherwise PO ± fludrocortisone.
Also	Acute infections: HIV, subacute bacterial endocarditis, parasites. Drugs: digoxin, metformin, levodopa. Neurological disease: stroke, Parkinson's disease, dementia. Connective tissue disease: SLE, scleroderma. Idiopathic or unknown.

Weight gain

In addition to usual details (speed of onset, etc.), assess the distribution of body fat. Is it mainly truncal or general (trunk and limbs)? Differentiate between increased oedema (pitting) and adiposity (non-pitting). Initial investigations (other tests in **bold** below): test urine for protein and glucose, do FBC, fasting glucose, U&E, TSH, and FT4.

Main differential diagnoses and typical outline evidence, etc.

Excessive caloric intake (by far the main cause: >95%), often with mild depression	*Suggested by:* gradual and progressive weight increase over months to years, no other associated symptoms. *Confirmed by:* history of overeating, all other investigations normal. *Finalized by the predictable outcome of management,* e.g. ↓calorie intake, ↑physical activity.
Drugs e.g. steroids, NSAIDs, sulphonylureas, insulin, oestrogen, etc.	*Suggested by:* history of medication. *Confirmed by:* weight decreasing following reduction or withdrawal of causative drug. *Finalized by the predictable outcome of management,* e.g. stop or reduce causative drugs.
Congestive cardiac failure	*Suggested by:* weight gain over days to months, dyspnoea, orthopnoea, paroxysmal nocturnal dyspnoea (PND), liver enlargement and tenderness, gallop rhythm, leg oedema. *Confirmed by:* **CXR** and **echocardiogram**. *Finalized by the predictable outcome of management,* e.g. furosemide, ACE inhibitor, spironolactone.
Hypothyroidism	*Suggested by:* weight gain over weeks to months, cold intolerance, constipation, lethargy, coarse and dry skin, puffy eyelids. *Confirmed by:* ↑TSH, ↓FT4, ↑**thyroid antibodies.** *Finalized by the predictable outcome of management,* e.g. thyroxine replacement.
Premenstrual fluid retention	*Suggested by:* premenstrual weight gain over days, breast swelling and tenderness, finger swelling. *Confirmed by:* oedema and weight decrease after menstruation. *Finalized by the predictable outcome of management,* e.g. weight reduction, salt reduction, spironolactone.
Polycystic ovary syndrome (associated with insulin resistance or sometimes type 2 diabetes mellitus)	*Suggested by:* weight gain over years, oligomenorrhoea or amenorrhoea, central obesity, hirsutism, acanthosis nigricans, acne. *Confirmed by:* ↑**testosterone,** ↓**SHBG,** ↑**LH, FSH** normal, **24h urinary free cortisol** normal, ovarian cysts on **US scan.** *Finalized by the predictable outcome of management,* e.g. weight reduction, metformin, oral contraceptive (with a low dose of oestrogen and a nonandrogenic progestin) to induce regular menses ± spironolactone for hirsutism and acne.

Pregnancy (common condtion but unusual to present as weight gain)	*Suggested by:* weight gain over weeks, amenorrhoea, and mass in pelvis (cannot get below it). *Confirmed by:* +ve **urine pregnancy test** or **plasma-hCG**. Also **abdominal/pelvic US scan**. *Finalized by the predictable outcome of management,* e.g. antenatal clinic follow-up.
Liver cirrhosis with ascites	*Suggested by:* weight gain over weeks to months, bilateral bulging flanks, shifting dullness, fluid thrill, sudden and rapid weight gain. *Confirmed by:* **US scan liver and abdomen**. *Finalized by the predictable outcome of management,* e.g. bed rest, salt restriction, fluid restriction if Na⁺ <120mmol/L, spironolactone ± furosemide, monitor daily weight. Ascitic tap—paracentesis if gross ascites and symptomatic, propranolol if portal hypertension.
Nephrotic syndrome	*Suggested by:* weight gain over weeks to months, generalized oedema, puffy eyelids, abdominal distension, weight gain may be sudden and rapid. *Confirmed by:* ↓serum albumin, 24h urine protein >3g. *Finalized by the predictable outcome of management,* e.g. salt restriction, furosemide ± metolazone, statins, ACE inhibitors, treat cause.
Cushing's syndrome due to ACTH-secreting pituitary tumour (Cushing's disease); adrenal adenoma; steroid therapy	*Suggested by:* weight gain over months to years, 'moon face', truncal obesity, hirsutism, 'buffalo hump', abdominal striae, proximal weakness, thin skin, bruising, purple striae. *Confirmed by:* **24h urinary free cortisol, ↑midnight serum or salivary cortisol** and/or failure to suppress cortisol after overnight 1 mg **dexamethasone suppression test**. *Finalized by the predictable outcome of management,* e.g. reduce any glucocorticoid if drug-induced, metyrapone to control cortisol prior to surgery, or ketoconazole for long-term use.
Also	Smoking cessation, alcohol excess, menopause, Klinefelter syndrome, Other endocrine disorders: hypopituitarism, acromegaly, insulinoma, hypogonadism. Hypothalamic disorder: craniopharyngioma, Congenital disorders: Prader–Willi syndrome, Laurence–Moon–Biedl syndrome.

Vomiting

Vomiting is not only a feature of GI disorders, but is also associated with a wide variety of local and systemic disorders. Therefore, look for better diagnostic leads. Ask about the amount, frequency, and nature of vomitus—red blood, 'coffee-ground', timing of vomit, i.e. in relation to meals, AND ask about weight loss, fever, headache, and abdominal pain. Initial investigations (other tests in **bold** below): test urine for protein and glucose, do FBC, fasting glucose, U&E, TSH, and FT4.

Try subdividing into
- Vomiting *with* weight loss
- Vomiting *without* weight loss
- Vomiting *(within hours)* of food
- Vomiting unrelated to food but *with abdominal pain AND fever*
- Vomiting unrelated to food *with abdominal pain but NO fever* (non-metabolic)
- Vomiting unrelated to food *with abdominal pain but NO fever* (metabolic)
- Vomiting unrelated to food *without abdominal pain but with headaches*
- Vomiting *unrelated* to food and *without* abdominal pain or headaches.

Vomiting with weight loss

Many causes are shared with weight loss alone. Initial investigations (other tests in **bold** below): test urine for sugar, request FBC, ESR or CRP, fasting blood glucose, U&E, calcium and bone profile, LFT, PSA, TSH, and FT4 before specific tests below.

Main differential diagnoses and typical outline evidence, etc.	
Oesophageal stricture	*Suggested by:* undigested solid food and fluid in vomitus, heartburn. *Confirmed by:* **barium swallow**, **oesophagogastroscopy** showing food residue and fixed narrowing. *Finalized by the predictable outcome of management,* e.g. small meals, avoiding fat, proton pump inhibitor (PPI). Severe: nasogastric (NG) tube + nil by mouth ± fluids IV, proton pump inhibitor (PPI). All: surgical intervention e.g. for endoscopic balloon dilatation, surgery.
Oesophageal carcinoma	*Suggested by:* dysphagia to solid food first, then semisolid, and finally fluid. *Confirmed by:* **barium swallow** showing filling defect, **fibreoptic gastroscopy** with biopsy of tumour. *Finalized by the predictable outcome of management,* e.g. NG tube, fluids IV ± antibiotic prophylaxis, endoscopic balloon dilatation or stent insertion.
Gastric carcinoma	*Suggested by:* satiety after small meal. *Confirmed by:* **oesophagogastroscopy** showing and allowing biopsy of visible tumour, **barium meal** showing filling defect. *Finalized by the predictable outcome of management,* e.g. if hypovolaemia and poor nutrition, NG tube ± fluids IV, surgical intervention.
Small intestinal tumour, e.g. lymphoma	*Suggested by:* abdominal pain, anorexia, bilious vomitus. *Confirmed by:* **small bowel follow-through, CT abdomen, flexible enteroscopy with biopsy**. *Finalized by the predictable outcome of management,* e.g. if hypovolaemia and poor nutrition, NG tube ± fluids IV, surgical intervention.
Achalasia	*Suggested by:* vomiting after large meals, undigested solid food and fluid, nocturnal regurgitation. *Confirmed by:* **barium swallow** demonstrating the absence of peristaltic contractions, **oesophagogastroscopy** showing dilatation. *Finalized by the predictable outcome of management,* e.g. smooth muscle dilator—nifedipine, verapamil, or isosorbide mononitrate. Endoscopic balloon dilatation or injection of botulinum toxin.

Vomiting without weight loss

Initial investigations (other tests in **bold** below): FBC, ESR or CRP, fasting blood glucose, U&E, calcium and bone profile, LFT, US scan abdomen before specific tests below.

Main differential diagnoses and typical outline evidence, etc.	
Oesophagitis and ulceration	*Suggested by:* retrosternal pain, heartburn, dyspepsia, 'waterbrash'. *Confirmed by:* **oesophagogastroscopy** showing inflammation and/or ulceration. *Finalized by the predictable outcome of management*, e.g. mild: small frequent meals long before bedtime, elevate head of bed, PPI. Severe: nil by mouth, fluids IV, PPI, antibiotics for any *Helicobacter* (*H.*) *pylori*.
Pharyngeal pouch	*Suggested by:* no pain, regurgitation of undigested food, aspiration ± pneumonia. *Confirmed by:* **barium swallow** showing saccular opacification outside pharynx. *Finalized by the predictable outcome of management*, e.g. fluids IV and NG tube + nil by mouth, if severe and/or aspiration, enteral feeding. Surgical intervention, e.g. stapling, diverticulotomy, crico-pharyngeal myotomy, or diverticulectomy if large.
Achalasia	*Suggested by:* vomiting after large meals, undigested solid food and fluid, dysphagia to fluid, nocturnal regurgitation. *Confirmed by:* **barium swallow** demonstrating the absence of peristaltic contractions, **oesophagogastroscopy** showing dilatation. *Finalized by the predictable outcome of management*, e.g. smooth muscle dilator, e.g. nifedipine, verapamil, or isosorbide mononitrate. Endoscopic balloon dilatation or injection of botulinum toxin.

Vomiting shortly after food

Initial investigations (other tests in **bold** below): test urine and request FBC, fasting blood glucose, U&E, calcium, etc., LFT, serum amylase, CXR, ECG, abdominal X-ray (AXR); specific tests depending on suspected diagnoses.

Main differential diagnoses and typical outline evidence, etc.

Gastritis/peptic ulcer disease: duodenal ulcer (DU) or gastric ulcer (GU)	*Suggested by:* vomiting during or soon after a meal, epigastric pain/discomfort (worse after food suggests GU, relieved by food suggests DU). *Confirmed by:* **oesophagogastroscopy, barium meal, and pH study**. *Finalized by the predictable outcome of management,* e.g. stop smoking, avoid NSAIDs and aspirin. Antacids. PPI for 4wk for DU, 8wk for GU + antibiotic regimen for any *H. pylori*.
Gastric outlet obstruction e.g. carcinoma, lymphoma, chronic scarring, congenital pyloric stenosis in newborn	*Suggested by:* intermittent vomiting ≥1h after eating, abdominal fullness or bloating, distended upper abdomen, succussion splash. *Confirmed by:* **oesophagogastroscopy** and **biopsy, double contrast barium meal** shows structural abnormality. *Finalized by the predictable outcome of management,* e.g. if hypovolaemia and poor nutrition: fluids IV, NG tube + nil by mouth. Surgical intervention.
Small intestinal tumour e.g. lymphoma	*Suggested by:* abdominal pain, anorexia, bilious vomitus, weight loss. *Confirmed by:* **small bowel barium meal** and **follow-through** showing filling defect, **CT abdomen** showing abnormal tumour in wall, **flexible enteroscopy** with biopsy showing abnormal histology. *Finalized by the predictable outcome of management,* e.g. if hypovolaemia and poor nutrition: fluids IV, NG tube + nil by mouth. Surgical intervention.
Gastroparesis due to diabetes mellitus	*Suggested by:* intermittent vomiting, occurs ≥1h after eating, abdominal fullness or bloating, distended upper abdomen, succussion splash, history of diabetes. *Confirmed by:* **oesophagogastroscopy, double contrast barium meal** showing normal mucosa but dilatation. *Finalized by the predictable outcome of management,* e.g. low-fat diet, frequent small meals; if severe, liquid meals + vitamins.
Acute cholecystitis due to cholelithiasis	*Suggested by:* nausea and vomiting after fatty food with colicky abdominal pain. Tenderness in the right upper quadrant (RUQ) or Murphy's sign +ve or jaundice. *Confirmed by:* **US scan** of biliary tree and gallbladder showing stones. *Finalized by the predictable outcome of management,* e.g. nil by mouth, fluids IV, pain relief with opioid analgesia, antibiotics IV, e.g. metronidazole + cephalosporin.

Acute pancreatitis	*Suggested by:* severe epigastric/central abdominal pain, jaundice, tachycardia, Cullen's sign (periumbilical discoloration) or Grey Turner's sign (discoloration at the flank).
	Confirmed by: ⇈**serum amylase**, ↓**Ca²⁺**, **CT pancreas**.
	Finalized by the predictable outcome of management, e.g. pain relief, e.g. pethidine, if abdominal distension due to paralytic ileus, NG tube + nil by mouth, fluids IV ± plasma expander/blood.

Vomiting with abdominal pain and fever

The vomiting is usually unrelated to eating. Also assess for consequences such as hypovolaemia. Initial investigations (other tests in **bold** below): test urine, examine stools (and send for culture, etc). Also request FBC, U&E, LFT, calcium, etc., serum amylase, CXR, AXR; specific tests depending on suspected diagnoses.

Main differential diagnoses and typical outline evidence, etc.	
Gastroenteritis (from live microbes, e.g. salmonella)	*Suggested by:* diarrhoea, ↑bowel sounds. *Confirmed by:* stools for culture. *Finalized by the predictable outcome of management,* e.g. oral rehydration solution (containing glucose and salt); if severe vomiting, fluids IV, etc.
Food poisoning (from toxins of dead microbes, e.g. staphylococci)	*Suggested by:* within hours of ingestion, associated with diarrhoea ± eating companions affected. *Confirmed by:* **stools for WBC and culture, cultures of vomitus, food and blood (–ve).** *Finalized by the predictable outcome of management,* e.g. oral rehydration solution (containing glucose and salt); if severe vomiting, fluids IV, etc.
Urinary tract infection ± pyelonephritis	*Suggested by:* dysuria, frequency, dipstick indicating blood, protein, and nitrites (if Gram –ve infection). *Confirmed by:* **MSU microscopy and culture** (± US scan showing anatomical abnormality). *Finalized by the predictable outcome of management,* e.g. hydration, provisional antibiotic (e.g. trimethoprim) then based on culture and sensitivity; antibiotic IV, e.g. cephalosporin if severe infection.
Acute appendicitis	*Suggested by:* right-lower quadrant (RLQ) pain, anorexia, nausea. *Confirmed by:* tenderness at McBurney's point, guarding ± rebound or right-sided rectal tenderness, US appendix or spiral CT. *Finalized by the predictable outcome of management,* e.g. nil by mouth, fluids IV, NG tube if vomiting, broad-spectrum antibiotic, e.g. cephalosporin, surgical, e.g. appendicectomy.
Mesenteric adenitis or non-specific abdominal pain (NSAP)	*Suggested by:* RLQ pain, anorexia, fever. *Confirmed by:* diffuse RLQ tenderness, no guarding, no rebound, no right-sided rectal tenderness, self-limiting outcome. *Finalized by the predictable outcome of management,* e.g. antipyretics, analgesia.
Hepatitis A or B	*Suggested by:* RUQ pain, jaundice. *Confirmed by:* ↑ALT, ↑bilirubin, **hepatitis serology**. *Finalized by the predictable outcome of management,* e.g. antipyretics, fluids IV, anti-emetics prn, colestyramine for pruritus.

Toxic shock syndrome	*Suggested by:* history of tampon use, nasal packing, high fever, vomiting, profuse watery diarrhoea, confusion, skin rash, hypotension, myalgia. FBC: ↑WCC, ↓platelets, ↑CPK.
	Confirmed by: **cultures of blood, stool, vaginal swab,** for staphylococcus and toxin.
	Finalized by the predictable outcome of management, e.g. ICU care, removal of tampon or nasal packings; fluids IV, dopamine IV if ↓↓BP; antibiotics IV, e.g. oxacillin or nafcillin.
Pneumonia (lower lobe)	*Suggested by:* productive cough, dyspnoea, fever, ↑WCC.
	Confirmed by: CXR shows consolidation. **Sputum and blood cultures. Serology** if atypical.
	Finalized by the predictable outcome of management, e.g. give O_2, monitor SpO_2, BP, pulse, fluids IV if dehydrated, paracetamol for fever. Provisional antibiotics, e.g. cephalosporin ± erythromycin or azithromycin, etc. pending sensitivities. Metronidazole if aspiration.
Pelvic inflammatory disease	*Suggested by:* lower abdominal pain, fever, vaginal discharge.
	Confirmed by: high vaginal swab, ↑ESR and CRP. FBC: leucocytosis, **pelvic US scan ± laparoscopy**.
	Finalized by the predictable outcome of management, e.g. analgesia, fluids IV if dehydrated, empirical antibiotics, e.g. cefoxitin or other 2nd generation cephalosporin + doxycycline 100mg bd, etc.
Haemolytic uraemic syndrome	*Suggested by:* diarrhoea, irritability, seizure, confusion, GI bleed, haematuria.
	Confirmed by: FBC: thrombocytopaenia, fragmented RBC on **blood film**, renal failure on U&E.
	Finalized by the predictable outcome of management, e.g. fluids IV, U&E, BP control, prophylaxis for seizures, dialysis, plasma exchange.
Malaria (Plasmodium (P.). vivax, P. ovale, P. malariae, P. knowlesi, P. falciparum)	*Suggested by:* recent travel to malaria zone, periodic paroxysms of rigors, fever, sweating, nausea.
	Confirmed by: Plasmodium in **blood smear**.
	Finalized by the predictable outcome of management, e.g. paracetamol for fever, blood transfusion if anaemic ++. Chloroquine+primaquine (or artemisinin based combination therapy if chloroquine-resistant) for *P. vivax, P. ovale, P. malariae, P. knowlesi*; artemisinin-based combination therapy for at least 3d, e.g. dihydroartemisinin+piperaquine for *P. falciparum*, artesunate IV if severe *P. falciparum*.
	Please refer to WHO guidelines for the up-to-date treatment regimens at ℘ http://www.who.int/topics/malaria/en

Vomiting with abdominal pain alone (unrelated to food and no fever)—non-metabolic causes

Look for better leads with the history and examination. Initial investigations (other tests in **bold** below): FBC, U&E, LFT, calcium, etc., serum amylase, CXR, ECG, AXR.

Main differential diagnoses and typical outline evidence, etc.

Large bowel obstruction, e.g. malignancy, strangulated hernia	*Suggested by:* faecal vomiting, abdominal distension. *Confirmed by:* **AXR** showing bowel dilation, **barium enema, colonoscopy.** *Finalized by the predictable outcome of management,* e.g. NG tube + nil by mouth, fluids IV, fluid balance, antibiotics, surgical.
Hepatic carcinoma, 1° or 2°	*Suggested by:* RUQ pain and mass, jaundice. *Confirmed by:* **weight loss over weeks to months,** ↑alpha-fetoprotein, **US scan/CT or MRI of liver** showing hepatic mass. *Finalized by the predictable outcome of management,* e.g. analgesia, surgical intervention
Mesenteric artery occlusion	*Suggested by:* wasting, periumbilical pain (postprandial), phagophobia, diarrhoea, melaena, absent bowel sounds. *Confirmed by:* CT abdomen, **mesenteric angiography** showing filling defect. *Finalized by the predictable outcome of management,* e.g. fluids IV, analgesia, antibiotics, surgical intervention.
Renal calculi	*Suggested by:* colicky loin pain, haematuria. *Confirmed by:* **plain AXR, US scan, abdominopelvic CT, intravenous urography (IVU).** *Finalized by the predictable outcome of management,* e.g. opioid analgesics + anti-emetics, urology intervention.
Ectopic pregnancy, miscarriage	*Suggested by:* cramping pain, spotting, PV bleeding. *Confirmed by:* +ve **pregnancy test, US scan of pelvis.** *Finalized by the predictable outcome of management,* e.g. analgesia, fluids IV, gynaecology intervention.
Acute inferior myocardial infarction	*Suggested by:* central chest pain, sweating, nausea. *Confirmed by:* ↑ST or ↓T wave on ECG **with↑cardiac enzymes,** e.g. CK-MB or **troponin.** *Finalized by the predictable outcome of management,* e.g. ECG monitor (best in CCU), O₂, GTN (IV if pain persists), morphine, aspirin 300mg, and clopidogrel 300mg stat, thrombolysis (if ST↑and <12h from the onset), LMW heparin or fondaparinux for unstable angina or NSTEMI.

Congestive cardiac failure (and liver congestion)	*Suggested by:* dyspnoea, orthopnoea, PND, liver enlargement and tenderness, leg oedema.
	Confirmed by: **CXR and echocardiogram**.
	Finalized by the predictable outcome of management, e.g. ECG monitor, O_2, slow furosemide IV, morphine or diamorphine, GTN (IV), dobutamine if hypotensive.

Vomiting with abdominal pain alone (unrelated to food and no fever)—metabolic causes

Look for better leads in the history and examination. Initial investigations (other tests in **bold** below): FBC, U&E, LFT, calcium, etc., serum amylase, CXR, ECG, AXR.

Main differential diagnoses and typical outline evidence, etc.	
Drugs overdose e.g. digoxin	*Suggested by:* drug history. *Confirmed by:* ↑**serum digoxin levels**. *Finalized by the predictable outcome of management,* e.g. O$_2$, ECG monitoring, IV access, stop digoxin, check U&E, digoxin. Fab antibody if severe, arrhythmias, or hyperkalaemia.
Diabetic ketoacidosis	*Suggested by:* polyuria, dehydration ± Kussmaul respiration. *Confirmed by:* ↑**blood glucose**, ↓**pH**, ketonaemia or **ketonuria** or ↓**plasma bicarbonate** <15mmol/L. *Finalized by the predictable outcome of management,* e.g. large volumes 0.9% saline IV with K$^+$, IV insulin sliding scale, hourly blood glucose, NG tube, bicarbonate if pH<7.0, treat any infection.
Hypercalcaemia	*Suggested by:* lethargy, confusion, constipation, muscle weakness, polydipsia and polyuria. *Confirmed by:* ↑↑**serum Ca^{2+}**. *Finalized by the predictable outcome of management,* e.g. large volumes 0.9% saline IV with K$^+$, furosemide IV, central venous pressure (CVP) monitoring; if severe, bisphosphonates, e.g. pamidronate disodium.
Addison's disease	*Suggested by:* lethargy, weakness, dizziness, pigmentation (buccal, scar), hypotension. *Confirmed by:* ↓9a.m. **plasma cortisol** and impaired response to **short Synacthen® test**. *Finalized by the predictable outcome of management,* e.g. if ↓BP, fluids IV or colloids, if ↓glucose, 10% glucose IV. If ill, hydrocortisone IV, otherwise PO ± fludrocortisone.
Acute intermittent porphyria	*Suggested by:* LFT, peripheral neuropathy, constipation, hypertension, psychosis, urine dark after standing. *Confirmed by:* ↑**urinary aminolevulinic acid and porphobilinogen, plasma porphyrins**. *Finalized by the predictable outcome of management,* e.g. fluids IV, haematin IV, analgesics, propranolol for tachycardia and hypertension, diazepam for seizures, high carbohydrate intake.

Phaeochromocytoma	*Suggested by:* headache, sweating, palpitations, pallor, nausea, hypertension (intermittent or persistent), tachycardia. *Confirmed by:* **↑24h urinary metanephrines, ↑serum catecholamines (adrenaline, noradrenaline), CT abdomen, MRI scan.** *Finalized by the predictable outcome of management,* e.g. fluids IV with CVP monitoring before α- and then β-blockade, e.g. phenoxybenzamine ± phentolamine, then β-blockade, e.g. propranolol. Endocrine surgical intervention.
Lead poisoning	*Suggested by:* anorexia, personality changes, headaches, metallic taste, loss of sensation. *Confirmed by:* **↑whole blood lead concentration** >2.4micromol/L. *Finalized by the predictable outcome of management,* e.g. stop exposure, analgesia, anti-emetic. If severe, 0.9% saline IV, NG tube + nil by mouth, intestinal irrigation with polyethylene glycol, diazepam IV for convulsion; if lead >2.16 micromol/L (45 micrograms/dL), chelation + supplements, including iron.
Vitamin A intoxication	*Suggested by:* ↑intracranial pressure, drowsiness, headache, irritability, muscle pain and weakness. *Confirmed by:* symptoms and signs go within 1–4wk after stopping vitamin A ingestion. *Finalized by the predictable outcome of management,* e.g. stop vitamin A, fluids IV if vomiting, diarrhoea or hypercalcaemia, O_2.

Vomiting with headache alone (unrelated to food and no abdominal pain)

Look for better leads with the history and examination. Initial investigations (other tests in **bold** below): FBC, U&E, LFT, CXR, ECG, CT scan.

Main differential diagnoses and typical outline evidence, etc.	
Migraine	*Suggested by:* throbbing headache with preceding visual auras or other transient sensory symptoms and 'trigger' factors, e.g. premenstrual, stress, foods. *Confirmed by:* history, but if in doubt, **MRI scan** to exclude anatomical abnormalities. *Finalized by the predictable outcome of management,* e.g. rest in dark and quiet; if mild, paracetamol, NSAIDs, dextropropoxyphene, or combinations; if worse, 5HT agonist, e.g. sumatriptan or ergot, e.g. ergotamine. Prevention: avoid 'trigger' factors, prescribe β-blocker, tricyclics, serotonergics.
Raised intracranial pressure	*Suggested by:* being worse in morning, on coughing and leaning forward, papilloedema, pupillary dilatation, bradycardia, increased pulse pressure. *Confirmed by:* **CT scan head** showing flattening of sulci and darkening of brain tissue. *Finalized by the predictable outcome of management,* e.g. ICU care, neuro obs, treat cause, hyperventilation to keep P_aCO_2 down, mannitol IV.
Meningitis (viral or bacterial)	*Suggested by:* photophobia, fever, neck stiffness, Kernig's sign, Brudzinski's sign. *Confirmed by:* **CT scan**—no signs of ↑intracranial pressure and **lumbar puncture** (LP): ↑lymphocytes and normal glucose in viral, ↑neutrophils and ↓glucose in bacterial + organisms on staining and culture. *Finalized by the predictable outcome of management,* e.g. paracetamol, nurse in dark and quiet room. Fluids IV. Antivirals if varicella or herpes. Bacterial—after LP: 3rd gen. cephalosporin, e.g. ceftriaxone or cefotaxime (+ vancomycin if high local prevalence of penicillin-resistant *pneumococci*); dexamethasone IV if Glasgow Coma Score 8–11.
Haemorrhagic stroke	*Suggested by:* sudden onset of headache, then hemiparesis, (but not upper face) dysarthria ± dysphasia, extensor plantar response. *Confirmed by:* **CT brain scan**—high attenuation area representing haemorrhage. *Finalized by the predictable outcome of management,* e.g. IV access, nil by mouth + NG tube, control BP, neurosurgical intervention.

Severe hypertension	*Suggested by:* continuous throbbing headache (non-severe hypertension is usually asymptomatic), but headache ± visual disturbance and papilloedema in malignant hypertension.
	Confirmed by: **serial BP measurement**: usually >140mmHg diastolic and/or >240mmHg systolic.
	Finalized by the predictable outcome of management, e.g. labetalol IV or sodium nitroprusside to lower diastolic BP to 100–105 in 2–6h.
Acute glaucoma	*Suggested by:* blurred vision, painful red eye, coloured haloes.
	Confirmed by: ↑**intraocular pressure** on measurement.
	Finalized by the predictable outcome of management, e.g. nurse supine, no eye covering ± analgesics ± anti-emetics. Pilocarpine 2–4% eyedrops ± oral acetazolamide. Ophthalmology intervention.
Epilepsy idiopathic or seceondary to brain tumour or cerebrovascular disease or acute hypotension or metabolic disturbance	*Suggested by:* aura, altered consciousness, abnormal movements.
	Confirmed by: **EEG** result—spikes and waves over focus.
	Finalized by the predictable outcome of management, e.g. BP and ECG monitoring, pulse oximetry ±intubation, fluids IV ±U&E, diazepam IV stat ±infusion for status ±phenytoin IV. CT brain to exclude intracranial pathology if first presentation.

Vomiting alone (unrelated to food and without abdominal pain or headaches)

Look for better leads with the history and examination Initial investigations (other tests in **bold** below): FBC, U&E, LFT, CXR, ECG.

Main differential diagnoses and typical outline evidence, etc.

Gastroenteritis	*Suggested by:* diarrhoea, ↑bowel sounds. *Confirmed by:* **stools for WBC and culture**. *Finalized by the predictable outcome of management,* e.g. oral rehydration solution (glucose + salt solution); fluids IV if severe vomiting; antibiotic if agent identified.
Acute viral labyrinthitis	*Suggested by:* vertigo, tinnitus, hearing loss, nystagmus. *Confirmed by:* being dehydrated over days. *Finalized by the predictable outcome of management,* e.g. bed rest. Fluids IV and anti-emetics (e.g. metoclopramide, prochlorperazine) if severe nausea and vomiting.
Drugs e.g. antibiotics, cytotoxics, metformin, any overdose, excessive alcohol ingestion, etc.	*Suggested by:* history of drug ingestion, vomiting soon after taking medication. *Confirmed by:* response of symptoms to avoidance of causative drug. *Finalized by the predictable outcome of management,* e.g. stop offending drug, no alcohol.
Sliding hiatus hernia	*Suggested by:* occasional chest pain precipitated by heavy meals, lying flat. *Confirmed by:* **barium meal** showing reflux, endoscopy. *Finalized by the predictable outcome of management,* e.g. reduce weight if overweight, avoid stooping, semi-sitting position for sleep, correct constipation, antacids, H$_2$ blockers or proton pump inhibitors for pain.
Chronic renal failure (CRF)	*Suggested by:* fatigue, pruritus, anorexia, nausea, 'lemon-tinged' skin. *Confirmed by:* **↑↑serum creatinine, ↓↓creatinine clearance or eGFR**. ↓**Hb** (if chronic), and small kidneys on **renal US scan**. *Finalized by the predictable outcome of management,* e.g. treat cause if possible. Low phosphate, low K$^+$ diet, fluid restriction. BP control, erythropoietin ± transfusion if ↓Hb, calcium carbonate to lower serum phosphate, calcium ± calcitriol if ↓serum Ca^{2+}; loop diuretics if overload. Renal replacement therapy.
Pregnancy— hyperemesis gravidarum	*Suggested by:* being worse soon after waking better later, amenorrhoea <3mo. *Confirmed by:* pregnancy test +ve. *Finalized by the predictable outcome of management,* e.g. fluids IV, anti-emetic, e.g. metoclopramide, obstetric intervention.

Ménière's disease	*Suggested by:* vertigo, tinnitus, deafness. *Confirmed by:* **audiometry**—sensory hearing loss. *Finalized by the predictable outcome of management,* e.g. acute—anticholinergics, antihistamine, and benzodiazepine; then salt restriction, diuretics ± betahistine.
Acute otitis media (in children)	*Suggested by:* fever, earache, decreased hearing, otorrhoea if eardrum is perforated, accompanying upper respiratory infection symptoms. *Confirmed by:* **otoscopy** or **tympanometry**. *Finalized by the predictable outcome of management,* e.g. analgesics ±amoxicillin, ENT intervention—?myringotomy.
Anaphylaxis	*Suggested by:* bronchospasm, laryngeal oedema, flushing, urticaria, angioedema. *Confirmed by:* relief with antihistamines or steroids. *Finalized by the predictable outcome of management,* e.g. adrenaline 0.5 mL 1 in 1,000 (1mg/mL) IM, repeat every 5–10min until pulse and BP normal; fluids IV if ↓BP, O$_2$, corticosteroids + nebulized salbutamol if bronchospasm ± intubation.
Addison's disease	*Suggested by:* lethargy, weakness, dizziness, pigmentation (buccal, scar), hypotension. *Confirmed by:* ↓9a.m. plasma cortisol and impaired response to **short Synacthen® test**. *Finalized by the predictable outcome of management,* e.g. if ↓BP, fluids IV or colloids; if ↓glucose, 10% glucose IV. If ill, hydrocortisone IV, otherwise PO ± fludrocortisone.
Functional	*Suggested by:* vomiting during or soon after a meal ± other psychological disturbance, and no symptoms and physical signs of organic disease. *Confirmed by:* response to psychotherapy. *Finalized by the predictable outcome of management,* e.g. psychotherapy.
Also	Diabetic gastroparesis, ↑intracranial pressure, oesophageal or pyloric obstruction, any viral or bacterial infection, etc.

Jaundice

This can be a symptom reported by the patient or a physical sign. It is confirmed by high bilirubin in the plasma. Yellow sclerae and skin usually becomes visible when serum bilirubin level is >35micromol/L, so urine tests may provide the first clue. First subdivide into the five leads below. Remember that haemolysis causes ↑urinary urobilinogen and decreased serum haptoglobin. Hepatic failure causes increased serum unconjugated bilirubin, but intrahepatic or extrahepatic biliary obstruction results in increased serum conjugated bilirubin. Initial investigations (other tests in **bold** below): FBC + reticulocyte count, U&E, LFT, clotting screen, viral antibodies.

Main differential diagnoses and typical outline evidence, etc.	
Carotinaemia	*Suggested by:* onset over months. Skin yellow with white sclerae, normal stools and normal urine. Diet rich in yellow vegetables/fruits).
	Confirmed by: no bilirubin, no **urobilinogen** in the urine, and normal **serum bilirubin**. Normal **LFT**. Response to diet change.
	Finalized by the predictable outcome of management, e.g. diet change.
'Pre-hepatic' jaundice due to haemolysis	*Suggested by:* jaundice and anaemia (the combination seen as 'lemon' or pale yellow). Normal dark stools and normal-looking urine.
	Confirmed by: ↑(unconjugated and thus insoluble) **serum bilirubin**, but normal (conjugated and soluble) bilirubin, and thus no ↑bilirubin in urine. **↑Urine urobilinogen** and **↓serum haptoglobin**. **↑Serum LDH**. **↑Reticulocyte count**, **↓Hb**.
	Finalized by the predictable outcome of management, e.g. stop drugs that can cause haemolysis, give folic acid, fluids IV if dehydrated. Corticosteroid if autoimmune haemolytic anaemia.
'Hepatic' jaundice due to congenital enzyme defect	*Suggested by:* normal-looking stools and normal-looking urine.
	Confirmed by: ↑**serum bilirubin** (unconjugated), but no (conjugated) bilirubin in urine. No **urobilinogen in urine** and normal **haptoglobin**. Normal **LFT**.
	Finalized by the predictable outcome of management, e.g. symptomatic treatment.
'Hepatocellular' jaundice ('hepatic' with element of 'obstructive' jaundice)	*Suggested by:* onset of jaundice over days or weeks, stools pale or normal, but dark urine.
	Confirmed by: ↑**serum** (conjugated) **bilirubin** and thus ↑**urine bilirubin**. Normal urine urobilinogen. LFT all abnormal especially ↑**ALT**.
	Finalized by the predictable outcome of management, e.g. fluids IV if dehydrated, treat underlying cause.

'Obstructive' jaundice	*Suggested by:* onset of jaundice over days or weeks with pale stools and dark urine. ↑Bilirubin (i.e. conjugated and thus soluble) in urine.
	Confirmed by: ↑**serum conjugated bilirubin** and thus ↑**urine bilirubin** but no ↑urobilinogen in urine. ↑↑**Alkaline phosphatase**, but less abnormal LFT and ↑GGT.
	Finalized by the predictable outcome of management, e.g. if dehydrated, fluids IV, give O_2, ECG monitor, NG suction, antibiotics IV; treatment of underlying cause.

Pre-hepatic jaundice due to haemolysis

Suggested by: jaundice and anaemia (the combination often seen as 'lemon' or pale yellow). Normal dark stools and normal-looking urine.

Confirmed by: ↑**serum bilirubin** (unconjugated and thus insoluble), but normal conjugated and thus soluble bilirubin, and in turn no bilirubin in urine. Evidence of haemolysis as: ↑**urinary urobilinogen** and ↓**serum haptoglobin**. ↑**Reticulocyte count**. ↑LDH, ↓**Hb**.

Main differential diagnoses and typical outline evidence, etc.

Hereditary haemolytic anaemia	*Suggested by:* LFT, anaemia, splenomegaly, leg ulcers. *Confirmed by:* above evidence of haemolysis, ↑osmotic fragility; enzyme deficiency, e.g. G6PD, **pyruvate kinase**. *Finalized by the predictable outcome of management*, e.g. no fava beans in G6PD deficiency, Transfusion, splenectomy if required (+ prior immunization for *H. influenza* and *S. pneumoniae*).
Acquired haemolytic anaemia	*Suggested by:* sudden onset, in later life, and on medication. *Confirmed by:* above evidence of haemolysis, **blood film, +ve Coombs' test** in autoimmune type. *Finalized by the predictable outcome of management*, e.g. stop drugs that cause immune haemolysis, prescribe folic acid ± blood transfusion.
Septicaemic haemolysis due to pneumonia, urinary tract infection (UTI), etc.	*Suggested by:* fever ± shock symptoms and signs of infection. *Confirmed by:* evidence of haemolysis, **blood culture** +ve. *Finalized by the predictable outcome of management*, e.g. fluids ± blood transfusion if ↓BP + active haemolysis; paracetamol if fever; antibiotics.
Malaria	*Suggested by:* recent travel to malaria zone, periodic paroxysms of rigors, fever, sweating, nausea. *Confirmed by:* *plasmodium* in **blood smear**. *Finalized by the predictable outcome of management*, e.g. paracetamol if fever, blood transfusion if severe anaemia; chloroquine+primaquine (or artemisinin based combination therapy if chloroquine-resistant) for *P. vivax, P. ovale, P. malariae, P. knowlesi*; artemisinin-based combination therapy for at least 3d, e.g. dihydroartemisinin+piperaquine for *P. falciparum*, artesunate IV if severe *P. falciparum*. Please refer to WHO guidelines for the up-to-date treatment regimens at ℘ http://www.who.int/topics/malaria/en

Hepatic jaundice due to congenital enzyme defect

Suggested by: jaundice. Normal-looking stools and normal-looking urine.

Confirmed by: ↑**serum bilirubin** (unconjugated), but no (conjugated) bilirubin in urine. No **urobilinogen in urine** and normal **haptoglobin**. Normal **LFT**.

Main differential diagnoses and typical outline evidence, etc.

Gilbert's syndrome (normal lifespan)	*Suggested by:* above evidence of impaired conjugation, asymptomatic. *Confirmed by:* demonstration of unconjugated hyperbilirubinaemia with normal LFT, no haemolysis. Rise in **bilirubin when fasting and after nicotinic acid**. *Finalized by the predictable outcome of management*, e.g. no treatment necessary. Reassure.
Crigler–Najjar syndrome (type I: severe, neonatal and often fatal; type II: normal lifespan)	*Suggested by:* above evidence of impaired conjugation. *Confirmed by:* unconjugated hyperbilirubinaemia with otherwise normal LFT, no haemolysis. No rise in **bilirubin when fasting or after nicotinic acid**. *Finalized by the predictable outcome of management*, e.g. type 1: phototherapy and plasmapheresis to lower serum bilirubin, definitive treatment, e.g. liver transplant; type 2: supportive therapy, no specific treatment for the hyperbilirubinaemia.

Hepatocellular jaundice (due to hepatitis or very severe liver failure)

> *Suggested by:* onset of jaundice over days or weeks, stools pale or normal but dark urine.
>
> *Confirmed by:* ↑serum (conjugated) **bilirubin** and thus ↑**urine bilirubin**. Normal urine urobilinogen. LFT all increasingly abnormal especially ↑**ALT**.

Main differential diagnoses and typical outline evidence, etc.

Drug-induced hepatitis e.g. paracetamol, halothane	*Suggested by:* drug history, recent surgery. *Confirmed by:* drug levels and improvement after stopping the offending drug. *Finalized by the predictable outcome of management,* e.g. withdrawal of the drug which causes hepatitis, supportive therapy—fluids, etc.
Acute (viral) hepatitis A	*Suggested by:* tender hepatomegaly. *Confirmed by:* presence of **hepatitis A IgM antibody** suggests acute infection. *Finalized by the predictable outcome of management,* e.g. antipyretics, fluids IV and anti-emetics if nausea and vomiting, colestyramine for pruritus.
Acute hepatitis B	*Suggested by:* history of IV drug user, blood transfusion, needle punctures, tattoos, tender hepatomegaly. *Confirmed by:* presence of **HBsAg in serum.** *Finalized by the predictable outcome of management,* e.g. antipyretics, colestyramine for pruritus; if acute hepatic failure, monitor blood glucose, U&E, LFT, coagulation profile. 5% glucose IV (10% if ↓blood glucose), NG tube + nil by mouth, neomycin PO, lactulose, vitamin K IV.
Acute hepatitis C	*Suggested by:* history of IV drug user, mild illness, blood transfusion, tender hepatomegaly. *Confirmed by:* presence of **anti-HCV antibody, HCV-PCR.** *Finalized by the predictable outcome of management,* e.g. antipyretics, colestyramine for pruritus, interferon may be effective at reducing the rate of chronicity; if acute hepatic failure, monitor blood glucose, U&E, LFT, coagulation profile. 5% glucose (10% if ↓blood glucose), NG tube + nil by mouth, neomycin PO, lactulose, vitamin K IV.
Alcoholic hepatitis	*Suggested by:* history of drinking, presence of spider naevi and other signs of chronic liver disease. **AST:ALT ratio** >2. *Confirmed by:* resolution with abstinence. *Finalized by the predictable outcome of management,* e.g. stop alcohol, give folic acid, thiamine, vitamin K IV if coagulopathy; if acute hepatic failure, monitor blood glucose, U&E, LFT, coagulation profile. 5% glucose IV (10% if ↓blood glucose), NG tube + nil by mouth, neomycin PO, lactulose, vitamin K IV.

Primary hepatoma	*Suggested by:* weight loss, abdominal pain, RUQ mass.
	Confirmed by: **US scan/CT or MRI liver**, **liver biopsy**, ↑alpha-fetoprotein.
	Finalized by the predictable outcome of management, e.g. surgical intervention, e.g. resection, and adjunct chemotherapy.
Right heart failure	*Suggested by:* ↑JVP, hepatomegaly, ankle oedema.
	Confirmed by: **CXR:** large heart. **Echocardiogram:** dilated right ventricle.
	Finalized by the predictable outcome of management, e.g. salt and fluid restriction, O_2, furosemide IV or PO ± K^+ supplement.
Glandular fever (infectious mononucleosis)	*Suggested by:* cervical lymphadenopathy, sharp edge hepatomegaly ± splenomegaly ± jaundice.
	Confirmed by: **Paul–Bunnell**, +ve **heterophil antibody test**.
	Finalized by the predictable outcome of management, e.g. gargles/lozenges, analgesics, paracetamol.
	No aspirin (associated with Reye syndrome).

Obstructive jaundice

Suggested by: jaundice with pale stools and dark urine. Bilirubin in urine (i.e. conjugated and thus soluble).

Confirmed by: ↑**conjugated bilirubin** and thus **urine bilirubin** but no ↑urobilinogen in urine. ↑↑**Alkaline phosphatase**, but less abnormal LFT and ↑GGT.

Main differential diagnoses and typical outline evidence, etc.

Common bile duct stones	*Suggested by:* pain or tenderness in RUQ ± Murphy's sign. *Confirmed by:* **US scan liver**—dilatation of biliary ducts. *Finalized by the predictable outcome of management,* e.g. acute—analgesic, anti-emetics, nil by mouth, fluids IV (no specific treatment for biliary colic, usually dehydration); antibiotic IV, e.g. cephalosporin if acute (infective) cholecystitis.
Cancer of head of pancreas	*Suggested by:* progressive painless jaundice, palpable gallbladder (Courvoisier's law), weight loss. *Confirmed by:* **US scan liver**—dilatation of biliary ducts. **CT pancreas; ERCP** or **MRCP**: obstruction within head of pancreas. *Finalized by the predictable outcome of management,* e.g. low fat, high-protein diet, pain control, pancreatic enzyme supplement, phenothiazine or colestyramine for pruritus, surgical intervention e.g. stenting, resection.
Sclerosing cholangitis	*Suggested by:* progressive fatigue, pruritus. *Confirmed by:* ↑**ALP. US scan liver**: no gallstones. ERCP (beading of the intra- and extrahepatic biliary ducts). *Finalized by the predictable outcome of management,* e.g. nil by mouth during acute phase, control sepsis—antibiotics for Gram –ve aerobes, enterococci and anaerobes, treatment of underlying cause.
Primary biliary cirrhosis	*Suggested by:* fatigue, pruritus, scratch marks, non-tender hepatomegaly ± splenomegaly, xanthelasmata and xanthomas, arthralgia. *Confirmed by:* +ve **anti-mitochondrial antibody,** ↑**serum IgM**, infiltrate around hepatic bile ducts, and cirrhosis on **liver biopsy**. *Finalized by the predictable outcome of management,* e.g. no alcohol, colestyramine or ursodeoxycholic acid for pruritus.
Drug-induced	*Suggested by:* drug history of oral contraceptive pill, phenothiazines, anabolic steroids, erythromycin, etc. *Confirmed by:* symptoms receding when drug discontinued. *Finalized by the predictable outcome of management,* e.g. stop offending drug(s).

Pregnancy (last trimester)	*Suggested by:* jaundice during pregnancy.
	Confirmed by: resolution following delivery.
	Finalized by the predictable outcome of management, e.g. antipruritics.
Alcoholic hepatitis or cirrhosis	*Suggested by:* history of excess alcohol intake, presence of spider naevi and other signs of chronic liver disease.
	Confirmed by: **US scan** or **CT liver, liver biopsy**, improvement if abstinence.
	Finalized by the predictable outcome of management, e.g. stop alcohol, no specific folate and thiamine, vitamin K IV if coagulopathy; if acute hepatic failure, monitor blood glucose, U&E, LFT, coagulation profile. 5% glucose IV (10% if ↓blood glucose), NG tube + nil by mouth, neomycin PO, lactulose, vitamin K IV.
Dubin–Johnson syndrome (decreased excretion of conjugated bilirubin)	*Suggested by:* intermittent jaundice and associated pain in the right hypochondrium. No hepatomegaly.
	Confirmed by: normal **ALP**, normal LFT, ↑**urinary bilirubin**. Pigment granules on **liver biopsy**.
	Finalized by the predictable outcome of management, e.g. analgesia as necessary.

Dysphagia for solids that stick

It is important to distinguish between oropharyngeal and oesophageal dysphagia. The patient is often able to point to a specific point where the food sticks. Dysphagia to solids alone is more likely to be due to a mechanical obstruction. Initial investigations (other tests in **bold** below): FBC, CRP or ESR, U&E, ECG, CXR.

Main differential diagnoses and typical outline evidence, etc.	
Oesophageal stricture	*Suggested by:* history of gastro-oesophageal reflux, ingestion of corrosives, radiation or trauma.
	Confirmed by: **barium swallow and meal, fibreptic endoscopy** show necrotic mucosa ± ulceration.
	Finalized by the predictable outcome of management, e.g. no fatty food, small slow meals, H_2-blocker or PPI. Severe: nil by mouth, fluids IV, PPI, endoscopic balloon dilatation or surgery.
Carcinoma of oesophagus	*Suggested by:* progressive dysphagia, weight loss.
	Confirmed by: **barium swallow** shows filling defect, **fibreptic endoscopy** with biopsy of mass.
	Finalized by the predictable outcome of management, e.g. fluids IV ± antibiotic prophylaxis, surgical intervention e.g. oesophageal dilatation or stent insertion by endoscopy.
Carcinoma of cardia of stomach	*Suggested by:* weight loss, epigastric pain, vomiting.
	Confirmed by: **barium swallow** shows filling defect, **fibreptic endoscopy** with biopsy of mass.
	Finalized by the predictable outcome of management, e.g. NG tube + nil by mouth, fluids IV, analgesics, surgical intervention.
External oesophageal compression	*Suggested by:* few other GI symptoms.
	Confirmed by: **barium swallow** shows filling defect, **endoscopy** shows normal mucosa, **CT thorax** shows extrinsic mass from retrosternal goitre, neoplasms (lung or mediastinal tumours, lymphoma), aortic aneurysm.
	Finalized by the predictable outcome of management, e.g. treatment of underlying cause.
Also	Pharyngeal carcinoma, foreign bodies, mediastinal lymphadenopathy, left atrial enlargement, substernal thyroid, etc.

Dysphagia for solids (that do not stick) > fluids

It is important to distinguish from odynophagia—painful swallowing. Initial investigations (other tests in **bold** below): FBC, CRP or ESR, U&E, ECG, CXR.

Main differential diagnoses and typical outline evidence, etc.	
Globus pharyngeus	*Suggested by:* feeling of a lump in the throat which needs to be swallowed, may be associated with anxiety.
	Confirmed by: normal **barium swallow/ endoscopy, resolution** with reassurance and/or **psychotheraphy.**
	Finalized by the predictable outcome of management, e.g. reassurance, treatment of underlying psychological disorder, psychotherapy.
Xerostomia **e.g. drugs, elderly, Sjögren's syndrome, post-parotidectomy**	*Suggested by:* dryness of mouth, elderly, especially females.
	Confirmed by: clinical appearance of atrophic, dry oral mucosa.
	Finalized by the predictable outcome of management, e.g. stop drugs that cause xerostomia, sips of water or sugar-free chewing gum, hypromellose or methylcellulose; pilocarpine or cevimeline.
Pharyngeal pouch **(pharyngo-oesophageal diverticulum)**	*Suggested by:* regurgitation of undigested food, a sensation of a lump in the throat, halitosis, neck bulge on drinking, aspiration into lungs.
	Confirmed by: **barium swallow** shows extra luminal collection (oesophagoscopy avoided).
	Finalized by the predictable outcome of management, e.g. fluids IV. NG tube + nil by mouth if vomiting or dysphagia to prevent aspiration and for enteral feeding. Surgical intervention, e.g. for endoscopic stapling, diverticulotomy, cricopharyngeal myotomy or diverticulectomy.
Post-cricoid web **congenital or Plummer–Vincent or Paterson–Kelly syndrome**	*Suggested by:* untreated, severe iron deficiency anaemia.
	Confirmed by: **barium swallow** shows a thin, horizontal shelf; **endoscopy** to exclude malignancy.
	Finalized by the predictable outcome of management, e.g. iron supplements, transfusion if severe anaemia, dilatation or resection.

Sore throat

Sore throat—pain in the throat that worsens with swallowing. Odynophagia—pain that occurs only with swallowing. Initial investigations (other tests in **bold** below): FBC, CRP or ESR, U&E, throat swab.

Main differential diagnoses and typical outline evidence. etc.

Viral pharyngitis	*Suggested by:* sore throat, pain on swallowing, fever, cervical lymphadenopathy and injected fauces. ↑Lymphocytes, normal or ↓leucocytes. *Confirmed by:* –ve **throat swab** for bacterial culture, dehydration: resolution within days. *Finalized by the predictable outcome of management,* e.g. gargles/lozenges, paracetamol, etc.
Acute follicular tonsillitis (streptococcal)	*Suggested by:* severe sore throat, pain on swallowing, fever, enlarged tonsils with white patches (like strawberries and cream). Cervical lymphadenopathy, especially in angle of jaw. Fever, ↑leucocytes in WCC. *Confirmed by:* **throat swab** for culture and sensitivities of organisms. *Finalized by the predictable outcome of management,* e.g. analgesic, antibiotics, e.g. phenoxymethylpenicillin or cephalosporin or co-amoxiclav.
Infectious mononucleosis (glandular fever) due to Epstein–Barr virus	*Suggested by:* very severe throat pain with enlarged tonsils covered with grey mucoid film. Petechiae on palate. Profound malaise. Generalized lymphadenopathy, hepatomegaly, splenomegaly. *Confirmed by:* ↑atypical lymphocytes in WBC. **Paul–Bunnell** or **Monospot® test** +ve. **Viral titres**. *Finalized by the predictable outcome of management,* e.g. gargles/lozenges, analgesics, e.g. paracetamol (amoxicillin causes rash, aspirin may cause Reye syndrome).
Candidiasis of buccal or oesophageal mucosa	*Suggested by:* painful dysphagia, white plaque, history of immunosuppression/diabetes/recent antibiotics. *Confirmed by:* **oesophagoscopy** showing erythema and plaques, **brush cytology ± biopsy** showing spores and hyphae. *Finalized by the predictable outcome of management,* e.g. analgesics, antifungal lozenges or solutions, e.g. nystatin suspension or oral fluconazole.
Agranulocytosis e.g. antithyroid drugs	*Suggested by:* sore throat, history of taking a drug (e.g. carbimazole) or contact with noxious substance. *Confirmed by:* low or absent neutrophil count. *Finalized by the predictable outcome of management,* e.g. stop offending drug, broad-spectrum antibiotics IV or PO, if febrile.

| Also with oropharyngeal ulceration; without oropharyngeal ulceration | Herpes zoster infection, herpes simplex infection, local herpangina, aphthous ulceration, etc. |
| | Reflux oesophagitis, epiglottitis, blood dyscrasia, etc. |

Dysphagia for fluids > solids

This implies that there is a neuromuscular as opposed to an obstructive cause. Initial investigations (other tests in **bold** below): FBC, CRP or ESR, U&E, CXR.

Main differential diagnoses and typical outline evidence, etc.	
Pseudobulbar palsy due to brainstem stroke, multiple sclerosis, motor neurone disease, etc.	*Suggested by:* nasal, 'Donald Duck'-like speech, small spastic tongue. *Confirmed by:* inhalation of **Gastrografin®** clinical features of brainstem stroke, multiple sclerosis, motor neurone disease, etc. *Finalized by the predictable outcome of management,* e.g. NG tube + nil by mouth initially, thickened fluids if swallowing mechanism adequate, if not, percutaneous gastrostomy (PEG).
Scleroderma	*Suggested by:* reflux symptoms: cough and inhalation of fluids, tight skin, hooked nose, mouth rugae. *Confirmed by:* **barium swallow**—diminished or absent peristalsis, **oesophageal manometry**—subnormal or absent lower oesophageal sphincter tone. *Finalized by the predictable outcome of management,* e.g. raise head of bed, small meals; physiotherapy, nifedipine for Raynaud's; antibiotics if bacterial overgrowth, fat-soluble vitamins for malabsorption.
Bulbar palsy	*Suggested by:* nasal, quiet, or hoarse speech; flaccid, fasciculating tongue. *Confirmed by:* clinical features of motor neurone disease/Guillain–Barré syndrome/brainstem tumour/syringobulbia/pontine demyelination. *Finalized by the predictable outcome of management,* e.g. NG tube + nil by mouth initially, thickened fluids if swallowing mechanism adequate; if not, PEG.
Myasthenia gravis	*Suggested by:* difficult start to swallowing movement, cough (inhalation) precipitated by swallowing, ptosis. *Confirmed by:* inhalation on **Gastrografin®** swallow. Response to **Tensilon® test, ↑anti-acetylcholine receptor antibody**. *Finalized by the predictable outcome of management,* e.g. stop drugs which exacerbate; e.g. β-aminoglycosides; pyridostigmine ± corticosteroids if severe. IV Ig if crisis. Monitor FVC; intubation if FVC <1L.
Motor neurone disease	*Suggested by:* combination of upper and lower motor neurone signs. *Confirmed by:* **EMG** and **nerve conduction studies.** *Finalized by the predictable outcome of management,* e.g. NG tube + nil by mouth initially, thickened fluids if swallowing mechanism adequate; if not, PEG.

Diffuse oesophageal spasm (intermittent)	*Suggested by:* intermittent crushing retrosternal pain. *Confirmed by:* **barium swallow**—sometimes 'corkscrew oesophagus', **oesophageal manometry** show abnormal pressure profiles. *Finalized by the predictable outcome of management,* e.g. calcium channel blocker, e.g. diltiazem, antidepressant, e.g. imipramine, or isosorbide dinitrate.
Achalasia (progressive)	*Suggested by:* dysphagia with almost every meal, regurgitation (postural and effortless, contains undigested food). *Confirmed by:* **barium swallow, oesophageal manometry, oesophagoscopy** demonstrate absence of progressive peristalsis. *Finalized by the predictable outcome of management,* e.g. symptomatic treatment with smooth muscle dilator, e.g. nifedipine, diltiazem or isosorbide mononitrate may be helpful. Endoscopic balloon dilatation of lower oesophageal sphincter or injection of botulinum toxin.
Also	Parkinson's disease (oropharyngeal dysphagia), cerebral palsy, amyotrophic lateral sclerosis, etc.

Acute pain in the upper abdomen

Trying to localize the pain to the right, left, or middle may be difficult for the patient. More information such as the site of tenderness will become available from examining the abdomen. Initial investigations (other tests in bold below): FBC, U&E, CXR, AXR.

Main differential diagnoses and typical outline evidence, etc.	
Gallstone colic (with no acute inflammation or infection)	*Suggested by:* jaundice, biliary colic, pain in epigastrium or RUQ radiating to right lower scapula. No fever. Tenderness in the RUQ. WCC normal. *Confirmed by:* **US scan of gallbladder and biliary ducts.** *Finalized by the predictable outcome of management,* e.g. pain relief, e.g. pethidine, nil by mouth, fluids IV, anti-emetic.
Acute cholecystitis	*Suggested by:* fever, guarding, and +ve Murphy's sign. WCC: leucocytosis. *Confirmed by:* **US scan gallbladder and biliary ducts.** *Finalized by the predictable outcome of management,* e.g. fluids IV, opioid analgesia, antibiotics IV, e.g. metronidazole + cephalosporin.
Acute pancreatitis	*Suggested by:* pain radiating straight through to the back, better on sitting up or leaning forward. General abdominal tendeness, reduced bowel sounds. *Confirmed by:* ⇈**serum amylase, CT pancreas.** *Finalized by the predictable outcome of management,* e.g. pethidine, fluids IV, NG tube + nil by mouth if ileus + colloid ± blood; monitor serum Ca^{2+} and glucose.
Acute cholangitis	*Suggested by:* fever, RUQ abdominal pain, and jaundice (Charcot's triad), hypotension. WCC: leucocytosis. *Confirmed by:* **US scan gallbladder and biliary ducts, blood cultures.** *Finalized by the predictable outcome of management,* e.g. fluids IV, opioid analgesia, antibiotics IV, e.g. metronidazole + cephalosporin, if severe, biliary decompression, e.g. percutaneous or endoscopic drainage.
Gastric carcinoma	*Suggested by:* marked anorexia, fullness, pain, Troisier's sign (a 'Virchow's' node, i.e. large lymph node in the left supraclavicular fossa). *Confirmed by:* **upper GI endoscopy with biopsy.** *Finalized by the predictable outcome of management,* e.g. NG tube + nil by mouth, fluids IV, analgesics, surgical intervention.
Gastritis	*Suggested by:* epigastric pain, dull or burning discomfort, nocturnal pain. *Confirmed by:* **oesophagogastroscopy, barium meal and pH study.** *Finalized by the predictable outcome of management,* e.g. antacids, H_2 blocker or PPI if symptoms persist.

Oesophagitis	*Suggested by:* retrosternal pain, heartburn.
	Confirmed by: **oesophagogastroscopy**.
	Finalized by the predictable outcome of management, e.g. small meal often, no food before bed, elevate head of bed, antacids; if severe: nil by mouth, fluids IV, H$_2$ blocker or PPI; if *H. pylori*, antibiotics to eradicate.
Hiatus hernia	*Suggested by:* heartburn, worsens with stooping or lying, relieved by antacids.
	Confirmed by: **oesophagogastroscopy, barium meal**.
	Finalized by the predictable outcome of management, e.g. lose weight, no stooping, semi-sitting for sleep, correct constipation, antacids, proton pump inhibitors or H$_2$ blockers if pain.
Acute coronary syndrome (unstable angina or infarction)	*Suggested by:* chest tightness or pain on exertion.
	Confirmed by: **ECG± coronary angiography** if troponin normal, or later if ↑troponin.
	Finalized by the predictable outcome of management, e.g. ECG monitor (best in CCU), O$_2$, GTN (IV if pain persists), morphine, aspirin 300mg and clopidogrel 300mg stat, if ↑ST thrombolysis (and <12h from the onset), LMW heparin or fondaparinux for unstable angina or NSTEMI.
Also	Pericarditis, pneumonia, empyema, herpes zoster, ruptured oesophagus (Boerhaave syndrome, preceded by forceful vomiting), subphrenic abscess, splenic infarction, early appendicitis, acute mesenteric lymphadenitis, acute intestinal obstruction, etc.

Acute central abdominal pain

Examination of the abdomen may provide better leads. Initial investigations (other tests in **bold** below): FBC, U&E, CXR, AXR.

Main differential diagnoses and typical outline evidence, etc.

Small bowel obstruction	*Suggested by:* vomiting, constipation with complete obstruction. *Confirmed by:* **AXR** shows small bowel loops and fluid levels. *Finalized by the predictable outcome of management*, e.g. NG tube + nil by mouth, fluids IV, surgical intervention.
Abdominal aortic dissection	*Suggested by:* tearing pain, hypertension, (hypotension and shock indicate grave prognosis). *Confirmed by:* **US scan** or **CT abdomen**. *Finalized by the predictable outcome of management*, e.g. pain control with morphine, group and crossmatch, IV access, reduce systolic BP to 100–120mmHg with labetalol IV or propranolol ± sodium nitroprusside. Surgical intervention.
Crohn's disease	*Suggested by:* chronic diarrhoea with abdominal pain, weight loss, palpable RLQ mass or fullness, mouth ulcers. *Confirmed by:* **colonoscopy with biopsy, barium studies** showing 'skip lesions', string sign in advanced cases. *Finalized by the predictable outcome of management*, e.g. antimotility or antidiarrhoeal drugs; acute: fluids IV, corticosteroids IV or PO, high dose 5-ASA analogues (e.g. mesalazine, sulfasalazine), analgesics, elemental diet ± parenteral nutrition.
Mesenteric artery occlusion	*Suggested by:* vomiting, bowel urgency, melaena, diarrhoea. *Confirmed by:* **mesenteric angiography, exploratory laparotomy**. *Finalized by the predictable outcome of management*, e.g. fluids IV ++ if ↓BP, analgesics, broad-spectrum antibiotics, surgical intervention.

Acute lateral abdominal pain

Examination of the abdomen may provide better leads. Initial investigations (other tests in **bold** below): FBC, U&E, CXR, AXR.

Main differential diagnoses and typical outline evidence, etc.	
Appendicitis	*Suggested by:* pain initially central, then radiating to RLQ, anorexia, low-grade fever, constipation. RLQ tenderness and guarding. *Confirmed by:* US appendix, inflamed appendix at **laparotomy.** *Finalized by the predictable outcome of management,* e.g. nil by mouth, fluids IV, NG tube + nil by mouth if vomiting, broad-spectrum antibiotic, surgical intervention.
Pyelonephritis	*Suggested by:* pain in loin (upper lateral), rigors, fever, vomiting, frequency of micturition, renal angle tenderness. *Confirmed by:* FBC: leucocytosis. **MSU:** pyuria, urine and blood culture and sensitivities. *Finalized by the predictable outcome of management,* e.g. fluids IV, analgesics, anti-emetic; provisional antibiotics pending sensitivities, e.g. ampicillin + gentamicin or 3rd generation cephalosporin.
Renal calculus	*Suggested by:* renal colic, mainly in loin (upper lateral), haematuria. *Confirmed by:* **urinalysis, renal US scan, IVU, CT/MRI.** *Finalized by the predictable outcome of management,* e.g. fluids IV, analgesic, anti-emetics, e.g. prochlorperazine.
Ureteric calculus	*Suggested by:* renal colic, moving from loin (upper lateral) down to RLQ, haematuria. *Confirmed by:* **urinalysis, renal US scan, IVU, CT/MRI.** *Finalized by the predictable outcome of management,* e.g. fluids IV, analgesic, anti-emetics, e.g. prochlorperazine.
Salpingitis	*Suggested by:* fever, nausea, vomiting, mucopurulent cervical discharge, irregular menses. Bilateral lower abdominal tenderness and guarding. *Confirmed by:* FBC: leucocytosis. **High vaginal swab, laparoscopy.** *Finalized by the predictable outcome of management,* e.g. analgesics, anti-emetics, antibiotics, e.g. cephalosporin, cefoxitin + doxycycline.
Also	Ruptured ovarian cyst or torsion, endometriosis, Meckel's diverticulitis, colonic diverticulitis, etc.

Acute lower central (hypogastric) abdominal pain

Examination of the abdomen may provide better leads. Initial investigations (other tests in **bold** below): FBC, U&E, CXR, AXR.

Main differential diagnoses and typical outline evidence, etc.

Cystitis due to bacterial infection	*Suggested by:* frequency, urgency, dysuria ± haematuria. *Confirmed by:* **MSU** for microscopy and culture. *Finalized by the predictable outcome of management,* e.g. fluids IV if dehydrated, antibiotics.
Pelvic inflammatory disease	*Suggested by:* vaginal discharge, dysuria, dyspareunia, pelvic tenderness on moving cervix, ↑ESR and CRP. WCC: leucocytosis. *Confirmed by:* **high vaginal swab** for culture and sensitivity, **pelvic US scan** ± **laparoscopy**. *Finalized by the predictable outcome of management,* e.g. analgesia, fluids IV if dehydrated, provisional antibiotic, e.g. cefoxitin pending sensitivities.
Pelvic endometriosis	*Suggested by:* dysmenorrhoea, ovulation pain, dyspareunia, infertility, pelvic mass. *Confirmed by:* **laparoscopy**. *Finalized by the predictable outcome of management,* e.g. analgesics, fluids IV for hypovolaemia, blood transfusion for severe bleeding, gynae intervention for large or ruptured endometriosis.
Ectopic pregnancy	*Suggested by:* constant unilateral pain ± referred shoulder pain, amenorrhoea, vaginal bleeding (usually less than normal period), faintness with an acute rupture. *Confirmed by:* **pregnancy test** +ve, bimanual examination finding enlarged uterus, **pelvic US scan** showing empty uterus with thickened decidua. *Finalized by the predictable outcome of management,* e.g. analgesics, fluids IV ++ if hypotension or shock, urgent gynae/surgical intervention.
Large bowel obstruction	*Suggested by:* severe distension, late vomiting, visible peristalsis, resonant percussion, increased bowel sounds. Supine AXR showing peripheral abdominal large bowel shadow (with haustra partly crossing the lumen). Fluid levels on erect film. *Confirmed by:* **US scan** and **laparotomy** findings. *Finalized by the predictable outcome of management,* e.g. NG tube, 'drip and suck', fluids IV, monitor intake/output, antibiotics, surgical intervention.
Infective or ulcerative colitis	*Suggested by:* abdominal pain, diarrhoea with blood and mucus. *Confirmed by:* **stool microscopy and culture, colonoscopy**. *Finalized by the predictable outcome of management,* e.g. nil by mouth, fluids IV with K supplement, corticosteroids IV, antibiotic prophylaxis, may need parenteral nutrition, surgical intervention if toxic megacolon.
Also	Diverticular disease, ovarian cysts, intussusceptions, inguinal hernia, etc.

Acute abdominal pain in children

Examination of the abdomen may provide better leads. Initial investigations (other tests in **bold** below): FBC, U&E, CXR, AXR.

Main differential diagnoses and typical outline evidence, etc.

Gastroenteritis (all ages)	*Suggested by:* crampy pain, low grade fever, diarrhoea, vomiting, symptoms resolve in 2wk. *Confirmed by:* virus in the **stool specimen**. *Finalized by the predictable outcome of management, e.g.* paracetamol for fever, oral rehydration solutions, fluids IV if severe dehydration.
Infantile colic (commonly between 2–16wk-old)	*Suggested by:* prolonged crying lasting >3h occurs during late afternoon and early evening >3d per week. *Confirmed by:* history and normal physical findings. *Finalized by the predictable outcome of management, e.g.* reassurance.
Mesenteric adenitis	*Suggested by:* symptoms and signs similar to early appendicitis, but without guarding or rectal tenderness. *Confirmed by:* spontaneous resolution (or findings at **laparotomy** or **laparoscopy**). *Finalized by the predictable outcome of management, e.g.* analgesia, monitoring.
UTI	*Suggested by:* vomiting, irritability, fever, poor feeding in baby; urgency, dysuria, suprapubic discomfort, fever in older children; (chills, nausea, loin pain in upper tract infection). *Confirmed by:* urine microscopy and culture. *Finalized by the predictable outcome of management, e.g.* antibiotics, e.g. oral amoxicillin or co-trimoxazole (>2mo old); 3rd generation cephalosporin IV if upper tract infection.
Intussusception (common between 6–9mo-old)	*Suggested by:* child, usually between 6–9mo of life, acute onset of colicky intermittent abdominal pain, redcurrant 'jelly' PR bleed ± a sausage-shaped mass in upper abdomen. *Confirmed by:* US scan, **barium or air enema**, may reduce the intussusceptions with appropriate hydrostatic pressure. *Finalized by the predictable outcome of management, e.g.* fluids IV, NG tube + nil by mouth, analgesics, surgical intervention, e.g. enema/hydrostatic reduction.
Acute appendicitis (mainly 5–15y)	*Suggested by:* vomiting, diarrhoea, pain initially central, then radiating to RLQ, anorexia, low-grade fever, constipation. RLQ tenderness and guarding. *Confirmed by:* inflamed appendix at **laparotomy.** *Finalized by the predictable outcome of management, e.g.* nil by mouth, fluids IV, NG tube + nil by mouth if vomiting, broad-spectrum antibiotic, surgical intervention.
Also	Diabetic ketoacidosis, infections—mumps, Epstein–Barr mononucleosis, pneumonia (especially right lower lobe), torsion of testes, Henoch–Schönlein purpura, sickle crisis, Meckel's diverticulitis.

Recurrent abdominal pain in children

Majority of cases of recurrent abdominal pain in children will not have organic pathology. However, organic disease is more likely if the pain is associated with vomiting, weight loss or failure to thrive, and may wake the child from sleep. Examination of the abdomen may provide better leads. Initial investigations (other tests in **bold** below): FBC, U&E.

Main differential diagnoses and typical outline evidence, etc.	
Recurrent viral illness	*Suggested by:* recurrent fever, malaise, diarrhoea and vomiting, blocked nose, etc. *Confirmed by:* WCC shows lymphocytosis, viral serology. *Finalized by the predictable outcome of management,* e.g. explanation, reassurance.
Psychosomatic cause e.g. stress, anxiety, depression, etc.	*Suggested by:* social withdrawal, irritability, poor attention, decreased activity, **school/home stress**, school avoidance. *Confirmed by:* **history**. *Finalized by the predictable outcome of management,* e.g. explanation, reassurance, consultation with child psychologist/psychiatrist.
Constipation	*Suggested by:* infrequent and/or painful bowel movements, hard stools. *Confirmed by:* history, **AXR** may show faeces and evidence of bowel obstruction ± barium enema. *Finalized by the predictable outcome of management,* e.g. high-fibre diet, increased fluid intake, regular toilet sitting; disimpaction, e.g. with phosphate enema, polyethylene glycol solution PO, or stool softener.
Recurrent UTI	*Suggested by:* vomiting, irritability, fever, poor feeding in baby; urgency, dysuria, suprapubic discomfort, fever in older children; (chills, nausea, loin pain in upper tract infection). *Confirmed by:* **urine microscopy and culture, US scan** to detect any abnormal urinary tract anatomy. *Finalized by the predictable outcome of management,* e.g. antibiotics, e.g. amoxicillin PO or co-trimoxazole (>2mo old); 3rd generation cephalosporin IV if upper tract infection.
Inflammatory bowel disease (in adolescents)	*Suggested by:* chronic diarrhoea with abdominal pain, weight loss, RLQ mass or fullness, mouth ulcers. *Confirmed by:* **colonoscopy with biopsy, barium studies** showing 'skip lesions', string sign (in advanced cases) in Crohn's; or loss of haustration, mucosal oedema, ulceration in ulcerative colitis. *Finalized by the predictable outcome of management,* e.g. antimotility drugs (e.g. loperamide) or antidiarrhoeal drugs; acute attack: fluids IV, corticosteroids PO or IV, high dose 5-ASA analogues (e.g. mesalazine, sulfasalazine), analgesics, elemental diet ± parenteral nutrition.
Also	Parasitic infestation of bowel, lactose intolerance, Hirschsprung's disease, ureteric reflux, lead poisoning, pica, etc.

Sudden diarrhoea, fever, and vomiting

Initial investigations (other tests in **bold** below): FBC, U&E, stool for culture and sensitivity. NB Measures to prevent cross infection.

Main differential diagnoses and typical outline evidence, etc.	
Viral gastroenteritis (usually Norwalk virus)	*Suggested by:* diarrhoea in older children and adults, symptoms resolve in 2wk. *Confirmed by:* **detection of virus in the stool**. *Finalized by the predictable outcome of management,* e.g. paracetamol, oral rehydration solutions or fluids IV, anti-emetic; antidiarrhoeals, e.g. loperamide for patient without 'dysentery'.
Rotavirus	*Suggested by:* diarrhoea in children <5y, symptoms resolving in a week. *Confirmed by:* detection of virus in the stool by immnunoassays or PCR. *Finalized by the predictable outcome of management,* e.g. paracetamol, oral rehydration solutions or fluids IV, anti-emetic; antidiarrhoeals, e.g. loperamide for patient without 'dysentery'.
Antibiotic-induced bacterial opportunists, e.g. *Clostridium (C.) difficile*	*Suggested by:* watery diarrhoea with a history of recent antibiotic therapy, abdominal cramps, ↑WCC. *Confirmed by:* **stool culture**, C. difficile toxins A and B in **stool.** *Finalized by the predictable outcome of management,* e.g. stop offending antibiotic, paracetamol for fever, fluids IV if dehydrated, oral metronidazole or vancomycin for 10–14d.
Food poisoning/ toxins *Salmonella typhimurium*	*Suggested by:* eating 'doubtful' meat, egg, poultry. Fever (with relative bradycardia), headache, dry cough. *Confirmed by:* **stool microscopy and culture**. *Finalized by the predictable outcome of management,* e.g. paracetamol for fever, oral rehydration solutions or fluids IV if dehydrated, ciprofloxacin or co-trimoxazole.
Clostridium perfringens	*Suggested by:* eating 'doubtful' meat, incubation period 8–16h, abdominal cramps, little vomiting, lasting 1–2d. *Confirmed by:* organism **isolation from faeces or suspected food**. *Finalized by the predictable outcome of management,* e.g. paracetamol for fever, oral rehydration solutions or fluids IV if dehydrated.
Staphylococcus (S.) aureus	*Suggested by:* eating 'doubtful' meat, incubation period <6h, marked vomiting. *Confirmed by:* isolation of S. aureus from **examination of suspected food**. *Initial management:* paracetamol for fever, oral rehydration solutions or fluids IV if dehydrated.

Bacillus cereus	*Suggested by:* eating 'doubtful' rice, incubation period <6h, marked vomiting. *Confirmed by:* **stool microscopy and culture**. *Finalized by the predictable outcome of management*, e.g. paracetamol for fever, oral rehydration solutions or fluids IV if dehydrated.
Vibrio para haemolyticus	*Suggested by:* 'doubtful' seafood, incubation period 16–72h. *Confirmed by:* **stool microscopy and culture**. *Finalized by the predictable outcome of management*, e.g. paracetamol for fever, oral rehydration solutions or fluids IV if dehydrated, tetracycline or doxycycline.
Botulism	*Suggested by:* eating 'doubtful' canned food, incubation period 18–36h (may vary from 4h to 8d), abdominal cramps, dry mouth, diplopia, progressive paralysis. *Confirmed by:* C. botulinum **toxin in serum or faeces**; C. botulinum **toxin isolation from suspected food**. *Finalized by the predictable outcome of management*, e.g. manage in ICU, monitor pulse, oximetry and spirometry, early intubation with ventilatory, botulinum antitoxin IV.

Recurrent diarrhoea with blood ± mucus—bloody flux

Initial investigations (other tests in **bold** below): FBC, U&E, stool for culture and sensitiviry. NB Measures to prevent cross infection.

Main differential diagnoses and typical outline evidence, etc.

Crohn's disease	*Suggested by:* chronic diarrhoea with abdominal pain, weight loss, RLQ mass or fullness, mouth ulcers. *Confirmed by:* **colonoscopy with biopsy, barium studies** showing 'skip lesions', string sign (in advanced cases). *Finalized by the predictable outcome of management,* e.g. antimotility drugs (e.g. loperamide) or antidiarrhoeal drugs; acute attack: fluids IV, corticosteroids PO or IV, high dose 5-ASA analogues (e.g. mesalazine, sulfasalazine), analgesics, elemental diet ± parenteral nutrition.
Ulcerative colitis	*Suggested by:* lower abdominal cramps, ↑urgency to defaecate, severe diarrhoea, ↑fever in acute attack. **FBC** showing ↑WCC, U&E; ↑urea and creatinine in dehydration. *Confirmed by:* **colonoscopy with biopsy, barium studies** show loss of haustration, mucosal oedema, ulceration. *Finalized by the predictable outcome of management,* e.g. nil by mouth, fluids IV with K⁺, corticosteroids IV, antibiotic prophylaxis ± parenteral nutrition; if toxic megacolon, surgical intervention.
Colonic carcinoma	*Suggested by:* alternate diarrhoea and constipation. *Confirmed by:* **barium enema** showing filling defect, **colonoscopy with biopsy** shows mass and malignant histology. *Finalized by the predictable outcome of management,* e.g. surgical intervention.
Colorectal carcinoma	*Suggested by:* sensation of incomplete evacuation. *Confirmed by:* **sigmoidoscopy with biopsy** showing mass and malignant histology, **barium enema** shows filling defect. *Finalized by the predictable outcome of management,* e.g. surgical intervention.
Diverticular disease/ diverticulitis	*Suggested by:* middle-aged or elderly, diarrhoea, LIF pain and tenderness, abdominal and rectal mass. *Confirmed by:* **barium enema** showing opaque filling diverticula, **colonoscopy** showing inflammatory foci. *Finalized by the predictable outcome of management,* e.g. clear liquids only, ciprofloxacin + metronidazole PO for 7–10d, high-fibre diet when acute phase is over; severe: hospitalization, fluids IV, nil by mouth, paracetamol for fever, metronidazole IV + a 3rd generation cephalosporin or a fluoroquinolone.

Acute bloody diarrhoea ± mucus—'dysentery'

Initial investigations (other tests in **bold** below): FBC, U&E, stool for culture and sensitiviry. NB Measures to prevent cross infection.

Main differential diagnoses and typical outline evidence, etc.	
Campylobacter enteritis	*Suggested by:* associated severe abdominal pain. *Confirmed by:* **stool microscopy and culture** of organism. *Finalized by the predictable outcome of management,* e.g. oral rehydration solution; fluids IV if severe vomiting, antidiarrhoeal, e.g. codeine, ciprofloxacin, or erythromycin.
Shigella (bacillary) dysenteriae	*Suggested by:* blood and mucus, fever, abdominal pain. *Confirmed by:* **stool microscopy** revealing red cells, pus cells, and appearance of organism. *Finalized by the predictable outcome of management,* e.g. oral rehydration solution; fluids IV if severe vomiting, antidiarrhoeal, ciprofloxacin or co-trimoxazole.
Enteroinvasive Escherichia (E.) coli	*Suggested by:* fever, watery diarrhea, later ± bloody diarrhoea. *Confirmed by:* **stool microscopy** and **culture** of organism. *Finalized by the predictable outcome of management,* e.g. paracetamol for fever, oral rehydration solutions or fluids IV if severe dehydration, antibiotic if frail or progressive.
Enterohaemorrhagic type 0157 E. coli	*Suggested by:* no fever, bloody diarrhoea ± haemolytic-uraemic syndrome. *Confirmed by:* **stool microscopy** and **culture** of organism. *Finalized by the predictable outcome of management,* e.g. oral rehydration solution or fluids IV if severe dehydration, correct electrolytes, watch for haemolytic-uraemic syndrome.
Entamoeba histolytica (amoebic) dysentery	*Suggested by:* abdominal discomfort, flatulence, frequent watery, bloody diarrhoea. *Confirmed by:* **stool microscopy** and **culture** of organism. *Finalized by the predictable outcome of management,* e.g. oral rehydration solution; fluids IV if severe vomiting, metronidazole PO for 10d.

Watery diarrhoea

Note that diarrhoea can result in severe dehydration. Initial investigations (other tests in **bold** below): FBC, U&E, stool for culture and sensitiviry. NB Measures to prevent cross infection.

Main differential diagnoses and typical outline evidence, etc.	
Traveller's diarrhoea	*Suggested by:* recent travel, no obvious ingestion of contaminated water or food. *Confirmed by:* rapid resolution or response to ciprofloxacin. *Finalized by the predictable outcome of management,* e.g. reassure that most cases are self-limited; oral rehydration solutions if severe diarrhoea; ciprofloxacin for 2d, or single dose of azithromycin; bismuth prep until diarrhoea resolves (up to x8); antimotility agents, e.g. loperamide or diphenoxylate.
Enterotoxigenic E. coli (commonest)	*Suggested by:* incubation period 12–72h in relation to contact to others with similar features. *Confirmed by:* **stool microscopy** and **culture**. *Finalized by the predictable outcome of management,* e.g. reassure that majority of cases are dehydration; oral rehydration solutions or fluids IV if severe dehydration.
Vibrio cholera	*Suggested by:* incubation period from a few hours to 5d, profuse watery diarrhoea, fever, vomiting. *Confirmed by:* **stool microscopy and culture**. *Finalized by the predictable outcome of management,* e.g. oral rehydration solutions, fluids IV if >10% bodyweight loss from dehydration, tetracycline for 3d or one dose of doxycycline.
Rotavirus	*Suggested by:* diarrhoea in children <5y and symptoms resolve in a week. *Confirmed by:* **detection of virus in the stool by immunoassays or PCR**. *Finalized by the predictable outcome of management,* e.g. paracetamol for fever, oral rehydration solutions or fluids IV if severe, no antimotility nor antispasmodics in children.
Norwalk virus	*Suggested by:* diarrhoea in older children and adults and symptoms resolve in 2wk. *Confirmed by:* detection of virus in **stool specimen**. *Finalized by the predictable outcome of management,* e.g. paracetamol to reduce fever, oral rehydration solutions or fluids IV if severe dehydration.

Recurrent diarrhoea with no blood in the stools, no fever

Initial investigations (other tests in **bold** below): FBC, U&E, LFT, random glucose, T4, TSH.

Main differential diagnoses and typical outline evidence, etc.	
Irritable bowel syndrome	*Suggested by:* no weight loss, intermittent daytime diarrhoea, pain relieved by defaecation, abdominal distension, mucus but no blood in the stool.
	Confirmed by: normal **colonoscopy and barium studies,** and no appearance of other cause of symptoms.
	Finalized by the predictable outcome of management, e.g. high-fibre diet; try metoclopramide, mebeverine, loperamide, lactulose; low dose tricyclic antidepressant and psychological therapy.
Faecal impaction with overflow	*Suggested by:* elderly patient and hard faeces on rectal examination.
	Confirmed by: **AXR** may show faecal impaction. Response to suppositories/removal of faeces.
	Finalized by the predictable outcome of management, e.g. laxatives and enemas ± gentle digital disimpaction.
Malabsorption due to coeliac disease, lactose intolerance, pancreatic disease, Whipple's disease	*Suggested by:* pale, bulky offensive stools, weight loss, signs of nutritional deficiencies.
	Confirmed by: **coeliac screen, small bowel biopsy** or **lactose tolerance test; intestinal biopsy** shows foamy macrophages containing PAS +ve glycoprotein in Whipple's.
	Finalized by the predictable outcome of management, e.g. nutritional support (treat cause).
Drug-induced	*Suggested by:* history of laxative abuse, magnesium alkalis, antibiotics, hypotensive agents, alcohol.
	Confirmed by: resolution on withdrawing drug.
	Finalized by the predictable outcome of management, e.g. stop offending drug.
HIV infection	*Suggested by:* weight loss, other opportunistic infection, lympadenopathy, Kaposi's sarcoma.
	Confirmed by: **HIV serology, stool microscopy and cultures** showing *Cryptosporidium*, microsporidia, *Isospora belli*, enteropathy, etc.
	Finalized by the predictable outcome of management, e.g. try loperamide, empirical antibiotics, e.g. ciprofloxacin + metronidazole (except if 0157 *E. coli* suspected).

Diabetic autonomic neuropathy	*Suggested by:* known diabetic, intermittent watery painless diarrhoea, postural hypotension, impotence, urinary retention. *Confirmed by:* lying and standing BP, loss of **beat-to-beat variation** during slow deep breathing. *Finalized by the predictable outcome of management,* e.g. loperamide or codeine for diarrhoea, co-amoxiclav + metronidazole for bacterial overgrowth, fludrocortisone for severe postural hypotension.
Thyrotoxicosis	*Suggested by:* heat intolerance, tremor, nervousness, palpitation, frequent bowel movements, goitre. *Confirmed by:* ↓**TSH**, ↑**FT4**, or ↑**FT3**. *Finalized by the predictable outcome of management,* e.g. propranolol 40–80 mg 8-hourly to control symptoms, carbimazole, or propylthiouracil to treat thyroid overactivity.
Carcinoid syndrome	*Suggested by:* facial flushing ± wheeze, abdominal pain. *Confirmed by:* ↑24h **urinary 5-HIAA**. *Finalized by the predictable outcome of management,* e.g. avoid precipitating factors, e.g. alcohol, physical activity. Codeine phosphate for diarrhoea, H_2 agonist or theophylline for asthma; octreotide; surgical, e.g. resection of tumour.

Chronic diarrhoea in children

Note that certain conditions that cause chronic diarrhoea in children require special attention. Initial investigations (other tests in **bold** below): FBC, U&E, LFT.

Main differential diagnoses and typical outline evidence, etc.	
Lactose intolerance	*Suggested by:* bloatedness, colicky abdominal pain, diarrhoea after digestion of lactose-containing food.
	Confirmed by: stool analysis shows presence of reducing substances in the liquid portion of stool, and pH of stool <5.5.
	Finalized by the predictable outcome of management, e.g. no lactose-containing products.
Cow's milk protein intolerance	*Suggested by:* crampy abdominal pain, diarrhoea after ingestion of cow's milk formula, onset of symptoms may be delayed.
	Confirmed by: response to withdrawal of cow's milk formula.
	Finalized by the predictable outcome of management, e.g. no cow's milk protein.
Chronic infection of bowel (e.g. Salmonella sp., Campylobacter, Giardia lambia, etc.)	*Suggested by:* abdominal discomfort, flatulence, frequent watery ±bloody diarrhoea.
	Confirmed by: **stool microscopy** and **culture** of organism.
	Finalized by the predictable outcome of management, e.g. oral rehydration solution; fluids IV if severe vomiting, no antidiarrhoeal drugs, treat underlying infection.
Coeliac disease (usually present at 9–18mo)	*Suggested by:* anorexia, irritability, frequent bulky offensive stools, failure to thrive, abdominal distension.
	Confirmed by: **coeliac screen, duodenal biopsy.**
	Finalized by the predictable outcome of management, e.g. gluten-free diet, nutritional supplements.
Cystic fibrosis (present in infancy)	*Suggested by:* LFT, meconium ileus in the neonate, fatty diarrhoea, malabsorption, recurrent chest infection, failure to thrive.
	Confirmed by: **sweat test**: Chloride >60mmol/L and genetic testing: (1 mutation = mild disease, 2 mutations = severe), response to pancreatic enzyme replacement.
	Finalized by the predictable outcome of management, e.g. pancreatic enzyme replacement, treatment of any chest infections, postural drainage.

Inflammatory bowel disease (adolescents)	*Suggested by:* chronic diarrhoea with abdominal pain, weight loss, RLQ mass or fullness, mouth ulcers.
	Confirmed by: **colonoscopy with biopsy, barium studies** showing 'skip lesions', string sign (in advanced cases) in Crohn's; or loss of haustration, mucosal oedema, ulceration in ulcerative colitis.
	Finalized by the predictable outcome of management, e.g. antimotility drugs (loperamide 2–4mg tds) or antidiarrhoeal drugs; acute attack: fluids IV, corticosteroids IV or PO, high dose 5-ASA analogues (e.g. mesalazine, sulfasalazine), analgesics, elemental diet ± parenteral nutrition.

Constipation

Constipation is defined as a change in a person's normal bowel habit to infrequent or more difficult defaecation. It is important to establish what the patient means by the term 'constipation', what his or her normal bowel habit is, and how the presenting problem differ from 'normal'. Initial investigations (other tests in **bold** below): FBC, U&E, LFT, serum calcium, T4, TSH, AXR, sigmoidoscopy.

Main differential diagnoses and typical outline evidence, etc.	
Change in diet, e.g. low-fibre diet	*Suggested by:* history of ↓diet fibre, ↓fluid intake. *Confirmed by:* normal **endoscopy** and response to diet change. *Finalized by the predictable outcome of management,* e.g. ↑dietary fibre and ↑fluid intake.
Change in the lifestyle or environment	*Suggested by:* history. *Confirmed by:* normal **sigmoidoscopy or colonoscopy** and constipation resolves when resuming prior lifestyle or environment. *Finalized by the predictable outcome of management,* e.g. resume lifestyle, ↑dietary fibre.
Immobility	*Suggested by:* history. *Confirmed by:* normal **sigmoidoscopy or colonoscopy** and history. *Finalized by the predictable outcome of management,* e.g. mobilization, ↑dietary fibre.
Drug-induced	*Suggested by:* constipating drugs (opioids, hypotensive agents, aluminium alkalis, etc.), purgative dependence. *Confirmed by:* normal **sigmoidoscopy or colonoscopy** and response to withdrawal of suspected agent. *Finalized by the predictable outcome of management,* e.g. stop offending drug.
Anal fissure	*Suggested by:* skin tag, pain on defaecation, staining of toilet paper following defaecation. *Confirmed by:* physical examination of anal region. *Finalized by the predictable outcome of management,* e.g. high-fibre diet, stool softeners. warm sitz baths, analgesic cream, glyceryl trinitrate ointment, oral or topical diltiazem, botulinum toxin injection near to the fissures, surgical intervention, e.g. sphincterotomy if medical therapy fails.
Haemorrhoids	*Suggested by:* rectal bleeding follows defaecation, perianal protrusion with pain. *Confirmed by:* anal inspection and **proctoscopy** (haemorrhoids drop over edge of proctoscope as it is withdrawn). *Finalized by the predictable outcome of management,* e.g. high-fibre diet, hydrocortisone suppositories to relieve irritation and pruritus ± surgical intervention.

Poor fluid intake	*Suggested by:* history of ↓fluid intake. *Confirmed by:* normal **sigmoidoscopy or colonoscopy** and response to increased fluid intake. *Finalized by the predictable outcome of management*, e.g. ↑fluid intake.
Hypothyroidism	*Suggested by:* cold intolerance, lethargy, weight gain, coarse and dry skin, puffy eyelids. *Confirmed by:* ↑TSH, ↓FT4 ± ↓FT3. *Finalized by the predictable outcome of management*, e.g. levothyroxine.
Rectal tumour	*Suggested by:* rectal bleeding with defaecation, blood limited to surface of stool. *Confirmed by:* **sigmoidoscopy with rectal biopsy**. *Finalized by the predictable outcome of management*, e.g. surgical intervention.
Colonic carcinoma	*Suggested by:* alternate diarrhoea and constipation, anaemia or weight loss. *Confirmed by:* **colonoscopy with biopsy, barium enema**. *Finalized by the predictable outcome of management*, e.g. surgical intervention.
Also	Hypercalcaemia, behavioural—'stool-holding' in children, external pelvic mass compression, intestinal pseudo-obstruction, Hirschsprung disease, Chagas disease, scleroderma, Parkinson's disease, dyssynergistic defaecation, etc.

Change in bowel habit

This may be an increase in constipation or diarrhoea or both alternating. Initial investigations (other tests in bold below): FBC, U&E, LFT, serum calcium, T4, TSH, AXR, sigmoidoscopy.

Main differential diagnoses and typical outline evidence, etc.	
Change in diet	*Suggested by:* history of ↓diet fibre, ↓fluid intake. *Confirmed by:* normal **sigmoidoscopy or colonoscopy** and response to diet change. *Finalized by the predictable outcome of management*, e.g. diet change—↑fibre and fluid intake.
Colonic carcinoma	*Suggested by:* alternate diarrhoea and constipation, anaemia or weight loss. *Confirmed by:* **colonoscopy with biopsy, CT abdomen, barium enema**. *Finalized by the predictable outcome of management*, e.g. surgical intervention.
Drug-induced	*Suggested by:* constipating drugs (opioids, hypotensive agents, aluminium alkalis, etc.), purgative dependence. *Confirmed by:* normal **sigmoidoscopy or colonoscopy** and response to stopping causal agent. *Finalized by the predictable outcome of management*, e.g. stop offending drug.
Depression	*Suggested by:* sleep disorders, social withdrawal, lack of interest in usual activities, etc. *Confirmed by:* normal **sigmoidoscopy or colonoscopy**, and response to lifting of depression. *Finalized by the predictable outcome of management*, e.g. psychiatric consultation and treatment.
Immobility	*Suggested by:* history. *Confirmed by:* normal **sigmoidoscopy or colonoscopy** and history. *Finalized by the predictable outcome of management*, e.g. mobilization, ↑fibre.
Cerebral or spinal cord lesion	*Suggested by:* neurological symptoms and signs ± abnormal sphincter tone and anal sensation. *Confirmed by:* **CT or MRI**. *Finalized by the predictable outcome of management*, e.g. rehabilitation programmes, ↑fibre.
Metabolic disturbances: hypothyroidism, hyperthyroidism, hypercalcaemia, hypokalaemia	*Suggested by:* symptoms of metabolic disturbance or absence of anatomical abnormality. *Confirmed by:* **TFT, serum calcium, potassium**, etc. *Finalized by the predictable outcome of management*, e.g. correction of electrolytes and metabolic disturbance, treatment of underlying cause.

Haematemesis ± melaena

Vomiting of bright red blood and/or passage of black tarry motions. This implies bleeding from the upper GI tract: oesophagus, stomach, and duodenum. Initial investigations (other tests in **bold** below): FBC, U&E, LFT, clotting screen, group and save, monitor Hb.

Main differential diagnoses and typical outline evidence, etc.	
Bleeding DU	*Suggested by:* epigastric pain and tenderness, nausea. *Confirmed by:* **oesophagogastroscopy** showing bleeding ulcer. *Finalized by the predictable outcome of management,* e.g. large-bore IV or central line, fluids IV—colloid initially ± transfusion, CVP monitoring, NG tube + irrigation, urinary catheter to monitor output, surgical referral. H₂ blocker or PPI for 4wk; *H. pylori* eradication therapy if *H. pylori* +ve.
Bleeding GU	*Suggested by:* epigastric pain, dull or burning discomfort, nocturnal pain. *Confirmed by:* appearance of ulcer on **oesophagogastroscopy** and **pH study** showing hyperacidity. *Finalized by the predictable outcome of management,* e.g. treatment of acute severe bleed as DU; antacid; H₂ blocker or PPI for 8wk; *H. pylori* eradication therapy if *H. pylori* +ve.
Gastric erosion	*Suggested by:* history of NSAIDs or alcohol ingestion, epigastric pain, dull or burning discomfort, nocturnal pain. *Confirmed by:* appearance of erosion on **oesophagogastroscopy** and **pH study** showing hyperacidity. *Finalized by the predictable outcome of management,* e.g. treatment of acute bleed as DU; stop aspirin, NSAIDs, alcohol; antacids, H₂ blocker, or PPI.
Oesophageal varices	*Suggested by:* liver cirrhosis, splenomegaly, prominent upper abdominal veins. *Confirmed by:* **oesophagogastroscopy** showing varicose mucosa and blood distally and in stomach. *Finalized by the predictable outcome of management,* e.g. if bleeding stopped, propranolol or long-acting nitrate. Still bleeding: large-bore IV or central line, fluids IV (colloid initially) ± transfusion, CVP monitoring, NG tube + irrigation, urinary catheter to monitor output, correct coagulopathy with FFP and vitamin K IV. Surgical or gastro intervention, e.g. banding or sclerotherapy.
Mallory–Weiss tear	*Suggested by:* preceding marked vomiting, later bright red blood. *Confirmed by:* **oesophagogastroscopy** showing tear. *Finalized by the predictable outcome of management,* e.g. monitor vital signs, Hb, fluids IV, nil by mouth, surgical intervention if persistent bleeding requiring blood transfusion, treatment of underlying cause.
Oesophageal carcinoma	*Suggested by:* progressive dysphagia with solids that stick, weight loss. *Confirmed by:* **barium swallow, fibreoptic gastroscopy with mucosal biopsy** showing malignant tissue. *Finalized by the predictable outcome of management,* e.g. treat severe bleed as DU. Nil by mouth, fluids IV, analgesics ± blood transfusion if bleeding continues ± antibiotic prophylaxis, surgical intervention, e.g. oesophageal dilatation or stent insertion by endoscopy.

Gastric carcinoma	*Suggested by:* marked anorexia, fullness, pain, Troisier's sign (enlarged left supraclavicular lymph (Virchow's) node). *Confirmed by:* **oesophagogastroscopy with biopsy** showing malignant tissue. *Finalized by the predictable outcome of management,* e.g. NG tube + nil by mouth, fluids IV, analgesics ± transfusion, treatment of severe bleed as DU, surgical intervention.
Gastro-oesophageal reflux	*Suggested by:* heartburn worse when lying flat, anorexia, nausea ± regurgitation of gastric content. *Confirmed by:* appearance of erosion on **oesophagoscopy, barium meal,** and **pH study** showing ↑acidity. *Finalized by the predictable outcome of management,* e.g. treatment of severe bleed as DU. Small meals, no food before bed, raise head of bed, antacids. Moderate to severe: nil by mouth, fluids IV, H_2 blocker or PPI, antibiotics to eradicate *H. pylori* if ulceration.
Hiatus hernia	*Suggested by:* heartburn, worse with stooping, relieved by antacids. *Confirmed by:* herniation of stomach into chest on plain X-ray or barium meal, appearance of erosion on **oesophagoscopy** and **pH study** showing hyperacidity. *Finalized by the predictable outcome of management,* e.g. treatment of severe bleed as DU. Reduce weight, avoid stooping, semi-sitting position for sleep, correct constipation, antacids, PPI, or H_2 blockers for pain.
Ingestion of corrosives	*Suggested by:* history of ingestion, etc. *Confirmed by:* **oesophagogastroscopy** showing severe erosions. *Finalized by the predictable outcome of management,* e.g. removal of offending agent, fluids IV ± blood transfusion if hypotension or bleeding, laryngoscopy ± tracheostomy if respiratory distress; broad-spectrum antibiotics infection, steroids to reduce stricture formation.
Meckel's diverticulum	*Suggested by:* no haematemesis, usually asymptomatic, anaemia, rectal bleeding. *Confirmed by:* **technetium-labelled red blood cell scan** showing isotopes in gut lumen and laparotomy. *Finalized by the predictable outcome of management,* e.g. fluids IV, nil by mouth ± NG tube, transfusion if significant bleeding, surgical intervention.
False haemate-mesis	*Suggested by:* swallowed nose bleed or haemoptysis. *Confirmed by:* normal **oesophagogastroscopy** and **bleeding source** identified in nose. *Finalized by the predictable outcome of management,* e.g. treatment of underlying cause.
Also	Angiodysplasia, bleeding disorders, vascular ectasia, arteriovenous malformations, Dieulafoy's lesion, hereditary haemorrhagic telangiectasia (Osler–Weber–Rendu), gallstone erosion, gastrinoma (Zollinger–Ellison syndrome), foreign bodies, etc.

Passage of blood per rectum

May not be noticed by the patient but only be discovered on rectal examination. Initial investigations (other tests in **bold** below): FBC, CRP or ESR, LFT, sigmoidoscopy or proctoscopy, AXR.

Main differential diagnoses and typical outline evidence, etc.	
Bleeding haemorrhoids	*Suggested by:* pain, discharge, pruritus, staining of toilet paper following defaecation. *Confirmed by:* physical and digital rectal examination, proctoscopy. *Finalized by the predictable outcome of management,* e.g. high-fibre diet, hydrocortisone suppositories for pruritus ± surgical intervention.
Anal fissure	*Suggested by:* skin tag, pain on defaecation, staining of toilet paper following defaecation, exquisite anal tenderness. *Confirmed by:* history and clinical examination. *Finalized by the predictable outcome of management,* e.g. high-fibre diet, stool softeners, warm sitz baths, analgesic cream, glyceryl trinitrate ointment, oral or topical diltiazem, botulinum toxin injection, surgical, e.g. sphincterotomy if above fails.
Diverticulitis	*Suggested by:* bloody 'splash in the pan', abdominal pain, usually LIF, diarrhoea and constipation. *Confirmed by:* **colonoscopy, barium enema**. *Finalized by the predictable outcome of management,* e.g. mild: clear liquids only, antibiotics, e.g. ciprofloxacin and metronidazole or co-amoxiclav for >7d, then high-fibre-diet. Severe: fluids IV, nil by mouth, metronidazole IV + a 3rd generation cephalosporin or a fluoroquinolone.
Carcinoma rectum	*Suggested by:* rectal bleeding with defaecation, unsatisfactory defaecation. *Confirmed by:* **sigmoidoscopy with biopsy**. *Finalized by the predictable outcome of management,* e.g. surgical intervention.
Colonic carcinoma	*Suggested by:* red blood mixed with stool and alternate diarrhoea and constipation. *Confirmed by:* **flexible colonoscopy with biopsy**. *Finalized by the predictable outcome of management,* e.g. surgical intervention.
Ulcerative colitis	*Suggested by:* lower abdominal pain, urgency to defaecate, severe bloody diarrhoea, fever in acute attack. *Confirmed by:* **colonoscopy with biopsy, barium studies** show loss of haustration, mucosal oedema, ulceration. *Finalized by the predictable outcome of management,* e.g. nil by mouth, fluids IV with K+ supplements, corticosteroids IV, antibiotics ± parenteral nutrition, surgical intervention if toxic megacolon.

Massive upper GI bleed	*Suggested by:* bright or dark red 'maroon'-coloured stool. *Confirmed by:* **upper GI endoscopy**. *Finalized by the predictable outcome of management,* e.g. stop aspirin or NSAIDs, large-bore IV or central line, group and crossmatch, fluids IV (colloid initially), transfusion, CVP monitoring, irrigate stomach, nil by mouth, correct coagulopathy with FFP and platelets, urine catheter to monitor output; gastro or surgical intervention.
Crohn's disease	*Suggested by:* chronic diarrhoea with abdominal pain, weight loss, palpable RLQ mass or fullness, mouth ulcers. *Confirmed by:* **colonoscopy with biopsy, barium studies** show 'skip lesions', string sign in advanced cases. *Finalized by the predictable outcome of management,* e.g. mild: antimotility drugs (e.g. loperamide); severe: fluids IV, corticosteroids IV or PO, 5-ASA analogues (e.g. mesalazine, sulfasalazine), analgesics, elemental diet ± parenteral nutrition.
Meckel's diverticulum	*Suggested by:* usually asymptomatic, anaemia, rectal bleeding. *Confirmed by:* **technetium-labelled red blood cell scan, laparotomy**. *Finalized by the predictable outcome of management,* e.g. fluids IV, nil by mouth ± NG tube, transfusion, surgical intervention if significant bleeding.
Trauma (in children, possible non-accidental injury)	*Suggested by:* fresh blood, sometimes external signs of trauma. *Confirmed by:* sensitive and careful history, possible surveillance, etc. *Finalized by the predictable outcome of management,* e.g. analgesia, comforting, etc.
Intussusception	*Suggested by:* child in first 6–18mo of life, acute onset of colicky intermittent abdominal pain, redcurrant 'jelly' PR bleed ± a sausage-shaped mass in upper abdomen. *Confirmed by:* **barium enema** ± reduction of intussusception with appropriate hydrostatic pressure. *Finalized by the predictable outcome of management,* e.g. fluids IV, NG tube for decompression, analgesics, therapeutic enemas, e.g. hydrostatic reduction.
Also	Ischaemic colitis, infectious colitis, angiodysplasia (lower bowel), stercoral ulcers, congenital polyps and hamartomas, etc.

Tenesmus

Intense desire to defaecate, but no stool. Initial investigations (other tests in **bold** below): FBC, CRP or ESR, LFT, sigmoidoscopy or proctoscopy, AXR.

Main differential diagnoses and typical outline evidence, etc.

Rectal inflammation (proctitis)	*Suggested by:* rectal bleeding, mucus discharge. *Confirmed by:* proctoscopy or **sigmoidoscopy** reveals inflamed rectal mucosa. *Finalized by the predictable outcome of management,* e.g. steroid suppositories or 5-ASA enemas or suppositories in mild disease; fluids IV if vomiting, antibiotics for infection, e.g. ceftriaxone, azithromycin, or doxycycline if *Chlamydia*.
Rectal tumour	*Suggested by:* rectal bleeding with defaecation, blood limited to surface of stool. *Confirmed by:* **sigmoidoscopy with rectal biopsy**. *Finalized by the predictable outcome of management,* e.g. surgical intervention.
Tumour of descending colon	*Suggested by:* alternate diarrhoea and constipation. *Confirmed by:* **colonoscopy with biopsy, barium enema**. *Finalized by the predictable outcome of management,* e.g. surgical intervention.
Pelvic inflammatory disease	*Suggested by:* lower abdominal pain, fever, vaginal discharge, dysuria, ↑ESR and CRP, leucocytosis. *Confirmed by:* **high vaginal swab, pelvic US scan ± laparoscopy**. *Finalized by the predictable outcome of management,* e.g. analgesia, fluids IV if dehydrated, empirical antibiotics, e.g. cefoxitin or other 2nd generation cephalosporin + doxycycline or clindamycin + gentamicin or ofloxacin + metronidazole.
Also	Haemorrhoids, rectal polyps, ulcerative colitis, infectious dysentery, etc.

Anorectal pain

Initial investigations (other tests in **bold** below): FBC, CRP or ESR, LFT, sigmoidoscopy or proctoscopy, AXR.

Main differential diagnoses and typical outline evidence, etc.

Anal fissure	*Suggested by:* skin tag, pain on defaecation, staining of toilet paper following defaecation. *Confirmed by:* physical examination of anal region. *Finalized by the predictable outcome of management,* e.g. high-fibre diet, stool softeners, warm sitz baths, analgesic cream, glyceryl trinitrate ointment, oral or topical diltiazem, botulinum toxin injection near to the fissures, surgical, e.g. sphincterotomy if medical therapy fails.
Haemorrhoids (thrombosed pile)	*Suggested by:* rectal bleeding following defaecation, perianal protrusion with pain. *Confirmed by:* digital rectal examination. *Finalized by the predictable outcome of management,* e.g. high-fibre diet, hydrocortisone for pruritus, surgical intervention.
Perianal abscess	*Suggested by:* severe constant throbbing pain, fever, tender lump, redness. *Confirmed by:* digital rectal examination. *Finalized by the predictable outcome of management,* e.g. analgesics, paracetamol for fever, surgical, e.g. drainage of abscess.
Proctalgia fugax, coccydynia	*Suggested by:* fleeting pain in rectum or coccyx which may be related to sitting but not defaecation, pain wakes patient at night. *Confirmed by:* physical examination, tenderness of levator muscle. *Finalized by the predictable outcome of management,* e.g. reassurance, analgesics.
Proctitis	*Suggested by:* rectal bleeding, mucus discharge. *Confirmed by:* proctoscopy or **sigmoidoscopy** revealing inflamed rectal mucosa. *Finalized by the predictable outcome of management,* e.g. steroid suppositories or 5-ASA enemas or suppositories in mild disease; fluids IV if nausea and vomiting, antibiotics for infection, e.g. ceftriaxone, azithromycin, or doxycycline if *Chlamydia*.
Prostatitis (referred pain)	*Suggested by:* rigor, fever, urinary frequency and urgency, dysuria, haemospermia. *Confirmed by:* tender prostate gland on PR examination, **urine microscopy**. *Finalized by the predictable outcome of management,* e.g. bed rest, NSAIDs for pain control, fluids IV, lactulose, antibiotics, e.g. cefotaxime or ceftriaxone ±aminoglycosides.
Also	Anal herpes, pilonidal sinus and abscess, caudal equine lesion, anal or rectal malignancy, trauma, referred pain from uterine disease, or pelvic inflammatory disease, faecal impaction, perianal fistula, levator ani syndrome, retained foreign body, etc.

Distended abdomen

Inspect the abdomen from a sitting position next to the bed or couch. Consider the general shape, then look at the skin. Next, consider movement of the abdomen. The causes are the traditional 6 'F's: Fat, Fluid, Flatus, Faeces, Fibroids, Foetus. Initial investigations (other tests in **bold** below): FBC, clotting screen, U&E, CRP or ESR, LFT, AXR, sigmoidoscopy or proctoscopy.

Main differential diagnoses and typical outline evidence, etc.	
Fat (obese)	*Suggested by:* usually sunken umbilicus, dullness to percussion throughout. *Confirmed by:* **CT abdomen**. *Finalized by the predictable outcome of management,* e.g. lifestyle changes—low-calorie diet, increased physical exercise.
Fluid (ascites)	*Suggested by:* bilateral bulging flanks, shifting dullness, fluid thrill. *Confirmed by:* **US scan liver and abdomen**. *Finalized by the predictable outcome of management,* e.g. salt restriction, fluid restriction if Na^+ <120mmol/L, spironolactone 100–400mg/d ± furosemide 40–120mg/d, thiamine 25–50mg od if alcoholic, daily weight; ascitic tap—paracentesis if gross ascites and symptomatic, treatment of underlying cause.
Flatus (gas) due to normal dietary variation	*Suggested by:* tympanic sound throughout. Often associated constipation. *Confirmed by:* **AXR** shows normal gas shadow. *Finalized by the predictable outcome of management,* e.g. diet change.
Small bowel obstruction ('flatus' again)	*Suggested by:* mild distension, early vomiting, central/upper abdominal pain, resonant percussion, increased bowel sounds. Supine AXR showing central gas but no peripheral abdominal large bowel shadow (i.e. without haustra partly crossing) but valvulae conniventes of small intestine entirely crossing the lumen. Fluid levels on erect film. *Confirmed by:* **abdominal US scan** and **laparotomy** findings. *Finalized by the predictable outcome of management,* e.g. NG tube + nil by mouth, fluids IV, surgical intervention.
Large bowel obstruction	*Suggested by:* severe distension, late vomiting, visible peristalsis, resonant percussion, increased bowel sounds. Supine AXR showing peripheral abdominal large bowel shadow (with haustra partly crossing the lumen). Fluid levels on erect film. *Confirmed by:* **abdominal US scan** and **laparotomy** findings. *Finalized by the predictable outcome of management,* e.g. NG tube with suction, nil by mouth, fluids IV, monitor intake and output, preop antibiotics, surgical intervention.

Splenic rupture (?delayed)	*Suggested by:* history of trauma (road traffic accident, fall onto left chest wall), bruising over left chest wall or upper abdomen, falling BP, rising pulse, abdominal tenderness, diminished bowel sounds, plain **AXR**—loss of left psoas shadow, **peritoneal tap** demonstrates free blood.
	Confirmed by: CT scan appearance.
	Finalized by the predictable outcome of management, e.g. large-bore IV access, group and crossmatch, fluids IV, colloid ± then blood. NG tube + nil by mouth, urethral catheter to monitor output, analgesics. Surgical, e.g. splenectomy, etc.
Faecal impaction	*Suggested by:* paucity of bowel movement and constipation. **AXR** shows stippled pattern of 'faecal loading'.
	Confirmed by: resolution of swelling with evacuation or partly with flatus tube.
	Finalized by the predictable outcome of management, e.g. laxatives, enemas ± gentle digital disimpaction.
Fibroids, large ovarian cyst	*Suggested by:* mass in pelvis in middle-aged female.
	Confirmed by: **abdominal US scan** or **CT**.
	Finalized by the predictable outcome of management, e.g. NSAIDs for pain, gynae intervention.
Foetus	*Suggested by:* amenorrhoea and mass in pelvis (cannot get below it).
	Confirmed by: +ve **urine pregnancy test** or ↑**plasma hCG**. Also **abdominal US scan.**
	Finalized by the predictable outcome of management, e.g. antenatal clinic follow-up.

Distended abdominal veins

This suggests that there is an obstruction to normal venous flow and that it is being diverted via superficial veins. Initial investigations (other tests in **bold** below): FBC, clotting screen, U&E, CRP or ESR, LFT, AXR.

Main differential diagnoses and typical outline evidence, etc.	
Portal hypertension	*Suggested by:* veins radiating out from umbilicus (caput medusa) ± ascites ± splenomegaly, other stigmata of chronic liver disease, venous hum over collaterals.
	Confirmed by: **US scan appearance** of liver which is small, cirrhotic with dilated portal veins.
	Finalized by the predictable outcome of management, e.g. β-blocker, e.g. propranolol, treat complications, e.g. oesophageal varices, ascites.
Superior vena cava obstruction (due to bronchogenic carcinoma, non-Hodgkin's lymphoma, etc.)	*Suggested by:* distended veins with blood flow from chest towards groin when compressed and one end released.
	Confirmed by: **CT thorax**.
	Finalized by the predictable outcome of management, e.g. elevate the head of the bed, O_2, corticosteroids and diuretics for laryngeal or cerebral oedema, treat underlying cause.
Inferior vena cava obstruction	*Suggested by:* distended veins with blood flow up from groin towards chest when compressed and one end released.
	Confirmed by: **CT abdomen**.
	Finalized by the predictable outcome of management, e.g. treat cause, e.g. DVT—anticoagulants or thrombolysis.

Abdominal bruising

Also consider the general causes of bruising as indicated in the general examination findings. Initial investigations (other tests in **bold** below): FBC, clotting screen, U&E, LFT, AXR.

Main differential diagnoses and typical outline evidence, etc.	
Retroperitoneal haemorrhage e.g. in acute pancreatitis	*Suggested by:* abdominal tenderness and rigidity, bruises in and around the umbilicus (Cullen's sign), on one or both flanks (Grey Turner's sign). *Confirmed by:* ↑**serum amylase, CT abdomen**. *Finalized by the predictable outcome of management,* e.g. pain relief, e.g. pethidine, nil by mouth, fluids IV, monitor glucose and Ca^{2+} (if acute pancreatitis), NG tube + nil by mouth for ileus, colloid ± blood.
Ruptured or dissecting abdominal aortic aneurysm	*Suggested by:* hypotension and abdominal pain, tenderness and rigidity, bruises in and around the umbilicus (Cullen's sign), on one or both flanks (Grey Turner's sign). Expansile pulsatile mass >3cm diameter, bruit over the mass. *Confirmed by:* **abdominal US scan** or **CT abdomen**. *Finalized by the predictable outcome of management,* e.g. pain control with morphine, group and crossmatch, IV access, reduce systolic BP to 100–120mmHg with labetalol IV or propranolol, nitroprusside may be added, intubate if haemodynamically unstable, refer for surgical repair.
Splenic rupture (?delayed)	*Suggested by:* history of trauma (road traffic accident, fall on to left chest wall), bruising over left chest wall or upper abdomen, falling BP, rising pulse, abdominal tenderness, diminished bowel sounds, plain AXR—loss of left psoas shadow, **peritoneal tap** demonstrates free blood. *Confirmed by:* **CT scan** appearance. *Finalized by the predictable outcome of management,* e.g. large-bore IV access, group and crossmatch, fluids IV, colloid then ± blood. NG tube + nil by mouth, urethral catheter to monitor output, analgesics. Surgical, e.g. splenectomy, etc.

Poor abdominal movement

From the sitting position, watch and ask about any areas of tenderness and begin furthest away, palpating gently looking at the patient's face to see if there is any reaction. 'Rigidity' is when there is no initial lack of resistance but reflex rigidity from the outset. Initial investigations (other tests in **bold** below): FBC, clotting screen, U&E, LFT, AXR.

Main differential diagnoses and typical outline evidence, etc.	
Small bowel obstruction	*Suggested by:* mild distension, early vomiting, central/upper abdominal pain, resonant percussion, increased bowel sounds. Supine AXR shows central gas but no peripheral abdominal large bowel shadow (i.e. without haustra partly crossing) but valvulae conniventes of small intestine crossing the entire lumen. Fluid levels on erect film. *Confirmed by:* **abdominal US scan** and **laparotomy** findings. *Finalized by the predictable outcome of management,* e.g. NG tube + nil by mouth, fluids IV, surgical intervention.
Large bowel obstruction	*Suggested by:* severe distension, late vomiting, visible peristalsis, resonant percussion, increased bowel sounds. Supine AXR shows peripheral abdominal large bowel shadow (with haustra partly crossing the lumen). Fluid levels on erect film. *Confirmed by:* **abdominal US scan** and **laparotomy** findings. *Finalized by the predictable outcome of management,* e.g. NG tube + suction, nil by mouth, fluids IV, monitor intake and output, preop antibiotics, surgical intervention.
Peritonitis from perforated stomach, duodenum, diverticulum; intraperitoneal haemorrhage, or bowel infarction	*Suggested by:* decreased or absent abdominal movement, generalized tenderness and rigidity, absent bowel sounds, and board-like rigidity. *Confirmed by:* **erect AXR** or **CXR** show gas under diaphragm and laparotomy. *Finalized by the predictable outcome of management,* e.g. analgesics, fluids IV, NG tube + nil by mouth for ileus, broad-spectrum antibiotics—2nd or 3rd generation cephalosporin or quinolone ± metronidazole.

Localized tenderness in the hypogastrium (suprapubic area)

Initial investigations (other tests in **bold** below): FBC, U&E, LFT, urine dip-stick testing, MSU culture, and sensitivity.

Main differential diagnoses and typical outline evidence, etc.	
Acute bladder distension (due to prostatic hypertrophy in males)	*Suggested by:* suprapubic mass (cannot get below), dull to percussion. *Confirmed by:* **bladder US scan**, **urethral catheterization** and drainage of high volume of urine (e.g. >1L). *Finalized by the predictable outcome of management,* e.g. urethral or suprapubic catheter, treat underlying cause, e.g. α-blocker for prostatic hypertrophy, urological intervention.
Cystitis	*Suggested by:* frequency of urine, dysuria, turbid urine, haematuria on dipstick. *Confirmed by:* excess **WBC** and organisms on microscopy and growth of 'significant' bacterial colonies on **MSU** culture. *Finalized by the predictable outcome of management,* e.g. fluids to rehydrate (IV if vomiting), provisional antibiotics, e.g. trimethoprim, pending sensitivities.

Localized tenderness in the right upper quadrant

Initial investigations (other tests in **bold** below): FBC, U&E, LFT, AXR.

Main differential diagnoses and typical outline evidence, etc.	
Acute cholecystitis	*Suggested by:* fever, guarding and +ve Murphy's sign (abrupt stopping of inspiration when the palpating hand meets the inflamed gallbladder descending with the liver from behind the subcostal margin on the right side—but not on the left side).
	Confirmed by: **US scan gallbladder and biliary ducts.**
	Finalized by the predictable outcome of management, e.g. nil by mouth, fluids IV, opioid analgesia, antibiotics IV, e.g. metronidazole + cephalosporin.
Acute alcoholic hepatitis	*Suggested by:* history of recent drinking binge, tender hepatomegaly, jaundice.
	Confirmed by: rise and fall in LFT to coincide with binge, –ve **hepatitis serology**.
	Finalized by the predictable outcome of management, e.g. stop alcohol, no specific treatment in mild illness, folate and thiamine supplements. If hepatic failure: monitor blood glucose, electrolytes, liver function and coagulation profile, IV infusion 5% glucose (10% if ↓blood glucose), NG tube + nil by mouth, neomycin PO, lactulose, vitamin K IV.
Acute viral hepatitis A (or hepatitis B, C, D, or E)	*Suggested by:* –ve history of recent binge drinking, fever, tender hepatomegaly, jaundice.
	Confirmed by: +ve **hepatitis serology A, B C, D, or E**.
	Finalized by the predictable outcome of management, e.g. antipyretics, fluids IV, anti-emetics, colestyramine for severe pruritus. If hepatic failure: manage as in acute alcoholic hepatitis.
Acute liver congestion	*Suggested by:* tender hepatomegaly, ↑JVP, leg oedema.
	Confirmed by: **CXR** showing large heart, **liver US scan** showing distension.
	Finalized by the predictable outcome of management, e.g. salt and fluid restriction, furosemide IV or PO ± K⁺ supplement, treat underlying cause.
Liver abscess pyogenic, amoebic, or fungal	*Suggested by:* fever, anorexia, malaise, ±tender hepatomegaly.
	Confirmed by: ↑WCC, **liver US or CT scan**.
	Finalized by the predictable outcome of management, e.g. percutaneous or surgical drainage + IV antibiotics e.g. carbapenem, or 2nd generation cephalosporin + metronidazole or clindamycin if pyogenic, metronidazole if amoebic, amphotericin B if fungal.

| Chlamydia peritonitis (Curtis–Fitz-Hugh syndrome) with generalized peritonitis and pelvic inflammatory disease | *Suggested by:* tenderness in right upper quadrant and in lower abdomen. Cervical and ovarian tenderness.

Confirmed by: **US scan ± CT scan** of gallbladder and remainder of the abdomen and pelvis showing 'violin string' adhesions. **High vaginal swab** showing chlamydia trachomatis.

Finalized by the predictable outcome of management, e.g. antibiotics according to culture and senstivity results. Possible division of adhesions and future management of infertiility. |

Localized tenderness in the left upper quadrant

Initial investigations (other tests in **bold** below): FBC, U&E, LFT, AXR.

Main differential diagnoses and typical outline evidence, etc.	
Pyelonephritis	*Suggested by:* fever, rigor, vomiting, loin pain, tenderness at renal angle, ↑**WCC**, proteinuria, haematuria, leucocytes on **urine testing**.
	Confirmed by: above clinical picture and 'significant' growth of organisms on **urine culture**. US scan for possible anatomical abnormality.
	Finalized by the predictable outcome of management, e.g. fluids IV, anti-emetic; provisional antibiotics: ampicillin + gentamicin or 3rd generation cephalosporin, e.g. ceftriaxone.
Splenic rupture (?delayed)	*Suggested by:* history of trauma (road traffic accident, fall on to left chest wall), bruising over left chest wall or upper abdomen, falling BP, rising pulse, abdominal tenderess, diminished bowel sounds, plain AXR—loss of left psoas shadow, **peritoneal tap** demonstrates free blood.
	Confirmed by: CT scan appearance.
	Finalized by the predictable outcome of management, e.g. large-bore IV access, group and crossmatch, fluids IV, colloid then ±blood. NG tube + nil by mouth, urethral catheter to monitor output, analgesics. Surgical, e.g. splenectomy, etc.
Splenic infarct	*Suggested by:* presence of predisposing cause, especially sickle cell disease and crisis.
	Confirmed by: **CT abdomen**.
	Finalized by the predictable outcome of management, e.g. pain control with opioid analgesics or NSAIDs, surgical intervention if abscess, haemorrhage, or pseudocyst develops.

Localized tenderness in the epigastrium or central abdomen

Initial investigations (other tests in **bold** below): FBC, U&E, LFT, AXR.

Main differential diagnoses and typical outline evidence, etc.

Gastritis

Suggested by: epigastric pain, dull or burning discomfort, nocturnal pain.

Confirmed by: **oesophagogastroscopy, barium meal,** and **pH study.**

Finalized by the predictable outcome of management, e.g. antacids, H₂ blocker or PPI if symptoms persist.

DU

Suggested by: epigastric pain, dull or burning discomfort, typically relieved by food, nocturnal pain.

Confirmed by: **oesophagogastroscopy, barium meal,** and **pH study. H. pylori** present in mucosa or **serology.**

Finalized by the predictable outcome of management, e.g. antacids, H₂ blocker or PPI for 4wk; H. pylori eradication therapy if H. pylori +ve: two antibiotics + one PPI, e.g. omeprazole or lansoprazole + metronidazole or amoxicillin + clarithromycin.

GU

Suggested by: epigastric pain, dull or burning discomfort, typically exacerbated by food.

Confirmed by: **oesophagogastroscopy, barium meal,** and **pH study.**

Finalized by the predictable outcome of management, e.g. antacids, H₂ blocker or PPI for 8wk; H. pylori eradication therapy if H. pylori +ve (as for DU).

Pancreatitis

Suggested by: rigidity or guarding ± bruises, e.g. Cullen or Grey Turner's signs.

Confirmed by: ↑↑**serum amylase, CT pancreas** showing enlargement cyst/pseudocyst.

Finalized by the predictable outcome of management, e.g. acute: pethidine, nil by mouth, fluids IV, monitor glucose and Ca²⁺, NG tube + nil by mouth if ileus, colloids and blood; chronic: analgesics, pancreatic supplements, monitor blood glucose—?onset diabetes.

Small bowel infarction

Suggested by: abdominal distension, absent bowel sounds. Predisposing cause, e.g. atrial fibrillation, extensive atheroma in diabetes.

Confirmed by: **AXR** showing dilated loop of small bowel with valvulae conniventes but no large bowel (with haustra etc.).

Finalized by the predictable outcome of management, e.g. fluids if hypovolaemia, analgesics, broad-spectrum antibiotics, surgical intervention.

Ruptured or dissecting abdominal aortic aneurysm

Suggested by: hypotension and abdominal pain, tenderness and rigidity, bruises in and around the umbilicus (Cullen's sign), on one or both flanks (Grey Turner's sign). Expansile pulsatile mass >3cm diameter, bruit over the mass.

Confirmed by: **abdominal US scan** or **CT abdomen.**

Finalized by the predictable outcome of management, e.g. morphine, group and crossmatch, reduce systolic BP to 100–120mmHg with IV labetalol or propranolol ± sodium nitroprusside, NG tube + nil by mouth, surgical intervention.

Localized tenderness in the left or right loin

Initial investigations (other tests in **bold** below): FBC, U&E, LFT, AXR.

Main differential diagnoses and typical outline evidence, etc.	
Pyelonephritis	*Suggested by:* fever, rigor, vomiting, loin pain, tenderness at renal angle, ↑**WCC**, proteinuria, haematuria, leucocytes on **urine testing**. *Confirmed by:* clinical picture and 'significant' growth of organisms on **urine culture**. **US scan** for possible anatomical abnormality. *Finalized by the predictable outcome of management,* e.g. fluids IV, analgesics, anti-emetic; provisional antibiotics pending sensitivities: ampicillin + gentamicin or 3rd generation cephalosporin, e.g. ceftriaxone.
Renal calculus	*Suggested by:* colicky pain beginning in loin and radiating down to lower abdomen. Tenderness at renal angle. *Confirmed by:* haematuria, dilated ureter on **renal US scan**, filling defect on **IVU**. *Finalized by the predictable outcome of management,* e.g. IV access, opioid analgesics and anti-emetic, urological intervention.
Ruptured or dissecting abdominal aortic aneurysm	*Suggested by:* hypotension and abdominal pain, tenderness and rigidity, bruises in and around the umbilicus (Cullen's sign), on one or both flanks (Grey Turner's sign). Expansile pulsatile mass >3cm diameter, bruit over the mass. *Confirmed by:* **abdominal US scan or CT abdomen.** *Finalized by the predictable outcome of management,* e.g. morphine, group and crossmatch, IV access, reduce systolic BP to 100–120mmHg with labetalol IV or propranolol ± sodium nitroprusside, NG tube + nil by mouth, surgical intervention.

Localized tenderness in left or right lower quadrant

Initial investigations (other tests in **bold** below): FBC, U&E, LFT, AXR.

Main differential diagnoses and typical outline evidence, etc.	
Appendicitis	*Suggested by:* abdominal pain, then localized to right lower quadrant (rarely to left in situs inversus), GUARDING +VE, +ve Rovsing's sign (tender on contralateral side), psoas sign (pain from passive extension of right hip), adductor pain (on passive internal rotation of flexed thigh); anterior tenderness on rectal exam.
	Confirmed by: macroscopic and microscopic appearances at **laparotomy**.
	Finalized by the predictable outcome of management, e.g. nil by mouth, fluids IV, NG tube + nil by mouth if vomiting, analgesics, broad-spectrum antibiotic, e.g. cephalosporin, surgical intervention.
Diverticulitis	*Suggested by:* LIF tenderness ± tender mass.
	Confirmed by: **flexible sigmoidoscopy, barium enema**.
	Finalized by the predictable outcome of management, e.g. mild: clear liquids only, ciprofloxacin PO + metronidazole PO for >7d, then high-fibre diet. Severe: fluids IV, nil by mouth, paracetamol for fever, metronidazole IV + a 3rd generation cephalosporin or a fluoroquinolone.
Mesenteric adenitis (or NSAP)	*Suggested by:* RLQ pain, anorexia, fever.
	Confirmed by: diffuse RLQ tenderness, no guarding, no rebound, no right-sided rectal tenderness, self-limiting outcome.
	Finalized by the predictable outcome of management, e.g. analgesia.
Ectopic pregnancy	*Suggested by:* enlarged uterus (but often small for dates), vaginal bleeding, faintness/shock in acute rupture.
	Confirmed by: pregnancy test +ve, mass on bimanual examination. **Pelvic US scan** shows empty uterus with thickened decidua.
	Finalized by the predictable outcome of management, e.g. analgesics, fluid resuscitation if hypotension or shock, urgent surgical intervention.

Hepatomegaly—smooth and tender

Initial investigations (other tests in **bold** below): FBC, coagulation profile, U&E, LFT, US scan.

Main differential diagnoses and typical outline evidence, etc.

Alcoholic hepatitis	*Suggested by:* history of drinking binge, ↑MCV, jaundice. *Confirmed by:* abnormal **LFT**: ↑AST, ↑ALP, **liver biopsy** later. *Finalized by the predictable outcome of management,* e.g. no alcohol, folate and thiamine supplements, vitamin K IV if coagulopathy; if acute hepatic failure, monitor blood glucose, U&E, LFT, and coagulation profile. IV infusion 5% glucose (10% if ↓blood glucose), NG tube + nil by mouth, neomycin PO, lactulose, vitamin K IV.
Infectious hepatitis	*Suggested by:* sharp edge, no or slight splenomegaly, jaundice. *Confirmed by:* abnormal LFT, hepatitis A serology +ve. *Finalized by the predictable outcome of management,* e.g. antipyretics, fluids IV and anti-emetics if vomiting, colestyramine for pruritus.
Glandular fever (infectious mononucleosis)	*Suggested by:* cervical lymphadenopathy, sharp edge ± splenomegaly ± jaundice. *Confirmed by:* **Paul–Bunnell**, +ve **heterophil antibody test**. *Finalized by the predictable outcome of management,* e.g. gargles/lozenges, analgesics, paracetamol; if neurological involvement, thrombocytopenia or haemolysis, no aspirin (causes Reye syndrome). Amoxicillin causes rash.
Right heart failure due to pulmonary hypertension. Acutely due to pulmonary embolus	*Suggested by:* leg oedema, ↑JVP. *Confirmed by:* large heart on **CXR** and associated large pulmonary arteries or pulmonary oedema if congestive cardiac failure, **echocardiogram**—dilated right ventricle. *Finalized by the predictable outcome of management,* e.g. stop smoking, salt and fluid restriction, O$_2$, furosemide IV or PO ± K+ supplement, treat underlying cause.
Tricuspid regurgitation with right heart failure	*Suggested by:* pulsatile liver ± jaundice, ↑JVP with big V waves, systolic murmur louder on inspiration. *Confirmed by:* **echocardiogram**—dilated right ventricle. *Finalized by the predictable outcome of management,* e.g. bed rest during acute phase, stop smoking, salt and fluid restriction, give O$_2$, furosemide IV or PO ± K$^+$ supplement, treat cause.
Also	Hepatic abscess, Budd–Chiari syndrome (hepatic vein thrombosis), etc.

Hepatomegaly—smooth but not tender

Initial investigations (other tests in **bold** below): FBC, coagulation profile, U&E, LFT, US scan.

Main differential diagnoses and typical outline evidence, etc.

Cirrhosis of the liver (early + fatty change)	*Suggested by:* firm, round edge ± splenomegaly, other stigmata of chronic liver disease (e.g. spider naevi). *Confirmed by:* small liver with abnormal parenchyma on **liver US scan and biopsy** appearance. *Finalized by:* the predictable outcome of management, e.g. stop alcohol, treat cause.
Lymphoma (Hodgkin's or non-Hodgkin's)	*Suggested by:* generalized lymphadenopathy, non-tender hepatomegaly, splenomegaly. *Confirmed by:* **lymph node biopsy, bone marrow biopsy, CT thorax/abdomen.** *Finalized by:* the predictable outcome of management, e.g. analgesics, transfusion if symptomatic anaemia, platelet transfusion if platelet count <20,000, broad-spectrum antibiotics IV if febrile and neutropaenia, staging + chemotherapy ± radiotherapy.
Leukaemia	*Suggested by:* anaemia, lymphadenopathy, splenomegaly. *Confirmed by:* abnormal WBC on blood film, **bone marrow examination**. *Finalized by:* the predictable outcome of management, e.g. analgesics, transfusion if symptomatic anaemia, platelet transfusion if platelet count <20,000, broad-spectrum antibiotics if fever and neutropaenia, paracetamol for fever. Oncology management.
Haemochromatosis	*Suggested by:* bronze skin pigmentation, evidence of diabetes mellitus, cardiac failure, arthropathy. *Confirmed by:* ↑**serum ferritin** (>500 micrograms/L), **liver biopsy with hepatic iron measurement.** *Finalized by:* the predictable outcome of management, e.g. regular venesection (prolongs life) e.g. 1 unit 1–2x per wk, then 1 unit per 3mo when serum iron and ferritin 'normal'.
Primary biliary cirrhosis	*Suggested by:* xanthelasmata and xanthomas, pruritus, scratch marks, arthralgia ± splenomegaly. *Confirmed by:* +ve **anti-mitochondrial antibody**, ↑**serum IgM, liver biopsy**. *Finalized by:* the predictable outcome of management, e.g. no alcohol, colestyramine to relieve pruritus (or ursodeoxycholic acid).

Amyloidosis in kidneys or heart, nerves, gut, liver, primary or secondary to rheumatoid, inflammatory bowel disease, TB, etc.	*Suggested by:* evidence of underlying chronic infective or inflammatory disease if secondary. *Confirmed by:* **biopsy of rectal mucosa,** stained with Congo red dye. *Finalized by the predictable outcome of management,* e.g. identify organ failure and treat, including associated illness, e.g. chronic infection, chronic inflammation, or myeloma.
Also	Fatty liver, human immunodeficiency virus (HIV) infection, sarcoidosis, emphysema (apparent hepatomegaly), etc.

Hepatomegaly—irregular, not tender

Initial investigations (other tests in **bold** below): FBC, coagulation profile, U&E, LFT, US scan.

Main differential diagnoses and typical outline evidence, etc.

Metastatic carcinoma	*Suggested by:* hard ±nodular liver, cachexia. *Confirmed by:* **liver US scan** or **CT ±biopsy**. *Finalized by the predictable outcome of management, e.g.* analgesics, packed cell transfusion if anaemia, hydration and bisphosphonate if hypercalcaemia, FFP and vitamin K for coagulopathy, nutritional support, treat primary.
Hepatoma	*Suggested by:* firm, nodular edge ± arterial bruit, weight loss, jaundice. *Confirmed by:* ↑ serum alpha-fetoprotein, **liver US scan** or CT and **biopsy**. *Finalized by the predictable outcome of management, e.g.* surgical intervention, adjunct chemotherapy.
Hydatid cyst	*Suggested by:* sometimes hard, nodular. *Confirmed by:* **liver US scan** or CT showing cyst and daughter cysts inside, eosinophilia, **serology** (Echinococcus granulosus), **Casoni intradermal test**. *Finalized by the predictable outcome of management, e.g.* albendazole for six 1-mo cycles separated by 14d interval, monitor FBC and LFT, surgical, e.g. resection of the cyst.
Also	Polycystic liver disease, macronodular cirrhosis, etc.

Splenomegaly—slight (<3 fingers)

Spleen enlarges diagonally downwards towards the RLQ. Begin there so as not to miss edge of massive enlargement. Initial investigations (other tests in **bold** below): FBC, coagulation profile, U&E, LFT, US scan.

Main differential diagnoses and typical outline evidence, etc.	
Glandular fever	Suggested by: cervical lymphadenopathy, hepatomegaly with sharp edge. Confirmed by: **Paul–Bunnell, +ve heterophil antibody test (Monospot®).** Finalized by the predictable outcome of management, e.g. gargles/lozenges, analgesics, paracetamol; if neurological involvement, thrombocytopenia, or haemolysis, no aspirin (causes Reye syndrome), amoxicillin causes rash.
Brucella	Suggested by: occupation, e.g. farmer, hepatomegaly. Confirmed by: **brucella serology.** Finalized by the predictable outcome of management, e.g. doxycycline + rifampicin for 6wk or doxycycline + streptomycin IM for 3wk for osteomyelitis, meningitis, or endocarditis. Prednisolone if CNS is involved.
Hepatitis A, B, C, or D	Suggested by: jaundice, tender hepatomegaly, lymphadenopathy. Confirmed by: abnormal **LFT, hepatitis A, B, C, and D serology.** Finalized by the predictable outcome of management, e.g. antipyretics, fluids IV and anti-emetics if vomiting, colestyramine for pruritus. In hepatic failure: monitor blood glucose, U&E, LFT, coagulation profile, IV infusion 5% glucose (10% if ↓blood glucose), NG tube + nil by mouth, neomycin PO, lactulose, vitamin K IV.
Bacterial endocarditis	Suggested by: splinter haemorrhages, heart murmur, anaemia, microscopic haematuria. Confirmed by: **blood cultures, trans-oesophageal echocardiography.** Finalized by the predictable outcome of management, e.g. antibiotics depending on organism and sensitivities, valve surgery.
Amyloidosis in kidneys or heart, nerves, gut, liver, 1° or 2° to rheumatoid, inflammatory bowel disease, TB, etc.	Suggested by: evidence of underlying chronic infective or inflammatory disease if secondary. Confirmed by: **biopsy of rectal mucosa,** stained with Congo red dye. Finalized by the predictable outcome of management, e.g. identify organ failure and treat, including associated illness, e.g. chronic infection, chronic inflammation or myeloma.

Haemolytic anaemia	*Suggested by:* anaemia, jaundice.
	Confirmed by: FBC showing reticulocytosis, anaemia, **LFT** showing ↑unconjugated bilirubin, ↑serum LDH, ↓haptoglobin.
	Finalized by the predictable outcome of management, e.g. avoid fava beans in G6PD deficiency ± blood transfusion; surgical, e.g. splenectomy. Immunization against *H. influenza* and *S. pneumoniae* procedure.
Also	Polycythaemia rubra vera, essential thrombocythaemia, megaloblastic anaemia, e.g. pernicious anaemia, chronic iron deficiency anaemia, idiopathic thrombocytopenic purpura, systemic lupus erythematosis, polyarteritis nodosa, Felty's syndrome, etc.

Splenomegaly—moderate (3–5 fingers)

Initial investigations (other tests in **bold** below): FBC, coagulation profile, U&E, LFT, US scan.

Main differential diagnoses and typical outline evidence, etc.	
Lymphoma (Hodgkin's or non-Hodgkin's)	*Suggested by:* generalized lymphadenopathy, non-tender hepatomegaly, splenomegaly. *Confirmed by:* **lymph node biopsy, bone marrow biopsy, CT thorax/abdomen.** *Finalized by the predictable outcome of management,* e.g. analgesics, transfusion if symptomatic anaemia, platelet transfusion if platelet count <20,000, broad-spectrum antibiotics if febrile and neutropaenia, staging + chemotherapy ± radiotherapy.
Chronic leukaemia	*Suggested by:* lymphadenopathy, non-tender hepatomegaly. *Confirmed by:* abnormal FBC and **blood film, bone marrow examination**. *Finalized by the predictable outcome of management,* e.g. supportive therapy includes analgesics, blood transfusion if symptomatic anaemia, platelet transfusion if platelet count <20,000, broad-spectrum antibiotics IV if febrile and neutropaenia, oncology management.
Cirrhosis ± portal hypertension	*Suggested by:* hard, round edge ± hepatomegaly, other stigmata of chronic liver disease. *Confirmed by:* small nodular **liver on US scan** ± biopsy. *Finalized by the predictable outcome of management,* e.g. no alcohol, propranolol if portal hypertension, treat underlying cause.
Also	Haemoglobinopathy, reticuloses e.g. lymphadenoma, storage disease e.g. Gaucher's disease, histiocytosis X e.g. Hand–Schuller–Christian, Letterer–Siwe syndrome, etc.

Splenomegaly—massive (>5 fingers)

Spleen enlarges diagonally downwards towards the RLQ. Begin there so as not to miss edge of massive enlargement. Initial investigations (other tests in **bold** below): FBC, coagulation profile, U&E, LFT, US scan.

Main differential diagnoses and typical outline evidence, etc.	
Chronic myeloid leukaemia	*Suggested by:* variable hepatomegaly, bruising, anaemia. *Confirmed by:* presence of **Philadelphia chromosome**, ⇈WCC. *Finalized by the predictable outcome of management,* e.g. hydration, avoid antiplatelets, e.g. aspirin, packed cell transfusion if symptomatic anaemia, platelet transfusion if platelet count <20,000, broad-spectrum antibiotics IV covering *Pseudomonas* and Gram +ve bacteria if febrile and neutropaenic. Specialist treatment—hydroxycarbamide to control WBC, imatinib 1st line therapy ± bone marrow transplant.
Myelofibrosis	*Suggested by:* anaemia ± **hepatomegaly** ± **lymphadenopathy**. *Confirmed by:* **bone marrow tap** is usually dry, **bone marrow biopsy** shows fibrosis. *Finalized by the predictable outcome of management,* e.g. analgesics, blood transfusion if symptomatic anaemia, platelet transfusion if platelet count <20,000, broad-spectrum antibiotics IV if febrile and neutropaenia, specialist treatment.
Malaria	*Suggested by:* anaemia, jaundice, hepatomegaly, paroxysmal rigors. *Confirmed by:* **thick and thin blood films** showing *Plasmodium*. *Finalized by the predictable outcome of management,* e.g. paracetamol for fever, transfusion for severe anaemia. Antimalarials: Chloroquine+primaquine (or artemisinin based combination therapy if chloroquine-resistant) for *P. vivax*, *P. ovale*, *P. malariae*, *P. knowlesi*; artemisinin-based combination therapy for at least 3d, e.g. dihydroartemisinin+piperaquine for *P. falciparum*, artesunate IV if severe *P. falciparum*. Please refer to WHO guidelines for the up to date treatment regimens at ✍ http://www.who.int/topics/malaria/en
Kala-azar (visceral leishmaniasis)	*Suggested by:* pancytopaenia, hepatomegaly. *Confirmed by:* demonstration of *Leishmania donovani* in **Giemsa-stained smears**, specific **serological test.** *Finalized by the predictable outcome of management,* e.g. transfusion for bleeding or anaemia, antibiotics for intercurrent infection; specific drugs: pentavalent antimonial compound, e.g. sodium stibogluconate or meglumine antimoniate; or for liposomal form: amphotericin B.

Bilateral masses in upper abdomen

The lower half of normal right kidney is often palpable. A renal mass is bimanually ballotable, moves slightly downwards on inspiration. Initial investigations (other tests in **bold** below): FBC, U&E, LFT, US scan.

Main differential diagnoses and typical outline evidence, etc.	
Polycystic renal disease	*Suggested by:* masses are bimanually ballotable, family history, hypertension. *Confirmed by:* **US scan/CT kidneys.** *Finalized by the predictable outcome of management,* e.g. keep BP <130/85 (125/75 if proteinuria is present) with ACE inhibitors or angiotensin receptor blockers, monitor renal function and renal US scan yearly, treat UTI, analgesics (avoid NSAIDs), dialysis if end-stage renal failure develops.
Bilateral hydronephroses	*Suggested by:* masses bimanually ballotable, renal impairment. *Confirmed by:* dilated ureters ± renal calyces on **abdominal US scan**. *Finalized by the predictable outcome of management,* e.g. analgesics, treat infection, urinary catheter if lower tract obstruction, urology intervention.
Amyloidosis in kidneys or heart, nerves, gut, liver, 1° or 2° to rheumatoid, inflammatory bowel disease, TB, etc	*Suggested by:* evidence of underlying chronic infective or inflammatory disease if secondary. *Confirmed by:* **biopsy of rectal mucosa,** stained with Congo red dye. *Finalized by the predictable outcome of management,* e.g. identify organ failure and treat, including associated illness, e.g. chronic infection, chronic inflammation, or myeloma.

Unilateral mass in right or left upper quadrant

Initial investigations (other tests in **bold** below): FBC, U&E, LFT, US scan.

Main differential diagnoses and typical outline evidence, etc.	
Renal carcinoma	*Suggested by:* haematuria, pyrexia of unknown origin (PUO) ± polycythaemia. *Confirmed by:* **renal US scan/CT with biopsy.** *Finalized by the predictable outcome of management,* e.g. surgical referral.
Unilateral hydronephrosis	*Suggested by:* no other symptoms and signs except bimanually ballotable mass. *Confirmed by:* unilateral dilated ureter ± **renal calyx on abdominal US scan.** *Finalized by the predictable outcome of management,* e.g. urology intervention e.g. insertion of nephrostomy tube or ureteric stent.
Renal cyst	*Suggested by:* tense, fluctuant feel. *Confirmed by:* cyst on **abdominal US scan**. *Finalized by the predictable outcome of management,* e.g. antibiotic if UTI is present.
Distended gallbladder (on right side)	*Suggested by:* right-sided, pear-shaped rounded mass that continues with the liver above (Courvoisier's sign—implies extrahepatic biliary obstruction). *Confirmed by:* **US scan gallbladder and biliary ducts.** *Finalized by the predictable outcome of management,* e.g. analgesics, fluids IV, NG drainage, broad-spectrum antibiotics, surgical intervention.

Mass in epigastrium (± umbilical area)

Initial investigations (other tests in **bold** below): FBC, U&E, LFT, US scan.

Main differential diagnoses and typical outline evidence, etc.	
Gastric carcinoma	*Suggested by:* anorexia, weight loss over weeks to months, hard, irregular mass, left supraclavicular node (Virchow's node giving Troisier's sign).
	Confirmed by: **gastroscopy with biopsy**.
	Finalized by the predictable outcome of management, e.g. NG tube, nil by mouth, fluids IV, analgesics, surgical intervention.
Carcinoma of pancreas	*Suggested by:* progressive painless jaundice ± abdominal or back pain later.
	Confirmed by: **ERCP** or **MRCP**.
	Finalized by the predictable outcome of management, e.g. low-fat and high-protein diet, analgesics, pancreatic supplement, phenothiazine or colestyramine to reduce pruritus; surgical intervention.
Aortic aneurysm	*Suggested by:* >3cm in diameter, pulsatile swelling with bruit.
	Confirmed by: **abdominal US scan** or **CT abdomen**.
	Finalized by the predictable outcome of management, e.g. BP control, surgical intervention.

Mass in right lower quadrant

Initial investigations (other tests in **bold** below): FBC, U&E, LFT, US scan.

Main differential diagnoses and typical outline evidence, etc.	
Appendix mass	*Suggested by:* recent history of fever and right iliac fossa (RIF) pain. *Confirmed by:* **US scan** or **CT abdomen** and findings at **laparotomy**. *Finalized by the predictable outcome of management,* e.g. fluids IV, NG tube + nil by mouth and suction if ileus, broad-spectrum antibiotic, surgical intervention.
Crohn's granuloma	*Suggested by:* aphthous ulcers, wasting, anaemia, tender mass, scars of previous surgery, anal fissures, fistulae. *Confirmed by:* **barium follow-through** and **small bowel enema, colonoscopy with biopsy.** *Finalized by the predictable outcome of management,* e.g. analgesics, haematinics, nutritional support.
Carcinoma of caecum	*Suggested by:* asymptomatic right iliac fossa mass, iron-deficiency anaemia. *Confirmed by:* **colonoscopy with biopsy.** *Finalized by the predictable outcome of management,* e.g. iron supplement, transfusion if severe anaemia; fluids IV, nil by mouth, NG tube + nil by mouth if bowel obstruction is present; surgical intervention.
Transplanted kidney	*Suggested by:* obvious history of transplant and scar over mass, usually in iliac fossa. *Confirmed by:* **abdominal US scan.**
Other causes	Intussusception, carcinoma of ascending colon, caecal volvulus, ileocaecal tuberculosis, right ovarian neoplasm, etc.

Mass in hypogastrium (suprapubic region)

Initial investigations (other tests in **bold** below): FBC, U&E, LFT, US scan.

Main differential diagnoses and typical outline evidence, etc.	
Distended bladder	*Suggested by:* suprapubic dullness, resonance in flank, tender mass and acute retention of urine. *Confirmed by:* mass disappears on **bladder US scan** and **catheterization, abdominal/pelvic US scan**. *Finalized by the predictable outcome of management,* e.g. urethral or suprapubic catheter to relieve retention, treat cause or urology intervention.
Pregnant uterus	*Suggested by:* suprapubic dullness, resonance in flank. *Confirmed by:* **pregnancy test** +ve, bimanual examination, **abdominal/pelvic US scan**. *Finalized by the predictable outcome of management,* e.g. antenatal clinic follow-up.
Uterine fibroid	*Suggested by:* asymptomatic, hard, rounded, non-tender mass on bimanual palpation. *Confirmed by:* **pelvic examination and US scan**. *Finalized by the predictable outcome of management,* e.g. analgesia, gynae intervention.
Uterine neoplasm	*Suggested by:* postmenopausal bleeding, bloodstained vaginal discharge, irregular bleeding. *Confirmed by:* pelvic examination and **pelvic US scan**. *Finalized by the predictable outcome of management,* e.g. gynae intervention.
Ovarian cyst	*Suggested by:* tense, fluctuant feel, fluid thrill if cyst is large. *Confirmed by:* pelvic examination and **US scan of ovary.** *Finalized by the predictable outcome of management,* e.g. analgesia, gynae intervention.

Mass in left lower quadrant

Initial investigations (other tests in **bold** below): FBC, U&E, LFT, US scan.

Main differential diagnoses and typical outline evidence, etc.	
Diverticular abscess	*Suggested by:* fever, tender mass. *Confirmed by:* **US scan/CT abdomen/pelvis**. *Finalized by the predictable outcome of management,* e.g. fluids IV, nil by mouth, paracetamol for pain and fever, antibiotics, e.g. metronidazole IV + a 3rd generation cephalosporin or a fluoroquinolone.
Carcinoma of descending or sigmoid colon	*Suggested by:* hard mass, not tender. *Confirmed by:* **barium enema, colonoscopy with biopsy.** *Finalized by the predictable outcome of management,* e.g. NG tube + nil by mouth with suction if obstructed, fluids IV, monitor intake and output, preop antibiotics; surgical intervention.
Faecal impaction	*Suggested by:* paucity of bowel movement and constipation. **AXR** shows stippled pattern of 'faecal loading'. *Confirmed by:* resolution of swelling with evacuation or partly with flatus tube. *Finalized by the predictable outcome of management,* e.g. laxatives, enemas ± digital disimpaction.
Also	Left ovarian neoplasm

Central dullness, resonance in flank

Initial investigations (other tests in **bold** below): FBC, U&E, LFT, US scan.

Main differential diagnoses and typical outline evidence, etc.	
Distended bladder	*Suggested by:* suprapubic mass, tender in acute retention of urine.
	Confirmed by: mass disappears on **bladder US scan and catheterization**.
	Finalized by the predictable outcome of management, e.g. urethral or suprapubic catheter to relieve retention, α-blocker for prostatism, treat cause, urology intervention.
Pregnant uterus	*Suggested by:* suprapubic mass.
	Confirmed by: **pregnancy test** +ve, pelvic/**abdominal US scan.**
	Finalized by the predictable outcome of management, e.g. antenatal clinic follow-up.
Massive ovarian cyst	*Suggested by:* tense, fluctuant feel, fluid thrill.
	Confirmed by: **pelvic/abdominal US scan.**
	Finalized by the predictable outcome of management, e.g. analgesia, gynae intervention.

Shifting dullness

Implies ascites. Initial investigations (other tests in **bold** below): FBC, U&E, LFT, US scan.

Main differential diagnoses and typical outline evidence, etc.	
Carcinomatosis with spread to peritoneum	*Suggested by:* cachexia. *Confirmed by:* **diagnostic paracentesis** including **cytology, liver US scan with biopsy.** *Finalized by the predictable outcome of management,* e.g. analgesia, paracentesis if massive ascites, packed cells if anaemia, hydration, FFP and vitamin K for coagulopathy, nutritional support, look for primary.
Cirrhosis	*Suggested by:* stigmata of chronic liver disease ± splenomegaly. *Confirmed by:* **paracentesis, liver US scan with biopsy.** *Finalized by the predictable outcome of management,* e.g. no alcohol, propranolol if portal hypertension, paracentesis if massive ascites, spironolactone PO ± furosemide PO, treat underlying cause.
Congestive cardiac failure	*Suggested by:* ↑JVP, leg oedema ± tender hepatomegaly. *Confirmed by:* **LFT,** FBC, **diagnostic paracentesis, CXR, echocardiogram.** *Finalized by the predictable outcome of management,* e.g. salt and fluid restriction, O_2, furosemide IV or PO ± K^+ supplement, spironolactone PO, look for cause.
Nephrotic syndrome	*Suggested by:* generalized oedema, including face on rising from bed. *Confirmed by:* **proteinuria >3g/d, hypoalbuminaemia.** *Finalized by the predictable outcome of management,* e.g. monitor BP, intake and output, fluid restriction to 1L/d, furosemide IV, monitor renal function; low protein, phosphate, and potassium diet; ACE inhibitor or ARB if hypertension. Establish cause, e.g. if glomerulonephritis, consider prednisolone.
Also	Pulmonary hypertension, tuberculosis, acute or chronic peritonitis, malnutrition, myxodema, Meig's syndrome, etc.

Silent abdomen with no bowel sounds

Initial investigations (other tests in **bold** below): FBC, U&E, LFT, AXR.

Main differential diagnoses and typical outline evidence, etc.	
Peritonitis e.g. due to bowel perforation	*Suggested by:* decreased or absent abdominal movement, generalized tenderness with 'board-like' rigidity. *Confirmed by:* **AXR**, erect **CXR** shows gas under diaphragm. *Finalized by the predictable outcome of management,* e.g. analgesia, fluids IV, NG tube + nil by mouth if ileus, broad-spectrum antibiotics, e.g. 2nd or 3rd generation cephalosporin or quinolone ± metronidazole. Surgical, e.g. repair of perforation.
Bowel infarction due to embolus, e.g. from fibrillating atrium or atheroma, e.g. in diabetic	*Suggested by:* decreased or absent abdominal movement, generalized tenderness with 'board-like' rigidity. *Confirmed by:* **AXR**, erect **CXR** shows no gas under diaphragm. *Finalized by the predictable outcome of management,* e.g. fluids IV if hypovolaemia, analgesia, broad-spectrum anibiotics. Surgical, e.g. possible resection of infarcted bowel.

High-pitched bowel sounds

Initial investigations (other tests in **bold** below): FBC, U&E, LFT, AXR.

Main differential diagnoses and typical outline evidence, etc.	
Small bowel obstruction	*Suggested by:* mild distension, early vomiting, central/upper abdominal pain, resonant percussion, increased bowel sounds. Supine AXR showing central gas but no peripheral abdominal large bowel shadow (i.e. without haustra partly crossing) but valvulae conniventes of small intestine entirely crossing the lumen. Fluid levels on erect film. *Confirmed by:* **abdominal US scan and laparotomy findings**. *Finalized by the predictable outcome of management,* e.g. NG tube + nil by mouth, fluids IV, surgical, e.g. initial defunctioning ileostomy.
Large bowel obstruction	*Suggested by:* severe distension, late vomiting, resonant percussion, increased bowel sounds. Supine AXR showing peripheral abdominal large bowel shadow (with haustra partly crossing the lumen). Fluid levels on erect film. *Confirmed by:* **abdominal US scan and laparotomy findings.** *Finalized by the predictable outcome of management,* e.g. NG tube + suction, nil by mouth, fluids IV, monitor intake and output, preop antibiotics, surgical, e.g. initial defunctioning colostomy.
Hernial orifice strangulation	*Suggested by:* hernia visible, not reducible, very ill, peritonism, **signs of bowel obstruction**. *Confirmed by:* **laparotomy** findings. *Finalized by the predictable outcome of management,* e.g. NG tube with suction, fluids IV, monitor intake and output, preop antibiotics, surgical intervention.
Sigmoid volvulus	*Suggested by:* **signs of severe bowel obstruction**. Supine AXR showing U-shaped gas shadow. *Confirmed by:* **sigmoidoscopy** and **reduction with flatus tube** and **laparotomy findings.** *Finalized by the predictable outcome of management,* e.g. analgesia, fluids IV, NG tube + nil by mouth; rigid sigmoidoscopic decompression, surgical, e.g. laparotomy and resection if gangrenous segment.
Irritable bowel syndrome	*Suggested by:* slight distension, history of abdominal pain and small hard motions. *Confirmed by:* abdominal US scan and spontaneous resolution. *Finalized by the predictable outcome of management,* e.g. high-fibre diet; symptomatic treatment, e.g. metoclopramide, mebeverine, loperamide, lactulose; reassurance.
Faecal impaction	*Suggested by:* paucity of bowel movement and constipation. Hard faeces on rectal examination. **AXR** shows stippled pattern of 'faecal loading'. *Confirmed by:* resolution of swelling with evacuation or partly with flatus tube. *Finalized by the predictable outcome of management,* e.g. laxatives and enemas ± digital disimpaction.

Abdominal/loin bruit

Initial investigations (other tests in **bold** below): FBC, U&E, LFT, US.

Main differential diagnoses and typical outline evidence, etc.	
Aortic aneurysm	*Suggested by:* systolic bruit in the epigastrium (over mass), expansile pulsatile swelling.
	Confirmed by: **US scan/CT abdomen.**
	Finalized by the predictable outcome of management, e.g. BP control, surgical repair.
Renal artery stenosis	*Suggested by:* systolic bruit in the RUQ, hypertension.
	Confirmed by: **renal arteriography—spiral CT or MR angiography.**
	Finalized by the predictable outcome of management, e.g. BP control (ACE inhibitors contraindicated), renal angioplasty ± stenting.
Dissecting aorta	*Suggested by:* tearing abdominal pain radiating to back, hypertension (severe hypotension is a grave prognostic indicator). Brachial–ankle gradient and pulse delay.
	Confirmed by: urgent **US scan/CT abdomen.**
	Finalized by the predictable outcome of management, e.g. BP control with oral propranolol, or labetalol IV, or sodium nitroprusside IV; surgical intervention.

Lump in the groin

Initial investigations (other tests in **bold** below): FBC, U&E, LFT, US scan.

Main differential diagnoses and typical outline evidence, etc.	
Lymph node inflammation	*Suggested by:* enlarged, tender, mobile, nodes, usually multiple. *Confirmed by:* above clinical examination. *Finalized by the predictable outcome of management,* e.g. analgesics, treat underlying cause.
Inguinal hernia	*Suggested by:* origin horizontally just above and medial to pubic tubercle, impulse on coughing or bearing down, reducible. *Confirmed by:* above clinical examination and surgery. *Finalized by the predictable outcome of management,* e.g. surgical intervention, e.g. herniorrhaphy.
Femoral hernia	*Suggested by:* origin horizontally just below and lateral to pubic tubercle, cough impulse rarely detectable, usually irreducible (because of narrow femoral canal). *Confirmed by:* above clinical examination and surgery. *Finalized by the predictable outcome of management,* e.g. surgical intervention, e.g. hernia repair.
Strangulated hernia	*Suggested by:* irreducible, tense and tender, red, followed by symptoms and signs of bowel obstruction. *Confirmed by:* above clinical examination and surgery. *Finalized by the predictable outcome of management,* e.g. analgesia, fluids IV, nil by mouth and NG tube + nil by mouth if obstruction, urgent surgical intervention.
Lymphoma (Hodgkin's or non-Hodgkin's)	*Suggested by:* fixed nodes when infiltrated by tumour. *Confirmed by:* **US scan, exploration of groin.** *Finalized by the predictable outcome of management,* e.g. analgesics, transfusion if symptomatic anaemia, platelet transfusion if platelet count <20,000, broad-spectrum antibiotics IV if febrile and neutropaenia, staging + chemotherapy ± radiotherapy.
Femoral artery aneurysm	*Suggested by:* lump lies below the midpoint of the inguinal ligament, expansile pulsation. *Confirmed by:* above clinical examination. **Duplex US scan.** *Finalized by the predictable outcome of management,* e.g. surgical, e.g. elective repair or reconstruction.
Saphena varix (dilatation of long saphenous vein in the groin)	*Suggested by:* soft and diffuse swelling that lies below inguinal ligament, empties with minimal pressure and refills on release, disappears on lying down, cough impulse. *Confirmed by:* above clinical examination. *Finalized by the predictable outcome of management,* e.g. avoid prolonged standing, avoid wearing anything that constricts the limb, treat complications, e.g. phlebitis, ulceration, etc.; treat underlying cause.

Cold abscess of psoas sheath	*Suggested by:* fluctuant, tender swelling arising below the inguinal ligament. *Confirmed by:* **US scan, exploration of groin.** *Finalized by the predictable outcome of management,* e.g. surgical drainage or by CT guided percutaneous catheter, followed by antibiotics.
Also	Sebaceous cyst, local abscess, retractile testicle, lipoma, etc.

Scrotal swelling

Initial investigations (other tests in **bold** below): FBC, U&E, LFT, US scan.

Main differential diagnoses and typical outline evidence, etc.

Inguinal hernia descended into scrotum	*Suggested by:* inability to get above it. Does not transilluminate.
	Confirmed by: above clinical examination.
	Finalized by the predictable outcome of management, e.g. surgical, e.g. hernia repair.
Hydrocoele	*Suggested by:* non-tender, unilateral mass in scrotal sac.
	Confirmed by: above clinical examination and demonstration of transillumination.
	Finalized by the predictable outcome of management, e.g. surgical intervention if it gets larger and causes discomfort.
Epididymal cyst	*Suggested by:* non-tender nodule in the head of epididymis, adjacent to inferior pole of testis and transillumination.
	Confirmed by: above clinical examination and demonstration of transillumination.
	Finalized by the predictable outcome of management, e.g. surgical, e.g. spermatocoelectomy if large or enlarges or causes discomfort.
Testicular torsion	*Suggested by:* exquisitely tender, unilateral mass in the scrotal sac, cord thickened, opposite testis lies horizontally (bell clapper testis).
	Confirmed by: above clinical examination, **US scan** reveals ↓blood flow.
	Finalized by the predictable outcome of management, e.g. emergency! Skilled manual detorsion of testicle immediately.
Haematocoele	*Suggested by:* history of trauma or scrotal surgery. Tenderness.
	Confirmed by: above history and examination, US scan.
	Finalized by the predictable outcome of management, e.g. surgical, e.g. exploration and evacuation of haematoma.
Varicocoele (90% on the left)	*Suggested by:* non-tender, unilateral fleshy mass that feels like a bag of worms, decreases in size with scrotal elevation.
	Confirmed by: above clinical examination (patient must be examined while standing).
	Finalized by the predictable outcome of management, e.g. scrotal support ± surgical, e.g. varicocoelectomy.

Acute epididymitis	*Suggested by:* diffuse tenderness in the epididymis, marked redness and oedema.
	Confirmed by: **urine microscopy and culture** (white cells and organisms).
	Finalized by the predictable outcome of management, e.g. elevation of scrotum, cold packs to the scrotum regularly, analgesia, antibiotic, e.g. doxycycline or a cephalosporin.
Acute orchitis	*Suggested by:* large and tender testes, fever.
	Confirmed by: above history and examination.
	Finalized by the predictable outcome of management, e.g. elevation of scrotum, cold packs for comfort, analgesia, e.g. NSAIDs or opiate, oral antibiotics, e.g. ciprofloxacin or a cephalosporin.
Chronic epididymitis	*Suggested by:* chronic, diffuse scrotal tenderness.
	Confirmed by: identification of infecting organism by **urine cultures or culture of urethral discharge** after prostatic massage.
	Finalized by the predictable outcome of management, e.g. analgesia, e.g. NSAIDs, antibiotics, e.g. doxycycline or a cephalosporin ± epididymectomy.
Spermatocoele	*Suggested by:* non-tender, small nodules posterior to the head of the epididymis.
	Confirmed by: above clinical examination, may or may not transilluminate.
	Finalized by the predictable outcome of management, e.g. surgical, e.g. spermatocoelectomy if enlarging or causes discomfort.
Seminoma	*Suggested by:* firm, non-tender, non-transilluminable nodule or mass adjacent to a testis.
	Confirmed by: **US scan of scrotal contents** showing a solid testicular mass, **direct surgical examination**, normal **serum alpha-fetoprotein**.
	Finalized by the predictable outcome of management, e.g. radiotherapy ± chemotherapy and orchidectomy.
Teratoma	*Suggested by:* firm, non-tender, non-transilluminable nodule or mass adjacent to a testis.
	Confirmed by: **US scan of scrotal contents** showing a solid testicular mass, **direct surgical examination**, ↑**serum alpha-fetoprotein.**
	Finalized by the predictable outcome of management, e.g. surgical, e.g. resection, followed by chemotherapy.

Anal swelling

The rectal examination (with a chaperone) begins with an examination of the anus by parting the buttocks with the patient lying in the left lateral position with knees flexed. Initial investigations (other tests in **bold** below): FBC, U&E, LFT.

Main differential diagnoses and typical outline evidence, etc.	
Prolapsed internal haemorrhoids	*Suggested by:* segmental, plum-coloured rectal protrusion. *Confirmed by:* proctoscopy. *Finalized by the predictable outcome of management,* e.g. high-fibre diet, hydrocortisone suppositories for pruritus, surgical intervention.
Acute anal fissure	*Suggested by:* acute pain during defaecation, exquisite anal tenderness. Mucosal fissure with skin tag if chronic (sentinel pile). *Confirmed by:* above history and clinical **examination under anaesthesia.** *Finalized by the predictable outcome of management,* e.g. high-fibre diet, stool softeners, warm sitz baths, analgesic cream, glyceryl trinitrate ointment, oral or topical diltiazem, botulinum toxin injection near to the fissures, surgical, e.g. sphincterotomy if medical therapy fails.
Spontaneous perianal haematoma	*Suggested by:* blue-black lump in the skin near the anal margin. *Confirmed by:* above history and examination. *Finalized by the predictable outcome of management,* e.g. ice or cold packs.
Perianal abscess	*Suggested by:* tender, fluctuant, perianal mass. *Confirmed by:* above clinical examination. *Finalized by the predictable outcome of management,* e.g. analgesics, paracetamol for fever, surgical intervention, e.g. for incision and drainage of abscess.
Rectal prolapse	*Suggested by:* smooth, elongated, rectal protrusion continuous with anal skin. *Confirmed by:* above clinical examination. *Finalized by the predictable outcome of management,* e.g. local perianal analgesia, reduction with digital pressure, treat constipation.

Enlargement of prostate

The rectal examination continues by feeling for a prostatic protrusion anteriorly and sweeping around for other masses including impacted faeces.
Initial investigations (other tests in **bold** below): FBC, U&E, LFT.

Main differential diagnoses and typical outline evidence, etc.	
Prostatitis	*Suggested by:* smooth, enlarged and tender.
	Confirmed by: +ve **urine culture, culture of prostatic secretions**.
	Finalized by the predictable outcome of management, e.g. fluids IV if vomiting and dehydration, analgesia, e.g. NSAIDs, stool softener, antibiotics, e.g. cephalosporins.
Benign prostatic hypertrophy	*Suggested by:* smooth, enlarged, firm, non-tender usually with a palpable median groove.
	Confirmed by: normal or slightly ↑**serum prostatic-specific antigen (PSA), prostatic biopsy**.
	Finalized by the predictable outcome of management, e.g. ↓fluid intake before bedtime, α-blocker, e.g. terazosin, alfuzosin to relieve symptoms, 5-α reductase inhibitor, e.g. finasteride, dutasteride, urology intervention if severe symptoms.
Prostatic carcinoma	*Suggested by:* irregular, hard, sometimes obliteration of median groove, non-tender.
	Confirmed by: ↑↑**serum PSA, prostatic biopsy**.
	Finalized by the predictable outcome of management, e.g. supportive therapy, urological consultation.

Melaena on finger

The rectal examination ends by inspecting the faecal smear on the examining gloved finger for colour, especially bright red blood or tarry melaena. Initial investigations (other tests in **bold** below): FBC, U&E, LFT.

Main differential diagnoses and typical outline evidence, etc.	
Bleeding DU	*Suggested by:* epigastric pain and tenderness, nausea.
	Confirmed by: **oesophagogastroscopy** showing bleeding ulcer.
	Finalized by the predictable outcome of management, e.g. large-bore IV or central line, fluids IV, colloid initially ± transfusion, CVP monitoring, NG tube + nil by mouth + irrigation, urinary catheter to monitor output, surgical intervention. H_2 blocker or PPI for 4wk; *H. pylori* eradication therapy if *H. pylori* +ve.
Bleeding GU	*Suggested by:* epigastric pain, dull or burning discomfort, nocturnal pain.
	Confirmed by: appearance of ulcer on **oesophagogastroscopy** and **pH study** showing hyperacidity.
	Finalized by the predictable outcome of management, e.g. treat acute severe bleed as DU; antacid; H_2 blocker or PPI for 8wk; *H. pylori* eradication therapy if *H. pylori* +ve.
Gastric erosion	*Suggested by:* history of NSAIDs or alcohol ingestion, epigastric pain, dull or burning discomfort, nocturnal pain.
	Confirmed by: appearance of erosion on **oesophagogastroscopy** and **pH study** showing hyperacidity.
	Finalized by the predictable outcome of management, e.g. treat acute bleed as DU; stop aspirin, NSAIDs, alcohol; antacids, H_2 blocker, or PPI.
Oesophageal varices	*Suggested by:* liver cirrhosis, splenomegaly, prominent upper abdominal veins.
	Confirmed by: **oesophagogastroscopy** showing varicose mucosa and blood, distally and in stomach.
	Finalized by the predictable outcome of management, e.g. if bleeding stopped, propranolol or long-acting nitrate. Still bleeding: large-bore IV or central line, fluids IV (colloid initially) ± transfusion, CVP monitoring, NG tube + nil by mouth + irrigation, urinary catheter to monitor output, correct coagulopathy with FFP and vitamin K IV. Surgical or gastro intervention, e.g. banding or sclerotherapy.
Mallory–Weiss tear	*Suggested by:* preceding marked vomiting, later bright red blood.
	Confirmed by: **oesophagogastroscopy** showing tear.
	Finalized by the predictable outcome of management, e.g. monitor vital signs, Hb, fluids IV, nil by mouth, surgical intervention if persistent bleeding requiring blood transfusion, treat underlying cause.

Oesophageal carcinoma	*Suggested by:* progressive dysphagia with solids that stick, weight loss.
	Confirmed by: **barium swallow, fibreoptic gastroscopy with mucosal biopsy** showing malignant tissue.
	Finalized by the predictable outcome of management, e.g. treat severe bleed as DU. Nil by mouth, fluids IV, analgesics ± blood transfusion if bleeding continues ± antibiotic prophylaxis, surgical, e.g. oesophageal dilatation or stent insertion by endoscopy.
Gastric carcinoma	*Suggested by:* marked anorexia, fullness, pain, Troisier's sign (enlarged left supraclavicular lymph (Virchow's) node).
	Confirmed by: **oesophagogastroscopy with biopsy** showing malignant tissue.
	Finalized by the predictable outcome of management, e.g. NG tube + nil by mouth, fluids IV, analgesics ± transfusion, treat severe bleed as DU, surgical intervention.
Gastro-oesophageal reflux	*Suggested by:* heartburn worse when lying flat, anorexia, nausea ± regurgitation of gastric content.
	Confirmed by: appearance of erosion on **oesophagoscopy, barium meal,** and **pH study** showing ↑acidity.
	Finalized by the predictable outcome of management, e.g. treat severe bleed as in DU. Small meals, no food before bed, raise head of bed, antacids; moderate to severe: nil by mouth, fluids IV, H_2 blocker or PPI, antibiotics to eradicate *H. pylori* if ulceration.
Hiatus hernia	*Suggested by:* heartburn, worse with stooping, relieved by antacids.
	Confirmed by: herniation of stomach into chest on plain X-ray or barium meal, appearance of erosion on **oesophagoscopy** and **pH study** showing hyperacidity.
	Finalized by the predictable outcome of management, e.g. treat severe bleed as DU. Reduce weight, avoid stooping, semi-sitting position for sleep, correct constipation, antacids, H_2 blockers, or PPI for pain.
Ingestion of corrosives	*Suggested by:* history of ingestion, etc.
	Confirmed by: **oesophagogastroscopy** showing severe erosions.
	Finalized by the predictable outcome of management, e.g. removal of offending agent, fluids IV ± blood transfusion if hypotension or bleeding, laryngoscopy ± tracheostomy if respiratory distress; broad-spectrum antibiotics if infection, steroids to reduce stricture formation.
Meckel's diverticulum	*Suggested by:* no haematemesis, usually asymptomatic, anaemia, rectal bleeding.
	Confirmed by: **technetium-labelled red blood cell scan**, showing isotopes in gut lumen and laparotomy.
	Finalized by the predictable outcome of management, e.g. fluids IV, nil by mouth ± NG tube, transfusion if significant bleeding, surgical intervention.

(Continued)

False haematemesis	*Suggested by:* swallowed nose bleed or haemoptysis.
	Confirmed by: normal **oesophagogastroscopy** and **bleeding source** identified in nose.
	Finalized by the predictable outcome of management, e.g. treat underlying cause.
Bleeding diathesis	*Suggested by:* symptoms or signs of bleeding elsewhere (or bruising), drug history of warfarin, etc.
	Confirmed by: abnormal clotting screen and/or low platelets and/or improvement on withdrawal of a potentially causal drug. (NB Possibility of another cause.)
	Finalized by the predictable outcome of management, e.g. discontinue warfarin, treat underlying cause.
Also	Angiodysplasia.

Fresh blood on finger on rectal examination

Usually suggestive of lower GI bleeding, but occasionally from massive upper GI bleeding passing through rapidly without alteration. Initial investigations (other tests in **bold** below): FBC, U&E, LFT.

Main differential diagnoses and typical outline evidence, etc.	
Haemorrhoids	*Suggested by:* rectal bleeding follows defaecation, perianal protrusion with pain.
	Confirmed by: anal inspection and **proctoscopy** (haemorrhoids drop over edge of proctoscope as it is withdrawn).
	Finalized by the predictable outcome of management, e.g. high-fibre diet, hydrocortisone suppositories for pruritus ± surgical intervention.
Rectal carcinoma	*Suggested by:* rectal bleeding with defaecation, blood often limited to surface of stool.
	Confirmed by: **sigmoidoscopy with rectal biopsy.**
	Finalized by the predictable outcome of management, e.g. surgical intervention, e.g. resection.
Colonic carcinoma	*Suggested by:* alternate diarrhoea and constipation with red blood.
	Confirmed by: **colonoscopy with biopsy, barium enema.**
	Finalized by the predictable outcome of management, e.g. surgical intervention.
Ulcerative colitis	*Suggested by:* loose bloodstained stools, anaemia ± arthropathy, uveitis, and iritis.
	Confirmed by: **colonoscopy with biopsy, barium studies.**
	Finalized by the predictable outcome of management, e.g. mild: prednisolone PO and mesalazine ± prednisolone enemas. Moderate: prednisolone + 5-ASA ± prednisolone enemas. Severe: fluids IV + hydrocortisone, antibiotics, NG tube + nil by mouth, transfusion if severe anaemia, surgical intervention if toxic megacolon.
Angiodysplasia	*Suggested by:* chronic recurrent GI bleeding.
	Confirmed by: **endoscopy, mesenteric angiography.**
	Finalized by the predictable outcome of management, e.g. fluids IV ± blood transfusion if symptomatic anaemia, correct coagulopathy, surgical intervention.
Diverticulitis	*Suggested by:* history of red 'splash' in the toilet pan, LIF tenderness ± tender mass.
	Confirmed by: **flexible sigmoidoscopy, barium enema.**
	Finalized by the predictable outcome of management, e.g. fluids IV, nil by mouth, transfusion if significant bleeding occurs, surgical intervention.

Ischaemic colitis	*Suggested by:* left-sided abdominal pain, loose stools, dark clots.
	Confirmed by: **barium enema** (may show 'thumb printing' sign), **colonoscopy**.
	Finalized by the predictable outcome of management, e.g. analgesia, fluids IV, nil by mouth, O_2, NG tube + nil by mouth if ileus ± broad-spectrum antibiotics. Surgical intervention.
Meckel's diverticulum	*Suggested by:* usually asymptomatic, anaemia, rectal bleeding.
	Confirmed by: **technetium-labelled red blood cell scan, laparotomy**.
	Finalized by the predictable outcome of management, e.g. fluids IV, nil by mouth, transfusion if significant bleeding, surgical intervention.
Intussusception (in children or elderly)	*Suggested by:* child, usually between 6–18mo of life, acute onset of colicky intermittent abdominal pain, redcurrant 'jelly' PR bleed ± a sausage-shaped mass in upper abdomen.
	Confirmed by: **barium or air enema**, may reduce the intussusceptions with appropriate hydrostatic pressure.
	Finalized by the predictable outcome of management, e.g. fluids IV, NG tube + nil by mouth for decompression, analgesics, therapeutic enemas, e.g. hydrostatic reduction.
Mesenteric infarction (acute occlusion)	*Suggested by:* acute abdominal pain, generalized tenderness, shock, profuse diarrhoea (patient often in atrial fibrillation).
	Confirmed by: **mesenteric angiography, exploratory laparotomy.**
	Finalized by the predictable outcome of management, e.g. fluids if hypovolaemia, analgesics, broad-spectrum antibiotics, surgical intervention.
Massive upper GI bleed	*Suggested by:* bright or dark red 'maroon'-coloured stool.
	Confirmed by: **upper GI endoscopy**.
	Finalized by the predictable outcome of management, e.g. stop aspirin or NSAIDs, large-bore IV or central line, group and crossmatch, fluids IV (colloid initially), transfusion, CVP monitoring, NG tube + nil by mouth, irrigate stomach, nil by mouth, correct coagulopathy with FFP and platelets, urine catheter to monitor output; gastro or surgical intervention.
Crohn's disease	*Suggested by:* aphthous ulcers, anaemia, tender mass, scars of previous surgery, anal fissures, fistulae.
	Confirmed by: **colonoscopy with biopsy, barium studies.**
	Finalized by the predictable outcome of management, e.g. mild: antimotility drugs (e.g. loperamide. Acute attack: fluids IV, corticosteroids IV or PO, high dose 5-ASA analogues (e.g. mesalazine, sulfasalazine), analgesics, elemental diet ± parenteral nutrition.
Trauma	*Suggested by:* pain, history, or physical signs of trauma (e.g. sexual assault).
	Confirmed by: sigmoidoscopy.
	Finalized by the predictable outcome of management, e.g. counselling if sexual assault.

Urological and gynaecological symptoms and physical signs

Urinary frequency ± dysuria 400
Incontinence of urine alone (not faeces) 401
Incontinence of urine and faeces 402
Painful haematuria (with dysuria) 403
Painless haematuria 404
Secondary amenorrhoea 406
Excessive menstrual loss—menorrhagia 408
Intermenstrual or post-coital bleeding 410
Vulval skin abnormalities 411
Ulcers and lumps of the vulva 412
Lumps in the vagina 413
Ulcers and lumps in the cervix 414
Tender or bulky mass (uterus, Fallopian tubes, or ovary)
    on pelvic examination 416
Vaginal discharge 420
Enlargement of prostate 422

Urinary frequency ± dysuria

This is a very common presentation and may pass unnoticed by the patient, especially in the elderly. A urine dipstick test should be peformed at the slightest suspicion. Initial investigations (other tests in **bold** below): urine dipstick ± MSU, FBC.

Main differential diagnoses and typical outline evidence, etc.	
Urinary tract infection with cystitis	*Suggested by:* vomiting, fever, abdominal pain, blood in urine, nitrites, white cells, and blood on urine dipstick. *Confirmed by:* **MSU** microscopy and culture. **US scan** for possible anatomical abnormality. *Finalized by the predictable outcome of management,* e.g. increased fluid intake, cranberry juice, and regular bladder emptying. Provisional 1st line antibiotic pending MSU result, e.g. trimethoprim, cefalexin for 3d; 2nd line, e.g. ciprofloxacin for 5d.
Bladder or urethral calculus	*Suggested by:* suprapubic pain, macroscopic or microscopic haematuria. *Confirmed by:* **US scan** of bladder showing urethral dilation, **plain X-ray** showing radio-opaque calculus, **IVU** showing filling defect. *Finalized by the predictable outcome of management:* immediate analgesia, e.g. diclofenac (IM or suppository), or pethidine IM with metoclopramide IM + antibiotics. Emergency surgery if renal tract obstruction was confirmed on imaging.
Uterine prolapse	*Suggested by:* incontinence of urine, 'feeling like something coming down'. *Confirmed by:* pelvic examination: cervix observed in lower vagina. *Finalized by the predictable outcome of management,* e.g. improvement after weight reduction, smoking cessation, and treating coexisting conditions, e.g. COPD, constipation. Ring pessary for frail patients. Surgical correction of prolapse.
Prostatic hypertrophy	*Suggested by:* hesitancy, poor stream, urgency, incontinence, nocturia, acute retention of urine, large prostate on rectal examination. *Confirmed by:* ↑prostatic-specific antigen (PSA), **US scan of prostate gland**, and response to transurethral resection of prostate (TURP). *Finalized by the predictable outcome of management,* e.g. catheter for acute retention. α-blockers, e.g. tamsulosin, then trial without catheter. 5α-reductase inhibitors, e.g. finasteride, TURP.
'Spastic' bladder due to upper motor neurone lesion	*Suggested by:* weakness, increased tone, and reflexes in lower limbs. *Confirmed by:* small bladder on **US scan**. *Finalized by the predictable outcome of management,* e.g. antibiotics for infections, catheterization.

Incontinence of urine alone (not faeces)

This symptom may be hidden because of embarrassment; a hint of ammonia smell on the patient's clothing during the examination should prompt gentle questioning. Initial investigations (other tests in **bold** below): urine dipstick ± MSU, FBC.

Main differential diagnoses and typical outline evidence, etc.	
Prostatic hypertrophy	*Suggested by:* hesitancy, poor stream, urgency, incontinence, nocturia, acute retention of urine, large prostate on rectal examination. *Confirmed by:* ↑PSA, **US scan of prostate gland**, and response to TURP. *Finalized by the predictable outcome of management,* e.g. catheter for acute retention. α-blockers, e.g. tamsulosin, then trial without catheter. 5α-reductase inhibitors, e.g. finasteride. TURP.
Uterine prolapse	*Suggested by:* incontinence of urine, 'feeling like something coming down'. *Confirmed by:* pelvic examination: cervix observed in lower vagina. *Finalized by the predictable outcome of management,* e.g. improvement after weight reduction, smoking cessation and treating coexisting conditions, e.g. COPD, constipation. Ring pessary for frail patients. Surgical correction of prolapse for suitable cases.
Urinary tract infection with cystitis	*Suggested by:* vomiting, fever, abdominal pain, blood in urine, nitrites, white cells, and blood on urine dipstick. *Confirmed by:* **MSU** microscopy and culture. US scan for possible anatomical abnormality. *Finalized by the predictable outcome of management,* e.g. increased fluid intake, cranberry juice, and regular bladder emptying. Provisional 1st line antibiotic pending MSU result, e.g. trimethoprim, cefalexin for 3d. 2nd line, e.g. ciprofloxacin bd for 5d.
Weakness of pelvic floor muscles	*Suggested by:* incontinence during coughing, sneezing, laughing. *Confirmed by:* **urodynamic studies**. *Finalized by the predictable outcome of management,* e.g. pelvic floor exercises.

Incontinence of urine and faeces

Again this symptom may be hidden because of embarrassment; a hint of ammonia or faecal soiling on the patient's clothing during the examination should prompt gentle questioning. Initial investigations (other tests in **bold** below): Urine dipstick ± MSU, FBC.

Main differential diagnoses and typical outline evidence, etc.	
'Neurogenic' bladder	*Suggested by:* paresis, low tone and diminished reflexes in lower limbs, sensory loss in anal region.
	Confirmed by: small and spastic bladder (upper motor neurone) or large and hypotonic bladder (lower motor neurone) on **US scan**.
	Finalized by the predictable outcome of management, e.g. treatment of infection. Wearing pads. Catheterization.
Epileptic fits	*Suggested by:* history of loss of consciousness, tongue biting, jerking movements (may be subtle).
	Confirmed by: clinical history, electroencephalogram (**EEG**).
	Finalized by the predictable outcome of management, e.g. carbamazepine, lamotrigine, or topiramate in focal fits; valproate or lamotrigine for generalized fit.
Dementia (Alzheimer's, cerebrovascular disease with multi-infarct dementia, B_{12} or folate deficiency, hypothyroidism)	*Suggested by:* chronic worsening confusion, especially in elderly, previous strokes.
	Confirmed by: low mental score with or without cerebral atrophy on **CT head scan**.
	Finalized by the predictable outcome of management, e.g. a care management plan and family support. Cholinesterase inhibitors for Alzheimer's disease. Treatment of any cause.
Severe depression	*Suggested by:* severe lack of motivation, low mood, tearfulness, precipitating event, e.g. bereavement.
	Confirmed by: continence improvement in response to treatment of depression.
	Finalized by the predictable outcome of management, e.g. counselling. Anti-depression agents.
Faecal impaction with 'overflow'	*Suggested by:* hard, rock-like faeces in rectum.
	Confirmed by: response to evacuation of faeces.
	Finalized by the predictable outcome of management, e.g. laxatives: large doses of compound macrogols (e.g. Movicol®, Laxido®), phosphate enema. Manual evacuation.

Painful haematuria (with dysuria)

Initial investigations (other tests in **bold** below): Urine dipstick, MSU, FBC, U&E.

Main differential diagnoses and typical outline evidence, etc.	
Urinary tract infection with cystitis	*Suggested by:* vomiting, fever, abdominal pain, blood in urine, nitrites, white cells, and blood on urine dipstick. *Confirmed by:* **MSU** microscopy and culture. US scan for possible anatomical abnormality. *Finalized by the predictable outcome of management,* e.g. increased fluid intake, cranberry juice, and regular bladder emptying. Provisional 1st line antibiotic pending MSU result, e.g. trimethoprim, cefalexin for 3d. 2nd line, e.g. ciprofloxacin bd for 5d.
Renal calculus	*Suggested by:* dysuria, spasmodic loin to groin pain, no fever. *Confirmed by:* **MSU** showing RBC, **renal US scan** showing ureteric dilatation, **IVU** showing filling defect in contrast medium. *Finalized by the predictable outcome of management,* e.g. immediate analgesia, e.g. diclofenac (IM or suppository) or pethidine IM with metoclopramide a IM + antibiotics. Emergency surgery if renal tract obstruction proved on imaging.
Trauma (due to urethral catheterization, traumatic sexual intercourse)	*Suggested by:* dysuria, history of urethral catheterization, or recent painful sexual intercourse. *Confirmed by:* history, normal **MSU**, **renal US scan**, **IVU**. *Finalized by the predictable outcome of management:* analgesia, e.g. paracetamol, alkalinization of urine (e.g. cranberry juice).

Painless haematuria

In females, care has to be taken to distinguish between haematuria, vaginal, and anorectal bleeding. This may depend on the result of pelvic and rectal examination. Initial investigations (other tests in **bold** below): FBC with platelets, clotting tests, US scan of abdomen.

Main differential diagnoses and typical outline evidence, etc.	
Renal tumour	*Suggested by:* palpable mass, fever (often previously of unknown origin). *Confirmed by:* **US scan or CT of abdomen/kidney**, **IVU** showing renal mass. *Finalized by the predictable outcome of management,* e.g. nephrectomy and tumour histology for local disease, Immunotherapy for metastatic disease.
Ureteric tumour	*Suggested by:* colicky pain if obstructed. *Confirmed by:* **US scan or CT abdomen/kidney**, **IVU** showing ureteric mass. *Finalized by the predictable outcome of management,* e.g. stenting to relieve obstruction with resection of the tumour with or without nephrectomy or cystectomy depending on site.
Bladder tumour	*Suggested by:* pelvic pain, pelvic mass, recurrent urine infections, dysuria, haematuria. *Confirmed by:* positive **urine cytology**, **cystoscopy**, **IVU** shows filling defects of bladder. *Finalized by the predictable outcome of management,* e.g. depends on staging. T1 local excision by transurethral cystoscopy and diathermy, followed by intravesicular chemotherapeutic agents, e.g. mitomycin. T2–3 radical cystectomy with post-operative chemotherapy. T4 palliative chemo- or radiotherapy.
Bleeding diathesis	*Suggested by:* anticoagulant therapy, easy bruising, or other bleeding sites. *Confirmed by:* abnormal **clotting screen** ± **FBC**: ↓platelets. *Finalized by the predictable outcome of management,* e.g. if on warfarin and INR >3.5, follow BNF protocol for the management of a raised INR, Otherwise, detailed assessment of clotting or platelet abnormality and appropriate treatment.
Urinary tract infection with cystitis	*Suggested by:* vomiting, fever, abdominal pain, blood in urine, nitrites, white cells, and blood on urine dipstick. *Confirmed by:* **MSU** microscopy and culture. **US scan** for possible anatomical abnormality. *Finalized by the predictable outcome of management,* e.g. increased fluid intake, cranberry juice and regular bladder emptying. Provisional 1st line antibiotic pending MSU result, e.g. trimethoprim, cefalexin for 3d. 2nd line, e.g. ciprofloxacin bd for 5d.

Secondary amenorrhoea

Absence of menstruation for >6mo in women with previously normal menstrual cycles. Initial investigations (other tests in **bold** below): pregnancy test, FSH, LH, testosterone, and sex hormone binding globulin (SHBG), prolactin.

Main differential diagnoses and typical outline evidence, etc.	
Pregnancy	*Suggested by:* presentation during childbearing age. *Confirmed by:* **pregnancy test** +ve, **pelvic US scan**. *Finalized by the predictable outcome of management,* e.g. community maternity health team for antenatal care and follow-up.
Normal menopause	*Suggested by:* >40y of age, hot flushes. *Confirmed by:* ↑**FSH**. *Finalized by the predictable outcome of management,* e.g. hormone replacement therapy (HRT) to ease menopausal symptoms and prevent osteoporosis after counselling the patient about benefits and risks.
Premature ovarian failure	*Suggested by:* hot flushes, <40y of age, and no signs of other endocrine disease (adrenal failure, hypothyroidism, etc.). *Confirmed by:* ↑**LH**, ↑**FSH**, ↓**oestradiol**, **ovarian biopsy**: atrophic. *Finalized by the predictable outcome of management,* e.g. HRT until the age of 50y, then review after counselling.
Polycystic ovary syndrome	*Suggested by:* oligo-/amenorrhoea, hirsutism, head hair thinning, acne, obesity, impaired fasting glucose or type 2 diabetes mellitus, acanthosis nigricans, skin tags, infertility. *Confirmed by:* ↑testosterone, ↓SHBG, ↑LH, LH>FSH, cystic ovaries on **pelvic US scan**. *Finalized by the predictable outcome of management,* e.g. co-cyprindiol (for hirsutism, acne) + cyclical progesterone (to induce monthly withdrawal bleed). Metformin for insulin resistance. Clomifene to induce ovulation.
Hyperprolactinaemia due to macro- or micro-adenoma, or idiopathic (no apparent adenoma)	*Suggested by:* galactorrhoea, amenorrhoea. Headache or bitemporal visual field defect (if large prolactinoma). *Confirmed by:* ↑serum prolactin. Expanded pituitary fossa on **skull X-ray** or **CT scan**. **MRI scan**: visible micro- (<10mm) or macro-adenoma (>10mm). *Finalized by the predictable outcome of management,* e.g. dopamine agonists, e.g. bromocriptine or cabergoline. Surgical resection if >10mm, field defect, pressure effects not changed by dopamine agonist, or pregnancy planned.

Thyrotoxicosis due to Graves' disease, single or multiple toxic nodules	*Suggested by:* amenorrhoea alone, anxious-looking, thin, lid retraction and lag, tremor, hyper-reflexic, diffuse goitre in Graves', visible or palpable nodule(s) if toxic nodules.
	Confirmed by: ↓**TSH** and ↑**T3** or ↑**T4** or both. **Thyroid antibodies** +ve if Graves'. **US scan** or **isotope scan** appearance.
	Finalized by the predictable outcome of management, e.g. propranolol 40–80mg 8-hourly to control symptoms. Carbimazole 40mg od, reduced to 5–15mg od over 1–3mo period with regular TFT monitoring; continue treatment for 6–18mo. Radioiodine therapy if hot nodule(s) or relapse of Graves' disease after full course of carbimazole.

Excessive menstrual loss—menorrhagia

Menorrhagia (in excess of 80mL per cycle) can be due to uterine or systemic disorders. Initial investigations (other tests in **bold** below): FBC, TSH, US scan of abdomen/pelvis.

Main differential diagnoses and typical outline evidence, etc.	
Fibroids	*Suggested by:* menorrhagia alone ± urinary frequency, pelvic pain, constipation, recurrent miscarriage, infertility. Mass on bimanual pelvic examination. *Confirmed by:* **US scan or CT** appearance. *Finalized by the predictable outcome of management,* e.g. antiprostaglandin agents, e.g. mefenamic acid, or antifibrinolytic agents, e.g. tranexamic acid to control bleeding. GnRH to shrink fibroids, e.g. prior to surgery (long-term use may cause osteoporosis). Hysterectomy in suitable patients or myomectomy to preserve fertility.
Endometrial carcinoma	*Suggested by:* abnormal uterine bleeding, bloodstained vaginal discharge, postmenopausal bleeding. *Confirmed by:* **pelvic US scan**, **hysteroscopy** with tissue sampling of endometrium. *Finalized by the predictable outcome of management,* e.g. depends on the stage of cancer and fitness of patient, e.g. total abdominal hysterectomy with bilateral salpingo-oophorectomy + radiotherapy if tumour stage >1b.
Pelvic endometriosis	*Suggested by:* dysmenorrhoea, heavy periods, abdominal pains, dyspareunia, infertility, pelvic mass. *Confirmed by:* appearance of peritoneal deposits at **laparoscopy**. *Finalized by the predictable outcome of management,* e.g. combined pill, e.g. norethisterone, danazol, etc., or GnRH analogues. Removal of deposits + abdominal hysterectomy + bilateral salpingo-oophorectomy.
Chronic pelvic inflammatory disease	*Suggested by:* lower abdominal pain, fever, vaginal discharge, dysuria. ↑ESR and ↑CRP, leucocytosis. *Confirmed by:* organisms on **high vaginal swab**, adhesions on **pelvic US scan** and **laparoscopy**. *Finalized by the predictable outcome of management,* e.g. long-term antibiotics with or without surgical restoration of normal anatomy.
Intrauterine contraceptive device (IUCD)	*Suggested by:* history of its insertion, painful periods. *Confirmed by:* symptoms subsiding after removal of IUCD.
1° hypothyroidism	*Suggested by:* menorrhagia alone ± cold intolerance, tiredness, constipation, bradycardia. *Confirmed by:* ↑TSH, ↓FT4. *Finalized by the predictable outcome of management,* e.g. thyroxine replacement.

Bleeding diathesis	*Suggested by:* anticoagulant therapy, easy bruising, or other bleeding sites.
	Confirmed by: abnormal **clotting screen. FBC**: ↓platelets.
	Finalized by the predictable outcome of management, e.g. if on warfarin and INR >3.5, follow the BNF protocol for the management of a raised INR, Otherwise, perform a detailed assessment of clotting or platelet abnormalities and treat appropriately.

Intermenstrual or post-coital bleeding

Expert pelvic examination is required. Initial investigations (other tests in **bold** below): pelvic US scan.

Main differential diagnoses and typical outline evidence, etc.	
Endometrial carcinoma of the uterus	*Suggested by:* abnormal uterine bleeding, bloodstained vaginal discharge, postmenopausal bleeding. *Confirmed by:* **pelvic US scan**, **hysteroscopy** with tissue sampling of endometrium. *Finalized by the predictable outcome of management,* e.g. depends on the stage of cancer and the fitness of patient, e.g. total abdominal hysterectomy with bilateral salpingo-oophorectomy + radiotherapy if tumour stage >1b.
Carcinoma of cervix	*Suggested by:* irregular vaginal bleeding, offensive, watery or bloodstained vaginal discharge, obstructive uropathy, and back pain in late stage. *Confirmed by:* appearance on vaginal speculum examination, **biopsy of cervix**. *Finalized by the predictable outcome of management,* e.g. if micro-invasive disease and incomplete family then cone biopsy and total hysterectomy after the completion of family. If invasive, radical hysterectomy and radiotherapy.
Cervical or intrauterine polyps	*Suggested by:* intermenstrual spotting or postmenstrual staining. *Confirmed by:* appearance on vaginal speculum examination, **hysteroscopy**, histology of resection specimen. *Finalized by the predictable outcome of management,* e.g. resection and histology.

Vulval skin abnormalities

Initial investigations (other tests in **bold** below): urine dipstick for glucose and blood, vulval swab for microsopy and culture.

Main differential diagnoses and typical outline evidence, etc.	
Thrush: *Candida albicans* (often in pregnancy, contraceptive, and steroids, immunodeficiencies, antibiotics, and diabetes mellitus)	*Suggested by:* vulva and vagina red, fissured, and sore. *Confirmed by:* mycelia or spores on **microscopy and culture**. *Finalized by the predictable outcome of management:* improvement with clotrimazole cream in addition to the treatment of any underlying condition.
Allergy	*Suggested by:* being worse after contact with some substances, e.g. nylon underwear, chemicals, and soap. *Confirmed by:* response to avoidance of precipitants. *Finalized by the predictable outcome of management,* e.g. emollient, with or without steroid creams or ointments.
Lichen sclerosis	*Suggested by:* being intensely itchy. Bruised, red, purpuric appearance. Bullae, erosions, and ulcerations. Later, white, flat, and shiny with an hourglass shape around the vulva and anus. *Confirmed by:* above clinical appearance and **biopsy**. *Finalized by the predictable outcome of management,* e.g. biopsy of any suspicious lesion. Topical steroids. Vulvectomy in advanced cases, if not responding to medical treatment. Follow-up to ensure resolution or to re-investigate.
Leukoplakia	*Suggested by:* itchiness and white vulval patches due to skin thickening and hypertrophy. *Confirmed by:* above clinical appearance and histology on **biopsy**. *Finalized by the predictable outcome of management,* e.g. if non-atrophic biopsy appearance: topical steroids. If atrophic histology: topical oestrogen or testosterone. Surgical treatment if suspicious histology.
Carcinoma of the vulva	*Suggested by:* an indurated ulcer with an everted edge. *Confirmed by:* appearance **biopsy**. *Finalized by the predictable outcome of management,* e.g. surgical resection (5y survival rate 95%).
Other rarer causes	Obesity, incontinence, diabetes mellitus, psoriasis, lichen planus, scabies, pubic lice, and threadworms.

Ulcers and lumps of the vulva

The diagnoses depend on examination and biopsy of lesions, and thus require specialist skills. Initial investigations (other tests in **bold** below): urine dipstick.

Main differential diagnoses and typical outline evidence, etc.	
Vulval warts (condylomata acuminata) due to human papilloma virus	*Suggested and confirmed by:* warts on vulva, perineum, anus, vagina, or cervix (florid in pregnancy or if immunosuppressed).
	Finalized by the predictable outcome of management, e.g. if a single wart in a non-pregnant lady, Podophyllin paint applied weekly by a nurse and washed after 6h (or liquid applied bd for 3d as a self-treatment).
	If multiple warts: cryotherapy, laser, or diathermy under general anaesthesia.
	Annual cervical smears, and checking of the vulva and anus.
Urethral carbuncle caused by meatal prolapse	*Suggested and confirmed by:* small, red swelling at the urethral orifice. Tender and pain on micturition.
	Finalized by the predictable outcome of management, e.g. topical oestrogen.
	Surgical resection if no resolution.
Bartholin's cyst and abscess caused by blocked duct	*Suggested and confirmed by:* extreme pain (cannot sit) and red, hot, swollen labium.
	Finalized by the predictable outcome of management, e.g. antibiotics in early stage.
	If no response, incision and drainage ('marsupialization').
Herpes simplex (herpes type II) complicated by urinary retention	*Suggested and confirmed by:* vulva ulcerated and exquisitely painful.
	Finalized by the predictable outcome of management, e.g. topical aciclovir, PO if severe. Topical or systemic antibiotics if 2° infection.
Other causes	Local varicose veins, boils, sebaceous cysts, keratoacanthomata, condylomata, latent syphilis, primary chancre, molluscum contagiosum, abscess, uterine prolapse or polyp, inguinal hernia, varicocoele, carcinoma. Also causes of vulval ulcers: syphilis, herpes simplex, chancroid, lymphogranuloma venereum, granuloma inguinale, TB, Behçet's syndrome, aphthous ulcers, Crohn's disease.

Lumps in the vagina

The clinical assessment depends on special examination techniques. Initial investigations (other tests in **bold** below): urine dipstick.

Main differential diagnoses and typical outline evidence, etc.

Cystocoele	*Suggested by:* frequency and dysuria. Bulging, upper front wall of the vagina. *Confirmed by:* **cystogram** showing residual urine within the cystocoele. *Finalized by the predictable outcome of management,* e.g. surgical anterior vaginal repair (colporrhaphy).
Urethrocoele	*Suggested by:* stress incontinence (e.g. 'leaks' when laughing or coughing). Bulging of the lower anterior vaginal wall. *Confirmed by:* **micturating cystogram** showing displaced urethra and impaired sphincter mechanisms. *Finalized by the predictable outcome of management,* e.g. surgical repair.
Rectocoele	*Suggested by:* patient may have to reduce herniation prior to defaecation by putting a finger in the vagina. Bulging, middle posterior wall. *Confirmed by:* **barium enema** or **MRI scan** showing rectum bulging through weak levator ani. *Finalized by the predictable outcome of management,* e.g. vaginal posterior repair (colporrhaphy).
Enterocoele	*Suggested by:* bulging of upper posterior vaginal wall. *Confirmed by:* **barium enema** or **MRI scan** showing loops of intestine in the pouch of Douglas. *Finalized by the predictable outcome of management,* e.g. vaginal posterior repair (colporrhaphy).
Uterine prolapse (made worse by obesity, chronic bronchitis, or COPD)	*Suggested by:* 'dragging' or 'something coming down', worse by day. Frequency, stress incontinence, and difficulty in defaecation. *Confirmed by:* cervix well down in the vagina (1st degree prolapse) or protruding from the introitus when standing or straining (2nd degree) or the keratinized uterus lying outside vagina, the cervix ulcerated (3rd degree prolapse or procidentia). *Finalized by the predictable outcome of management,* e.g. improvement after weight reduction and smoking cessation. Ring pessary for frail patients. Surgical correction of prolapse. Treat aggravating factors.
Vaginal carcinoma	*Suggested by:* vaginal bleeding, mass in the upper third of the vagina. *Confirmed by:* squamous cell carcinoma on **biopsy**. *Finalized by the predictable outcome of management,* e.g. surgical treatment in early cases, otherwise radiotherapy.

Ulcers and lumps in the cervix

The clinical assessment depends on special examination techniques. Initial investigations (other tests in **bold** below): urine dipstick.

Main differential diagnoses and typical outline evidence, etc.	
Cervical ectropion ('erosion' innocuous)	*Suggested by:* red ring of soft glandular tissue around cervical opening often found with puberty, combined pill, during pregnancy ± bleeding, producing excess mucus, or infected. *Confirmed by:* (in cases of doubt) **histology** showing columnar epithelium. *Finalized by the predictable outcome of management,* e.g. cauterization.
Nabothian cysts	*Suggested and confirmed by:* appearance of smooth spherical cyst (mucus retention). *Finalized by the predictable outcome of management,* e.g. cauterization.
Cervical polyps	*Suggested by:* increased mucus discharge or post-coital bleeding. *Confirmed by:* **histology** of resected, pedunculated, benign tumour arising from endocervical junction. *Finalized by the predictable outcome of management,* e.g. resection.
Cervicitis	*Suggested by:* increased mucus discharge or post-coital bleeding. Very red swollen cervix with overlying mucus and blood. *Confirmed by:* **histology** showing follicular or mucopurulent changes. Vesicles in herpes. **Culture** showing *Chlamydia,* gonococci, etc. *Finalized by the predictable outcome of management,* e.g. antibiotics for *chlamydia* or gonococcus. Cauterization.
Cervical intraepithelial neoplasia (CIN)	*Suggested by:* overlying cervicitis, in older woman, smoker, underprivileged background, prolonged pill use, high parity, many sexual partners or a partner having many other partners, early first coitus, past sexually transmitted diseases. *Confirmed by:* **papanicolaou smear** showing dyskaryosis; no malignancy on **cervical biopsy**. *Finalized by the predictable outcome of management,* e.g. small localized lesions of CIN1 and CIN2: cryocautery. More severe lesions: laser or loop wedge excision. Cone biopsy is for more advanced lesions. Hysterectomy if symptomatic, recurrent abnormal smears, and the family is completed.

Carcinoma of cervix	*Suggested by:* irregular vaginal bleeding, offensive, watery or bloodstained vaginal discharge, obstructive uropathy, and back pain in late stage. Firm or friable mass which bleeds on contact.
	Confirmed by: appearance on vaginal speculum examination, **biopsy of cervix**.
	Finalized by the predictable outcome of management, e.g. if it is micro-invasive disease and the family is not completed then cone biopsy followed by, total hysterectomy after the completion of the family. If invasive, radical hysterectomy and radiotherapy.

Tender or bulky mass (uterus, Fallopian tubes, or ovary) on pelvic examination

The clinical assessment depends on special examination techniques. Initial investigations (other tests in **bold** below): urine dipstick, pregnancy tests, US scan of pelvis.

Main differential diagnoses and typical outline evidence, etc	
Pregnancy	*Suggested by:* amenorrhoea in sexually active woman. Uterus at 6wk of pregnancy is like an egg, at 8wk like a peach, at 10wk like a grapefruit, and at 14wk, it fills the pelvis. *Confirmed by:* **pregnancy test** +ve, pregnancy sac seen on abdominal or **transvaginal US scan**. *Finalized by the predictable outcome of management*, e.g. community midwife for antenatal care and follow-up.
Ovarian mass (benign tumour, functional cysts, theca lutein cysts, epithelial cell tumours (serous and mucinous), cystadenomas, mature teratomas, fibromas malignant cystadenomas, germ cell or sex cord malignancies, 2°s from the uterus or stomach, Krukenberg tumours spreading via the peritoneum)	*Suggested by:* painless pelvic mass, often to one side and amenorrhoea. *Confirmed by:* **abdominal** or **transvaginal US scan** appearances. *Finalized by the predictable outcome of management*, e.g. analgesia, provisional antibiotics for associated infections. Surgical intervention.
Endometritis (uterine infection) after abortion and childbirth, IUCD insertion, or surgery. May involve Fallopian tubes and ovaries. Low-grade infection is often due to chlamydia	*Suggested by:* lower abdominal pain and fever, uterine tenderness on bimanual palpation. *Confirmed by:* **transvaginal US scan, endocervical swabs**, and **blood cultures**. *Finalized by the predictable outcome of management*, e.g. analgesics for pain, provisional broad spectrum antibiotics first, then change according to the results of culture and sensitivity.

Endometrial proliferation due to oestrogen stimulation	*Suggested by:* heavy menstrual bleeding and irregular bleeding (dysfunctional uterine bleeding), and polyps. *Confirmed by:* 'cystic glandular hyperplasia' in specimen after **dilatation and curettage**. *Finalized by the predictable outcome of management,* e.g. combined contraceptive pill for the young age group; antiprostaglandin agents, e.g. mefenamic acid or antifibrinolytic agents, e.g. tranexamic acid, to control bleeding. Endometrial ablation, hysterectomy.
Pyometra (uterus distended by pus, associated with salpingitis or 2° to outflow blockage)	*Suggested by:* lower abdominal pain and fever, uterine tenderness on bimanual palpation. *Confirmed by:* **transvaginal US scan, cervical swabs, and blood cultures.** *Finalized by the predictable outcome of management,* e.g. analgesia. Antibiotic according to culture and sensitivity; surgical evacuation + total hysterectomy + bilateral salpingo-oophorectomy.
Haematometra due to imperforate hymen in the young, carcinoma, iatrogenic cervical stenosis after cone biopsy	*Suggested by:* lower abdominal pain and uterine tenderness on bimanual palpation. *Confirmed by:* no fever, WCC normal. **Transvaginal US scan** appearance. *Finalized by the predictable outcome of management,* e.g. surgical evacuation.
Endometrial tuberculosis (also affects the Fallopian tubes with pyosalpinx)	*Suggested by:* infertility, pelvic pain, amenorrhoea, oligomenorrhoea. *Confirmed by:* **transvaginal US scan, cervical swabs,** and +ve smear or **cultures for AFB.** *Finalized by the predictable outcome of management,* e.g. antituberculosis treatment, e.g. isoniazid + rifampicin + pyrazinamide + ethambutol for 2/12 (initial phase), followed by combined isoniazid + rifampicin for another 4/12 (continuation phase).
Ectopic pregnancy	*Suggested by:* abdominal pain or bleeding in a sexually active woman with a history of a missed period. Gradually increasing vaginal bleeding, shoulder-tip pain (diaphragmatic irritation), and pain on defecation and passing water (due to pelvic blood). Sudden severe pain, peritonism, and shock with rupture. *Confirmed by:* **hCG** >6,000IU/L and an intrauterine gestational sac not seen on pelvic US scan, or if hCG 1,000–1,500IU/L and no sac is seen on **transvaginal US scan.** *Finalized by the predictable outcome of management,* e.g. IV access, crossmatch blood, correct shock and Hb. Emergency laparotomy with or without a preliminary laparoscopy.

(Continued)

Fibroids (uterine leiomyomata)

Suggested by: heavy and prolonged periods, infertility, pain, abdominal swelling, urinary frequency, oedematous legs and varicose veins, or cause retention of urine.

Confirmed by: normal **hCG** and **transvaginal US scan** showing discrete lump(s) in the wall of the uterus or bulging out to lie under the peritoneum (subserosal) or under the endometrium (submucosal) or pedunculated.

Finalized by the predictable outcome of management, e.g. if menorrhagia, small fibroids, and subfertility, then GnRH analogues short term. Hysterectomy in suitable cases or myomectomy if retaining fertility is an issue.

Acute salpingitis often associated with endometritis, peritonitis, abscess, and chronic infection

Suggested by: being unwell, with pain, fever, spasm of lower abdominal muscles (more comfortable lying on back with legs flexed). Cervicitis with profuse, purulent or bloody vaginal discharge. Cervical excitation and tenderness in the fornices bilaterally, but worse on one side. Symptoms vague in subacute infection.

Confirmed by: **laparoscopy**.

Finalized by the predictable outcome of management, e.g. analgesia. Fluids IV. Provisional broad-spectrum antibiotics to cover *Chlamydia trachomatis* and *Neisseria gonorrhoea*. Contact tracing and treatment of the sexual partner.

Chronic salpingitis (unresolved, unrecognized, or inadequately treated acute salpingitis) leading to fibrosis and adhesions, pyosalpinx, or hydrosalpinx

Suggested by: pelvic pain, menorrhagia, secondary dysmenorrhoea, discharge, deep dyspareunia, depression. Palpable tubal masses, tenderness, and fixed retroverted uterus.

Confirmed by: **laparoscopy** to differentiate between infection and endometriosis.

Finalized by the predictable outcome of management, e.g. analgesia. Surgical treatment in selected patients.

Vaginal discharge

The clinical assessment depends on special examination techniques. Initial investigations (other tests in **bold** below): urine dipstick, high vaginal swab.

Main differential diagnoses and typical outline evidence, etc.	
Excessive normal secretion	*Suggested by:* women of reproductive age, milky white, or mucoid discharge. *Confirmed by:* normal investigations. *Finalized by the predictable outcome of management,* e.g. explanation and reassurance.
Vaginal thrush	*Suggested by:* pruritis vulvae with a white discharge in a well patient. *Confirmed by:* **high vaginal swab**. *Finalized by the predictable outcome of management,* e.g. clotrimazole cream or pessaries or fluconazole orally (not in pregnancy).
Bacterial vaginosis	*Suggested by:* fishy odour discharge, itching, irritation. *Confirmed by:* **high vaginal swab + wet saline microscopy** shows presence of cells. *Finalized by the predictable outcome of management,* e.g. oral or vaginal metronidazole, amoxicillin in pregnancy.
Cervical erosions (ectropion)	*Suggested by:* no other obvious symptoms. *Confirmed by:* **speculum examination**. *Finalized by the predictable outcome of management,* e.g. colposcopy and cryo- or electrocautery of the affected area.
Endocervicitis (gonococcus, Chlamydia)	*Suggested by:* symptoms in partner of urethritis. *Confirmed by:* inflamed cervix on **speculum examination** and **endocervical swab** result. *Finalized by the predictable outcome of management,* e.g. broad-spectrum antibiotics. Contact tracing and treatment of sexual partner. Genitourinary medical team follow-up.
Carcinoma of cervix	*Suggested by:* bloodstained discharge, irregular vaginal bleeding, obstructive uropathy, and back pain in late stage. *Confirmed by:* **cervical smear, cytology, colposcopy with biopsy**. *Finalized by the predictable outcome of management,* e.g. pain relief. Cone biopsy for stage 1a if family is not yet completed (applies to squamous cell carcinoma only), otherwise radical surgery + radiotherapy.

Foreign body	*Suggested by:* bloodstained discharge, use of ring pessary, intrauterine contraceptive device, tampon. *Confirmed by:* **speculum examination** or colposcopy or hysteroscopy. *Finalized by the predictable outcome of management,* e.g. removal of foreign body.
Endometrial polyp	*Suggested by:* bloodstained discharge, intermenstrual spotting, postmenstrual staining. *Confirmed by:* **hysteroscopy**. *Finalized by the predictable outcome of management,* e.g. surgical excision.
Trichomonas vaginitis	*Suggested by:* profuse, greenish yellow, frothy discharge, dysuria, dyspareunia. *Confirmed by:* protozoa and WBC on **smear**. *Finalized by the predictable outcome of management,* e.g. metronidazole for 1wk. If pregnant, lower dose for 5d. Treat the partner.
Gonococcal cervicitis	*Suggested by:* purulent discharge, lower abdominal pain, fever, cervix appears red and bleeds easily. *Confirmed by:* **Gram stain of cervical or urethral exudates** shows intracellular Gram –ve diplococci. *Finalized by the predictable outcome of management,* e.g. cefixime or ciprofloxacin. Azithromycin or doxycycline for possible associated *Chlamydia*. Trace contacts and treat sexual partner. No alcohol or intercourse during treatment.
Chlamydia cervicitis	*Suggested by:* purulent discharge, lower abdominal pain, fever, cervix appears red and bleeds easily. *Confirmed by:* **endocervical swab**. *Finalized by the predictable outcome of management,* e.g. doxycycline or erythromycin at standard doses for 7–10d. Higher doses in addition to metronidazole for complicated infections. Trace contacts and treat sexual partner. No intercourse and alcohol for 4wk.

Enlargement of prostate

The rectal examination includes feeling for a prostatic protrusion anteriorly and sweeping around for other masses, including impacted faeces. Initial investigations (other tests in **bold** below): urine dipstick, MSU, FBC, PSA.

Main differential diagnoses and typical outline evidence, etc.	
Prostatitis	*Suggested by:* smooth, enlarged, and tender. *Confirmed by:* +ve **urine culture**, **culture of prostatic secretions**. *Finalized by the predictable outcome of management,* e.g. ciprofloxacin for 4wk.
Prostatic hypertrophy	*Suggested by:* hesitancy, poor stream, urgency, incontinence, nocturia, acute retention of urine, smooth, enlarged, firm, non-tender, usually with a palpable median groove. *Confirmed by:* ↑ **serum PSA**, **US scan of prostate gland**, and response to TURP. *Finalized by the predictable outcome of management,* e.g. catheter for acute retention. α-blockers, e.g. tamsulosin, then trial without catheter. 5α-reductase inhibitors, e.g. finasteride, TURP.
Prostatic carcinoma	*Suggested by:* irregular, hard, sometimes obliteration of median groove, non-tender. *Confirmed by:* ↑↑ **serum PSA**, **prostatic biopsy**. *Finalized by the predictable outcome of management,* e.g. for local disease, radical prostatectomy or radiotherapy combined with hormonal treatment. For metastatic disease, endocrine therapy.

Joint, limb, and back symptoms and physical signs

Muscle stiffness or pain 424
Monoarthritis 426
Polyarthritis 428
Pain or limitation of movement
    in the hand 430
    at the elbow 432
    at the shoulder 434
    at the neck 436
    of the back: with sudden onset over seconds to hours
        originally 438
    of the back: with onset over days to months originally 440
    of the back: with onset over years 441
    of the hip 442
    of the knee 446
    of the foot 450

Muscle stiffness or pain

Usually worse in the early morning, often with pain and stiffness. Initial investigations (others in **bold** below): FBC, ESR, or CRP.

Main differential diagnoses and typical outline evidence, etc.	
Normal response to strenuous exercise	*Suggested by:* fit, healthy, unaccustomed exercise 1–2d before. *Confirmed by:* spontaneous resolution. *Finalized by the predictable outcome of management*, e.g. rest improves symptoms.
Polymyalgia rheumatica	*Suggested by:* abrupt onset of symptoms, severe morning stiffness and limb girdle pain, tender proximal muscles. Fatigue, night sweats, and fever in elderly person. *Confirmed by:* ↑↑**ESR** and **CRP**, ↓**Hb**, **rheumatoid factor** –ve, prompt response to prednisolone, no other cause (e.g. infection on follow-up). *Finalized by the predictable outcome of management,* e.g. NSAIDs if not contraindicated, analgesics, advise exercises, low dose prednisolone, e.g. 20–30mg daily—reduced gradually over a period of weeks or months. Can resolve spontaneously, even without treatment.
Rheumatoid arthritis	*Suggested by:* early morning stiffness, fatigue, and joint pain, and swelling. Fingers showing 'swan neck' or 'boutonnière' deformities. Thumbs show Z-deformities. Metacarpophalangeal (MCP) joints and wrists—subluxed giving ulnar deviation. Knees—valgus or varus deformity and popliteal 'Baker's' cysts. Feet—subluxation of metatarsal heads with hallux valgus, clawed toes. *Confirmed by:* **rheumatoid factor** +ve, **anti-IgG auto-antibody**, **cryoglobulins**. **FBC**: normochromic anaemia, ↑**ESR** and ↑**CRP** when active. *Finalized by the predictable outcome of management,* e.g. supportive physiotherapy and occupational therapy, NSAIDs with gastric protection, analgesics. Disease-modifying drugs, e.g. methotrexate. Immunotherapy, e.g. infliximab.
Ankylosing spondylitis	*Suggested by:* onset over months or years. Spinal pain and stiffness with progressive loss of spinal movement. Kyphosis and spinal extension. *Confirmed by:* 'bamboo' spine on **back X-ray** and loss of sacroileal joint space. **Rheumatoid factor** –ve, **HLA-B27** +ve. ↑IgA. *Finalized by the predictable outcome of management,* e.g. exercise, physiotherapy, NSAIDs, and analgesics. Dramatic response to immunotherapy using anti-tumour necrosis factor (TNF) drugs, e.g. infliximab.

1° muscle disease	*Suggested by:* onset over weeks to years. Predominant weakness of proximal muscles mainly, seasonal variation of symptoms ± symptoms of an associated malignancy. *Confirmed by:* ↑**CPK**, **electromyography (EMG)**, **MRI scan**, and **muscle biopsy.** *Finalized by the predictable outcome of management*, e.g. possible diagnosis of an underlying malignancy. Physiotherapy, high-dose steroids, immunosuppressants, e.g. methotrexate.
1° hypothyroidism	*Suggested by:* onset over weeks to months. Predominant fatigue. Also cold intolerance, depression. *Confirmed by:* ↑**TSH**, ↓**FT4**. *Finalized by the predictable outcome of management*, e.g. thyroid replacement treatment.
Early manifestation of occult malignancy	*Suggested by:* onset over weeks or months. Weight loss, anorexia. *Confirmed by:* subsequent appearance of malignancy, especially spinal 2° deposits.
Fibromyalgia	*Suggested by:* variable onset—weeks to years. Fatigue, diffuse pain, muscles stiffness, and tender points, but no features of specific diagnosis. *Confirmed by:* no 'subsequent' development of features of another diagnosis, normal **ESR**, **rheumatoid factor** –ve, **CPK** normal, **TSH** and **FT4** normal. *Finalized by the predictable outcome of management*, e.g. education and reassurance, exercise, relaxation techniques, tricyclic antidepressants (e.g. amitriptyline), selective serotonin reuptake inhibitors—SSRIs (e.g. fluoxetine), muscle relaxants (e.g. tizanidine).

Monoarthritis

One joint affected by pain, swelling, overlying erythema, stiffness, and local heat (± fever). Initial investigations (others in **bold** below): FBC, ESR or CRP, rheumatoid factor.

Main differential diagnoses and typical outline evidence, etc.	
Acute septic arthritis	*Suggested by:* extremely painful, red hot joint, high fever. *Confirmed by:* ↑↑WCC. Joint **aspiration**: synovial fluid turbid. **Culture** growing *Staphylococcus* or *Streptococcus* or *Pseudomonas* or gonococci or TB, etc. *Finalized by the predictable outcome of management,* e.g. aspiration of joint, culture, and sensitivity, analgesics, NSAIDs, antimicrobial according to culture and sensitivity results, urgent orthopaedic referral for possible washout.
Gout	*Suggested by:* one acutely inflamed joint (usually small, esp. big toe) at a time, but other joints in hands, arms, legs, and feet deformed. Tophi on ears and tendon sheaths. *Confirmed by:* ↑**serum urate** (not always). Urate crystals (negatively birefringent in plane-polarized light) present on **joint aspiration**. **X-rays** show damage to cartilage and bones. *Finalized by the predictable outcome of management,* e.g. appropriate diet, avoid food high in purines, plenty of fluids, reduce alcohol consumption, lose weight, analgesics, NSAIDs, colchicine. Allopurinol to prevent future attacks.
Pseudogout (Ca²⁺ pyrophosphate arthropathy/ chondrocalcinosis) hyperparathyroidism, myxoedema, osteoarthritis, dialysis or trauma, haemochromatosis, acromegaly	*Suggested by:* one painful joint (usually knee), especially in elderly or history of associated condition. Occasionally, family history of the condition. *Confirmed by:* **X-rays of joint show chondrocalcinosis. Joint aspiration:** synovial calcium pyrophosphate crystal deposits, positively birefringent in plane-polarized light. *Finalized by the predictable outcome of management,* e.g. joint aspiration to ease pain, analgesics, NSAIDs, intra-articular joint injection, colchicine, and in severe cases, systemic steroids.
Reiter's disease	*Suggested by:* monoarthritis, urethritis, conjunctivitis— especially in a young man—or a history of diarrhoea (dysentery). Also suggested by associated iritis, keratoderma blenorrhagica (brown, aseptic abscesses on soles and palms), mouth ulcers, circinate balanitis (painless, serpiginous penile rash), plantar fasciitis, Achilles' tendonitis, and aortic incompetence. *Confirmed by:* **rheumatoid factor** –ve (i e. 'seronegative'), ↑**ESR**, +ve culture for *Chlamydia*. **X-rays** show spondylitis and sacroiliitis. Urinalysis: first glass of a 2-glass urine test shows debris in urethritis. *Finalized by the predictable outcome of management,* e.g. bed rest, exercise, analgesics, NSAIDs, local intra-articular steroid injections, antibiotics for proved infections, e.g. *Chlamydia*. Immunosuppression in severe cases.

Psoriasis	*Suggested by:* acutely inflamed terminal interphalangeal (IP) joint, but other joints deformed, especially terminal IP joints, and pitting and thickening of fingernails. *Confirmed by:* psoriatic plaques on elbows and extensor surfaces of limbs, scalp, behind ears, and around navel. **Rheumatoid factor** −ve (i.e. 'seronegative'). *Finalized by the predictable outcome of management,* e.g. analgesics, NSAIDs, and in intractable cases, immunosuppressants, e.g. methotrexate.
Rheumatoid arthritis	*Suggested by:* early morning stiffness. Fingers: 'swan neck' or 'boutonnière' deformities. Thumbs have Z-deformities. MCP joints and wrists: subluxation acquiring ulnar deviation. Knees: valgus or varus deformity and popliteal 'Baker's' cysts. Feet: subluxation of metatarsal heads with hallux valgus, clawed toes, and calluses. *Confirmed by:* **rheumatoid factor** +ve (i. e. 'seropositive'), ↑**anti-IgG autoantibody**. **FBC:** normochromic anaemia, ↑ESR when active. *Finalized by the predictable outcome of management,* e.g. supportive physiotherapy and occupational therapy, NSAIDs with stomach protection, analgesics. Disease-modifying drugs, e.g. methotrexate. Immunotherapy, e.g. infliximab.
Traumatic haemarthrosis	*Suggested by:* acutely inflamed joint after trauma. *Confirmed by:* **joint aspiration:** aspiration of blood from joint. *Finalized by the predictable outcome of management,* e.g. analgesia ± joint aspiration.
Leukaemic joint deposits	*Suggested by:* acutely inflamed joint. *Confirmed by:* leukaemic picture on **peripheral film** and **bone marrow**. *Finalized by the predictable outcome of management,* e.g. analgesics, NSAIDs, and treatment of the original problem.
Reactive arthritis (aseptic) due to venereal or enteric infection, *Yersinia, Chlamydia trachomatis, Campylobacter, Salmonella/Shigella,* and *Chlamydia pneumoniae,* HIV, *Vibrio parahaemolyticus, Borrelia burgdorferi, Clostridium difficile*	*Suggested by:* asymmetric mono- or oligoarthritis developing about 1wk after infection elsewhere. Previous history of food poisoning or another intestinal illness. *Confirmed by:* ↑ESR, HLA-B27 +ve, microbiological investigations. *Finalized by the predictable outcome of management,* e.g. heat–cold application for temporary easing of pain, analgesics, NSAIDs, appropriate antibiotics, exercise, and in severe cases, DMARDs.

Polyarthritis

Several joints affected by pain, swelling, overlying redness, stiffness, and local heat (± fever). Initial investigations (others in **bold** below): FBC, ESR or CRP, rheumatoid factor.

Main differential diagnoses and typical outline evidence, etc.

Viruses	*Suggested by:* several acutely inflamed joints. History of recent rubella or mumps or hepatitis A or Epstein–Barr viral infection or Parvovirus B19 infection, etc.
	Confirmed by: ↑**viral titres**, **rheumatoid factor** −ve ('seronegative').
	Finalized by the predictable outcome of management, e.g. analgesia and reassurance.
Rheumatoid arthritis	*Suggested by:* history of early morning stiffness. Fingers: 'swan neck' or 'boutonnière' deformities. Thumbs have Z-deformities. MCP joints and wrists: subluxation acquiring ulnar deviation. Knees: valgus or varus deformity and popliteal 'Baker's' cysts. Feet: subluxation of metatarsal heads with hallux valgus, clawed toes, and calluses.
	Confirmed by: **rheumatoid factor** +ve, ↑**anti-IgG autoantibody**. ↑**ESR** when active.
	Finalized by the predictable outcome of management, e.g. supportive physiotherapy and occupational therapy, NSAIDs with stomach protection, analgesics. DMARDs, e.g. methotrexate. Immunotherapy, e.g. infliximab.
Sjögren's syndrome associated diabetes mellitus, hypothyroidism	*Suggested by:* several acutely inflamed joints and diminished lacrimation, causing dry eyes and dry mouth. Enlarged salivary glands.
	Confirmed by: Schirmer's test +ve (ability to wet a small test strip put under the eye), **rheumatoid factor** +ve, and **anti-Ro** (SS-A) and **anti-La** (SS-B) antibodies present. Salivary gland biopsy.
	Finalized by the predictable outcome of management, e.g. symptomatic. For dry eyes, artificial tears, eye lubricants, or ciclosporin eye drops. For dry mouth, artificial saliva, lemon drops, and salivary gland stimulants, e.g. pilocarpine—if not contraindicated ± hydroxychloroquine. For severe cases with vasculitis, immunosuppressants, e.g. prednisolone or azathioprine.
Rheumatic fever (reactive arthritis to earlier infection with Lancefield Group A β-haemolytic streptococci)	*Suggested by:* flitting polyarthritis (a major 'Jones criterion').
	Confirmed by: evidence of recent streptococcal infection plus 1 more major revised Jones criterion or 2 more minor criteria. Evidence of streptococcal infection = scarlet fever or positive throat swab or increase in **ASOT** >200 or ↑**DNase B** titre. (Major criteria = carditis or flitting polyarthritis or subcutaneous nodules or erythema marginatum or Sydenham's chorea. Minor criteria = fever or ↑**ESR/CRP**, arthralgia (but not if arthritis is one of the major criteria), prolonged PR interval on ECG (but not if carditis is a major criterion), previous rheumatic fever.) **Rheumatoid factor** −ve.
	Finalized by the predictable outcome of management, e.g. bed rest, penicillin to eradicate streptococcal infection, NSAIDs. Treat chorea with benzodiazepines or haloperidol.
Systemic lupus erythematosus	*Suggested by:* polyarthritis with periarticular and tendon involvement, muscle pain, proximal myopathy.
	Confirmed by: ↑↑**double-stranded DNA antibodies** titre. **ANA** +ve and **rheumatoid factor** +ve.
	Initial management: analgesics and NSAIDs, sunscreens to protect skin, oral steroids for acute exacerbations, hydroxychloroquine to improve joint and skin symptoms, immunosuppressants, e.g. methotrexate, for resistant cases.

Ulcerative colitis	*Suggested by:* large joint polyarthritis, sacroiliitis, ankylosing spondylitis, background of gradual onset of diarrhoea with blood and mucus, and crampy abdominal discomfort. *Confirmed by:* **rheumatoid factor** −ve. **FBC:** ↓Hb and ↑**ESR**. Inflamed, friable mucosa on **sigmoidoscopy** and biopsy shows inflammatory infiltrate, goblet cell depletion, etc. *Finalized by the predictable outcome of management*, e.g. analgesics and antidiarrhoeic agents, topical anti-inflammatory agents (e.g. mesalazine), systemic anti-inflammatory agents (e.g. oral steroids), and immunosuppressants (e.g. azathioprine and methotrexate) for the more severe cases. Surgical intervention after many years when risk of colon cancer increases.
Crohn's disease	*Suggested by:* large joint polyarthritis, sacroiliitis, ankylosing spondylitis, background of gradual onset of diarrhoea, abdominal pain, weight loss. *Confirmed by:* **rheumatoid factor** −ve. **Contrast studies** showing ileal strictures, proximal dilatation, inflammatory mass or fistula, e.g. **barium enema**: 'cobblestoning', 'rose thorn' ulcers, colonic strictures with rectal sparing. *Finalized by the predictable outcome of management*, e.g. advise healthy, balanced and high-fibre content diet. Analgesics and antidiarrhoeic agents, oral anti-inflammatory agents (e.g. mesalazine, oral prednisolone) or immunosuppressants (e.g. azathioprine) in more severe cases. Surgical intervention for intractable symptoms not controlled medically.
Drug reaction	*Suggested by:* several acutely inflamed joints. History of suspicious drug. *Confirmed by:* **rheumatoid factor** −ve and improvement on withdrawing drug. *Finalized by the predictable outcome of management*, e.g. withdrawing suspect drug(s).
Reiter's syndrome	*Suggested by:* polyarthritis, urethritis, conjunctivitis—especially in a young man—or a history of diarrhoea (dysentery). Also suggested by associated iritis, keratoderma blenorrhagica (brown, aseptic abscesses on soles and palms), mouth ulcers, circinate balanitis (painless, serpiginous penile rash), plantar fasciitis, Achilles' tendonitis, and aortic incompetence. *Confirmed by:* **rheumatoid factor** −ve. **Urinalysis:** first glass of a 2-glass urine test shows debris in urethritis. *Finalized by the predictable outcome of management*, e.g. bed rest, exercise, analgesics, NSAIDs, local intra-articular steroid injections, antibiotics for proved infections, e.g. *Chlamydia*. Immunosuppression in severe cases.
Psoriasis	*Suggested by:* several acutely inflamed joints (usually terminal IP and other joints deformed, especially terminal IP joints, with pitting and thickening of fingernails. *Confirmed by:* psoriatic plaques on elbows and extensor surfaces of limbs, scalp, behind ears, and around navel. Rheumatoid factor −ve. *Finalized by the predictable outcome of management*, e.g. analgesics, NSAIDs, or immunosuppressants, e.g. methotrexate.

Pain or limitation of movement in the hand

Ask patient to flex and extend fingers, and then wrists. Observe opening and closing of buttons, range of movement, any limitation, or pain. Initial investigations (others in **bold** below): X-ray hand and wrist.

Main differential diagnoses and typical outline evidence, etc.

Carpal tunnel syndrome associated hypothyroidism, acromegaly, or pregnancy.	*Suggested by:* pain, numbness, and weakness of hand. Symptoms worse early hours of morning, waking up patient from sleep. Shaking the hand eases symptoms. *Confirmed by:* nerve conduction studies showing a delay at the wrist. *Finalized by the predictable outcome of management,* e.g. analgesics, night splints, local injection of steroids, or surgery.
Dupuytren's contracture usually familial or associated with alcohol, anti-epileptic therapy, or diabetes mellitus	*Suggested by:* progressive flexion deformity of ring and little fingers, mainly with palmar fibrosis (often bilateral, familial). *Confirmed by:* fixed flexion at MCP joints first, then IP joints (inability to place hand on flat surface = severe). *Finalized by the predictable outcome of management,* e.g. wait and see if the palm only is affected. Surgical intervention if fingers affected.
Ganglion	*Suggested by:* painless, spherical swelling around wrist. *Confirmed by:* fluctuant, soft sphere. Disappears spontaneously leave alone, if persists or after blow, e.g. from a book. *Finalized by the predictable outcome of management,* e.g. aspiration and local steroid injection.
Rheumatoid arthritis	*Suggested by:* 'swan neck' or 'boutonnière' deformities of fingers. Thumbs have Z-deformities. MCP joints and wrists: subluxation acquiring ulnar deviation. Nodules on elbows and extensor tendons. *Confirmed by:* **rheumatoid factor** +ve. †**anti-IgG autoantibody**. *Finalized by the predictable outcome of management,* e.g. supportive physiotherapy and occupational therapy, NSAIDs with stomach protection, analgesics. DMARDs, e.g. methotrexate. Immunotherapy, e.g. infliximab.
Psoriasis	*Suggested by:* several acutely inflamed joints (usually terminal IP) and other joints deformed, especially terminal IP joints with pitting and thickening of fingernails. *Confirmed by:* psoriatic plaques on extensor surfaces of limbs, scalp, behind ears, and around navel. **Rheumatoid factor** –ve. *Finalized by the predictable outcome of management,* e.g. analgesics, NSAIDs or immunosuppressants, e.g. methotrexate.

Trigger finger due to nodule sticking in tendon sheath	*Suggested by:* fixed flexion at the ring or little finger with no fibrosis in palm. Patient unable to extend finger spontaneously. *Confirmed by:* 'click' as fingers passively extended. Nodule, then palpable on flexor surface of finger. *Finalized by the predictable outcome of management*, e.g. orthopaedic intervention, e.g. division of the sheath at the level of MP joint.
De Quervain's syndrome— stenosing tenosynovitis	*Suggested by:* pain at the wrist, e.g. when lifting teapot. History of forceful hand use, e.g. wringing clothes. Weakness of grip. *Confirmed by:* pain over radial styloid process, made worse by forced adduction and flexion of thumb into palm. *Finalized by the predictable outcome of management*, e.g. orthopaedic intervention, e.g. dividing of lateral wall of tendon sheath.
Volkmann's ischaemic contracture due to ischaemia flexor muscles of thumb and fingers (supplied by brachial artery)	*Suggested by:* flexion deformity at the thumb, fingers, wrist, and elbow with forearm pronation. History of trauma or surgery near to brachial artery, or plaster of Paris applied too tightly to forearm. *Confirmed by:* cold, dark, ischaemic arm, no pulse at the wrist, and pain when fingers extended. *Finalized by the predictable outcome of management*, e.g. surgical release of pressure.
Soft tissue injury or fracture	*Suggested by:* history of recent impact and acute pain and/or loss of function, tenderness, deformity, swelling, crepitus. *Confirmed by:* acute pain and deformity clinically and on **X-ray**. *Finalized by the predictable outcome of management*, e.g. analgesia; orthopaedic intervention if fracture ± physiotherapy.

Pain or limitation of movement at the elbow

Ask the patient to straighten arms, and compare for deformity and deviation from the normal valgus angle. Ask the patient to flex elbow, and to supinate and rotate normally over 90°. Note degree of **bold** movement, any limitation, or pain. Initial investigations (others in below): FBC, ESR, rheumatoid factor, X-ray elbow.

Main differential diagnoses and typical outline evidence, etc.	
Epicondylitis: tennis elbow (tenoperiostitis)	*Suggested by:* preceding repetitive strain, e.g. use of screwdriver, tennis racquet. Pain worse when patient asked to flex fingers and wrist, and pronate hand. Difficulty in holding a heavy object at arm's length. The arm feels stiff, heavy, and weak. *Confirmed by:* pain when patient's extended wrist pulled. Improvement after avoidance of preceding repetitive movement. *Finalized by the predictable outcome of management,* e.g. avoid suspected triggering activity, analgesics, and NSAIDs. RICE (**R**est, **I**ce, **C**ompression, and **E**levation), physiotherapy, arm brace or tape, or local injections.
Osteoarthritis	*Suggested by:* joint deformity, intermittent pain and swelling, past history of injury, e.g. fracture or dislocation. 'Locking' if loose bodies. *Confirmed by:* impairment of flexion and extension, but rotation full. **Elbow X-ray** showing osteoarthritic changes and might show loose bodies. *Finalized by the predictable outcome of management,* e.g. analgesics, NSAIDs, physiotherapy, local injections of steroids or hyaluronic acid. Arthroscopy to remove inflammatory tissues or loose bodies, and to smooth out irregular surfaces. Joint replacement if severe.
Old trauma	*Suggested by:* history of impact, fracture, deformity. *Confirmed by:* deformity and related **elbow X-ray**. *Finalized by the predictable outcome of management,* e.g. analgesia and physiotherapy.
Soft tissue injury or fracture	*Suggested by:* recent impact and acute pain and/or loss of function, tenderness, deformity, swelling, crepitus. *Confirmed by:* X-ray appearance. *Finalized by the predictable outcome of management,* e.g. analgesia; orthopaedic intervention if fracture ± physiotherapy.

Pain or limitation of movement at the shoulder

Ask patients to put their arms behind their head, and note angle at which any restriction and pain occurs. Initial investigations (others in **bold** below): FBC, ESR or CRP, X-ray shoulder.

Main differential diagnoses and typical outline evidence, etc.	
Impingement syndrome	*Suggested by:* pain on shoulder abduction, e.g. when throwing. Pain worse at night.
	Confirmed by: painful arc of movement between 70° and 120° abduction. Neer's impingement test: pain is triggered when forcibly internally rotating the shoulder while flexed to 90°. **MRI** studies of shoulder joint.
	Finalized by the predictable outcome of management, e.g. rest and reduced activities, analgesics and NSAIDs, physiotherapy, local injection of steroids. Surgery with decompression of subacromial space in non-responding cases.
Rotator cuff tears of the supraspinatus tendon or adjacent subscapularis or infraspinatus tendons	*Suggested by:* limitation and/or pain on abduction at the shoulder to the first 60° range (achieved by scapular rotation), the pain is recurrent for several months. History of trauma at the time of onset.
	Confirmed by: passive movement pain-free and spontaneous above 90°. **MRI** showing connection between joint capsule and subacromial bursa.
	Finalized by the predictable outcome of management, e.g. analgesics, NSAIDs, and physiotherapy. Surgical repair in selected cases.
Chronic supraspinatus inflammation ± calcification	*Suggested and confirmed by:* acute and continued limitation and/ or pain on abduction at the shoulder in the final 60° to 90° range. Acutely painful, tender, swollen, and warm shoulder.
	Further confirmation by: any calcification in muscle on **shoulder X-ray**.
	Finalized by the predictable outcome of management, e.g. analgesics and NSAIDs. Joint aspiration and local injection.
Cervical spondylosis (pain is referred to shoulder), very common cause of shoulder pain	*Suggested by:* pain and tenderness on the same side of the neck, occipital headache.
	Confirmed by: any positive neurological signs, e.g. absent arm reflexes, muscle weakness, and sensory impairment. **Neck X-ray and MRI scan**.
	Finalized by the predictable outcome of management, e.g. analgesics, NSAIDs, cervical collar, and physiotherapy. Surgical decompression of nerve root if intractable pain.
Biceps tendonitis	*Suggested by:* repetitive overhead activity, pain in front of the shoulder aggravated by contraction of the biceps.
	Confirmed by: above clinical findings.
	Finalized by the predictable outcome of management, e.g. resting arm, change of activity or sport, NSAIDs, physiotherapy. Orthopaedic intervention, e.g. arthroscopic surgery.

Rupture of long head of biceps	*Suggested by:* sudden pain in front of the shoulder during an activity, a snapping sensation felt. *Confirmed by:* pain aggravated by contraction of the biceps, and a lump (contracting muscle belly) appears between the shoulder and elbow, possibly with some bruising. *Finalized by the predictable outcome of management*, e.g. a sling to rest shoulder, NSAIDs, occupational therapy and physiotherapy, surgical repair for patients who need arm strength.
Frozen shoulder— adhesive capsulitis	*Suggested by:* pain worse at night, marked reduction in active and passive movement with less than 90° abduction. Difficulty in brushing hair or putting on shirts or bra. *Confirmed by:* above clinical findings and normal **shoulder X-ray**. *Finalized by the predictable outcome of management*, e.g. NSAIDs, analgesics, exercises, physiotherapy, and intra-articular steroid injections. Surgical intervention, e.g. manipulation under anaesthesia and arthroscopic capsular release.
Osteoarthritis of acromio-clavicular (AC) joint	*Suggested by:* pain and swelling at the AC joint. *Confirmed by:* very well localized tenderness to the AC joint. Positive **X-ray** and **MRI** appearance. *Finalized by the predictable outcome of management*, e.g. analgesics, NSAIDs, physiotherapy. Surgical intervention if intractable.
Rheumatoid arthritis	*Suggested by:* history of early morning stiffness. Multiple joint involvement, small joints affected, 'swan neck' or 'boutonnière' deformities of fingers. Z-deformities of thumbs. *Confirmed by:* **rheumatoid factor** +ve, ↑**anti-IgG autoantibody**. ↑**ESR** when active. *Finalized by the predictable outcome of management*, e.g. supportive physiotherapy and occupational therapy, NSAIDs with gastric protection, e.g. PPI. DMARDs, e.g. methotrexate. Immunotherapy, e.g. infliximab.
Soft tissue injury or fracture	*Suggested by:* recent impact and acute pain and/or loss of function, tenderness, deformity, swelling, crepitus. *Confirmed by:* **X-ray** appearance. *Finalized by the predictable outcome of management*, e.g. analgesia; support and immobilize. Orthopaedic intervention if fractured ± physiotherapy.
Septic arthritis	*Suggested by:* acutely, painful, red hot joint, with very restricted movements. High temperature with sweats and shivering. *Confirmed by:* ↑**WCC**, ↑**ESR**, ↑**CRP**, joint aspirate positive for culture and sensitivity. *Finalized by the predictable outcome of management*, e.g. antibiotics as per culture and sensitivity results.
Osteoarthritis of the glenohumeral joint. Very rare	*Suggested by:* history of avascular necrosis of head of humerus, following an injury to the proximal humerus. *Confirmed by:* X-ray appearance, arthroscopy. *Finalized by the predictable outcome of management*, e.g. analgesics, e.g. NSAIDs, local injection of steroids, joint replacement for severe cases.

Pain or limitation of movement at the neck

Look from the side to see if there is normal cervical (and lumbar) lordosis. Ask the patient to tilt head: move ear towards shoulder. Note angle at which any restriction and pain occurs. Initial investigations (others in **bold** below): FBC, ESR, X-ray of cervical spine.

Main differential diagnoses and typical outline evidence, etc.	
Neck pain due to an abnormal posture	*Suggested by:* a sedentary job, long hours on computer or driving. Loss of normal neck curvature. *Confirmed by:* history, full range of neck movements, and normal **cervical X-rays**. *Finalized by the predictable outcome of management,* e.g. analgesics, NSAIDs, postural exercises for the neck, eliminating bad posture, and a good support neck pillow for sleeping.
Whiplash (rapid extension and flexion movement) and extension injuries	*Suggested by:* history of road traffic accident (RTA) (rear end car crashes) with rapid extension and flexion movement of neck. Pain and stiffness of neck and the arms. *Confirmed by:* typical history. *Finalized by the predictable outcome of management,* e.g. soft cervical collar, analgesics, NSAIDs, and physiotherapy. Encourage early return to work.
Spasmodic torticollis (cervical dystonia) anterocollis (tilts forwards), retrocollis (tilts backwards), laterocollis (tilts to one side)	*Suggested by:* recurrent involuntary contraction of neck muscles causing pain and the turning of the head to one side. *Confirmed by:* presence of tremor, stiffness of neck muscles, and elevation of shoulder on the affected side. Absence of root compression pattern pain or paresis. *Finalized by the predictable outcome of management,* e.g. analgesics for pain. GABA-regulating drugs (e.g. lorazepam or baclofen), dopamine agonists (e.g. bromocriptine), or anticonvulsants (e.g. carbamazepine), all used individually or in combination. Botulinum toxin or surgery for non-responding cases.
Infantile torticollis due to birth damage of sternomastoid	*Suggested by:* onset early childhood (up to 3y). Head tilted to shoulder with restricted neck movements, and retarded growth of the cranium or face on the affected muscle side (plagiocephaly). Presence of associated muscle or skeletal disorder, e.g. hip dysplasia. *Confirmed by:* palpable nodule in muscle on affected side. **Biopsy of nodule:** fibrous only and no gangliocytoma. *Finalized by the predictable outcome of management,* e.g. physiotherapy consisting of positioning, gentle range of movements, and strengthening by the stimulation of head and trunk muscles. Cervical collars and cranial remoulding orthosis in cases of plagiocephaly. Botulinum toxin and surgery for intractable cases.

Cervical rib with compression of lower brachial plexus affecting median and ulnar nerves, and brachial artery (thoracic outlet syndrome)	*Suggested by:* weakness and numbness in forearm and hand, usually on ulnar side. Wasting of the intrinsic hand muscles. Arm cyanosis and absent pulse. *Confirmed by:* symptoms exacerbated by abduction and external rotation of shoulder. **Cervical rib neck X-ray** (may be no rib—fibrous band instead). *Finalized by the predictable outcome of management,* e.g. analgesics, NSAIDs, physiotherapy, and local injections of trigger points. Surgical intervention.
Cervical spondylosis	*Suggested by:* pain and stiffness of neck. Occipital headache, shoulder and arm pain due to radiation. Symptoms of nerve root or spinal cord involvement. *Confirmed by:* **X-ray** and **MRI** appearances. *Finalized by the predictable outcome of management,* e.g. analgesics and NSAIDs, physiotherapy, and local injections. Trial of traction. Surgical intervention for intractable symptoms.
Posterior prolapsed (cervical disc, usually C5/C6 disc and C6/C7 disc pressure on nerve roots)	*Suggested by:* torticollis, stiffness and pain in neck over side of disc lesion. Pain, numbness in arm and tip of little or middle finger or thumb. *Confirmed by:* loss of biceps or supinator reflexes. Loss of sensation in medial or lateral borders of hand. **MRI scan** shows posterior protrusion. *Finalized by the predictable outcome of management,* e.g. analgesics and NSAIDs, physiotherapy, and local injections. Trial of traction. Surgical intervention if weakness, severe pain, or suspected cord compression.
Anterior prolapsed cervical disc (usually C5/C6 disc and C6/C7 disc pressure on spinal cord)	*Suggested by:* torticollis, stiffness and pain in neck over side of disc lesion. Numbness and weakness in leg. Unsteadiness of gait, walking problems, and impaired bladder and bowel function. *Confirmed by:* flaccid first, then spastic paresis of leg. Loss of knee, ankle reflexes, and extensor plantar response. Loss of vibration sense, touch and pain with sensory level. MRI scan shows protrusion. *Finalized by the predictable outcome of management,* e.g. analgesics and NSAIDs, physiotherapy, and local injections. Trial of traction. Surgical intervention if weakness, severe pain, or suspected cord compression.

Pain or limitation of movement of the back: with sudden onset over seconds to hours originally

Look from the side to see if there is normal lumbar lordosis. Ask patients to touch their toes and watch for movement of spine and hips. Ask the patient to arch backwards, bend to each side, and rotate trunk from side to side. Lie patient down and measure length of legs. Raise each straight leg for any restriction before 45°. Initial investigations (others in **bold** below): FBC, ESR or CRP, rheumatoid factor.

Main differential diagnoses and typical outline evidence, etc.	
Mechanical pain (strains, tear, or crushing of ligaments, discs, vertebrae with normal healing)	*Suggested by:* recent onset over minutes of pain and restriction of movement in lower back in a young person. History of lifting a heavy weight or a head-on impact RTA. *Confirmed by:* recovery with minimal loss of function over days or weeks. *Finalized by the predictable outcome of management,* e.g. analgesics, NSAIDs, and physiotherapy. Encourage back to work early.
Posterior lumbar disc prolapse	*Suggested by:* onset over seconds of severe back pain on coughing, sneezing, or twisting after earlier strain. Radiation to buttock, thigh, or calf if prolapse compresses posterior root. *Confirmed by:* back flexed and extension restricted. Straight leg raising stopped before 45° by pain. Loss of sensation lateral foot (L4/5). Loss of ankle jerk and sensation sole of foot (S1). **MRI scan**. *Finalized by the predictable outcome of management,* e.g. bed rest, analgesics, NSAIDs, muscle relaxants, and physiotherapy. If these fail, then surgical intervention.
Anterior lumbar disc prolapsed	*Suggested by:* onset over seconds of severe back pain on coughing, sneezing, or twisting after earlier strain (if large, prolapse compresses cauda equina, with leg weakness, incontinence, and numbness around perineum). *Confirmed by:* flaccid paresis of leg(s). Loss of knee, ankle reflexes, and extensor plantar response. Loss of vibration sense, touch, and pain with sensory level. **MRI scan** shows protrusion. *Finalized by the predictable outcome of management,* e.g. bed rest, analgesics, NSAIDs, muscle relaxants, and physiotherapy. If these fail, then surgical intervention.

Spondylolisthesis due to spondylolysis, congenital malformation of articular process, osteoarthritis of posterior facet joints	*Suggested by:* positive family history. Sudden onset over minutes of back pain with or without sciatica in adolescence. *Confirmed by:* **plain back X-ray** shows forward displacement of vertebra over one below. *Finalized by the predictable outcome of management, e.g.* analgesics, NSAIDs, avoidance of sports, and the use of a corset support. Surgical intervention if intractable symptoms.
Central disc protrusion	*Suggested by:* sudden onset over minutes or hours with bilateral sciatica, disturbance of bladder or bowel function. Saddle or perineal anaesthesia. *Confirmed by:* history and compression of cord visible on MRI scan. *Finalized by the predictable outcome of management, e.g.* pain control and neurosurgery.

Pain or limitation of movement of the back: with onset over days to months originally

Look from the side to see if there is normal lumbar lordosis. Ask the patient to touch toes, and watch for movement of spine and hips. Ask patient to arch backwards, bend to each side, and rotate trunk from side to side. Lie patient down and measure length of legs. Raise each straight leg for any restriction before 45°. Initial investigations (others in **bold** below): FBC, ESR, rheumatoid factor.

Main differential diagnoses and typical outline evidence, etc.

Lumbar spinal stenosis due to facet joint osteoarthrosis	*Suggested by:* onset of pain over months, worse on walking with ache and weakness in one leg.
	Confirmed by: pain on extension of back. Straight leg raising normal. Few CNS signs (but may appear shortly after exercise). **MRI scan**.
	Finalized by the predictable outcome of management, e.g. analgesics. Spinal decompression if intractable pain.
Spinal tumours (1° or 2° to carcinoma of lung, breast, prostate, thyroid, kidney, myeloma)	*Suggested by:* onset of back pain over months with progressive pain or paresis in one or both legs. (Physical signs depend on part of cord or nerve roots affected.)
	Confirmed by: 'hot spot' on bone scan with erosion or sclerosis on **plain X-ray** of 'hot spot'. Space-occupying lesion on **MRI** or **CT scan** and **histology on biopsy**.
	Finalized by the predictable outcome of management, e.g. effective analgesia and control of other symptoms, e.g. vomiting. Radiotherapy, chemotherapy, and surgery, individually or in combination.
Pyogenic spinal infection usually of disc space due to Staphylococcus, Salmonella typhi, etc.	*Suggested by:* onset of pain over days or weeks. Little or no fever, tenderness or ↑WCC. ↑ESR. Background debilitation, surgery, or diabetes.
	Confirmed by: bone rarefaction or erosion with joint space narrowing on **back X-ray**. 'Hot spot' on **isotope bone scan** and space-occupying lesion on **MRI** or **CT scan**.
	Finalized by the predictable outcome of management, e.g. analgesics, NSAIDs, and antibiotics.
Spinal TB with abscesses and cord compression (Pott's paraplegia), psoas abscess	*Suggested by:* onset of weeks or months. Low-grade fever, tenderness or ↑WCC. ↑ESR. Background debilitation, diabetes.
	Confirmed by: bone rarefaction or erosion with joint space narrowing, then wedging of vertebrae. Space-occupying lesion on MRI and CT scan. Tubercle baccilli on stains or culture of drainage material.
	Finalized by the predictable outcome of management, e.g. standard anti-tuberculous treatment.

Pain or limitation of movement of the back: with onset over years

This is a notoriously poor lead. Look from the side to see if there is normal lumbar lordosis. Ask the patient to touch toes and watch for movement of spine (?rounded) and hips. Ask the patient to arch backwards, bend to each side, and rotate trunk from side to side. Lie patient down and measure length of legs. Raise each straight leg for any restriction before 45°. Initial investigations (others in **bold** below): FBC, ESR, rheumatoid factor, back X-ray (A–P and lateral).

Main differential diagnoses and typical outline evidence, etc.	
Kyphotic pain	*Suggested by:* poor posture with a hump appearance of the back (hunchback). Onset over years usually, exacerbated over days with wedge fracture. Spinal curvature visible from the side. Associated neuromuscular disease.
	Confirmed by: **back X-ray** appearance suggestive of congenital deformity, Scheuermann's or Calve's osteochondritis, wedge fracture from osteoporosis or carcinoma, ankylosing spondylitis.
	Finalized by the predictable outcome of management, e.g. analgesics and OBAS (Observation, Bracing, And Surgery).
Scoliotic pain, poliomyelitis, syringomyelia, etc. (see under 'Suggested by', this Table)	*Suggested by:* lateral curvature visible from the back and associated rib prominence apparent from the front. Head appears off centre, and a hip or shoulder is higher than the other side. Known to have past poliomyelitis, syringomyelia, torsion dystonia, spinal tumours, spondylolisthesis, arthrogryposis, enchondromatosis, osteogenesis imperfecta, neurofibromatosis, Chiari malformation, Duchenne muscular dystrophy, Friedreich's ataxia, Marfan's syndrome, Pompe's disease.
	Confirmed by: history and **X-ray** appearance of bony congenital anomaly.
	Finalized by the predictable outcome of management, e.g. treat underlying causes. Otherwise analgesics and OBAS.
Idiopathic scoliosis of thoracic or lumbar spine	*Suggested by:* progressive loss over years of horizontal alignment of shoulders and hips with age, usually in adolescent girls more than boys.
	Confirmed by: **X-ray** appearance. Increased scoliosis with growth.
	Finalized by the predictable outcome of management, e.g. OBAS.

Pain or limitation of movement of the hip

Assess activity. Test flexion (normal >120°) by grasping ankle in one hand and iliac crest in the other to eliminate pelvic rotation. Test abduction (normal 30–40°), preventing pelvic tilt. Test abduction in flexion (normal >70°) and adduction (normal >30°) by moving one foot over the other, internal and external rotation (normal >30°). Measure true length of legs from anterior superior iliac spines to medial malleoli. Trendelenburg test is positive if hip drops when foot on that same side is lifted from ground. Initial investigations (others in bold below): FBC, ESR, X-ray (A–P and lateral).

Main differential diagnoses and typical outline evidence, etc.	
Osteoarthritis	*Suggested by:* elderly, overweight, and overwork. Onset over months or years. Pain, often causing a disturbed sleep, with stiffness and limitation of movement, initially of internal rotation. Difficulties in putting on stockings and cutting the toenails.
	Confirmed by: **A–P and lateral X-rays of hips** show loss of joint space, deformity of head and acetabulum with osteophytes and sclerosis.
	Finalized by the predictable outcome of management, e.g. advise weight reduction, analgesics, NSAIDs, physiotherapy. Hip replacement/resurfacing in severe cases.
Coxa vara caused by congenital slipped upper femoral epiphyses, fracture with malunion or non-union, osteomalacia or Paget's disease	*Suggested by:* pain and stiffness, limp with Trendelenburg 'dip' to affected side. True shortening of leg.
	Confirmed by: angle between neck and femur <125° on **X-ray**.
	Finalized by the predictable outcome of management, e.g. surgical correction.
Transient synovitis (most common cause of hip pain in children)	*Suggested by:* hip pain in a child, usually a boy, with a limp and sometimes history of a preceding minor trauma. Restricted extension and internal rotation of hip. Usually no temperature.
	Confirmed by: **X-ray** and **US scan** showing synovitis.
	Finalized by the predictable outcome of management, e.g. symptomatic treatment with analgesics and NSAIDs ± bed rest for up to 6wk. If slow to respond, check stool culture for *Campylobacter*, and treat accordingly.
Soft tissue injury or fracture	*Suggested by:* recent impact and acute pain and/ or loss of function, tenderness, deformity, swelling, crepitus.
	Confirmed by: **A–P and lateral X-ray** appearance.
	Finalized by the predictable outcome of management, e.g. analgesia; surgical intervention if fracture ± physiotherapy.

Perthes' disease	*Suggested by:* pain in hip or knee with limp with onset over months from age 3–11y. Limitation of hip movement in all ranges ± thin affected leg.
	Confirmed by: **A–P and lateral X-rays** of hips show widening of joint space and ↓size of femoral head, patchy density and later, collapse. **US scan** shows capsular distension due to synovial thickening, usually bilateral.
	Finalized by the predictable outcome of management, e.g. analgesics, NSAIDs, rest and traction + physiotherapy. If it is difficult to preserve mobility, then plaster casts, bracing, and surgery (to put the femoral head back in the socket).
Slipped femoral epiphysis sometimes associated with 1° hypothyroidism	*Suggested by:* typically an overweight boy with pain in groin, front of thigh or knee, and limping with onset over minutes (if acute) or weeks to months. Limitation of flexion, abduction, and medial rotation. Pain usually comes with exercise and sports. Affected leg turns outwards and might be shorter than other side. Both hips might be affected.
	Confirmed by: displacement of growth plate visible on **lateral X-ray view of hip** (not A–P) or avascular necrosis and chondrolysis.
	Finalized by the predictable outcome of management, e.g. exclude associated conditions, e.g. hypothyroidism. If suspected, admit straight away. Traction initially; early surgical intervention.
Tuberculous arthritis	*Suggested by:* fever and night sweats. Pain and limp in 2–5y old, especially from poor country. Pain at night. Pain and spasm in all directions of movement with progressive muscle wasting.
	Confirmed by: rarefaction of bone on **X-ray,** then fuzziness of joint margin, then erosions. AFB in **biopsy ± culture of synovial membrane** (or in cultures from aspirates).
	Finalized by the predictable outcome of management, e.g. rifampicin + isoniazid + pyrazinamide + ethambutol for 2mo, followed by rifampicin and isoniazid for another 4mo in addition to bed rest and traction. Surgical intervention if deformity.

(Continued)

Developmental dysplasia (still referred to as congenital dislocation of the hip)	*Suggested by:* pain, stiffness and ↓movement in childhood or adolescence; undiagnosed hip dislocation early in life. Waddling gait with hyperlordosis in bilateral hip involvement. *Confirmed by:* positive Ortolani test (palpable clunk when hip is reduced in and out of acetabulum) or Barlow test (clunk is felt when gentle pressure is applied to the adducted hip) in the newborn. Shallow acetabulum with or without current dislocation on **A–P and lateral X-ray of hips** (ultrasound in neonate). *Finalized by the predictable outcome of management,* e.g. bracing (Pavlick harness) if under 6y-old. Closed reduction preceded by traction for the 'over 6y-old'. If >2y or failed previous treatment, open reduction or various procedures depending on age.
Post-total hip replacement problems (dislocation, prosthesis failure, prosthesis loosening, and infection)	*Suggested by:* pain, difficult or impossible weight-bearing. Limb shorter and externally rotated in the case of dislocation. General ill heath, high temperature, and night sweats in cases of infection. *Confirmed by:* radiological appearances. +ve culture and sensitivity if infection. *Finalized by the predictable outcome of management,* e.g. analgesia. Antibiotics. Re-replacement of hip if indicated.

Pain or limitation of movement of the knee

Look for quadriceps wasting, ability to weight bear, deformity of the knee, or swelling. Feel for swelling with palm of other hand pressing above patella. Compare flexion and extension on both sides. Abduct and adduct tibia with knee flexed at 30° to test medial and lateral ligaments. With knee flexed at 90°, pull and push tibia to test anterior and posterior cruciate ligaments. Initial investigations (others in **bold** below): FBC, ESR, or CRP, X-ray of knee (P–A and lateral).

Main differential diagnoses and typical outline evidence, etc.	
Osteoarthritis	*Suggested by:* old age, overweight, or overwork. Onset of months or years, worse in cold and damp. Deformity (especially varus—bow-legged) and swelling. Crepitus on passive movement. *Confirmed by:* above history and examination. Loss of joint space on **X-ray** with deformity, osteophytes, and sclerosis. *Finalized by the predictable outcome of management,* e.g. weight reduction, analgesics, NSAIDs, physiotherapy. Orthopaedic intervention, e.g. for total knee replacement in advanced cases.
Chondromalacia patellae	*Suggested by:* patella aching after sitting or walking on slopes or stairs in a young adult, typically females. Patellar tenderness. *Confirmed by:* above history and examination, and 'fibrillation' of patellar cartilage on **arthroscopy or MRI**. *Finalized by the predictable outcome of management,* e.g. restrict activities that aggravate symptoms, analgesics, and physiotherapy. Surgical intervention if no response.
Recurrent patella subluxation	*Suggested by:* jumping-type sports, e.g. basketball or volleyball. Knee often giving way (especially in knock-kneed girls). *Confirmed by:* increased lateral movement of patella. *Finalized by the predictable outcome of management,* e.g. surgical intervention for joint stabilization.
Patella tendinopathy (jumper's knee)	*Suggested by:* jumping-type sports. Pain on forceful movement of knee in sport. *Confirmed by:* tenderness over patellar tendon. **X-rays** show normal bones. *Finalized by the predictable outcome of management,* e.g. rest, NSAIDs, analgesics, physiotherapy to build up quadriceps, hamstrings, and calf muscles. Orthopaedic intervention if no response.

Iliotibial band syndrome	*Suggested by:* long distant runners and cyclists, pain when active. Rest eases the pain.
	Confirmed by: tenderness over lateral femoral condyle.
	Finalized by the predictable outcome of management, e.g. RICER regime (Rest, Ice, Compression, Elevation and Referral). If no response, advise different sporting activity.
Medial shelf syndrome	*Suggested by:* repetitive stress, single blunt trauma, anterior knee pain, knee clicking or brief locking. Symptoms made worse by activity, prolonged standing or stair climbing.
	Confirmed by: inflamed synovial fold above medial meniscus on **arthroscopy**.
	Finalized by the predictable outcome of management, e.g. analgesics, NSAIDs, and physiotherapy. If no response, possible arthroscopic resection of inflamed medial band.
Hoffa's fat pad syndrome	*Suggested by:* history of major acute or chronic repetitive trauma. Brief locking of knee with pain and swelling under patella.
	Confirmed by: hypertrophic pad between articular surfaces on **MRI** or **arthroscopy**.
	Finalized by the predictable outcome of management, e.g. analgesics, NSAIDs, ice, and rest in the acute stage ± physiotherapy. If no response, arthroscopic resection of inflamed fat pad.
Acute arthritis due to sepsis, gout or rheumatoid arthritis	*Suggested by:* onset hours, days of pain and swelling.
	Confirmed by: aspiration, microscopy, and culture. ↑**urate** in gout. **Rheumatoid factor** +ve in rheumatoid arthritis.
	Finalized by the predictable outcome of management, e.g. analgesics, NSAIDs; treat cause, e.g. antibiotics, and arthroscopic drainage if septic arthritis with no response to antibiotics.
Medial collateral ligament (MCL) tear	*Suggested by:* a blow on the outer surface of the knee or an injury forcing the leg outwards. Pain and swelling over the injured ligament. Pain triggered by stretching ligament. Unstable knee, feeling that the knee may give way or buckle.
	Confirmed by: pain and excessive laxity when gentle pressure is applied to the outside of the knee. **X-ray** and **MRI scan**.
	Finalized by the predictable outcome of management, e.g. rest, ice, compression, analgesics, and NSAIDs. Wearing knee immobilizer; avoid weight-bearing. Surgical repair for very severe injuries.

(Continued)

Lateral collateral ligament (LCL) tear	*Suggested by:* an injury causing a direct impact to the inner surface of the knee. Pain and swelling over the injured ligament. Pain is triggered or made worse by stretching the ligament. In severe injuries, the knee is very unstable. *Confirmed by:* pain and laxity when gentle pressure is applied to the inside of the knee. **X-ray** and **MRI scan**. *Finalized by the predictable outcome of management,* e.g. rest, ice, compression, analgesics, and NSAIDs. Wearing of a knee immobilizer and avoiding weight-bearing for about 2wk in more severe injuries. Surgical repair for very severe injuries with persisting instability.
Anterior cruciate ligament (ACL) tears	*Suggested by:* history of a posterior blow or a rotational force when foot fixed to ground. Sudden swelling and pain in the knee. Hearing a 'pop' at the time of the injury and/ or a sensation that the knee will 'give way'. *Confirmed by:* tibia moves forward when pulled after effective analgesia or anaesthesia (Lachman's test). **X-ray** and **MRI scan**. *Finalized by the predictable outcome of management,* e.g. RICE, analgesics, and NSAIDs. Reconstruction of ACL if instability persists.
Posterior cruciate ligament (PCL) tears	*Suggested by:* history of a direct impact on the shin when the knee is bent. Pain and swelling with a feeling that the knee will 'give way'. *Confirmed by:* tibia moves backward when pulled after effective analgesia or anaesthesia (reverse Lachman's test). **X-ray** and **MRI scan**. *Finalized by the predictable outcome of management,* e.g. RICE, analgesics, and NSAIDs. Reconstruction of PCL if persistent instability.
Meniscal tears	*Suggested by:* history of twisting, pivoting, and decelerating of the knee. Stiffness, swelling, locking, and buckling of the knee. A popping sensation at the time of injury. *Confirmed by:* **X-ray** and **MRI scan**. *Finalized by the predictable outcome of management,* e.g. RICE, analgesics, and NSAIDs. Arthroscopic trimming of damaged meniscus.
Meniscal cyst	*Suggested by:* history of a blow on the side of the knee. Variable swelling, worse when knee flexed to 60°, less when flexed further. Knee clicking and giving way. *Confirmed by:* cyst present on **MRI scan**. *Finalized by the predictable outcome of management,* e.g. aspiration to give temporary relief. Definitive treatment is excision with or without meniscectomy.

Osteochondritis dessicans (juvenile and adult types)	*Suggested by:* history of repetitive stress as in competitive sports. Pain and swelling of knee. A snapping, catching feeling, or locking when the knee is moved. *Confirmed by:* defect on articular surface with or without a loose body on **X-ray**. *Finalized by the predictable outcome of management,* e.g. in the juvenile, suspending exercise and sports, using crutches, or wearing a cast for 2mo (until symptoms subside) followed by physiotherapy. Surgical correction if bone growth ceased.
Loose bodies due to osteochondritis dessicans, osteoarthritis, chip fractures, synovial chondromatosis	*Suggested by:* locking of knee during extension and flexion. Swelling and effusion. *Confirmed by:* seeing loose bodies on **arthroscopy**. *Finalized by the predictable outcome of management,* e.g. arthroscopic or open surgical removal if symptomatic.
Bursitis (without or with infection) due to prepatellar bursitis (housemaid's knee), etc.	*Suggested by:* localized pain and swelling over site of bursa (e.g. below patella). *Confirmed by:* localized pain and swelling over site of bursa. Improvement with rest, analgesia, and physiotherapy. *Finalized by the predictable outcome of management,* e.g. analgesics and antibiotics if infected. Aspiration and local steroid injection if no infection. Surgical excision.

Pain or limitation of movement of the foot

Observe gait, examine wear on shoe sole and print on floor of damp foot. Ask to extend or dorsiflex (normal >25°), flex (normal 30°). Evert and invert. Ask to extend toes (normal >60°) and stand on tiptoe. Initial investigations (others in **bold** below): FBC, ESR, rheumatoid factor, X-ray.

Main differential diagnoses and typical outline evidence, etc.	
Hallux valgus associated with bunion and osteoarthritis	*Suggested by:* the first metatarsal is deviated medially and the big toe deviated laterally. Painful motion of joint and/or difficulty with footwear. *Confirmed by:* above clinical appearance (big toe deviated laterally). **X-ray** to assess joint pathology and measure angular deformity. *Finalized by the predictable outcome of management,* e.g. analgesics, NSAIDs, adapting footwear, and functional orthotic therapy. Surgical correction of the deformity.
Pes planus	*Suggested by:* loss of medial foot arch (appearance of damp surface in contact with floor, normal in early childhood) causing the foot to roll inwards. Pain if foot and heel everted. *Confirmed by:* above clinical appearance and response to exercises, and medial heel shoe wedges in some cases. *Finalized by the predictable outcome of management,* e.g. use of orthotics (special insoles), combined with supportive footwear that fit the foot correctly and contains a firm low heel. Surgical correction if these measures fail.
Pes cavus normal variant, hereditary, idiopathic, or due to spina bifida, past polio	*Suggested and confirmed by:* accentuated foot arches and other neurological disorders, e.g. spina bifida. The ankle may be rolled out slightly and the toes may appear clawed. *Confirmed by:* above clinical appearance. *Finalized by the predictable outcome of management,* e.g. foot orthotics (insoles), pads to get pressure off painful areas, proper fitting of footwear, treatment of associated corns and calluses.
Hammer toes	*Suggested by:* tip of a lesser toe points downwards. *Confirmed by:* toe extended at the metatarsophalangeal (MTP) joint, flexed at the proximal IP joint but extended at the distal IP joint. *Finalized by the predictable outcome of management,* e.g. wide fitted, low-heeled shoes, non-medicated pads to take pressure off corns and hard skin, moisturizing creams to keep skin soft, silicon toe prop to prevent further contracture. In rigid deformities, surgical interventions, e.g. arthroplasty or arthrodesis.

Claw toes	*Suggested by:* tip of a lesser toe points down and back.
	Confirmed by: toe extended at the MTP joint, flexed at the proximal IP and distal IP joint.
	Finalized by the predictable outcome of management, e.g. same as in hammer toes.
Mallet toes	*Suggested by:* tip of a lesser toe points downwards.
	Confirmed by: toe is extended at the MTP and proximal IP joints, and flexed at the distal IP joint.
	Finalized by the predictable outcome of management, e.g. same as in hammer toes.
Trigger toe	*Suggested by:* tip of the big toe points downwards.
	Confirmed by: big toe is extended at MTP joint and flexed at the IP joint.
	Finalized by the predictable outcome of management, e.g. same as in hammer toes.
Hallux rigidus	*Suggested by:* pain and stiffness localized to big toe, aggravated by cold damp weather. Difficulties with running and squatting.
	Confirmed by: tenderness and swelling of 1st MTP joint. **X-ray** may show a distal ring of osteophytes.
	Finalized by the predictable outcome of management, e.g. shoe modifications, e.g. wide-fitting shoes, orthotic devices, analgesics, NSAIDs, physiotherapy, local steroid injections. Surgical intervention in advanced cases.
Metatarsalgia due to shoe pressure, previous trauma, rheumatoid arthritis, sesamoid fracture, synovitis	*Suggested by:* pain in the ball of the foot, the part of the sole just behind the toes worse on standing or running. Feeling as if walking on pebbles. Patient typically does high impact sport or overweight.
	Confirmed by: tenderness of heads of metatarsals. **X-ray** to exclude other conditions, e.g. stress fracture.
	Finalized by the predictable outcome of management, e.g. rest, ice packs on the affected areas, analgesics, and NSAIDs, proper shoes, shock-absorbing insoles, metatarsal pads. Surgical intervention if these measures fail.
Morton's metatarsalgia due to interdigital neuroma	*Suggested by:* intermittent pain, burning sensation or numbness on the bottom of the foot radiating to the 3rd and 4th toes. A description of 'as if walking on marbles'.
	Confirmed by: tenderness on compression of site of neuroma between metatarsals (e.g. squeezing the forefoot together triggers pain) and massaging offers significant relief.
	Finalized by the predictable outcome of management, e.g. soft-soled shoes with a wide toe box and low heel. Plantar pad to elevate metatarsal head adjacent to neuroma preventing compression. Surgical intervention if refractory case.

(Continued)

March fracture	*Suggested by:* localized foot pain after excessive walking.
	Confirmed by: tenderness of 2nd or 3rd metatarsals. **X-ray** showing fracture.
	Finalized by the predictable outcome of management, e.g. analgesics, NSAIDs.
Calcaneum disease; arthritis of subtalar joint; tear of calcaneal tendon; post calcaneal bursitis; plantar fasciitis, etc.	*Suggested by:* localized heel pain.
	Confirmed by: **X-ray** and **MRI scan** appearance.
	Finalized by the predictable outcome of management, e.g. analgesics, NSAIDs, physiotherapy. Surgical intervention if refractory.
Soft tissue injury or fracture	*Suggested by:* recent impact and acute pain and/or loss of function, tenderness, deformity, swelling, crepitus.
	Confirmed by: X-ray appearance.
	Finalized by the predictable outcome of management, e.g. analgesia; surgical intervention if fracture ± physiotherapy.

Psychiatric and neurological symptoms and physical signs

Neurological and psychiatric symptoms and signs 455
Inability to carry out the activities of daily living 456
Acute anxiety 458
Depression 462
Delusions 464
Acute confusion 466
Chronic confusion or cognitive impairment 468
Headache—acute, new onset 470
Headache—subacute onset 472
Headache—chronic and recurrent 473
Stroke 474
Dizziness 476
Vertigo 478
'Fit' 480
Transient neurological deficit 482
Fatigue, 'tired all the time' 484
Examining the nervous system 486
Disturbed consciousness 487
Best verbal response 487
Best motor response 488
Eye opening 488
Speech disturbance 489
Dysarthria 490
Absent sense of smell 491
Abnormal ophthalmoscopy appearance 492
Ophthalmoscopy appearance in the diabetic 494
Ophthalmoscopy appearances in the hypertensive 496
Sudden loss of central vision and acuity 497
Gradual onset of visual loss 498
Peripheral visual field defect 499
Ptosis 500
Large (mydriatic) pupil with no ptosis 502
Small (miotic) pupil with no ptosis 503
Squint and diplopia: ocular palsy 504
Loss of facial sensation 506
Jaw muscle weakness 507
Facial muscle weakness 508
Loss of hearing 510
Abnormal tongue, uvula, and pharyngeal movement 511

Multiple cranial nerve lesions 512
Odd posture of arms and hands at rest 514
Fine tremor of hands 515
Coarse tremor of hands 516
Wasting of some small muscles of hand 518
Wasting of arm and shoulder 520
Abnormalities of arm tone 521
Weakness around the shoulder and arm without pain 522
Incoordination (on rapid wrist rotation or hand tapping) 523
Muscle wasting 524
Weakness around one lower limb joint 526
Bilateral weakness of all foot movements 528
Spastic paraparesis 529
Hemiparesis (weakness of arm and leg) 530
Disturbed sensation in upper limb 532
Diminished sensation in arm dermatome 533
Diminished sensation in the hand 534
Disturbed sensation in lower limb 536
Brisk reflexes 538
Diminished reflexes 539
Gait abnormality 540
Difficulty in rising from chair or squatting position 542

Neurological and psychiatric symptoms and signs

Neurological and psychiatric symptoms (e.g. stroke and depression) are more damaging to self-confidence than symptoms in the other systems. Self-confidence is central to the way in which we interact with our environment, both social and physical. It was emphasized in ➲ Dynamic diagnoses, p.20 that there are three areas over which our bodies try to exercise control:

- the internal milieu;
- the structure of our bodies; and
- our environment, social, and physical.

We are unaware of the first two when we are healthy, but when we become ill, we become actively involved in supplementing them. We are aware of the third from our earliest experience. Difficulties with the way we interact with people and our environment blend into a continuum with neurological and mental illness. The diagnosis and treatment of neurological and psychiatric conditions has to focus on how patients can learn how to adapt to their circumstances and how those around them can help, including those who work in health and social services.

Psychiatric signs may have been noted during the history and examination. The patient may have complained of 'anxiety' or 'depression', but in order to arrive at diagnoses, a number of attributes have to be present, some of which are observed rather than reported by the patient.

The idea that a diagnosis is an envelope that encloses patients with different requirements, which share a common mechanism, is particularly applicable to psychiatry. For example patients within the 'envelope' of depression will contain subgroups, many of whom recover without help, some of whom benefit from cognitive therapy alone, others who benefit from antidepressant medication (especially if the depression is moderate); in severe cases, they may require electroconvulsive treatment (ECT).

Inability to carry out the activities of daily living

This is the patient's failure to exercise the most basic control over his or her personal space and immediate environment due to mental or physical disability. The patient's family, neighbours, or community may provide support to compensate (which can place enormous demands and burdens upon them). Failing this, it has to be provided by salaried personnel from a funded source. Each disability will then need to be identified specifically so that it can be supported properly.

Main differential diagnoses and typical outline evidence, etc.	
Mildly impaired activities of daily living	*Suggested by:* inability without assistance to: get out of bed or chair or dress or use toilet or wash or bathe or prepare food or eat it or shop or maintain a home or go outside or earn a living. *Confirmed by:* formal documentation of **at least one** of the above disabilities. *Finalized by the predictable outcome of management,* e.g. assistance for each specific disability in patient's own home.
Moderately impaired activities of daily living	*Suggested by:* inability without assistance to: get out of bed or chair, or dress or use toilet, or wash or bathe, or prepare food or eat it, or shop, or maintain a home, or go outside or earn a living. *Confirmed by:* formal documentation of **many of the above** disabilities, which require **constant supervision** but no additional skilled nursing assistance. *Finalized by the predictable outcome of management,* e.g. admission to residential home or constant supervision in patient's home.
Severely impaired activities of daily living	*Suggested by:* inability without assistance to: get out of bed or chair, or dress or use toilet, or wash or bathe, or prepare food or eat it, or shop, or maintain a home, or go outside or earn a living. *Confirmed by:* formal documentation of many of the above disabilities, which require constant supervision **and additional skilled nursing assistance.** *Finalized by the predictable outcome of management,* e.g. admission to institution providing skilled nursing or constant supervision and skilled nursing assistance in patient's home.

Acute anxiety

Anxiety is a common experience but when patients or their family or friends seek urgent advice, it is usually because it has been unusually severe and prolonged, or because of associated physical symptoms, e.g. palpitations. There may be associated physical illnesses that have precipitated the anxiety state (e.g. heart failure), as opposed to being direct causes (e.g. thyrotoxicosis). It may also be part of an underlying psychiatric illness. The direct causes are considered here. The history, examination, and tests are directed at confirming or excluding such direct or indirect causes. Initial investigations: FBC, U&E, LFT, TSH, FT4.

Main differential diagnoses and typical outline evidence, etc.	
Exacerbation of generalized anxiety disorder	*Suggested by:* background of recurrent tension, agitation, feelings of impending doom, trembling, a sense of collapse, insomnia, poor concentration, 'goose flesh', 'butterflies in the stomach', hyperventilation, tinnitus, tingling, tetany, chest pains, headaches, sweating, palpitations, poor appetite, nausea, inability to swallow but no physical abnormaility ('globus hystericus'), difficulty in getting to sleep, exessive concern about self or bodily functions, repetitive thoughts and activities (thumb sucking, nail biting, bed-wetting, food fads in children). *Confirmed by:* recognized criteria, e.g. the ICD-10.* *Finalized by the predictable outcome of management,* e.g. listening, reassurance about nature of symptoms, regular exercise, meditation, cognitive-behaviour therapy, progressive relaxation training, hypnosis, anxiolytics (e.g. diazepam), or antidepressants, e.g. selective serotonin reuptake inhibitors (SSRIs), e.g. paroxetine, azapirones, β-blockers, anti-histamines.
Panic disorder	*Suggested by:* intense feeling of apprehension or impending disaster. Developing quickly and unexpectedly without a recognizable trigger. Shortness of breath and sensation of smothering, nausea, abdominal pain, depersonalization and derealization, choking, numbness, tingling, palpitations, flushes, trembling, shaking, chest discomfort, fear of dying, sweating, dizziness, faintness. *Confirmed by:* recognized criteria, e.g. the ICD-10.* *Finalized by the predictable outcome of management,* e.g. reassurance about nature of symptoms, cognitive behaviour therapy, anxiolytics (e.g. diazepam), or antidepressants (e.g. SSRIs).

Agitated depression	*Suggested by:* such as agitation, anxiety, fatigue, guilt, impulsiveness, irritability, morbid or suicidal ideation, panic, paranoia, pressured speech and rage, occur simultaneously. *Confirmed by:* recognized criteria, e.g. the ICD-10.* *Finalized by the predictable outcome of management,* e.g. reassurance, cognitive behavioural therapy. Antidepressant, especially if somatic symptoms. ECT if severely depressed, especially with delusions and poor response to medications alone. Admission if suicidal ideas and isolation.
Alcohol withdrawal	*Suggested by:* recent heavy alcohol intake (usually superimposed on habitually high level). Visual hallucinations imply 'delirium tremens', tremor, agitations, paranoid delusions, and intense fright, sleep disturbance, ↑**MCV**, abnormal **LFT**, **EEG** changes. *Confirmed by:* alcohol history, subsequent episodes in similar circumstances, and recognized criteria, e.g. the ICD-10.* *Finalized by the predictable outcome of management,* e.g. sedation and alcohol detoxification (e.g. chlordiazepoxide or diazepam) with tailing off over days, thiamine IV.
Thyrotoxicosis usually to be excluded	*Suggested by:* heat intolerance, tremor, nervousness, palpitations, frequent bowel movements, proptosis, lid retraction, goitre. *Confirmed by:* ↓**TSH**, ↑**FT4**. *Finalized by the predictable outcome of management,* e.g. non-selective β-blocker, e.g. propranolol, to control symptoms if no contraindication, e.g. asthma, carbimazole, or propylthiouracil to suppress thyroid hormone production.
Phaeochromocytoma rare but to be considered and discounted if other symptoms are absent	*Suggested by:* abrupt episodes of anxiety, fear, chest tightness, sweating, headaches, and marked rises in BP. *Confirmed by:* catecholamines (↑**VMA**, ↑**HMMA**) or ↑free **metadrenaline** in urine and blood soon after episode. *Finalized by the predictable outcome of management,* e.g. α-blocker followed by β-blocker and then surgery.
Simple (specific) phobia	*Suggested by:* evoked anxiety in specific situations, avoidance of phobic situation, symptoms and signs of generalized anxiety disorder. *Confirmed by:* recognized criteria, e.g. the ICD-10.* *Finalized by the predictable outcome of management,* e.g. behavioural therapy, e.g. systematic desensitization therapy, exposure, flooding, implosion therapy, anti-anxiety medications, or antidepressant.

(Continued)

Obsessive–compulsive disorder	*Suggested by:* anxiety associated with history of compulsion to perform actions, rituals, or to repeat phrases that come to mind, which are understood to be senseless, e.g. handcleaning, checking that doors are locked. *Confirmed by:* recognized criteria, e.g. the ICD-10.* *Finalized by the predictable outcome of management,* e.g. behavioural or cognitive therapy, anti-depressants, e.g. clomipramine or SSRI, e.g. fluoxetine.
Social phobia (social anxiety)	*Suggested by:* anxiety with intense and persistent fear of being scrutinized or negatively evaluated by others in comparatively small groups, resulting in fear and avoidance of social situations (e.g. meeting people in authority, using a telephone). Fear of specific social situations. *Confirmed by:* recognized criteria, e.g. the ICD-10.* *Finalized by the predictable outcome of management,* e.g. cognitive behavioural therapy ± antidepressants, e.g. SSRI, paroxetine, fluoxetine.
Agoraphobia	*Suggested by:* fear of open spaces, crowds, or situations where escape is difficult. Staying at home, will not visit doctors ± depression, ± obsessional thought. *Confirmed by:* recognized criteria, e.g. the ICD-10.* *Finalized by the predictable outcome of management,* e.g. cognitive behavioural therapy ± anti-anxiety medications, antidepressants, e.g. SSRI.
Post-traumatic stress disorder caused by experiencing a traumatic event, e.g. major accident, fire, assault, military combat	*Suggested by:* memories, nightmares, flashbacks, numbing of emotions, anxiety and irritability, insomnia, poor concentration, hypervigilance, and depression, anxiety, and alcohol/other substance abuse and dependence. Delayed response arising within 6mo of an exceptional traumatic event. *Confirmed by:* recognized criteria, e.g. the ICD-10.* *Finalized by the predictable outcome of management,* e.g. psychotherapy, trauma-focused cognitive therapy, antidepressants, e.g. paroxetine if depressive component and with somatic symptoms.

Anorexia nervosa	*Suggested by:* self-induced weight loss, body image distortion, intense fear of gaining weight though underweight. Amenorrhoea in women for ≥3mo. and diminished sexual interest. Bingeing and vomiting, purging, or excessive exercise. Depression and social withdrawal, sensitivity to cold, delayed gastric emptying, constipation, low BP, bradycardia, hypothermia. *Confirmed by:* recognized criteria, e.g. the ICD-10.* *Finalized by the predictable outcome of management,* e.g. if no cooperation with keeping food diary, restoration of nutritional balance, correction of electrolyte and other deficiencies, admission to specialist unit. Cognitive behavioural therapies, analytic therapy, interpersonal therapy, supportive therapy, family therapy, antidepressants (e.g. SSRIs), specialist feeding.
Bulimia nervosa	*Suggested by:* preoccupation with eating and irresistible craving for food, fear of gaining weight, recurrent episodes of binge eating far beyond normally accepted amounts of food, self-induced vomiting, use of laxatives, diuretics ± appetite suppressants, often previous history of anorexia nervosa. *Confirmed by:* recognized criteria, e.g. the ICD-10.* *Finalized by the predictable outcome of management,* e.g. keeping food diary, cognitive behavioural therapy, SSRI antidepressants, fluoxetine.
Somatization disorder (Briquet's syndrome)	*Suggested by:* long history of numerous unsubstantiated physical complaints with no adequate physical explanation and refusal to be reassured. *Confirmed by:* recognized criteria, e.g. the ICD-10.* *Finalized by the predictable outcome of management,* e.g. reassurance that no serious underlying illness, explanation of mechanisms of symptoms, treatment of any underlying psychiatric disorder, e.g. antidepressants if indicated by other features, cognitive behaviour therapy.

*The ICD-10 Classification of Mental and Behavioural Disorders.

⅁ http://www.who.int/classifications/icd/en/bluebook.pdf

NB The diagnostic criteria are freely accessible on this URL but qualified with a caveat that the findings are elicited by someone trained to do so.

Depression

Depression is a common experience; it is its duration and severity that make patients to seek advice. This is also what is used to select the appropriate treatment. The diagnosis and selection of treatment is based on the history and mental state examination. Mild depression is usually self-limiting and the patient is supported by familiy and friends. Depression often presents as self-harm, which may be a serious suicide attempt or a 'cry for help'. It is usually a matter of professional judgement to predict that the illness has features that indicate that recovery will be spontaneous or prolonged and distressing unless there is intervention.

Main differential diagnoses and typical outline evidence, etc.	
Major depression	*Suggested by:* depressed mood ± loss of interest and enjoyment, reduced energy causing easy tiredness and reduced activity, change in appetite or weight, psychomotor agitation or retardation, insomnia or hypersomnia, sense of worthlessness or guilt, fatigue or loss of energy, diminished appetite, recurrent thoughts of death, low self-esteem, poor attention and concentration, hopelessness, suicidal and self-harm preoccupations.
	Confirmed by: recognized criteria, e.g. the ICD-10.*
	Finalized by the predictable outcome of management, e.g. reassurance, cognitive behavioural therapy, and shared decision with patient: antidepressant suggested if somatic symptoms. ECT if severely depressed, especially with delusions and poor response to medications alone. Admission if suicidal ideas and isolation.
Mild to moderate depression	*Suggested by:* depressed mood ± loss of interest in pleasure, change in appetite or weight, psychomotor agitation or retardation, insomnia or hypersomnia, sense of worthlessness or guilt, fatigue, loss of energy, recurrent thoughts of death or suicide.
	Confirmed by: recognized criteria, e.g. the ICD-10.*
	Finalized by the predictable outcome of management, e.g. cognitive behavioural therapy. Antidepressants.
Depression 2° or partly due to other conditions	*Suggested by:* history of any other illness that undermines self-confidence, e.g. stroke or physical illness.
	Confirmed by: resolution when underlying condition alleviated.
	Finalized by the predictable outcome of management, e.g. treatment of identifiable cause. Antidepressant, especially if somatic symptoms.

Depression 2° or partly due to medication	*Suggested by:* history of taking β-blockers, α-blockers, methydopa, statins, anticonvulsants, calcium channel blockers, corticosteroids, oral contraceptives, opiates, drugs used for Parkinson's disease (e.g. levodopa).
	Confirmed by: improvement if drug stopped or changed.
	Finalized by the predictable outcome of management, e.g. stopping potential causal drug.
Seasonal affective disorder	*Suggested by:* 'winter blues'—depression of mood + ↑sleep, ↑food intake (with carbohydrate craving), and weight gain, opposite mood swings in summer.
	Confirmed by: recognized criteria, e.g. the ICD-10.*
	Finalized by the predictable outcome of management, e.g. reassurance, antidepressant, especially if somatic symptoms.

*The ICD-10 Classification of Mental and Behavioural Disorders.

℘ http://www.who.int/classifications/icd/en/bluebook.pdf

NB The diagnostic criteria described are qualified with a caveat that the findings are elicited by someone trained to do so.

Delusions

Delusions are firmly held beliefs, held in the absence of supporting evidence or recognized shared cultural (e.g. religious) conventions. They may be depressive (in major depression), opitimistic (in mania), or neutral (in schizophrenia) in nature.

Main differential diagnoses and typical outline evidence, etc.	
Schizophrenia with acute presentation	*Suggested by:* primary delusions (usually bizarre), somatic or auditory hallucinations, thought disorder, e.g. insertion ± withdrawal, thought broadcasting, passivity feelings, thought echo, or hearing voices referring to the patient in the 3rd person), including blunting of emotions. *Confirmed by:* recognized criteria, e.g. the ICD-10.* *Finalized by the predictable outcome of management,* e.g. antipsychotics, e.g. olanzapine, risperidone to avoid side-effects. Typical antipsychotics, e.g. chlorpromazine or haloperidol (if extrapyramidal side effects, reducing dose, adding anticholinergic, e.g. procyclidine, or using atypical antipsychotics, e.g. clozapine—specialist treatment). Admission for supervision of care if danger to self or others.
Mania and hypomania unipolar or bipolar disorder (i.e. manic depression)	*Suggested by:* highly optimistic delusions, persistently high or euphoric mood out of keeping with circumstances, pressure of speech, no insight, over-assertiveness, ↑energy and activity, grandiose delusions, spending spree, ↑appetite, hallucinations, disinhibition, ↑sexual desire, labile mood, elation, self-important ideas, ↓pain threshold, irritability, poor concentration, hostility when thwarted, ↓desire or need for sleep. *Confirmed by:* recognized criteria, e.g. the ICD-10.* *Finalized by the predictable outcome of management,* e.g. antipsychotics (e.g. olanzapine) or mood stabilizer (e.g. valproate or lithium), admission for supervision of care if danger to self or others, treatment of potential precipitating cause, e.g. infection, hyperthyroidism, etc. Stopping potential precipitating drug, e.g. amphetamine, cocaine, antidepressants, glucocorticoids, etc.

Major psychotic depression	*Suggested by:* pessimistic delusions, depressed mood ± loss of interest in pleasure, change in appetite or weight, psychomotor agitation or retardation, insomnia or hypersomnia, sense of worthlessness or guilt, fatigue or loss of energy, recurrent thoughts of death, poor concentration, suicide. Concurrent psychotic symptoms, e.g. delusions and unpleasant auditory hallucinations.
	Confirmed by: recognized criteria, e.g. the ICD-10.*
	Finalized by the predictable outcome of management, e.g. combined antipsychotic and antidepressant medication. Admission to hospital if symptoms are severe, suicidal ideas, and isolation. Consider adding ECT if poor response to medication.

*The ICD-10 Classification of Mental and Behavioural Disorders.

🕮 http://www.who.int/classifications/icd/en/bluebook.pdf

NB The diagnostic criteria described are qualified with a caveat that the findings are elicited by someone trained to do so.

Acute confusion

Onset over hours/days, fluctuating conscious level (typically worse at night), impaired memory, disorientation in time and place, drowsy ± withdrawn or hyperactive and agitated, disordered thinking, (slow and muddled ± delusions, e.g. accusing relatives of taking things), hallucinations (particularly visual), mood swings.

Diagnostic approach: look for other leads in history and examination. Initial investigations (other tests in **bold** below): FBC, U&E, ABG, blood glucose, urine and blood cultures, LFT, CXR, ECG, CT scan.

Main differential diagnoses and typical outline evidence, etc.	
Bacteraemia or septicaemia due to urinary tract infection (UTI), upper respiratory tract infection (URTI)	*Suggested by:* fever, rigors, associated cough, chest signs, dysuria, frequency, urine dipstick +ve if UTI, ↑WCC. *Confirmed by:* blood or urine culture growing bacteria. Resolution of confusion on antibiotics. *Finalized by the predictable outcome of management,* e.g. provisional antibiotics depending on suspected source (e.g. trimethoprim for UTI), then definitive antibiotics depending on sensitivities.
Hypoxia	*Suggested by:* history or signs of lung or heart disease. Central cyanosis. *Confirmed by:* ↓P_aO_2, ↓P_aCO_2 on **blood gas analysis** in type 1 respiratory failure or right-to-left pulmonary shunt, ↑P_aCO_2 in type 2 respiratory failure. *Finalized by the predictable outcome of management,* e.g. controlled O_2 <28% if ↑P_aCO_2.
Alcohol withdrawal	*Suggested by:* tremor, visual hallucinations, ↑MCV, abnormal LFT. *Confirmed by:* history of heavy alcohol intake with sudden decrease. *Finalized by the predictable outcome of management,* e.g. sedation (e.g. chlordiazepoxide or diazepam) with tailing off over days.
Post-ictal state	*Suggested by:* history of previous fits, evidence of injury from clonic movements, tongue biting, incontinence. *Confirmed by:* recovery of minutes to hours and subsequent history of fit from witness. *Finalized by the predictable outcome of management,* e.g. neurological observations. Restoration of anti-epileptic treatment of already established, manage as 'first fit' if not.
Thiamine deficiency	*Suggested by:* history of poor diet, ataxia, nystagmus, ocular palsies. *Confirmed by:* ↓**red cell ketolase activity**, response to treatment. *Finalized by the predictable outcome of management,* e.g. thiamine IV initially, then PO.

Hypothyroidism	*Suggested by:* puffy features, sleepy, cold intolerant, slow-relaxing ankle (and other) jerks.
	Confirmed by: ↓T4, ↑TSH (if primary thyroid failure), ↓TSH or normal (if 2° to pituitary failure).
	Finalized by the predictable outcome of management, e.g. low-dose liothyronine initially if severe.
Thyrotoxicosis	*Suggested by:* tremor, sweating, lid retraction, or lag, ± goitre, tachycardia, hyper-reflexia.
	Confirmed by: ↑T4 or ↑T3, ↓TSH.
	Finalized by the predictable outcome of management, e.g. non-selective β-blocker, e.g. propranolol, followed by carbimazole or propylthiouracil.
Hypoglycaemia due to insulin errors usually, rarely insulinoma or adrenal failure	*Suggested by:* confusion, ataxia, sweating, tachycardia, known diabetes.
	Confirmed by: ↓blood glucose (<2mmol/L).
	Finalized by the predictable outcome of management, e.g. if unconscious, 10% glucose IV or glucagon IM or buccal glucose gel. If safe to swallow, glucose by mouth, then carbohydrate snack.
Adrenal failure due to 1° adrenal disease (Addison's disease) or 2° to ACTH deficiency	*Suggested by:* lethargy, weakness, dizziness, buccal and scar pigmentation if Addison's, hypotension.
	Confirmed by: ↓9a.m. plasma cortisol and impaired response to **short Synacthen® test.**
	Finalized by the predictable outcome of management, e.g. if ↓BP, fluids IV or colloids; if glucose, 10% glucose IV. If ill, hydrocortisone IV, (otherwise PO) + fludrocortisone.
Frontal lobe lesion: ischaemia, tumour, abscess	*Suggested by:* personality change, emotional lability, features of dementia, recent epilepsy.
	Confirmed by: **CT** or **MRI scan** of brain.
	Finalized by the predictable outcome of management, e.g. assess for feasibility of surgical removal.
Drug effect	*Suggested by:* presence drug which can potentially cause acute confusion.
	Confirmed by: resolution by stopping drug.
	Finalized by the predictable outcome of management, e.g. stopping drug.

Chronic confusion or cognitive impairment

Patient admitting to 'being a bit forgetful', but relatives complain of loss of short-term memory and inability to perform normally simple tasks, or failure to cope at home, or self-neglect. Established with Mini Mental State Examination (MMSE) with scores: place and date (10), registering three named objects (3), calculation (5), recall above three objects (3), naming two objects (2), repeating a phrase (1), three-stage command (3), reading (1), writing (1), copying (1), interpretation: <10/30—severe cognitive impairment, <17/30—moderate, <23/30—mild.

Diagnostic approach: history and examination for more diagnostic leads.

Initial investigations (other tests in **bold** below): FBC, ESR or CRP, LFT, calcium etc., TSH, FT4, CT scan.

Main differential diagnoses and typical outline evidence, etc.	
Alzheimer's disease	*Suggested by:* MMSE <10 with dysphasia, dyspraxia, agnosia, and inability to plan strategically. *Confirmed by:* by absence of features of vascular (multi-infarct) dementia or parkinsonism. CT: reduced brain mass and ↑ventricles. *Finalized by the predictable outcome of management,* e.g. provision of care requirements at home or need for institutional care.
Vascular (multi-infarct) dementia	*Suggested by:* stepwise progression of dementia with each infarct. Associated neurological defects, e.g. hemiparesis, pseudobulbar palsy, etc. *Confirmed by:* by multiple lacunar infarcts or larger strokes on CT scan. *Finalized by the predictable outcome of management,* e.g. aspirin, statin, control of BP to prevent progression, provision of care requirements.
Lewy body dementia	*Suggested and confirmed by:* fluctuating but persistent dementia with Parkinsonism ± hallucinations. CT scan unremarkable. *Finalized by the predictable outcome of management,* e.g. provision of care requirements. Treatment of associated Parkinsonism, etc.
Huntington's disease	*Suggested and confirmed by:* cognitive impairment in 3rd or 4th decade with psychomotor slowing, personality change, apathy, and depression. Involuntary choreiform movements of the face, shoulders, upper limbs, and gait. *Finalized by the predictable outcome of management,* e.g. provision of care requirements.

Creutzfeldt–Jakob disease (CJD) and variant CJD (even rarer since control of BSE)	*Suggested by:* progressive dementia, myoclonus, depression, diplopia, supranuclear palsy, field defects, hallucinations, cortical blindness. Aged <50 and slower progress suggests variant CJD. *Confirmed by:* clinical progress, tonsillar biopsy, **MRI scan** appearance. *Finalized by the predictable outcome of management, e.g.* provision of care requirements.

Headache—acute, new onset

Onset over seconds to hours. Initial investigations (other tests in **bold** below): FBC, ESR or CRP, CT scan.

Main differential diagnoses and typical outline evidence, etc.

Meningitis viral or bacterial	*Suggested by:* photophobia, fever, neck stiffness, vomiting, Kernig's sign. Petechial or purpuric rash (in meningococcal meningitis).
	Confirmed by: **CT brain** to exclude abscess if neurological signs present, **lumbar puncture**—viral meningitis: CSF clear, ↑lymphocytes, ↑protein, normal glucose. Bacterial meningitis: CSF ↑neutrophils, ↑protein, ↓glucose ↑visible bacteria on Gram stain.
	Finalized by the predictable outcome of management, e.g. benzylpenicillin IM or IV while awaiting confirmation of diagnosis, culture and sensitivity. Analgesia.
Low CSF pressure	*Suggested by:* worsening or recurrence of headache after lumbar puncture (usually for suspected meningitis) made worse by sitting up.
	Confirmed by: spontaneous resolution after few days.
	Finalized by the predictable outcome of management, e.g. bed rest for 24h until CSF reforms. Analgesia.
Subarachnoid haemorrhage	*Suggested by:* sudden occipital headache (often described as 'like a blow to the head'), variable degree of consciousness ± neck stiffness, subhyaloid haemorrhage ± focal neurological signs.
	Confirmed by: **CT or MRI brain scan. Lumbar puncture:** bloodstained CSF that does not clear in successive bottles, presence of xanthochromia in CSF (up to 2wk after the haemorrhage).
	Finalized by the predictable outcome of management, e.g. neuro obs until stable enough for neurosurgery if indicated by imaging results. Analgesia. Dexamethasone if ↑intracranial pressure.
Intracranial haemorrhage	*Suggested by:* focal neurological signs.
	Confirmed by: **CT/MRI brain scan.**
	Finalized by the predictable outcome of management, e.g. endotracheal intubation and ventilation if decreased level of consciousness and poor airway protection. Nil by mouth and fluids IV if dysphagia. Speech and language therapist (SALT) assessment. Treatment of severe hypertension (systolic >200mmHg), neuro obs until stable enough for neurosurgery (if indicated by imaging results). Analgesia. Dexamethasone or mannitol if ↑intracranial pressure.

Head injury with cerebral contusion	*Suggested by:* history of trauma, cuts/bruises, ↓conscious level, lucid period, amnesia.
	Confirmed by: **skull X-ray, CT head** normal or showing oedema but no subdural haematoma or extradural haemorrhage.
	Finalized by the predictable outcome of management, e.g. neuro obs until stable enough for neurosurgery if indicated by imaging results. Analgesia. Dexamethasone or mannitol if ↑intracranial pressure.
Acute closed angle glaucoma	*Suggested by:* red eyes, haloes, ↓visual acuity due to corneal clouding, pupil abnormality.
	Confirmed by: ↑**intra-ocular pressure.**
	Finalized by the predictable outcome of management, e.g. pilocarpine 2–4% eye drops 1 hourly. Acetazolamide PO or IV. Stepwise analgesia.
Sinusitis	*Suggested by:* fever, facial pain, mucopurulent nasal discharge, tender over sinuses ± URTI. ↑WCC suggest bacterial infection.
	Confirmed by: **X-ray of sinuses or CT scan:** mucosal thickening, a fluid level or opacification.
	Finalized by the predictable outcome of management, e.g. analgesia. Antibiotic if strong suspicion of bacterial infection.
Tension headache	*Suggested by:* generalized or bilateral, continuous, tight bandlike, worsens as the day progresses, associated with stress or tension ± aggravated by eye movement.
	Confirmed by: spontaneous improvement with simple analgesia.
	Finalized by the predictable outcome of management, e.g. reassurance regarding benign nature. Simple analgesia.
Bilateral migraine	*Suggested and confirmed by:* bilateral, throbbing ± vomiting, aura ± visual or other neurological disturbances with precipitating factor, e.g. premenstrual.
	Finalized by the predictable outcome of management, e.g. simple analgesia. Bed rest in darkened room. Prophylaxis.

Headache—subacute onset

Onset over hours to days. Initial investigations (other tests in **bold** below): FBC, ESR or CRP, CT scan.

Main differential diagnoses and typical outline evidence, etc.	
Raised intracranial pressure due to tumour, hydrocephalus, cerebral abscess, etc.	*Suggested by:* dull headache, worse on waking, vomiting, aggravated by, for example, cough, sneezing, bending; look for papilloedema, ↑BP, ↓pulse rate progressive focal neurological signs. *Confirmed by:* **CT/MRI brain scan.** *Finalized by the predictable outcome of management,* e.g. analgesia. Dexamethasone or mannitol for ↑intracranial pressure.
Encephalitis	*Suggested by:* fever, confusion, ↓conscious level. *Confirmed by:* CSF microscopy, serology, or PCR. *Finalized by the predictable outcome of management,* e.g. analgesia. Provisional antibiotics after discussion with microbiologist while awaiting culture results. Aciclovir if virus suspected. Dexamethasone or mannitol if ↑intracranial pressure.
Temporal/ giant cell or cranial arteritis	*Suggested by:* scalp tenderness, jaw claudication, loss of temporal arterial pulsation, sudden loss of vision, ↑↑ESR. *Confirmed by:* **temporal artery biopsy** (may be done shortly after starting prednisolone). *Finalized by the predictable outcome of management,* e.g. high dose prednisolone.

Headache—chronic and recurrent

Onset over weeks to months. Initial investigations (other tests in **bold** below): FBC, ESR or CRP, U&E, LFT, CT scan.

Main differential diagnoses and typical outline evidence, etc.

Tension headache	*Suggested and confirmed by:* generalized or bilateral, continuous, tight bandlike, worsens as the day progresses, associated with stress or tension, often aggravated by eye movement.
	Finalized by the predictable outcome of management, e.g. simple analgesia.
Migraine	*Suggested and confirmed by:* typically unilateral, throbbing ± vomiting, aura ± visual disturbances, precipitating factors.
	Finalized by the predictable outcome of management, e.g. simple analgesia. Bed rest in darkened room. Prophylaxis.
Cluster headache	*Suggested by:* episodic, typically nightly pain in one eye for wks with nasal stuffiness on same side.
	Confirmed by: episodes resolving over hours (like migraine).
	Finalized by the predictable outcome of management, e.g. simple analgesia.
Cervical root headache	*Suggested by:* occipital and back of the head, temples, vertex and frontal regions, worse on neck movement or restricted neck movements.
	Confirmed by: **cervical X-ray** showing degenerative changes (or normal) and response to NSAIDs.
	Finalized by the predictable outcome of management, e.g. simple analgesia, NSAIDs.
Eye strain	*Suggested by:* headaches worse after reading. Refractory error.
	Confirmed by: improvement with appropriate spectacles.
	Finalized by the predictable outcome of management, e.g. simple analgesia, appropriate spectacles.
Drug side-effect	*Suggested by:* drug history (e.g. nitrates).
	Confirmed by: improvement on drug withdrawal.
	Finalized by the predictable outcome of management, e.g. drug withdrawal.

Stroke

This is a sudden onset of a neurological deficit. Initial investigations (other tests in **bold** below): FBC, ESR or CRP, U&E, CT scan.

Main differential diagnoses and typical outline evidence, etc.	
Cerebral infarction	*Suggested by:* onset over minutes to hours of hemiparesis or major neurological defect that lasts >24h.
	Confirmed by: **CT scan** apparently normal initially, ↓ attenuation after days.
	Finalized by the predictable outcome of management, e.g. nil by mouth and fluids IV if dysphagia. SALT assessment. DVT prophylaxis: stockings/LMW heparin (if no bleed). If infarct: stat high dose and daily regular dose aspirin. Thrombolysis if initial event <4h previously. Dipyridamole if stroke occurred whilst on aspirin.
Transient cerebral ischaemic attack due to carotid artery stenosis, etc. (see ⊅ Transient neurological deficit, p.482)	*Suggested by:* onset over seconds to minutes of a neurological deficit that is improving already.
	Confirmed by: deficit resolving within 24h. **CT scan** showing no area of low attenuation and Carotis doppler.
	Finalized by the predictable outcome of management, e.g. aspirin 75mg daily.
Cerebral embolus due to atheroma, atrial fibrillation, myocardial infarction	*Suggested by:* onset over seconds of hemiparesis or other neurological defect that lasts >24h.
	Confirmed by: **CT scan** and **lumbar puncture** showing little change initially. Evidence of a potential source for an embolus, e.g. echocardiogram showing intracardiac thrombus.
	Finalized by the predictable outcome of management, e.g. withholding anticoagulation for weeks. Fluids IV if ability to swallow suspect. Dexamethasone for cerebral oedema. Rehabilitation. Anticoagulation later.
Cerebral haemorrhage due to atheromatous degeneration, cerebral tumour	*Suggested by:* onset over seconds of hemiparesis or major neurological defect that lasts >24h.
	Confirmed by: **CT** showing high attenuation ± 'low' (dark) 'oedema' area ± high density 'blood' in ventricles.
	Finalized by the predictable outcome of management, e.g. fluids IV if ability to swallow suspect. Dexamethasone for cerebral oedema. ±evacuation of haematoma by neurosurgeons. Rehabilitation.

Subdural haemorrhage due to blunt head injury	*Suggested by:* onset over hours, days, or weeks of a fluctuating hemiaparesis following history of head injury or fall (but often not) especially in elderly or alcoholic. *Confirmed by:* **CT** showing low attenuation parallel to skull if chronic but high attenuation if acute. *Finalized by the predictable outcome of management,* e.g. plan craniotomy to remove substantial thrombus. Fluids IV if ability to swallow suspect. Dexamethasone if cerebral oedema. Rehabilitation.
Extradural haemorrhage due to skull fracture lacerating middle meningeal artery	*Suggested by:* onset over minutes or hours of confusion, disturbed consciousness and hemiaparesis after 'lucid interval' of hours following head injury. *Confirmed by:* **CT head** showing high attenuation adjacent to skull ± midline shift. *Finalized by the predictable outcome of management,* e.g. craniotomy to remove thrombus. Fluids IV if ability to swallow suspect.
Subarachnoid haemorrhage from berry aneurysm	*Suggested by:* sudden onset over seconds of headache ± disturbance of consciousness (usually under 45y of age), neck stiffness. *Confirmed by:* **CT head** showing high attenuation area on surface of brain. **Lumbar puncture** showing blood. *Finalized by the predictable outcome of management,* e.g. fluids IV if ability to swallow suspect. Dexamethasone if cerebral oedema. Clipping of aneurysm if feasible.
Cerebellar stroke	*Suggested by:* sudden onset of ataxia. *Confirmed by:* **MRI scan** (**CT head** poorly visualizes hindbrain). *Finalized by the predictable outcome of management,* e.g. fluids IV if ability to swallow suspect. Dexamethasone if cerebral oedema. Rehabilitation.
Pontine stroke	*Suggested by:* sudden loss of consciousness. Cheyne–Stokes breathing (speeding up and slowing down over minutes) pinpoint pupils, hemiparesis, and eyes deviated towards paresis. *Confirmed by:* above clinical findings ± **MRI scan.** *Finalized by the predictable outcome of management,* e.g. fluids IV if ability to swallow suspect. Rehabilitation.

Dizziness

Dizziness is often self-limiting or 'non-specific' (nothing significant is ever found), but one of the following will be discovered in a proportion of patients. Distinguish between dizziness and vertigo (which has a sensation of movement), the latter being more 'specific' of an identifiable lesion. Initial investigations (other tests in **bold** below): FBC, ESR or CRP, U&E, CXR.

Main differential diagnoses and typical outline evidence, etc.	
Hyperventilation due to anxiety, panic attacks	*Suggested by:* associated anxiety and claustrophobia. Finger and lip paraesthesia of hyperventilation. Resting tachypnoea, no hypoxia. *Confirmed by:* **ABG:** normal or ↑O_2, ↓CO_2; **CXR:** normal; **spirometry** normal; **VQ scan** normal. Nijmegen score > 23 out of 64. *Finalized by the predictable outcome of management,* e.g. reassurance, anxiolytics, and breathing exercises.
Postural hypotension due to drugs to lower BP, loss of circulating volume, dehydration, diabetic autonomic neuropathy, old age + heavy meal, dopamine agonists, Addison's disease	*Suggested by:* associated palpitations, loss of consciousness. Supine and standing BP after 1min: >10mm drop. *Confirmed by:* response of BP changes to treatment of cause. *Finalized by the predictable outcome of management,* e.g. correction of underlying cause, then if necessary, fludrocortisone to raise BP.
Anaemia	*Suggested by:* subconjunctival pallor (± face, nail, and hand pallor). *Confirmed by:* **FBC:** ↓Hb. *Finalized by the predictable outcome of management,* e.g. treatment of underlying cause, e.g. recent blood loss with transfusion, iron deficiency with ferrous compound.
Hypoxic (with or without CO_2 retention)	*Suggested by:* blue hands and tongue (central cyanosis), restlessness, confused, drowsy, or unconscious. *Confirmed by:* **ABG:** ↓P_aO_2 <8kPa on blood gas analysis or **pulse oximetry** of <90% saturation (mild) or <80% (severe). *Finalized by the predictable outcome of management,* e.g. O_2 <28% if CO_2 retention, high flow (>28%) if no CO_2 retention.
Carotid sinus hypersensitivity	*Suggested by:* onset on head turning or shaving neck. *Confirmed by:* reproduction of symptoms while turning neck or pressure on carotid sinus. *Finalized by the predictable outcome of management,* e.g. advice about avoiding precipitating neck movements and/or soft collar.

Epilepsy	*Suggested by:* aura followed by other 'positive' neurological symptoms.
	Confirmed by: **EEG:** focal abnormality or 'spike and wave', etc.
	Finalized by the predictable outcome of management, e.g. anti-epileptic medication.
Drug effect	*Suggested by:* history of taking sedative or hypotensive drug, including alcohol.
	Confirmed by: resolution of symptom after stopping drug.

Vertigo

Vertigo is a sensation of movement of self ± the environment, especially rotation or oscillation. Initial investigations (other tests in **bold** below): FBC, ESR or CRP, U&E, ECG.

Main differential diagnoses and typical outline evidence, etc.	
Vertebrobasilar insufficiency (brainstem ischaemia)	*Suggested by:* visual disturbances, other signs of cerebral ischaemia, e.g. dysarthria, faint. *Confirmed by:* **carotid Doppler**—evidence of arterial disease. **MR angiogram** of brain and neck vessels. *Finalized by the predictable outcome of management,* e.g. antiplatelet drug (e.g. aspirin), BP, cholesterol, stop smoking, controlling risk factors.
Benign positional vertigo	*Suggested by:* attacks with duration of minutes only. *Confirmed by:* **Hallpike head tilt test:** nystagmus after 5s, lasting a minute. Shorter duration when repeated. *Finalized by the predictable outcome of management,* e.g. histamine analogues (e.g. betahistine) or sedatives (e.g. prochlorperazine), reassurance, positional physiotherapy. Canalith repositioning procedure.
Ménière's disease	*Suggested by:* attacks with duration of hours often incapacitating. Tinnitus ± progressive deafness in older patient. *Confirmed by:* **audiometry:** hearing loss with loudness recruitment. *Finalized by the predictable outcome of management,* e.g. histamine analogues (e.g. betahistine) or sedatives (e.g. prochlorperazine), surgical decompression of saccus endolymphaticus.
Vestibular neuronitis (associated with viral illness)	*Suggested by:* sudden, single prostrating attack, usually with nystagmus with resolution over weeks. *Confirmed by:* **caloric testing.** *Finalized by the predictable outcome of management,* e.g. histamine analogues (e.g. betahistine) or sedatives (e.g. prochlorperazine), reassurance regarding resolution within days to weeks.
Middle ear disease	*Suggested by:* painful ear, recurrent attacks, or persistent vertigo and nystagmus. *Confirmed by:* **audiometry:** conductive deafness. Otoscopic appearance of otitis media or cholesteatoma. *Finalized by the predictable outcome of management,* e.g. histamine analogues (e.g. betahistine) or sedatives (e.g. prochlorperazine), antibiotic for bacterial infection, surgical intervention.
Wernicke's encephalopathy due to thiamine deficiency, usually in alcoholism)	*Suggested by:* persistence of vertigo, ataxia, slurring of speech, and nystagmus despite withdrawal of alcohol. *Confirmed by:* resolution or improvement on thiamine treatment. *Finalized by the predictable outcome of management,* e.g. thiamine IV, then PO.

Ototoxic drugs	*Suggested by:* recurrent attacks or persistent vertigo and little nystagmus, history of streptomycin, gentamicin, kanamycin, phenytoin, quinine, or salicylates, etc.
	Confirmed by: bilateral loss of response to **caloric tests.** No signs of disease in brainstem, ears, or cerebellum.
	Finalized by the predictable outcome of management, e.g. stop potentially ototoxic drug.
Brainstem ischaemia or infarction	*Suggested by:* sudden onset and associated with peripheral vascular disease.
	Confirmed by: associated cranial nerve palsies, long tract signs (e.g. spastic paresis, extensor plantar response, sensory loss).
	Finalized by the predictable outcome of management, e.g. fluids IV if swallowing defect, antiplatelet agents after stabilization, nursing support.
Posterior fossa tumour	*Suggested by:* onset of vertigo over months, nystagmus. Bilateral papilloedema. Ipsilateral absent corneal reflex. Cranial nerve lesions V, VI, VII, X, and XI. Ipsilateral cerebellar and contralateral pyramidal signs.
	Confirmed by: **MRI scan** showing tumour.
	Finalized by the predictable outcome of management, e.g. histamine analogues (e.g. betahistine) or sedatives (e.g. prochlorperazine), surgical intervention.
Multiple sclerosis	*Suggested by:* sudden onset and central type nystagmus (occurs equally in both directions and sometimes vertically) in young person, other neurological disturbances, scanning speech, optic atrophy.
	Confirmed by: other similar neurological episodes 'disseminated in time and space' and multiple, enhancing lesions in various parts of nervous system on **MRI scan.**
	Finalized by the predictable outcome of management, e.g. histamine analogues (e.g. betahistine) or sedatives (e.g. prochlorperazine), methylprednisolone IV or immunoglobulin IV.
Migraine	*Suggested by:* associated headache (vertigo instead of visual aura).
	Confirmed by: resolution and recurrence in episodic manner.
	Finalized by the predictable outcome of management, e.g. simple analgesia. Bed rest in darkened room. Prophylaxis e.g. with clonidine.
Temporal lobe epilepsy	*Suggested by:* associated temporal lobe symptoms, e.g. odd taste, smells, visual hallucinations.
	Confirmed by: **EEG** findings and details of history.
	Finalized by the predictable outcome of management, e.g. anti-epileptic agent (e.g. carbamazepine, sodium valproate).
Ramsay Hunt syndrome due to herpes zoster	*Suggested by:* associated ear pain, lower motor neurone facial palsy.
	Confirmed by: Zoster vesicles at the external auditory meatus or fauces.
	Intial management: histamine analogues (e.g. betahistine) or sedatives (e.g. prochlorperazine), aciclovir.

'Fit'

History of aura, loss of consciousness, tonic and clonic movements. Initial investigations (other tests in **bold** below): FBC, ESR or CRP, U&E, blood glucose, calcium, ECG.

Main differential diagnoses and typical outline evidence, etc.	
Febrile convulsion	*Suggested by:* young age, especially in childhood and associated with a febrile illness. *Confirmed by:* normal **EEG** and **CT scan,** and no subsequent recurrence without febrile illness on follow-up. *Finalized by the predictable outcome of management,* e.g. lowering temperature with fan, oral or fluids IV, antipyretics (e.g. paracetamol).
Idiopathic epilepsy—new presentation	*Suggested by:* young age, especially in teens. *Confirmed by:* abnormal or normal **EEG,** and normal **CT scan** but subsequent recurrence. *Finalized by the predictable outcome of management,* e.g. if status epilepticus—benzodiazepine IV (e.g. lorazepam). If previous fit, anti-epileptic agent (e.g. carbamazepine, sodium valproate).
Known idiopathic epilepsy	*Suggested by:* history of previous fits. *Confirmed by:* past medical history of past investigations and on treatment. *Finalized by the predictable outcome of management,* e.g. if status epilepticus—benzodiazepine IV (e.g. lorazepam). Review ± adjusting existing dose in light of drug levels.
Brain tumour	*Suggested by:* older age (but any age), headaches, papilloedema. *Confirmed by:* **CT or MRI scan** showing cerebral mass. *Finalized by the predictable outcome of management,* e.g. if status epilepticus—benzodiazepine IV (e.g. lorazepam). If previous fit, anti-epileptic agent (e.g. carbamazepine, sodium valproate). Brain surgery.
Epilepsy due to meningitis	*Suggested by:* fever, neck stiffness. *Confirmed by:* **CT scan** and lumbar puncture. *Finalized by the predictable outcome of management,* e.g. if status epilepticus—benzodiazepine IV (e.g. lorazepam). Benzylpenicillin IM or IV while awaiting confirmation of diagnosis, culture, and sensitivity.
Epilepsy due to old brain scar tissue	*Suggested by:* past history of serious head injury or stroke. *Confirmed by:* abnormal **EEG, CT** or **MRI brain scan.** *Finalized by the predictable outcome of management,* e.g. if status epilepticus—benzodiazepine IV (e.g. lorazepam). If previous fit, anti-epileptic agent (e.g. carbamazepine).

Alcohol withdrawal	*Suggested by:* recent heavy alcohol intake (usually superimposed on habitually high intake).
	Confirmed by: subsequent episodes in similar circumstances.
	Finalized by the predictable outcome of management, e.g. if status epilepticus—benzodiazepine IV (e.g. diazepam) followed by oral sedative (e.g. chlordiazepoxide 15–50mg 6-hourly).
Hypoglycaemia due to too much insulin with too little food in diabetic, or insulinoma	*Suggested by:* sweating, hunger, known diabetic on insulin or medication.
	Confirmed by: ↓blood sugar (<2mmol/L) during episode.
	Finalized by the predictable outcome of management, e.g. buccal glucose gel if concious (e.g. GlucoGel®) or 50% glucose IV or glucagon 1mg IV or IM if unconscious.
Sudden severe hypotension (especially cardiac arrest)	*Suggested by:* peripheral and central cyanosis, no pulse or BP.
	Confirmed by: **ECG** shows asystole or ineffectual fast or slow rhythm (or electromechanical dissociation).
	Finalized by the predictable outcome of management, e.g. saline IV and/or plasma expander under central venous pressure (CVP) control. Cardiopulmonary resuscitation if cardiac arrest.
Severe electrolyte disturbance due to very high or low sodium, calcium, magnesium, etc.	*Suggested by:* abnormality on serum biochemistry.
	Confirmed by: no recurrence of fits after metabolic abnormality treated.
	Finalized by the predictable outcome of management, e.g. normal saline IV, then correction of hypertonicity or hypotonicity, and replacement of deficiencies.
'Functional' (pseudo-fit)	*Suggested by:* always occurring in front of audience, eyes closed during episode.
	Confirmed by: normal EEG when episode documented on video-recording. Normal **CT scan.**
	Finalized by the predictable outcome of management, e.g. counselling, psychotherapy.

Transient neurological deficit

Sudden dysphasia, facial or limb weakness resolving within 24h. Initial investigations (other tests in **bold** below): FBC, ESR or CRP, U&E, blood glucose, ECG, CT scan.

Main differential diagnoses and typical outline evidence, etc.	
Transient cerebral ischaemic attack (TIA) from platelet embolus? due to carotid artery stenosis or vasculitic process	*Suggested by:* onset over minutes, and then immediate improvement with prospect of complete resolution within 24h ± carotid bruit. *Confirmed by:* resolution within 24h, absence of previous fit, no throbbing migrainous headache, no chest pain, normal **ECG** and **troponin** after 12h, normal **blood sugar**, no witnessed fits and normal **CT. Doppler ultrasound** of carotids (to seek operable stenosis). ↑**ESR** or ↑**CRP** (if there is a vasculitic process, e.g. cranial arteritis). *Finalized by the predictable outcome of management,* e.g. aspirin 75mg daily, cholesterol-lowering agent (e.g. simvastatin).
Atrial fibrillation with cerebral embolus	*Suggested by:* irregularly irregular pulse. *Confirmed by:* irregularly irregular QRS complexes, no P wave on **ECG**. Echocardiogram showing intracardiac thrombus. *Finalized by the predictable outcome of management,* e.g. wait for weeks to avoid bleed into infarcted tissue, then anticoagulation (e.g. warfarin).
Intracerebral space-occuping lesion: tumour, aneurysm haematoma, arterio-venous malformation	*Suggested by:* associated headache. *Confirmed by:* **CT** or **MRI scan** appearance. *Finalized by the predictable outcome of management,* e.g. dexamethasone to reduce any oedema, planning for possible surgery.
Transient hypotension due to arrhythmia or myocardial infarction	*Suggested by:* history of chest pain or past medical history of ischaemic heart disease. *Confirmed by:* **ECG:** ST changes. ↑**troponin. 24h ECG:** recurrence of arrhythmia. *Finalized by the predictable outcome of management,* e.g. aspirin 75mg daily, cholesterol-lowering agents (e.g. simvastatin).
Todd's paralysis (following focal epileptic fit)	*Suggested by:* witness's history of fitting. *Confirmed by:* **EEG** changes. *Finalized by the predictable outcome of management,* e.g. if previous fit, anti-epileptic agent (e.g. carbamazepine, sodium valproate).

Migraine	*Suggested by:* associated throbbing headache (neurological deficit instead of visual aura).
	Confirmed by: resolution over minutes to hours. Normal **CT** and **MRI scan.**
	Finalized by the predictable outcome of management, e.g. simple analgesia for associated headache. Full recovery.
Hypoglycaemic episode	*Suggested by:* a known diabetic and associated sudden hunger, sweating, confusion, loss of consciousness.
	Confirmed by: **blood sugar** <2mmol/L.
	Finalized by the predictable outcome of management, e.g. oral glucose gel if conscious, 50% glucose IV bolus if unconscious.
Hyponatraemia	*Suggested by:* ↓↓sodium concentration (e.g. <120mmol/L) and ↓↓serum osmolality. Associated confusion.
	Confirmed by: resolution of deficit as **sodium concentration** and **osmolality** abnormality corrected.
	Finalized by the predictable outcome of management, e.g. normal saline IV or fluid restriction, depending on cause. Investigation and correction of underlying cause.
Multiple sclerosis (MS)	*Suggested by:* sudden onset and central type nystagmus (occurs equally in both directions and sometimes vertically) in young person, other neurological disturbances, scarring speech, optic atrophy.
	Confirmed by: other similar neurological episodes, 'disseminated in time and space' and multiple, enhancing lesions in various parts of nervous system on **MRI scan.**
	Finalized by the predictable outcome of management, e.g. methylprednisolone or immunoglobulin IV, physiotherapy, multidisciplinary (MDT) care.
Psychological	*Suggested by:* past history of similar episodes from young (<30y) age.
	Confirmed by: absence of any objective evidence of physical cause of deficit on follow-up.
	Finalized by the predictable outcome of management, e.g. counselling, assessment and psychotherapy.

Fatigue, 'tired all the time'

A poor lead—but consider the following possibilities during the history and examination. Initial investigations (other tests in **bold** below): FBC, U&E, fasting blood glucose, TSH, FT4.

Main differential diagnoses and typical outline evidence, etc.

Depression	*Suggested by:* early morning wakening, fatigue worse in the morning that never goes during the day, anhedonia, poor appetite. *Confirmed by:* recognized criteria, e.g. the ICD-10.* *Finalized by the predictable outcome of management,* e.g. response to psychotherapy or antidepressants.
Anaemia— microcytic, macrocytic, or normocytic	*Suggested by:* pale palms or conjunctivae. *Confirmed by:* ↓Hb, ↓MCV (microlytic)/↑MCV (microlytic)/ normal MCV (normolytic). *Finalized by the predictable outcome of management,* e.g. investigate with ferritin, folate, and vitamin B₁₂, treatment of cause.
1° hypothyroidism	*Suggested by:* cold intolerance, tiredness, constipation, bradycardia. *Confirmed by:* ↑**TSH**, ↓**FT4** and +ve **thyroid antibodies.** *Finalized by the predictable outcome of management,* e.g. thyroxine replacement therapy.
Sleep apnoea syndrome	*Suggested by:* frequent awakening at night, snoring and breathing pauses during sleep (history from a sleeping partner), and sleepiness during the day. *Confirmed by:* multiple dips in O₂ levels whilst asleep during home or hospital monitoring. *Finalized by the predictable outcome of management,* e.g. continuous positive airway pressure (CPAP) while asleep.
Drug-induced	*Suggested by:* taking sedating drug, including anti-epileptic treatment. *Confirmed by:* improvement by stopping or changing drug.
Post-viral fatigue	*Suggested by:* history of recent viral illness, especially glandular fever. *Confirmed by:* resolution after weeks or months. *Finalized by the predictable outcome of management,* e.g. reassurance.
Type 2 Diabetes mellitus	*Suggested by:* thirst polyuria, polydipsia, family history (but all may be absent). *Confirmed by:* **fasting blood glucose** ≥7.0mmol/L OR **random glucose** ≥11.1mmol/L on two occasions or during **GTT** in combination with symptoms. *Finalized by the predictable outcome of management,* e.g. education on diabetes, controlled carbohydrate, high-fibre diet ± metformin, sulphonylurea, insulin, etc.

Chronic fatigue syndrome (CFS)	*Suggested by:* (1) impaired memory/concentration unrelated to drugs or alcohol use, (2) unexplained muscle pain, (3) polyarthralgia, (4) unrefreshing sleep, (5) post-exertional malaise lasting over 24h, (6) persisting sore throat not caused by glandular fever, (7) unexplained tender cervical or axillary nodes.
	Confirmed by: recognized criteria, e.g. the ICD-10.*
	Finalized by the predictable outcome of management, e.g. reassurance and counselling.
Poor sleep habit	*Suggested by:* long working hours, little sleep, insomnia.
	Confirmed by: sleep diary and improvement with better sleep habits.
	Finalized by the predictable outcome of management, e.g. counselling.
Parasomnias	*Suggested by:* cataplexy, narcolepsy, and daytime somnolence.
	Confirmed by: response of symptoms to stimulant medication, e.g. methylphenidate.

*The ICD-10 Classification of Mental and Behavioural Disorders.

🔎 http://www.who.int/classifications/icd/en/bluebook.pdf

NB The diagnostic criteria are freely accessible on this URL but qualified with a caveat that the findings are elicited by someone trained to do so.

Examining the nervous system

If there were no symptoms at all suggestive of neurological disease, it is usual to perform a quick examination of the nervous system, and if this examination is normal, then the nervous system is not examined further. There will have been an opportunity to note the patient's posture and gait in the consulting room (or as the patient moves around the bed on the ward). If the patient's face looks normal and moves normally during speech, then there is unlikely to be a cranial nerve abnormality. The patient is then asked to hold both arms out to assess posture, to perform a 'finger-nose' test, to tap each hand on the other in turn, to 'unscrew door knobs', to tap each foot on the floor (or the examiner's hand if in bed), and then to do a 'heel-shin' test with each leg. Finally, reflexes are tested in the arms and legs. If all these are normal (and as emphasized already, there are no symptoms of neurological disorder), then the nervous system is not examined further. If there is a symptom or sign of neurological disorder, then the nervous system has to be examined carefully perhaps beginning with the territory under suspicion.

Disturbed consciousness

Consciousness assessed using Glasgow Coma Scale (GCS) based on adding score for (a) best verbal response (see ➔ Best verbal response, p.487), (b) best motor response (see ➔ Best motor response, p.488), and (c) eye opening (see ➔ Eye opening, p.488).

Main differential diagnoses and typical outline evidence, etc.	
Probably no current brain damage	*Suggested by:* GCS = 15 (patient complying with all requests, oriented in time and place, opening eyes spontaneously). *Confirmed by:* neurological observation.
Probable minor brain injury	*Suggested by:* GCS of 13–15. *Confirmed by:* neurological observation or **CT or MRI scan** appearance.
Probable moderate brain injury	*Suggested by:* GCS of 9–12. *Confirmed by:* neurological observation or **CT or MRI scan** appearance.
Probable severe brain injury	*Suggested by:* GCS of 3–8. *Confirmed by:* neurological observation or **CT or MRI scan** appearance.
Probable very severe brain injury	*Suggested by:* GCS = 3 (no response to pain, no verbalization, and no eye opening). *Confirmed by:* neurological observation or **CT or MRI scan** appearance.

Best verbal response

Differential diagnosis	
Oriented: score 5	*Confirmed by:* knowing own name, the place, why there, year, season and month.
Confused conversation: score 4	*Confirmed by:* conversation, but does not know name, not the place, not why there, nor year, season or month.
Inappropriate speech: score 3	*Confirmed by:* no conversation, but random speech or shouting.
Incomprehensible speech: score 2	*Confirmed by:* moaning but no words.
No speech at all: score 1	*Confirmed by:* silence.

Best motor response

Differential diagnosis

Carrying out verbal requests: score 6	*Confirmed by:* doing simple things that you ask (ignore grasp reflex).
Localizing response to pain: score 5	*Confirmed by:* purposeful movement in response to pressure on fingernail, supra-orbital ridges and sternum.
Withdraws to pain: score 4	*Confirmed by:* pulling limb away from painful stimulus.
Flexor response to pain— 'decorticate posture': score 3	*Confirmed by:* flexion of limbs to painful stimulus.
Extensor response to pain— 'decerebrate posture': score 2	*Confirmed by:* pain causing adduction and internal rotation of shoulder, and pronation of forearm.
No response to pain: score 1	*Confirmed by:* no response to painful stimulus.

Eye opening

Comment: to be used to give GCS score.

Spontaneous eye opening: score 4	*Confirmed by:* eyes open and fixing on objects.
Eye opening in response to speech: score 3	*Confirmed by:* response to specific request or a shout.
Eye opening in response to pain: score 2	*Confirmed by:* response to pain.
No eye opening at all: score 1	*Confirmed by:* no response to pain.

Speech disturbance

Inability to converse can be due to disturbance in any part of the process due to deafness, poor attention, receptive dysphasia, motor dysphasia, dysarthria, dysphonia or aphonia, or combinations of these. Initial investigations (other tests in **bold** below): FBC, ESR or CRP, CT scan.

Main differential diagnoses and typical outline evidence, etc.	
Deafness due to ear disease or 8th cranial nerve lesions	*Suggested by:* no reaction to speech or noises. *Confirmed by:* conductive or nerve deafness on Rinne or Weber tests. *Finalized by the predictable outcome of management,* e.g. hearing aid for conductive deafness.
Inattention due to dementia, depression, etc.	*Suggested by:* normal reaction (e.g. startling) to noise or speech, but no interest in source of noise or speech. *Confirmed by:* low MMSE score ± **CT** or **MRI** of brain showing cerebral atrophy.
Sensory dysphasia due to lesion in Wernicke's area	*Suggested by:* inability to understand or comprehend speech (as if a foreign language is being spoken to patient). Worse for vocabulary or language acquired later in life. *Confirmed by:* **CT** or **MRI scan** showing lesion in Wernicke's area in dominant temporal lobe.
Motor dysphasia (or aphasia) due to lesion in dominant frontal-parietal lobe	*Suggested by:* inability to find words or names of things (nominal dysphasia). *Confirmed by:* **CT** or **MRI** scan showing lesion in Broca's area in frontal lobe. *Finalized by the predictable outcome of management,* e.g. speech therapy.
Dysarthria (or anarthria) due to cerebellar connections, upper or lower motor neurone lesion	*Suggested by:* inability to coordinate speech with slurring, mumbling, failure to initiate or sustain speech. *Confirmed by:* associated features of weakness or in-coordination of oral muscles. *Finalized by the predictable outcome of management,* e.g. speech therapy.
Dysphonia (or aphonia) due to vocal cord dysfunction	*Suggested by:* hoarseness, voice loss or weakness, inability to cough properly. *Confirmed by:* indirect laryngoscopy (using mirror) to show vocal cord dysfunction or paresis. *Finalized by the predictable outcome of management,* e.g. treatment of underlying cause.

Dysarthria

Difficulty with articulation and incoordination of speech muscles. Initial investigations (other tests in **bold** below): FBC, ESR or CRP, U&E, CT scan.

Main differential diagnoses and typical outline evidence, etc.	
Cortical cerebral lesion (due to bleed, infarction, or tumour)	*Suggested by:* slow, stiff speech (and dysphasia if extensive lesion in dominant hemisphere, i.e. most dextrous hand is also affected) and other 'cortical' signs. *Confirmed by:* **CT** or **MRI scan** of brain. *Finalized by the predictable outcome of management,* e.g. speech therapy.
Internal capsule cerebral lesion (due to bleed, infarction, or tumour)	*Suggested by:* slow, stiff speech, and other internal capsule signs (e.g. spastic hemiparesis). *Confirmed by:* **CT** or **MRI scan** of brain. *Finalized by the predictable outcome of management,* e.g. speech therapy.
Upper motor neurone brainstem (pseudobulbar palsy due to ischaemia, motor neurone disease, MS)	*Suggested by:* slow, stiff nasal quality, slurred, and other brainstem signs (e.g. spastic hemiparesis, dysphagia). *Confirmed by:* **MRI scan** of brainstem. *Finalized by the predictable outcome of management,* e.g. speech therapy.
Lower motor neurone brain stem (bulbar) palsy due to ischaemia, motor neurone disease, 'polio' syringobulbia, MS)	*Suggested by:* nasal ('Donald Duck' quality) and other brainstem signs (e.g. spastic hemiparesis, dysphagia). *Confirmed by:* **MRI scan** of brain stem. *Finalized by the predictable outcome of management,* e.g. speech therapy.
Extrapyramidal dysarthria (due to Parkinson's disease)	*Suggested by:* difficulty in initiating speech, which is slow with other signs of Parkinsonian syndrome. *Confirmed by:* response to dopaminergic drugs. *Finalized by the predictable outcome of management,* e.g. speech therapy.
Cerebellar lesion (due to MS, ischaemia, tumour, hereditary ataxias)	*Suggested by:* staccato, undulating, broken flow, slurred, and other cerebellar signs (e.g. ataxia). *Confirmed by:* **MRI scan** of cerebellum. *Finalized by the predictable outcome of management,* e.g. speech therapy.
Drug effect (e.g. alcohol, sedatives)	*Suggested by:* dysarthria (slurred) and other drug effects. *Confirmed by:* response to removal of drug. *Finalized by the predictable outcome of management,* e.g. await metabolism of alcohol.

Absent sense of smell

This is not tested routinely, but ask the patient if there is anything abnormal about their smell or taste. Test using bottles with familiar essences. Initial investigations (other tests in **bold** below): skull X-ray, FSH, LH.

Main differential diagnoses and typical outline evidence, etc.	
Coryza (common cold)	*Suggested by:* runny nose, fever, headache, sporadic, perhaps with contact history. *Confirmed by:* history and nasal speculum examination. *Finalized by the predictable outcome of management,* e.g. awaiting resolution of infection.
Nasal allergy	*Suggested by:* runny nose, fever, headache, recurrent and recognizable precipitant. *Confirmed by:* history and nasal speculum examination. *Finalized by the predictable outcome of management,* e.g. nasal glucocorticoid spray.
Skull fracture	*Suggested by:* history of facial or head injury. *Confirmed by:* history or **skull X-ray** in acute phase. *Finalized by the predictable outcome of management,* e.g. await recovery from fracture.
Frontal lobe tumour	*Suggested by:* personality change, features of dementia, recent epilepsy. *Confirmed by:* **CT** or **MRI scan** of brain. *Finalized by the predictable outcome of management,* e.g. surgical removal.
Kallman's syndrome	*Suggested by:* delayed puberty or poor secondary sexual characteristics and libido, infertility. 1° amenorrhoea in females. (As condition is congenital, patient may be unaware of absent sense of smell (i.e. only detected on formal testing with scents). *Confirmed by:* ↓**oestrogens** or ↓**testosterone**, and normal or ↓**FSH**, and normal or ↓**LH**.

Abnormal ophthalmoscopy appearance

Start with high positive (+) numbers for the eye surface and use the lowest light level possible. Look for the red reflex, and zoom into the eye until the red reflex fills the field of view. Examine the retina by rotating down to negative (−) numbers. Start with the disc, found by looking towards the patient's midline, and then follow the four main arteries out and back. Examine the macula by asking the patient to look at the light.

Main differential diagnoses and typical outline evidence, etc.	
Corneal opacity in quiet eye (old ulcer due to past trauma, trachoma—tropical countries)	*Suggested by:* grey opacity in the clear cornea without dilated blood vessels, gradual loss of vision. *Confirmed by:* absence of staining with fluorescein. *Finalized by the predictable outcome of management,* e.g. corneal replacement surgery.
Cataract (due to ageing (75%), diabetes, trauma, steroids, radiation, intra-uterine rubella or toxoplasmosis, or rubella, hypocalcaemia, etc.)	*Suggested by:* history of gradual onset of visual blurring, and lens opacity visible during the red reflex examination with the ophthalmoscope. Usually >65y or history of underlying condition (often already known and cataract develops later). *Confirmed by:* ophthalmoscopical appearance. *Finalized by the predictable outcome of management,* e.g. mydriatic eye drops, sunglasses, phaco-emulsion with lens implantation.
Optic nerve swelling or (eventually) atrophy (due to papillitis from MS, or papilloedema or optic nerve infarction in temporal arteritis and retinal artery occlusion)	*Suggested by:* raised pink optic disc with blurred margins ± distended capillaries, and adjacent streak haemorrhages progressing to pale white disc with pale margins. Gradual loss of vision after initial disturbance. *Confirmed by:* visual field charting. Ophthalmoscopical appearance. *Finalized by the predictable outcome of management,* e.g. treatment of underlying cause, e.g. dexamethasone for ↑intracranial pressure, prednisolone for cranial arteritis.
Peripheral retinal damage (e.g. due to laser therapy for diabetic retinopathy)	*Suggested by:* irregular pale patches of depigmentation with central black areas of pigment clumping. *Confirmed by:* ophthalmoscopical appearance and history. *Finalized by the predictable outcome of management,* e.g. counselling regarding permanence.
'Wet' age-related macular degeneration (about 10% of MD)	*Suggested by:* rapid loss of central vision. *Confirmed by:* ophthalmoscopical and fluorescein angiographic appearance of neovascular vessel formation at the macula with exudates. *Finalized by the predictable outcome of management,* e.g. intraocular injection of anti-VEGF (vascular endothelial growth factor), e.g. ranibizumab or laser photocoagulation or photodynamic laser therapy.

'Dry' age-related macular degeneration (about 90% of MD)	*Suggested by:* gradual loss of central vision, large, central, yellowish white scar or haemorrhage when patient looks at ophthalmoscope light. *Confirmed by:* ophthalmoscopical ± and fluorescein angiographic appearance. *Finalized by the predictable outcome of management,* e.g. supportive measures.
Retinal vein occlusion	*Suggested by:* sudden vision loss, often in upper or lower half only. *Confirmed by:* extensive superficial retinal haemorrhages following the nerve fibre layer in the upper or lower half of the retina. *Finalized by the predictable outcome of management,* e.g. argon laser grid photocoagulation.
Retinal artery occlusion	*Suggested by:* sudden loss of vision—total or partial upper or lower field. *Confirmed by:* in the first few days retinal pallor. Later, a white, thready, thin artery. *Finalized by the predictable outcome of management,* e.g. prevention of further episodes, e.g. aspirin, lipid-lowering drugs.
Primary optic atrophy (prior inflammation not seen—due to MS or optic nerve infarction)	*Suggested by:* gradual visual loss in a quiet eye and pale disc with sharp margins. *Confirmed by:* ophthalmoscopical appearance of pale, white, featureless disc ± thin thready vessels. *Finalized by the predictable outcome of management,* e.g. prevention of further episodes, e.g. aspirin, lipid-lowering drugs.
Glaucoma	*Suggested by:* gradual loss of vision, deeply cupped disc. *Confirmed by:* ophthalmoscopical appearance of deep cupping with visible cribriform plate and nasal displacement of vessels. Loss of peripheral field. ↑intra-ocular pressure. *Finalized by the predictable outcome of management,* e.g. pilocarpine eye drops + betaxolol, or timolol.
Retinitis pigmentosa	*Suggested by:* loss of peripheral and night vision. *Confirmed by:* visual field charting. Pale disc, thin thready blood vessels, and fine star-shaped pigment without patches of depigmentation. Visual field charting. *Finalized by the predictable outcome of management,* e.g. counselling regarding prognosis.
Choroidoretinitis	*Suggested by:* gradual loss of vision or blurring (in acute phases), and 'patchy' visual loss—scotoma. *Confirmed by:* visual field charting showing irregular patchy areas of visual loss. Corresponding areas in the eye of irregular depigmentation with dense areas of pigment in the centre. Tests results for underlying cause: CXR, serology, sputum, lung biopsy, etc. *Finalized by the predictable outcome of management,* e.g. treatment of underlying cause, e.g. for toxoplasmosis, cytomegalovirus infection, TB.

Ophthalmoscopy appearance in the diabetic

Red-free or green light of ophthalmoscope very useful for retinopathy. NB Serial visual acuity measurements to detect early maculopathy.

Main differential diagnoses and typical outline evidence, etc.	
'Diabetic' cataract	*Suggested by:* gradual visual loss in a diabetic. *Confirmed by:* ophthalmoscopical appearance. *Finalized by the predictable outcome of management,* e.g. mydriatic eye drops, sunglasses, phaco-emulsion with lens implantation.
'Diabetic' glaucoma	*Suggested by:* pale, deeply cupped disc with sharp margins. *Confirmed by:* ophthalmoscopical appearance and visual field test. ↑intraocular pressure. *Finalized by the predictable outcome of management,* e.g. pilocarpine eye drops + betaxolol, or timolol.
Diabetic micro-aneurysm and bleeding into retina	*Suggested by:* dots (micro-aneurysms or deep haemorrhages) and blots or flames (deep and superficial haemorrhages). *Confirmed by:* regular retinal photography for progress. *Finalized by the predictable outcome of management,* e.g. strict BP and diabetic control, laser photocoagulation.
Venous irregularity preceding haemorrhage	*Suggested by:* localized widening of veins (e.g. sausage-shaped). *Confirmed by:* regular retinal photography for progress. *Finalized by the predictable outcome of management,* e.g. strict BP and diabetic control, laser photocoagulation.
Diabetic hard exudates	*Suggested by:* round and small pale area (after a single, serous leak), circular with central red dot (indicating a continuous leak), enlarging circle with time. *Confirmed by:* regular retinal photography for progress. *Finalized by the predictable outcome of management,* e.g. strict BP and diabetic control, laser photocoagulation.
Diabetic macular exudates (leading to visual loss)	*Suggested by:* star-shaped pallor (as the exudates follow the radial nerve fibre arrangement) and loss of visual acuity. *Confirmed by:* regular retinal photography for progress. *Finalized by the predictable outcome of management,* e.g. laser photocoagulation.
Diabetic soft exudates (nerve fibre infarct preceding new vessels)	*Suggested by:* pale grey area with indistinct margins. *Confirmed by:* regular retinal photography for progress. *Finalized by the predictable outcome of management,* e.g. strict BP and diabetic control, laser photocoagulation.

Diabetic new vessel formation (leads to haemorrhage)	*Suggested by:* 'frond' growing forwards into the vitreous (seen by adjusting focus) or like a net growing on the surface of the retina, arising from disc or larger peripheral veins. *Confirmed by:* three-dimensional clinical appearance. *Finalized by the predictable outcome of management,* e.g. laser photocoagulation.
Retinal haemorrhage and detachment	*Suggested by:* subhyaloid haemorrhage obscuring underlying vessels, often forming 'nest shape'—flat top and round bottom. *Confirmed by:* three-dimensional clinical appearance. *Finalized by the predictable outcome of management,* e.g. sclera silicone implants, or cryotherapy, or argon or laser coagulation.
Vitreous haemorrhage	*Suggested by:* sudden loss of vision in a diabetic and a poor red reflex on ophthalmoscopy. *Confirmed by:* retinal photography. *Finalized by the predictable outcome of management,* e.g. vitrectomy.
Retinal vein occlusion	*Suggested by:* sudden vision loss, often in upper or lower half only. *Confirmed by:* extensive superficial retinal haemorrhages following the nerve fibre layer which may be in only the upper or lower half of the retina. *Finalized by the predictable outcome of management,* e.g. argon laser grid photocoagulation.

Ophthalmoscopy appearances in the hypertensive

Main differential diagnoses and typical outline evidence, etc.

Grade I hypertensive retinopathy	*Suggested by:* ↑BP on three occasions typically >90mmHg diastolic or >140mmHg systolic. *Confirmed by:* segmental narrowing and tortuosity of arteries. *Finalized by the predictable outcome of management,* e.g. control of BP.
Grade II hypertensive retinopathy	*Suggested by:* moderately ↑BP on three occasions typically >100mmHg diastolic or >160mmHg systolic. *Confirmed by:* segmental narrowing and tortuosity of arteries, and arterio-venous nipping. *Finalized by the predictable outcome of management,* e.g. control of BP.
Grade III hypertensive retinopathy	*Suggested by:* severely ↑BP on three occasions typically >120mmHg diastolic or >180mmHg systolic. *Confirmed by:* segmental narrowing and tortuosity of arteries, and arterio-venous nipping, and haemorrhages and exudates. *Finalized by the predictable outcome of management,* e.g. control of BP.
Grade IV hypertensive retinopathy	*Suggested by:* severely ↑BP, typically >140mmHg diastolic or >200mmHg systolic. *Confirmed by:* segmental narrowing and tortuosity of arteries, and arterio-venous nipping, and haemorrhages, exudates, and papilloedema. *Finalized by the predictable outcome of management,* e.g. control of BP.

Sudden loss of central vision and acuity

Visual acuity is tested in each eye with a Snellen chart at 6m: 6/6 = 100% acuity and 6/60 = 10% acuity (letters normally read at 60m only readable at 6m). Fields are tested by facing patient 1m away and patient closing matching eyes. Wag your finger, moving in from the periphery horizontally and diagonally, changing hands. Test for scotoma with red marker pen top, moving horizontally, and asking for change of colour and disappearance. The rate of onset is important, sudden loss of vision is an emergency. Investigations in **bold** below.

Main differential diagnoses and typical outline evidence, etc.	
Optic nerve swelling or (eventually) atrophy (due to papillitis from MS or papilloedema or optic nerve infarction in temporal arteritis and retinal artery occlusion)	*Suggested by:* raised pink optic disc with blurred margins ± distended capillaries, and adjacent streak haemorrhages progressing to pale white disc with pale margins. Gradual loss of vision after initial disturbance. *Confirmed by:* visual field charting. Ophthalmoscopical appearance. *Finalized by the predictable outcome of management,* e.g. treatment of underlying cause, e.g. dexamethasone for ↑intracranial pressure, prednisolone for temporal arteritis.
Temporal/giant cell or cranial arteritis	*Suggested by:* scalp tenderness, jaw claudication, loss of temporal arterial pulsation, sudden loss of vision, ↑↑ESR. *Confirmed by:* **temporal artery biopsy** (may be done shortly after starting prednisolone). *Finalized by the predictable outcome of management,* e.g. prednisolone 40–60mg daily initially.
Retinal artery occlusion	*Suggested by:* sudden loss of vision—total or partial upper or lower field. *Confirmed by:* in the first few days, retinal pallor. Later a white, thready, thin artery. *Finalized by the predictable outcome of management,* e.g. prevention of further episodes, e.g. aspirin, lipid-lowering drugs.
Retinal vein occlusion	*Suggested by:* sudden vision loss, often in upper or lower half only. *Confirmed by:* extensive superficial retinal haemorrhages following the nerve fibre layer in the upper or lower half of the retina. *Finalized by the predictable outcome of management,* e.g. argon laser grid photocoagulation.
Vitreous haemorrhage	*Suggested by:* sudden loss of vision in a diabetic and a poor red reflex on ophthalmoscopy. *Confirmed by:* retinal photography. *Finalized by the predictable outcome of management,* e.g. vitrectomy.

Gradual onset of visual loss

Investigations in **bold** below.

Main differential diagnoses and typical outline evidence, etc.

Cataract (due to ageing (75%), diabetes, trauma, steroids, radiation, intra-uterine rubella or toxoplasmosis, or rubella, hypocalcaemia, etc.)	*Suggested by:* gradual onset of visual blurring and lens opacity visible during the red reflex examination with the ophthalmoscope. Usually >65y or history of underlying condition (often already known and cataract develops later). *Confirmed by:* ophthalmoscopical appearance. *Finalized by the predictable outcome of management,* e.g. mydriatic eye drops, sunglasses, phaco-emulsion with lens implantation.
Macular degeneration (age-related)	*Suggested by:* gradual loss of central vision, large, central, yellowish white scar or haemorrhage when patient looks at ophthalmoscope light. *Confirmed by:* ophthalmoscopical appearance. *Finalized by the predictable outcome of management,* e.g. laser photocoagulation or photodynamic laser therapy.
Choroidoretinitis	*Suggested by:* gradual loss of vision, or blurring (in acute phases), and 'patchy' visual loss—scotomata. *Confirmed by:* visual field charting showing irregular patchy areas of visual loss. Corresponding areas in the eye of irregular depigmentation with dense areas of pigment in the centre. Tests results for underlying cause: **CXR, serology, sputum, lung biopsy.** *Finalized by the predictable outcome of management,* e.g. treatment of underlying cause, e.g. for toxoplasmosis, cytomegalovirus infection, TB.
Glaucoma	*Suggested by:* gradual loss of vision, deeply cupped disc. *Confirmed by:* ophthalmoscopical appearance of deep cupping with visible cribriform plate and nasal displacement of vessels. Loss of peripheral field. ↑intra-ocular pressure. *Finalized by the predictable outcome of management,* e.g. pilocarpine eye drops + betaxolol, or timolol.
Primary optic atrophy (prior inflammation not seen—due to MS or optic nerve infarction)	*Suggested by:* gradual visual loss in a quiet eye and pale disc with sharp margins. *Confirmed by:* ophthalmoscopical appearance of pale, white, featureless disc, and may have thin thready vessels. *Finalized by the predictable outcome of management,* e.g. treatment of underlying cause.

Peripheral visual field defect

An upper or lower half defect is due to ocular pathology. Lesions between eye and chiasm cause unilateral defects, but those from chiasma to brain are homonymous, i.e. affecting same area in each eye. Investigations in **bold** below.

Main differential diagnoses and typical outline evidence, etc.	
Psychogenic field defect	*Suggested by:* 'TUNNEL vision' (same diameter at all distances). Normal optic disc, visual acuity, and colour vision. *Confirmed by:* no progression on follow-up. *Finalized by the predictable outcome of management*, e.g. reassurance about prognosis.
Retinitis pigmentosa	*Suggested by:* funnel vision with good visual acuity in light, with inability to navigate around objects, and virtually blind in the dark. *Confirmed by:* pale atrophic disc, thin thready vessels, and asterisk or reticular type pigment in the retina without pale patches of depigmentation. Visual field charting. *Finalized by the predictable outcome of management*, e.g. counselling regarding prognosis.
Choroiditis (choroido-retinitis) (due to TB, sarcoid, toxoplasmosis, toxacara)	*Suggested by:* gradual loss vision or blurring (in acute phases), grey white raised patch on retina, vitreous opacities, muddiness in the anterior chamber, then white patch with pigmentation around on retina (choroidoretinal scarring). *Confirmed by:* tests results for underlying cause—**CXR, serology, sputum, lung biopsy.** *Finalized by the predictable outcome of management*, e.g. treatment of underlying cause, e.g. anti-TB therapy.
Optic chiasm lesion (due to pituitary tumour, craniopharyngioma, aneurysm)	*Suggested by:* bitemporal hemianopia (or sometimes bitemporal upper quadrantinopia from tumour pushing up). *Confirmed by:* visual field charting. **CT or MRI scan** appearance. *Finalized by the predictable outcome of management*, e.g. treatment of underlying cause, e.g. surgical removal or reduction.
Optic tract lesion (due to middle cerebral artery thrombosis of contralateral side)	*Suggested by:* homonymous hemianopia. *Confirmed by:* visual field charting. **MRI scan** appearance. *Finalized by the predictable outcome of management*, e.g. treatment of underlying cause, prevention of recurrence, e.g. aspirin.
Visual cortex lesion (due to posterior cerebral artery occlusion, tumour)	*Suggested by:* homonymous hemianopia or occasionally quadrantanopia. May have macular sparing (visual acuity normal). Funnel vision if bilateral. *Confirmed by:* visual field charting. **CT or MRI scan** appearance. *Finalized by the predictable outcome of management*, e.g. treatment of underlying cause and prevention of recurrence, e.g. aspirin.

Ptosis

Drooping of one or both upper eyelids. Investigations in **bold** below.

Main differential diagnoses and typical outline evidence, etc.	
Oculomotor (3rd nerve) lesion due to pituitary tumour, intra-cavernous or posterior communicating artery aneurysm, meningioma, tentorial pressure cone, diabetes mellitus, syphilis, and brainstem ischaemia	*Suggested by:* ptosis, diplopia, and squint maximal on looking up and in; but therefore, in total loss, eye looks down and out. **Dilated pupil (except in diabetes mellitus, syphilis, and brainstem ischaemia when pupil not dilated)**; other cranial nerve lesions that form a pattern (see ➔ Multiple cranial nerve lesions, p.512). *Confirmed by:* **CT** or **MRI scan** appearance. *Finalized by the predictable outcome of management,* e.g. treatment of underlying cause.
Horner's syndrome due to neck trauma or tumours, cervical rib pancoast tumour (in lung apex), syringomyelia (in cervical spine), lateral medullary syndrome (in brainstem), hypothalamic lesion	*Suggested by:* ptosis and constricted (miotic) pupil, recessed globe of the eye, and diminished sweating on same side of face. *Confirmed by:* history of trauma or onset over week or months suggestive of tumour, or years suggestive of MS or syrinx. Other cranial nerve signs that form a pattern of cervical plexus lesion or brainstem lesion. X-ray of upper chest, ribs, or neck. **CT** of neck or upper chest or **MRI scan** of brainstem. *Finalized by the predictable outcome of management,* e.g. treatment of underlying cause.
Myasthenia gravis	*Suggested by:* bilateral partial ptosis worsening as day progresses. *Confirmed by:* eyes begin to droop after 15min of upgaze. +ve **Tensilon test** (edrophonium results in improvement in ptosis). *Finalized by the predictable outcome of management,* e.g. pyridostigmine, prednisolone, plasmapheresis, immunoglobulin, thymectomy.
Myopathy (dystrophia myotonica)	*Suggested by:* bilateral partial ptosis with evidence of weakness in other muscle groups. Frontal balding, inability to release hand grip. *Confirmed by:* biopsy histology of other affected muscle. *Finalized by the predictable outcome of management,* e.g. mexiletine, phenytoin, acetazolamide; genetic counselling.
Congenital ptosis	*Suggested by:* unilateral or bilateral partial ptosis present since birth. Compensatory head posture. *Confirmed by:* absence of other neurological signs. *Finalized by the predictable outcome of management,* e.g. explanation, reassurance.

Large (mydriatic) pupil with no ptosis

Main differential diagnoses and typical outline evidence, etc.

Holmes–Adie pupil due to ciliary ganglion degeneration	*Suggested by:* dilated pupil (often widely) that only reacts slowly to light by constricting in well-lit room after 30min. Reacts to accommodation. Absent knee jerks. Females > male. Unilateral > bilateral. *Confirmed by:* benign outcome with no action necessary. *Finalized by the predictable outcome of management,* e.g. explanation, reassurance.
Traumatic iridoplegia	*Suggested by:* history of direct trauma. Dilated, fixed irregular pupil that does not accommodate nor react to light. *Confirmed by:* slit-lamp examination of anterior eye chamber. *Finalized by the predictable outcome of management,* e.g. explanation, reassurance.
Drug effect due to cocaine, amphetamines, tropicamide, atropine	*Suggested by:* bilateral pupil dilation. *Confirmed by:* drug history and resolution with withdrawal. *Finalized by the predictable outcome of management,* e.g. withdrawal of drug.
Severe brainstem dysfunction (or death)	*Suggested by:* bilateral pupil dilation with no reaction to light, comatose, long tract pyramidal signs. *Confirmed by:* absent corneal reflex response, no vestibulo-ocular reflexes, no cranial motor response to stimulation, no gag reflex, insufficient respiratory effort when P_aCO_2 >6.7kPa to prevent further ↑of P_aCO_2 and ↓P_aO_2. *Finalized by the predictable outcome of management,* e.g. management of terminal illness.

Small (miotic) pupil with no ptosis

Investigations in **bold** below.

Main differential diagnoses and typical outline evidence, etc.	
Argyll Robinson pupil (due to syphilis and diabetes mellitus, rarely)	*Suggested by:* unilateral, small, irregular pupil that 'accommodates' by constricting when focusing on near finger, but does not react to light. *Confirmed by:* **syphilis serology** or **fasting blood glucose** ≥7mmol/L and random or **GTT glucose** ≥11.0mmol/L. *Finalized by the predictable outcome of management,* e.g. treatment of underlying cause.
Anisocoria (normal variation)	*Suggested by:* unilateral, small, miotic pupil that reacts normally to light and accommodation. *Confirmed by:* no change with time, benign outcome with no action necessary. *Finalized by the predictable outcome of management,* e.g. explanation, reassurance.
Age-related miosis (due to autonomic degeneration)	*Suggested by:* bilateral, small, miotic pupils that react normally to light and accommodates normally. *Confirmed by:* discovery in old age, no change with time, benign outcome with no action. *Finalized by the predictable outcome of management,* e.g. explanation, reassurance.
Drug effect due to opiates, pilocarpine	*Suggested by:* bilateral, small pupils. Not reacting to light. *Confirmed by:* drug history and resolution with withdrawal. *Finalized by the predictable outcome of management,* e.g. withdrawal of drug.
Pontine haemorrhage	*Suggested by:* bilateral, small, miotic pupils that react to light. Patient comatose, bilaterally or unilaterally, hyper-reflexic, and high or fluctuating temperature. *Confirmed by:* evolution of signs to localize to brainstem. **MRI scan.** *Finalized by the predictable outcome of management,* e.g. treatment of underlying cause and complications.

Squint and diplopia: ocular palsy

Elicited by asking the patient to follow the examiner's finger and asking if this results in 'seeing double', and looking for development of a convergent or divergent squint. Cover test: fix focus in the distance and alternately cover either eye in quick succession. As cover is lifted, observe the eye. If the uncovered eye now moves in, this indicates a divergent squint. If the eye moves out, this indicates a convergent squint. Initial investigations (other tests in **bold** below): FBC, ESR or CRP, CT or MRI scan.

Main differential diagnoses and typical outline evidence, etc.	
Oculomotor (3rd nerve) paresis intra-cavernous or posterior communicating artery aneurysm, meningioma, tentorial pressure cone, diabetes mellitus, syphilis, and brainstem ischaemia	*Suggested by:* ptosis, diplopia, and squint maximal on looking up and in; but therefore, in total loss, eye looks down and out. **Dilated pupil (except in diabetes mellitus, syphilis, and brainstem ischaemia when pupil not dilated).** *Confirmed by:* other cranial nerve lesions that form pattern (see ⊃ Multiple cranial nerve lesions, p.512), **skull X-ray P–A and lateral, CT or MRI scan** appearance. *Finalized by the predictable outcome of management,* e.g. treatment of underlying cause and complications.
Trochlear (4th cranial nerve) paresis	*Suggested by:* diplopia and squint maximal on looking down and in. Double-vision for reading and walking down stairs. *Confirmed by:* other cranial nerve lesions that form pattern (see ⊃ Multiple cranial nerve lesions, p.512). **MRI scan** appearance. *Finalized by the predictable outcome of management,* e.g. treatment of underlying cause.
Abducent (6th cranial nerve) paresis	*Suggested by:* **double-vision looking in direction of the affected muscle.** Head turn in direction of affected muscle. *Confirmed by:* other cranial nerve lesions that form pattern (see ⊃ Multiple cranial nerve lesions, p.512). **MRI scan** appearance. *Finalized by the predictable outcome of management,* e.g. treatment of underlying cause.
Myasthenia gravis, Graves' disease, orbital cellulitis, or tumour	*Suggested by:* diplopia and squint in all directions of gaze. *Confirmed by:* **CT or MRI scan** of orbit or +ve Tensilon test (edrophonium results in less diplopia and squint in myasthenia). *Finalized by the predictable outcome of management,* e.g. pyridostigmine, prednisolone, consider plasmapheresis, immunoglobulin, thymectomy.

| Internuclear ophthalmoplegia due to lesion in the medial longitudinal bundle, usually due to MS or sometimes vascular | *Suggested by:* impaired conjugate gaze (slowness of adducting eye and nystagmus in abducting eye). *Confirmed by:* other signs of brainstem lesion. *Finalized by the predictable outcome of management,* e.g. treatment of underlying cause. |

Loss of facial sensation

Investigations in **bold** below.

Main differential diagnoses and typical outline evidence, etc.	
Ophthalmic branch of trigeminal nerve lesion	*Suggested by:* absent corneal reflex (present corneal reflex excludes lesion) with diminished touch and pain sensation in upper face above the line of the eye.
	Confirmed by: other cranial nerve lesions that form pattern (see ⊃ Multiple cranial nerve lesions, p.512). **MRI scan** appearance.
	Finalized by the predictable outcome of management, e.g. treatment of underlying cause.
Maxillary branch of trigeminal nerve lesion	*Suggested by:* diminished touch and pain sensation in midface between line of mouth and line of eye.
	Confirmed by: other cranial nerve lesions that form pattern (see ⊃ Multiple cranial nerve lesions, p.512). **MRI scan** appearance.
	Finalized by the predictable outcome of management, e.g. treatment of underlying cause.
Mandibular branch of trigeminal nerve lesion	*Suggested by:* diminished touch and pain sensation in lower face below line of mouth.
	Confirmed by: other cranial nerve lesions that form pattern (see ⊃ Multiple cranial nerve lesions, p.512). **MRI scan** appearance.
	Finalized by the predictable outcome of management, e.g. treatment of underlying cause.

Jaw muscle weakness

Investigations in **bold** below.

Main differential diagnoses and typical outline evidence, etc.	
Motor branch of trigeminal nerve (5th cranial): lower motor neurone type on same (ipsilateral) side	*Suggested by:* weakness of jaw movement. Deviation of jaw when opening against resistance and poor contraction of masseter on clenching. Decreased jaw jerk. *Confirmed by:* other cranial nerve lesions that form pattern (see ➔ Multiple cranial nerve lesions, p.512). **MRI scan** appearance. *Finalized by the predictable outcome of management*, e.g. treatment of underlying cause.
Motor branch of trigeminal nerve (5th cranial): upper motor neurone type on other (contralateral) side.	*Suggested by:* weakness of jaw movement. Deviation of jaw when opening against resistance and poor contraction of masseter on clenching. Increased jaw jerk. *Confirmed by:* other cranial nerve lesions that form pattern (see ➔ Multiple cranial nerve lesions, p.512). **MRI scan** appearance. *Finalized by the predictable outcome of management*, e.g. treatment of underlying cause.

Facial muscle weakness

Distinguish between upper (forehead muscles movement preserved) and lower (forehead movement weak) motor neurone type. Investigations in **bold** below.

Main differential diagnoses and typical outline evidence, etc.	
Facial nerve palsy (7th cranial): *upper motor neurone type* on other (contralateral) side due to internal capsule lesion—cerebrovascular accident, tumour	*Suggested by:* **able** to raise eyebrows and close eye but **unable** to grimace nor smile symmetrically; other cranial nerve lesions that form pattern (see ➔ Multiple cranial nerve lesions, p.512). *Confirmed by:* **MRI scan.** *Finalized by the predictable outcome of management,* e.g. treatment of underlying cause.
Facial nerve palsy (7th cranial): *lower motor neurone type* on same (ipsilateral) side	*Suggested by:* inability to raise eyebrows nor close eye (rolls upwards to hide iris revealing the white of the eye) nor grimace nor smile symmetrically; other cranial nerve lesions that form pattern (see ➔ Multiple cranial nerve lesions, p.512). *Confirmed by:* **MRI scan.** *Finalized by the predictable outcome of management,* e.g. treatment of underlying cause.
Bell's palsy	*Suggested and confirmed by:* lower motor neurone 7th nerve palsy. Prior ache behind ear. No other physical signs. (NB Corneal reflex present, and no deafness or vertigo.) *Finalized by the predictable outcome of management,* e.g. prednisolone within 5d of onset. Protective dark glasses and 'artificial tears'. Manual closure of eyelid ± tape.
Ramsay Hunt syndrome	*Suggested by:* lower motor neurone 7th nerve palsy. Taste diminished on same side. Vesicles in external auditory meatus. *Finalized by the predictable outcome of management,* e.g. analgesia, e.g. paracetamol initially. Aciclovir.
Facial nerve palsy from parotid swelling	*Suggested by:* lower motor neurone 7th nerve palsy. Swelling in midface on same side. *Confirmed by:* above clinical features and **MRI scan.** *Finalized by the predictable outcome of management,* e.g. surgical decompression, release of nerve ± repair with nerve tissue taken from lateral cutaneous nerve of thigh.

Cerebello-pontine lesion (e.g. tumour)	*Suggested by:* lower motor neurone 7th nerve palsy. Associated 5th (loss of corneal reflex) and 7th cranial nerve lesion. *Confirmed by:* above clinical features. **MRI scan** appearance of space-occupying lesion in or near internal auditory canal. *Finalized by the predictable outcome of management, e.g.* excision.
Cholesteatoma	*Suggested by:* lower motor neurone 7th nerve palsy. Also deafness and vertigo. *Confirmed by:* above clinical features. **MRI scan** appearance. *Finalized by the predictable outcome of management, e.g.* surgical clearance.
Facial nerve palsy from demyelination	*Suggested by:* lower motor neurone 7th nerve palsy. Other focal neurological signs and symptoms disseminated in time and space. *Confirmed by:* above clinical features. **MRI scan** appearance. *Finalized by the predictable outcome of management, e.g.* methylprednisolone to hasten remission.
Facial nerve palsy from brain stem ischaemia	*Suggested by:* lower motor neurone 7th nerve palsy. Signs of adjacent dysfunction, e.g. nystagmus, long tract signs, e.g. spastic hemiparesis. *Confirmed by:* above clinical features. **MRI scan** appearance. *Finalized by the predictable outcome of management, e.g.* aspirin and 'statin' to prevent/ reduce risk of recurrence.

Loss of hearing

Inability to hear whispering or ticking watch, and test with tuning fork held near ear (testing air and bone conduction together). Investigations in **bold** below.

Main differential diagnoses and typical outline evidence, etc.

8th nerve conduction defect on side X due to wax, foreign body, otitis externa, recurrent otitis media, injury to tympanic membrane, otosclerosis, cholesteatoma	*Suggested by:* forehead vibration heard louder on side X than on side Y (Weber's test), and mastoid vibration on side X louder than for air (Rinne's test). *Confirmed by:* auroscope appearance, formal audiometry, and other cranial nerve lesions that form pattern (see ⮞ Multiple cranial nerve lesions, p.512). **MRI scan** appearance. *Finalized by the predictable outcome of management,* e.g. treatment of underlying cause.
Sensorineural (8th cranial) lesion on side Y due to old age, noise trauma, Paget's disease, Meniere's disease, drugs, viral infections (e.g. measles), congenital rubella, meningitis, acoustic neuroma, meningioma	*Suggested by:* forehead vibration heard louder on side X than on side Y (Weber's test), and mastoid vibration same for both sides (Rinne's test). *Confirmed by:* other cranial nerve lesions that form pattern (see ⮞ Multiple cranial nerve lesions, p.512), formal audiometry, and **MRI scan** appearance. *Finalized by the predictable outcome of management,* e.g. treatment of underlying cause.

Abnormal tongue, uvula, and pharyngeal movement

9th, 10th (not 11th), and 12th cranial nerve lesions. Investigations in **bold** below.

Main differential diagnoses and typical outline evidence, etc.	
Glossopharyngeal (9th cranial) nerve lesion	*Suggested by:* loss of gag reflex and taste on posterior one third of tongue; other cranial nerve lesions that form pattern (see ➲ Multiple cranial nerve lesions, p.512). *Confirmed by:* **MRI scan.** *Finalized by the predictable outcome of management*, e.g. treatment of underlying cause.
Vagus (10th cranial) nerve lesion due to jugular foramen lesion, bulbar palsy	*Suggested by:* deviation of uvula away from affected side when saying 'ah'; nasal regurgitation of water. Dysarthria; other cranial nerve lesions that form pattern (see ➲ Multiple cranial nerve lesions, p.512). *Confirmed by:* **MRI scan.** *Finalized by the predictable outcome of management*, e.g. treatment of underlying cause only.
Lower motor neurone hypoglossal (12th cranial) nerve lesion on same (ipsilateral) side of deviation	*Suggested by:* deviation of tongue to side of lesion on protrusion. Fasciculation and wasting; other cranial nerve lesions that form pattern (see ➲ Difficulty in rising from chair or squatting position, p.542). *Confirmed by:* **MRI scan.** *Finalized by the predictable outcome of management*, e.g. treatment of underlying cause.
Upper motor neurone hypoglossal (12th cranial) nerve lesion on other (contralateral) side of deviation	*Suggested by:* deviation of tongue to opposite side of lesion on protrusion. Small stiff tongue and cortical or internal capsule signs. *Confirmed by:* **CT or MRI scan.** *Finalized by the predictable outcome of management*, e.g. treatment of underlying cause.
Tardive dyskinesias due to dopamine agonist	*Suggested by:* vacuous chewing and grimacing movements. *Confirmed by:* clinical appearance. *Finalised by the predictable outcome of management:* stopping dopamine agonist.

Multiple cranial nerve lesions

Investigations in **bold** below.

Main differential diagnoses and typical outline evidence, etc.	
Pituitary tumour	*Suggested by:* optic tract or chiasm lesion. 3rd cranial nerve lesion. *Confirmed by:* **CT or MRI scan** appearance. *Finalized by the predictable outcome of management,* e.g. surgical decompression or hypophysectomy, radiotherapy or (dopamine agonist if prolactinoma).
Anterior communicating artery aneurysm (cerebral artery aneurysm)	*Suggested by:* optic nerve lesion, 3rd and 4th cranial nerve lesions. *Confirmed by:* **CT or MRI scan** appearance. *Finalized by the predictable outcome of management,* e.g. surgical clipping.
Posterior communicating artery aneurysm (cerebral artery aneurysm)	*Suggested by:* 4th and 5th cranial nerve lesions. *Confirmed by:* **CT** or **MRI scan** appearance. *Finalized by the predictable outcome of management,* e.g. surgery.
Gradenigo's syndrome (lesion in petrous temporal bone)	*Suggested by:* 5th and 6th cranial nerve lesions. *Confirmed by:* **MRI scan** appearance. *Finalized by the predictable outcome of management,* e.g. surgery.
Facial canal lesion, e.g. cholesteatoma	*Suggested by:* 7th and 8th cranial nerve lesions alone (no 5th or 6th). *Confirmed by:* **CT or MRI scan** appearance. *Finalized by the predictable outcome of management,* e.g. surgical clearance.
Cerebello-pontine angle lesion, e.g. tumour	*Suggested by:* 5th, 7th, and 8th ± 6th cranial nerve lesions. *Confirmed by:* **CT or MRI scan** appearance. *Finalized by the predictable outcome of management,* e.g. surgery.
Jugular foramen syndrome due to tumour, tuberculoma	*Suggested by:* 9th, 10th, and 11th cranial nerve lesions. *Confirmed by:* **MRI scan** appearance. *Finalized by the predictable outcome of management,* e.g. surgery or anti TB treatment.
Lateral medullary syndrome	*Suggested by:* vertigo, nystagmus, 5th cranial nerve lesion, Horner's syndrome, contralateral spinothalamic loss on trunk. *Confirmed by:* above clinical features. **MRI scan** appearance. *Finalized by the predictable outcome of management,* e.g. aspirin and 'statin' to reduce risk of progression or recurrence after 1–2wk to avoid risk of bleeding into infarcted tissue.

Weber's syndrome	*Suggested by:* ipsilateral 3rd cranial nerve lesion and contralateral hemiparesis.
	Confirmed by: above clinical features. MRI scan appearance.
	Finalized by the predictable outcome of management, e.g. treatment of underlying cause.

Odd posture of arms and hands at rest

Investigations in **bold** below.

Main differential diagnoses and typical outline evidence, etc.	
Internal capsule bleed, infarct, or tumour (or pre-central gyrus and connections, or lower pyramidal tract, i.e. upper motor neurone)	*Suggested by:* arms flexed at elbow and wrist, and weak. Increased tone and reflexes. Upper motor neurone facial weakness. *Confirmed by:* brain **CT or MRI scan** appearance. *Finalized by the predictable outcome of management*, e.g. treatment of any remediable underlying cause.
T1 anterior root lesion	*Suggested by:* **claw hand**, wasting of all small muscles of the hand. Loss of sensation of ulnar 1½ fingers and ulnar border of forearm. *Confirmed by:* nerve conduction study result. MRI scan appearance of neck showing root compression. *Finalized by the predictable outcome of management*, e.g. treatment of any remediable underlying cause.
Ulnar nerve lesion (below elbow)	*Suggested by:* **claw hand**, wasting of hypothenar eminence and dorsal guttering, especially first. Weakness of finger abduction and adduction. Loss of sensation of ulnar 1½ fingers. *Confirmed by:* nerve conduction studies. *Finalized by the predictable outcome of management*, e.g. treatment of any remediable underlying cause.
Radial nerve lesion (or C7 anterior root lesion)	*Suggested by:* **wrist drop**. Inability to extend wrist and grip. Loss of sensation over 1st dorsal interosseous muscle. *Confirmed by:* nerve conduction study result. *Finalized by the predictable outcome of management*, e.g. treatment of any remediable underlying cause.

Fine tremor of hands

Elicited by asking patient to hold arms out straight in front and placing sheet of paper to rest on them (to amplify fine tremor). Investigations in **bold** below.

Main differential diagnoses and typical outline evidence, etc.	
Thyrotoxicosis	*Suggested by:* fine tremor, anxiety, tachycardia, sweating, weight loss, goitre, increased reflexes. *Confirmed by:* **↑FT4** or **FT3**, and **↓↓TSH.** *Finalized by the predictable outcome of management,* e.g. β-blocker, e.g. propranolol to control any intolerable symptoms for few weeks, antithyroid drug, e.g. carbimazole or propylthiouracil for 6–18mo (± block and replacement with thyroxine). Radio-iodine for hot nodule or recurrence.
Anxiety state	*Suggested by:* fine tremor, anxiety, tachycardia, sweating, weight loss. *Confirmed by:* normal thyroid function tests. Improvement with sedation, psychotherapy, etc. *Finalized by the predictable outcome of management,* e.g. β-blocker or minor tranquilizer.
Alcohol withdrawal	*Suggested by:* fine or coarse tremor, history of high alcohol intake and recent withdrawal, anxiety. *Confirmed by:* improvement with sedation, etc. e.g. chlordiazepoxide in reducing dose.
Sympathomimetic drugs	*Suggested by:* fine tremor, drug history. *Confirmed by:* improvement with withdrawal of drug.
Benign essential tremor	*Suggested by:* usually coarse tremor, long history, no other symptoms or signs. *Confirmed by:* normal **thyroid test results**. Improvement with β-blocker. *Finalized by the predictable outcome of management,* e.g. β-blocker, e.g. propranolol.

Coarse tremor of hands

Elicited by asking patient to hold arms out straight in front and extending wrists (for asterixis or flap), then asking the patient to touch their own nose and then the examiner's finger with arm extended—repetitively (for intention tremor). Investigations in **bold** below.

Main differential diagnoses and typical outline evidence, etc.	
Hepatic failure	*Suggested by:* flapping tremor (asterixis), aggravated when wrists extended. Spider naevi. Jaundice. *Confirmed by:* abnormal **LFT** and prolonged **prothrombin time.** *Finalized by the predictable outcome of management,* e.g. avoid sedatives, 20° bed head uptilt, lactulose (for 2–3 stool/d).
Carbon dioxide retention	*Suggested by:* flapping tremor (asterixis), aggravated when wrists extended. Muscle twitching, bounding pulse, warm peripheries. *Confirmed by:* **ABG** show ↑P_aCO_2. *Finalized by the predictable outcome of management,* e.g. if on O_2, reduce %, **bi-level positive airway pressure (BiPAP)**.
Cerebellar disease	*Suggested by:* intention tremor (past pointing) when patient attempts to touch examiner's finger. *Confirmed by:* **MRI scan.** *Finalized by the predictable outcome of management,* e.g. treatment of any remediable underlying cause.
Parkinsonism due to Parkinson's disease, Lewy body dementia; drug-induced (chlorpromazine, haloperidol, metoclopramideprochlorperazine); post-encephalitis, normal pressure hydrocephalus	*Suggested by:* **resting** coarse tremor, ('pill-rolling'), 'lead-pipe rigidity', expressionless face, paucity of movement, small hand writing, rapid, shuffling ('festinant') gait with small steps. *Confirmed by:* clinical findings, e.g. persistent blinking when forehead tapped (e.g. 'glabellar tap'). *Finalized by the predictable outcome of management,* e.g. withdrawal of potentially causative drug or antimuscarinic, e.g. procyclidine. Counselling, explain long-term strategy, MDT planning, low dose levodopa with dopa-decarboxylase inhibitor.
Benign essential tremor	*Suggested by:* usually coarse tremor, long history, no other symptoms or signs. *Confirmed by:* normal **thyroid test** results. Improvement with β-blocker. *Finalized by the predictable outcome of management,* e.g. β-blocker, e.g. propranolol.

Wasting of some small muscles of hand

Inter-metacarpal grooves are prominent due to muscle wasting.
Investigations in **bold** below.

Main differential diagnoses and typical outline evidence, etc.	
Median nerve palsy usually due to carpal tunnel syndrome	*Suggested by:* wasting of thenar eminence. Weakness of thumb flexion, abduction, and opposition. **Unable** to lift thumb with palm upwards, but **able** to press with index finger. Loss of sensation over palmar aspect of radial 3½ fingers of hand. *Confirmed by:* **nerve conduction study** results. *Finalized by the predictable outcome of management,* e.g. surgery to decompress nerve.
Ulnar nerve lesion from elbow (high) to wrist (low)	*Suggested by:* wasting of hypothenar eminence. **Able** to lift thumb with palm upwards, but **unable** to press with index finger. Weakness of finger abduction and adduction. Loss of sensation in ulnar aspect 1½ fingers of hand. Claw hand (in lower lesions). *Confirmed by:* **nerve conduction study** results. *Finalized by the predictable outcome of management,* e.g. treatment of any remediable underlying cause, e.g. surgical decompression.
T1 lesion: anterior horn cell or root lesion	*Suggested by:* wasting of all small muscles of hand. **Unable** to lift thumb with palm upwards, and **unable** to press with index finger. *Confirmed by:* **nerve conduction study** results. **MRI scan** appearance around T1 level. *Finalized by the predictable outcome of management,* e.g. treatment of any remediable underlying cause, e.g. NSAID to reduce swelling around inflamed root canal, surgical decompression.
Motor neurone disease	*Suggested by:* signs of T1 lesion, prominent fasciculation, spastic paraparesis, wasted fasciculating tongue, no sensory signs. *Confirmed by:* clinical presentation and absence of structural abnormality on **MRI scan** appearance. *Finalized by the predictable outcome of management,* e.g. care by MDT, propantheline for drooling, analgesic ladder for pain, blending food, NG tube for dysphagia, non-invasive ventilation for early breathing difficulty.
Syringomyelia	*Suggested by:* **signs of T1 lesion**, fasciculation **not** prominent, burn scars, dissociated sensory loss, Horner's syndrome, nystagmus. History over months to years. *Confirmed by:* **MRI scan** appearances. *Finalized by the predictable outcome of management,* e.g. surgical decompression of foramen magnum, care by MDT.

Any prolonged systemic illness	*Suggested by:* global muscle wasting, general weight loss. *Confirmed by:* improvement in muscle wasting if primary disease treatable.
Cervical spondylosis compressing nerve root	*Suggested by:* **signs of T1 lesion**, neck pain and stiffness, and referred pain. *Confirmed by:* **MRI scan** showing root canal compression. *Finalized by the predictable outcome of management*, e.g. physiotherapy, NSAIDs to reduce swelling around root canal, surgical decompression if intractible pain.
Tumour compressing nerve root	*Suggested by:* **signs of T1 lesion**, referred pain. Progressing over months. *Confirmed by:* **MRI scan** showing root canal compression. *Finalized by the predictable outcome of management*, e.g. radiotherapy or surgical decompression.
Brachial plexus lesion	*Suggested by:* **signs of T1 lesion**, and history of trauma to shoulder area or birth injury. *Confirmed by:* **nerve conduction study** results. *Finalized by the predictable outcome of management*, e.g. treatment of underlying cause.
Cervical rib	*Suggested by:* **signs of T1 lesion** aggravated by movement or posture. *Confirmed by:* **neck and chest X-ray**—presence of cervical rib. *Finalized by the predictable outcome of management*, e.g. physiotherapy, rib removal, or band division.
Pancoast tumour	*Suggested by:* **signs of T1 lesion**, Horner's syndrome, features of lung cancer (clubbing, chest signs, etc.). *Confirmed by:* **CXR** and **CT scan** appearances. *Finalized by the predictable outcome of management*, e.g. radiotherapy.

Wasting of arm and shoulder

Loss of rounded contour of deltoid and biceps muscle. Fasciculation is localized twitching of muscle. Note facial expression. Investigations in **bold** below.

Main differential diagnoses and typical outline evidence, etc.	
Progressive muscular atrophy	*Suggested by:* bilateral wasting of hand, arm, and shoulder girdle with fasciculation. *Confirmed by:* **EMG** results. *Finalized by the predictable outcome of management,* e.g. care by MDT, especially occupational and physiotherapy.
Motor neurone disease (amyotrophic lateral sclerosis) with anterior horn cell degeneration	*Suggested by:* initially unilateral wasting of shoulder abductor and biceps. Weakness of speech, swallowing. No sensory signs. *Confirmed by:* **EMG** results. *Finalized by the predictable outcome of management,* e.g. MDT care, propantheline for drooling, analgesic ladder for pain, blending food, NG tube for dysphagia, non-invasive ventilation early breathing difficulty.
1° muscle disease	*Suggested by:* bilateral wasting of shoulder abductor, and biceps. *Confirmed by:* **EMG** findings or **muscle biopsy.** *Finalized by the predictable outcome of management,* e.g. MDT care, especially occupational and physiotherapy.

Abnormalities of arm tone

Elicited by supporting elbow in one hand, and asking patient to allow you to flex and extend arm at the elbow without assistance. Investigations in **bold** below.

Main differential diagnoses and typical outline evidence, etc.	
Cerebellar lesion	*Suggested by:* **tone diminished**, no wasting. Diminished reflexes. Past pointing, truncal ataxia, nystagmus. *Confirmed by:* **CT or MRI scan** appearance of cerebellum. *Finalized by the predictable outcome of management,* e.g. treatment of any remediable underlying cause. MDT care, especially occupational and physiotherapy.
1° muscle disease	*Suggested by:* **tone diminished** with wasting ± fasciculation. *Confirmed by:* **EMG** findings or **muscle biopsy.** *Finalized by the predictable outcome of management,* e.g. MDT care, especially occupational and physiotherapy.
Upper motor neurone	*Suggested by:* **tone increased**. Brisk reflexes below lesion. *Confirmed by:* **CT or MRI scan** of brain or spinal cord. *Finalized by the predictable outcome of management,* e.g. care by MDT, especially occupational and physiotherapy.
Parkinson's disease	*Suggested by:* **tone increased** with cogwheel effect (superimposed tremor). Poor facial movement, shuffling, hesitant, 'festinant' gait, coarse tremor. *Confirmed by:* response to drug therapy. *Finalized by the predictable outcome of management,* e.g. withdrawal of potentially causative drug or antimuscarinic, e.g. procyclidine. Counselling, care by MDT, low dose levodopa initially with dopa-decarboxylase inhibitor.

Weakness around the shoulder and arm without pain

Elicited by asking the patient to flex and extend wrist and elbow against resistance, and to abduct, adduct, flex and extend shoulder against resistance, comparing both sides. Investigations in **bold** below.

Main differential diagnoses and typical outline evidence, etc.	
C4–5 root lesion	*Suggested by:* weakness of abduction at the shoulder only (**not elbow or wrist**). *Confirmed by:* **nerve conduction studies** and **MRI scan** of neck. *Finalized by the predictable outcome of management,* e.g. physiotherapy, treatment of any remediable underlying cause.
C5–6 root lesion Erb's palsy	*Suggested by:* weakness of flexion at the shoulder and elbow, but not wrist. Arm externally rotated and adducted behind back ('porter's tip' position). History of birth trauma. *Confirmed by:* **nerve conduction studies** and **MRI scan** of neck. *Finalized by the predictable outcome of management,* e.g. physiotherapy.
C7 root lesion	*Suggested by:* wrist drop or weakness of grip, and extension at the **elbow and wrist.** *Confirmed by:* **nerve conduction studies** and **MRI scan** of neck. *Finalized by the predictable outcome of management,* e.g. physiotherapy.
Radial nerve lesion	*Suggested by:* wrist drop or weakness of grip and extension at the wrist but **not** at the elbow. *Confirmed by:* **nerve conduction studies** and history of trauma. *Finalized by the predictable outcome of management,* e.g. physiotherapy, surgical repair.
C8–T1 root lesion (Klumpke's paralysis)	*Suggested by:* arm held in adduction, paralysis/paresis of the small muscles of the hand, loss of sensation over ulnar border of the hand. History of birth trauma. *Confirmed by:* **nerve conduction studies** and **MRI scan** of neck. *Finalized by the predictable outcome of management,* e.g. physiotherapy.

Incoordination (on rapid wrist rotation or hand tapping)

Comment: this is often used as a 'screening' test (i.e. if normal, you can discount any significant neuromuscular condition of the upper limbs in the absence of other symptoms or signs). Investigations in **bold** below.

Main differential diagnoses and typical outline evidence, etc.

Upper motor neurone paresis	*Suggested by:* spastic weakness (i.e. with increased tone) in upper limb. *Confirmed by:* **CT scan** of brain or **MRI scan** of neck. *Finalized by the predictable outcome of management*, e.g. physiotherapy.
Lower motor neurone paresis	*Suggested by:* flaccid weakness (i.e. with decreased tone) in upper limb. *Confirmed by:* **nerve conduction studies** and **MRI scan** of neck. *Finalized by the predictable outcome of management*, e.g. physiotherapy.
Ipsilateral cerebellar lesion	*Suggested by:* decreased tone, past pointing, diminished reflexes. *Confirmed by:* **CT or MRI scan** of cerebellum. *Finalized by the predictable outcome of management*, e.g. physiotherapy, treatment of any remediable underlying cause.
Loss of proprioception	*Suggested by:* loss of joint position sense and vibration sense. *Confirmed by:* **nerve conduction studies.** *Finalized by the predictable outcome of management*, e.g. physiotherapy, treatment of any remediable underlying cause.

Muscle wasting

Comment: has to be assessed in context of the bulk of other muscles. Investigations in **bold** below.

Main differential diagnoses and typical outline evidence, etc.	
Adjacent bone, joint or muscle disease	*Suggested by:* wasting with pain and limitation of movement. Visible swelling or deformity of bone or joint. *Confirmed by:* **X-ray of affected part. EMG.** *Finalized by the predictable outcome of management,* e.g. physiotherapy, treatment of any remediable underlying cause.
Lower motor neurone lesion	*Suggested by:* wasting and fasciculation. Tone decreased. Weakness and diminished reflexes. *Confirmed by:* **nerve conduction studies.** *Finalized by the predictable outcome of management,* e.g. physiotherapy, treatment of any remediable underlying cause.
Muscle disease	*Suggested by:* wasting. Tone decreased. Weakness and diminished reflex. *Confirmed by:* **EMG.** *Finalized by the predictable outcome of management,* e.g. physiotherapy, treatment of any remediable underlying cause.

Weakness around the lower limb joint

Weakness around one lower limb joint

These weaknesses may point strongly to one nerve root lesion. Test by asking the patient to perform the movement against your resistance. Initial investigations (other tests in **bold** below).

Main differential diagnoses and typical outline evidence, etc.	
L1/2 root lesion or femoral nerve	*Suggested by:* weakness of hip flexion alone. *Confirmed by:* **X-ray of lumbar spine and sacrum**. **Nerve conduction studies**. **MRI scan** if lesion can be localized clinically. *Finalized by the predictable outcome of management, e.g.* physiotherapy, treatment of any remediable underlying cause.
L2/3 root lesion or obturator nerve	*Suggested by:* weakness of hip adduction alone. *Confirmed by:* **X-ray of lumbar spine and sacrum**. **Nerve conduction studies**. **MRI scan** if lesion can be localized clinically. *Finalized by the predictable outcome of management, e.g.* physiotherapy, treatment of any remediable underlying cause.
L3/4 root lesion or femoral nerve	*Suggested by:* weakness of knee extension alone. *Confirmed by:* **X-ray of lumbar spine and sacrum**. **Nerve conduction studies**. **MRI scan** if lesion can be localized clinically. *Finalized by the predictable outcome of management, e.g.* physiotherapy, treatment of any remediable underlying cause.
L4/5 root lesion or tibial nerve	*Suggested by:* weakness of foot dorsiflexion and inversion at the ankle. *Confirmed by:* **X-ray of lumbar spine and sacrum**. **Nerve conduction studies**. **MRI scan** if lesion can be localized clinically. *Finalized by the predictable outcome of management, e.g.* physiotherapy, treatment of any remediable underlying cause.
L5/S1 root lesion or common peroneal nerve	*Suggested by:* weakness of knee flexion alone. *Confirmed by:* **X-ray of lumbar spine and sacrum**. **Nerve conduction studies**. **MRI scan** if lesion can be localized clinically. *Finalized by the predictable outcome of management, e.g.* physiotherapy, treatment of any remediable underlying cause.
S1/2 root lesion or sciatic nerve	*Suggested by:* weakness of toe flexion alone. *Confirmed by:* **X-ray of lumbar spine and sacrum**. **Nerve conduction studies**. **MRI scan** if lesion can be localized clinically. *Finalized by the predictable outcome of management, e.g.* physiotherapy, treatment of any remediable underlying cause.

Lateral popliteal nerve palsy (usually traumatic)	*Suggested by:* flaccid 'foot drop with weakness of eversion and dorsiflexion of the foot, and a sensory loss over lateral aspect of leg. *Confirmed by:* **nerve conduction study** result. *Finalized by the predictable outcome of management, e.g.* physiotherapy, possible surgical repair.

Bilateral weakness of all foot movements

Initial investigations (other tests in **bold** below): FBC, ESR or CRP, U&E, CT scan.

Main differential diagnoses and typical outline evidence, etc.	
Guillain–Barré syndrome.	*Suggested by:* onset over days preceding viral illness. *Confirmed by:* nerve conduction studies, ↑**CSF protein**. Progressive course then variable recovery. *Finalized by the predictable outcome of management,* e.g. monitor breathing and ventilation in ITU as necessary.
Lead poisoning	*Suggested by:* gradual onset over weeks to months. *Confirmed by:* **nerve conduction studies**, and history of exposure. **Serum lead** levels. *Finalized by the predictable outcome of management,* e.g. identify and remove source of poisoning, EDTA (e.g. if levels >45 micrograms/dL).
Porphyria	*Suggested by:* onset over months to years. Usually known to have porphyria. *Confirmed by:* **EMG** and ↑urine or **faecal porphobilinogens.** *Finalized by the predictable outcome of management,* e.g. stopping potentially precipitating drug, fluids IV, ↑carbohydrate intake, haematin IV.
Charcot–Marie–Tooth disease	*Suggested by:* onset over years. Associated with foot drop and peroneal atrophy upper limbs affected later. *Confirmed by:* **EMG.** *Finalized by the predictable outcome of management,* e.g. MDT planning, especially occupational and physiotherapy. Assessment for possible nerve release.

Spastic paraparesis

Bilateral lower limb paresis with increased tone. This is a *medical emergency*, if acute. Initial investigations (other tests in **bold** below): FBC, ESR or CRP, U&E, MRI scan.

Main differential diagnoses and typical outline evidence, etc.	
Prolapsed disc (anteriorly thus compressing spinal cord)	*Suggested by:* sudden onset often associated with change in spinal posture. *Confirmed by:* **MRI scan** appearance. *Finalized by the predictable outcome of management,* e.g. urgent spinal cord decompression surgery.
Traumatic vertebral displacement or fracture	*Suggested by:* sudden onset associated with violent injury. *Confirmed by:* **MRI scan** appearance. *Finalized by the predictable outcome of management,* e.g. urgent spinal cord decompression surgery.
Collapsed vertebra (due to 2° carcinoma or myeloma)	*Suggested by:* sudden onset over minutes or hours. Other symptoms suggestive of neoplasia over months. *Confirmed by:* **nerve conduction studies**. **MRI scan** appearance. *Finalized by the predictable outcome of management,* e.g. urgent spinal cord decompression surgery.
Spondylitic bone formation compressing spinal cord	*Suggested by:* onset over months to years. Often past history of spondylitic back pain. *Confirmed by:* **MRI scan** appearance. *Finalized by the predictable outcome of management,* e.g. spinal cord decompression surgery.
MS affecting spinal cord	*Suggested by:* this and other intermittent neurological symptoms disseminated in site and time. *Confirmed by:* **MRI scan** appearance. *Finalized by the predictable outcome of management,* e.g. methyl-prednisolone, physiotherapy, MDT care.
Infective space-occupying lesion e.g. TB or abscess	*Suggested by:* onset over days or weeks with fever from low grade to spiking. *Confirmed by:* **MRI scan** and findings at surgery, **histology**, and **microbiology.** *Finalized by the predictable outcome of management,* e.g. urgent surgery.
Glioma or ependymoma in spinal cord	*Suggested by:* gradual onset over months. *Confirmed by:* **MRI scan** and findings at surgery, **histology.** *Finalized by the predictable outcome of management,* e.g. surgery.
Parasagittal cerebral meningioma or other tumour	*Suggested by:* gradual onset over months. *Confirmed by:* **MRI scan** and findings at surgery, **histology.** *Finalized by the predictable outcome of management,* e.g. surgery.

Hemiparesis (weakness of arm and leg)

During the history and examination, other leads may appear, e.g. dysphagia, cough, and breathlessness, limited or no support at home, ipsilateral facial weakness, cognitive impairment, raised urea and creatinine, opacification on the CXR. Some of these may lead to additional diagnoses, which are causes and complications of one of those below. Initial investigations (other tests in **bold** below): FBC, ESR or CRP, U&E, CT scan.

Main differential diagnoses and typical outline evidence, etc.	
Occlusion of upper branch of middle cerebral artery with infarction, including Broca's area	*Suggested by:* expressive dysphasia and contralateral lower face and arm weakness. *Confirmed by:* **MRI or CT scan** appearance. *Finalized by the predictable outcome of management,* e.g. nil by mouth, fluids IV until swallowing assessed, attention to pressure areas, MDT care esp. physiotherapy and occupational therapy and social services.
Occlusion of perforating branch of middle cerebral artery with lacunar infarction	*Suggested by:* hemiparesis alone with subsequent spasticity (or receptive dysphasia alone or hemi-anaesthesia alone). *Confirmed by:* **MRI or CT scan** appearance. *Finalized by the predictable outcome of management,* e.g. nil by mouth, fluids IV until swallowing assessed, attention to pressure areas, MDT care esp. physiotherapy and occupational therapy and social services.
Total middle cerebral artery territory infarction (usually embolic)	*Suggested by:* contralateral flaccid hemiplegia (with little subsequent spasticity) and hemi-anaesthesia with deviation of eyes to side of lesion. Also homonymous hemianopia with aphasia if dominant hemisphere affected or 'neglect' if non-dominant hemisphere affected. *Confirmed by:* **MRI or CT scan** appearance. *Finalized by the predictable outcome of management,* e.g. nil by mouth, fluids IV until swallowing assessed, attention to pressure areas, MDT care esp. physiotherapy and occupational therapy and social services.
Posterior cerebral artery infarction	*Suggested by:* contralateral homonymous hemianopia or upper quadrantinopia, mild contralateral hemiparesis and sensory loss, ataxia and involuntary movement, memory loss, dyslexia, and ipsilateral 3rd nerve palsy. *Confirmed by:* **MRI or CT scan** appearance. *Finalized by the predictable outcome of management,* e.g. nil by mouth, fluids IV until swallowing assessed, attention to pressure areas, MDT care esp. physiotherapy and occupational therapy and social services.

Anterior cerebral artery infarction	*Suggested by:* paresis of contralateral leg, rigidity, perseveration, grasp reflex in opposite hand, urinary incontinence, and dysphasia if in dominant hemisphere.
	Confirmed by: **MRI or CT scan** appearance.
	Finalized by the predictable outcome of management, e.g. nil by mouth, fluids IV until swallowing assessed, attention to pressure areas, MDT care for physiotherapy and occupational therapy and social services.

Disturbed sensation in upper limb

Elicit by testing touch (a piece of cotton wool), heat (a cold metal object), and pain (pinprick with a sterile needle) in each dermatome distribution. Note any discrepancy between these modalities of sensation. In the palm, examine the radial 3 ½ fingers and the ulnar 1 ½ fingers. Test joint position sense (by holding digits at their sides) and vibration with a tuning fork over bony prominences. Then use a two-pointed device (2-point discrimination) placing objects into the patient's hand and asking to guess what they are with eyes closed, e.g. a 20-pence piece (stereognosis), and drawing figures on the palm (graphaesthesia). Consider if you have discovered any of the patterns described below. Investigations in **bold** below.

Main differential diagnoses and typical outline evidence, etc.	
Contralateral cortical (pre-central gyrus) lesion	*Suggested by:* astereognosis, diminished 2-point discrimination, and graphaesthesia. *Confirmed by:* **CT or MRI scan** of brain. *Finalized by the predictable outcome of management,* e.g. treatment of any remediable underlying cause, e.g. surgical removal of tumour.
Peripheral neuropathy	*Suggested by:* loss of touch and pinprick sensation worse in hand progressing upwards. *Confirmed by:* **nerve conduction studies.** *Finalized by the predictable outcome of management,* e.g. treatment of any remediable underlying cause, e.g. stop drug, better control of diabetes.
Spinothalamic tract damage (no dorsal column loss) due to syringomyelia in cervical cord	*Suggested by:* loss of pinprick and temperature sensation, normal or disturbed touch, but normal joint position and vibration sense in hand. *Confirmed by:* **nerve conduction studies**. **MRI** of cervical cord. *Finalized by the predictable outcome of management,* e.g. treatment of underlying cause, e.g. surgical decompression of foramen magnum, MDT care.
Cervical or thoracic nerve root lesion	*Suggested by:* loss of sensation in dermatome distribution in hand or forearm or upper arm. *Confirmed by:* **nerve conduction studies**. **X-ray** and **MRI scan** of neck. *Finalized by the predictable outcome of management,* e.g. treatment of any remediable underlying cause, e.g. NSAIDs to reduce swelling around inflamed root canal, surgical decompression.
Peripheral nerve lesions in arm	*Suggested by:* loss of sensation localized to the forearm, upper arm or radial 3 ½ fingers or ulnar 1 ½ fingers in the palm. *Confirmed by:* **nerve conduction studies.** *Finalized by the predictable outcome of management,* e.g. treatment of any remediable underlying cause by surgical decompression.

Diminished sensation in arm dermatome

Investigations in **bold** below.

Main differential diagnoses and typical outline evidence, etc.	
C5 posterior root lesion	*Suggested by:* loss of sensation of **lateral aspect of upper arm.** *Confirmed by:* **nerve conduction studies. MRI scan** appearance. *Finalized by the predictable outcome of management,* e.g. treatment of any remediable underlying cause, e.g. NSAIDs to reduce swelling around inflamed root canal, surgical decompression.
C6 posterior root lesion	*Suggested by:* loss of sensation of **lateral forearm and thumb.** *Confirmed by:* **nerve conduction studies. MRI scan** appearance. *Finalized by the predictable outcome of management,* e.g. treatment of any remediable underlying cause, e.g. NSAIDs to reduce swelling around inflamed root canal, surgical decompression.
C8 posterior root lesion	*Suggested by:* loss of sensation of **palmar and dorsal aspect of ulnar 1½ fingers** and the ulnar border of the wrist. *Confirmed by:* **nerve conduction studies. MRI scan** appearance. *Finalized by the predictable outcome of management,* e.g. treatment of any remediable underlying cause, e.g. NSAIDs to reduce swelling around inflamed root canal, surgical decompression.
T1 posterior root lesion	*Suggested by:* loss of sensation of **ulnar border of the forearm.** *Confirmed by:* **nerve conduction studies. MRI scan** appearance. *Finalized by the predictable outcome of management,* e.g. treatment of any remediable underlying cause, e.g. NSAIDs to reduce swelling around inflamed root canal, surgical decompression.
T2 posterior root lesion	*Suggested by:* loss of sensation of **inner aspect of upper arm and breast.** *Confirmed by:* **nerve conduction studies. MRI scan** appearance. *Finalized by the predictable outcome of management,* e.g. treatment of any remediable underlying cause, e.g. NSAIDs to reduce swelling around inflamed root canal, surgical decompression.

Diminished sensation in the hand

Investigations in **bold** below.

Main differential diagnoses and typical outline evidence, etc.

Median nerve lesion due to carpal tunnel syndrome, 'pill', pregnancy, hypothyroidism, acromegaly, rheumatoid arthritis, or nerve trauma	*Suggested by:* loss of sensation of **palmar aspect of radial 3½ fingers** (in carpal tunnel syndrome, also discomfort in forearm and tingling if front of wrist tapped). If nerve severed, wasting of thenar eminence and thumb opposition. *Confirmed by:* **X-ray wrist and elbow. Nerve conduction studies** and **thyroid function tests, rheumatoid factor**, etc. *Finalized by the predictable outcome of management,* e.g. treatment of any remediable underlying cause, e.g. thyroid hormone replacement, surgical decompression of carpal tunnel.
Ulnar nerve lesion due to compression of deep palmar branch from trauma or ulnar groove at elbow from trauma or osteoarthritis	*Suggested by:* loss of sensation of **palmar and dorsal aspect of ulnar 1½ fingers** *but* not the ulnar border of the wrist. *Confirmed by:* **nerve conduction studies. X-ray wrist and elbow.** *Finalized by the predictable outcome of management,* e.g. surgical decompression.
Radial nerve lesion due to local compression (e.g. arm left hanging over chair)	*Suggested by:* loss of sensation of **dorsal aspect of radial 3½ fingers.** *Confirmed by:* **nerve conduction studies.** *Finalized by the predictable outcome of management,* e.g. physiotherapy if cause self-limiting.
C7 posterior root lesion due to cervical osteophytes	*Suggested by:* loss of sensation of **middle finger alone.** *Confirmed by:* **nerve conduction studies. MRI scan** appearances. *Finalized by the predictable outcome of management,* e.g. NSAIDs to reduce swelling around inflamed root canal, physiotherapy, surgical decompression.
C8 posterior root lesion due to cervical osteophytes	*Suggested by:* loss of sensation of **palmar and dorsal aspect of ulnar 1½ fingers** and the ulnar border of the wrist. *Confirmed by:* **nerve conduction studies. MRI scan** appearances. *Finalized by the predictable outcome of management,* e.g. NSAIDs to reduce swelling around inflamed root canal, physiotherapy, surgical decompression.

Disturbed sensation in lower limb

Look for specific patterns as indicated below. Investigations in **bold** below.

Main differential diagnoses and typical outline evidence, etc.	
Contralateral cortical (pre-central gyrus) lesion	*Suggested by:* graphaesthesia. *Confirmed by:* **CT or MRI scan** of brain. *Finalized by the predictable outcome of management,* e.g. treatment of any remediable underlying, e.g. surgical removal of tumour.
Peripheral neuropathy (due to diabetes mellitus, carcinoma, vitamin B$_{12}$ deficiency, drugs therapy, heavy metal, or chemical exposure	*Suggested by:* loss of touch and pinprick sensation worse in foot (e.g. stocking distribution) progressing upwards. *Confirmed by:* **nerve conduction studies. MRI scan** appearance. *Finalized by the predictable outcome of management,* e.g. treatment of any remediable underlying cause, e.g. stop drug, better control of diabetes.
Spinothalamic tract damage (no dorsal column loss) due to contralateralhemisection of the cord	*Suggested by:* loss of pinprick and temperature sensation, normal or disturbed touch, but normal joint position and vibration sense in foot. *Confirmed by:* **nerve conduction studies. MRI** of cervical cord. *Finalized by the predictable outcome of management,* e.g. treatment of any remediable underlying cause.
Dorsal column loss due to vitamin B$_{12}$ deficiency, ipsilateral hemisection of the cord, rarely tabes dorsalis	*Suggested by:* loss of joint position and vibration sense in foot. Pinprick and temperature sensation normal. *Confirmed by:* **nerve conduction studies.** Vitamin B$_{12}$ levels. *Finalized by the predictable outcome of management,* e.g. treatment of any remediable underlying cause, e.g. vitamin B$_{12}$ injections.
L1 posterior root lesion	*Suggested by:* loss of sensation in **inguinal region.** *Confirmed by:* **nerve conduction studies.** X-ray of lumbar spine and sacrum. *Finalized by the predictable outcome of management,* e.g. NSAIDs to reduce swelling around inflamed root canal, physiotherapy.
L2/3 posterior root lesion	*Suggested by:* loss of sensation in **anterior thigh.** *Confirmed by:* **nerve conduction studies.** X-ray of lumbar spine and sacrum. *Finalized by the predictable outcome of management,* e.g. NSAIDs to reduce swelling around inflamed root canal, physiotherapy.

L4/5 posterior root lesion	*Suggested by:* loss of sensation in **anterior shin.**
	Confirmed by: **nerve conduction studies**. X-ray of lumbar spine and sacrum.
	Finalized by the predictable outcome of management, e.g. NSAIDs to reduce swelling around inflamed root canal, physiotherapy.
S1 posterior root lesion	*Suggested by:* loss of sensation in **lateral border of foot.**
	Confirmed by: **nerve conduction studies**. X-ray of lumbar spine and sacrum.
	Finalized by the predictable outcome of management, e.g. NSAIDs to reduce swelling around inflamed root canal, physiotherapy.

Brisk reflexes

Investigations in **bold** below.

Main differential diagnoses and typical outline evidence, etc.	
Thyrotoxicosis	*Suggested by:* brisk reflexes in all limbs with normal flexor plantar responses.
	Confirmed by: ↑**FT4** and ↓↓**TSH** levels.
	Finalized by the predictable outcome of management, e.g. β-blocker, e.g. propranolol to control distressing symptoms, carbimazole or propylthiouracil to block thyroid hormone production.
High level pyramidal tract lesion (cervical cord, brainstem, bilateral internal capsule, or diffuse bilateral cortical lesion)	*Suggested by:* brisk reflexes in all limbs with **extensor** plantar responses.
	Confirmed by: normal **FT4** and **TSH** levels. **MRI scan** appearances.
	Finalized by the predictable outcome of management, e.g. physiotherapy, identification of any underlying treatable cause, e.g. tumour or removable haematoma.
Contralateral pyramidal tract lesion in internal capsule, primary cortex, brainstem, or cervical cord	*Suggested by:* unilateral brisk reflexes in upper and lower limb.
	Confirmed by: **MRI** of brain or cervical cord.
	Finalized by the predictable outcome of management, e.g. physiotherapy, identification of any underlying treatable cause, e.g. tumour or removable haematoma.

Diminished reflexes

Investigations in **bold** below.

Main differential diagnoses and typical outline evidence, etc.	
Sensory neuropathy	*Suggested by:* diminished reflexes, most marked peripherally. Normal muscle power. Normal plantar responses. *Confirmed by:* **nerve conduction studies.** *Finalized by the predictable outcome of management,* e.g. protection of vulnerable areas, e.g. feet from neuropathic trauma.
Motor neuropathy	*Suggested by:* diminished reflexes, muscle wasting, fasciculation and weakness. *Confirmed by:* **nerve conduction studies** and normal EMG. *Finalized by the predictable outcome of management,* e.g. physiotherapy to optimize function.
1° muscle disease	*Suggested by:* diminished reflexes, muscle wasting and weakness. No fasciculation. *Confirmed by:* **nerve conduction studies** and abnormal EMG and muscle biopsy. *Finalized by the predictable outcome of management,* e.g. physiotherapy to optimize function.
Cerebellar disease	*Suggested by:* unilateral diminished brisk reflexes in upper and lower limb. *Confirmed by:* **CT** and **MRI** of brain posterior fossa. *Finalized by the predictable outcome of management,* e.g. identification of any underlying treatable cause, e.g. tumour or removable haematoma.
Posterior root lesion in C7/C8	*Suggested by:* loss of **triceps** jerk. *Confirmed by:* **MRI** of disc space. *Finalized by the predictable outcome of management,* e.g. NSAIDs to reduce swelling around inflamed root canal, physiotherapy.
Posterior root lesion in C5/C6	*Suggested by:* loss of **biceps** jerk. *Confirmed by:* **MRI** of disc space. *Finalized by the predictable outcome of management,* e.g. NSAIDs and physiotherapy.
Posterior root lesion in L3/L4	*Suggested by:* loss of **knee** jerk. *Confirmed by:* **MRI** of disc space. *Finalized by the predictable outcome of management,* e.g. NSAIDs and physiotherapy.
Posterior root lesion in S1/S2	*Suggested by:* loss of **ankle** jerk. *Confirmed by:* **MRI** of disc space. *Finalized by the predictable outcome of management,* e.g. NSAIDs and physiotherapy.

Gait abnormality

Initial investigations (other tests in **bold** below).

Main differential diagnoses and typical outline evidence, etc.	
Somatomization 'functional' cause	*Suggested by:* **bizarre gait with exaggerated delay on affected limb**. No other physical signs of a lesion. *Confirmed by:* careful follow-up. *Finalized by the predictable outcome of management,* e.g. reassurance.
Contralateral pyramidal tract lesion (in cerebral hemisphere, internal capsule, brainstem or spinal cord)	*Suggested by:* **stiff leg swung in arc**. Other motor (± sensory) localizing signs indicating level of lesion. *Confirmed by:* **CT scan** or **MRI** of probable site. *Finalized by the predictable outcome of management,* e.g. identification of any underlying treatable cause, e.g. tumour or removable haematoma.
Parkinsonism	*Suggested by:* **shuffling festinant gait**, paucity of facial expression and movement, stiffness, tremor, etc. *Confirmed by:* response to treatment by dopamine agonist drugs, etc. *Finalized by the predictable outcome of management,* e.g. counselling, explain long-term strategy, MDT care, low dose levodopa with dopa-decarboxylase inhibitor.
Cerebellar lesion (tumour, ischaemia, etc.)	*Suggested by:* **wide-based gait**, inability to stand with feet together, falling to one side (truncal ataxia). Loss of tone and reflexes on same side as lesion. *Confirmed by:* **MRI** of posterior fossa of brain. *Finalized by the predictable outcome of management,* e.g. identification of any underlying treatable cause, e.g. tumour or removable haematoma.
Dorsal column loss or peripheral neuropathy (due to vitamin B$_{12}$ deficiency, etc.)	*Suggested by:* **bilateral stamping**, **high-stepping gait**, unsteadiness made worse by closing eyes (positive Rombergism). *Confirmed by:* **nerve conduction studies** and response to treatment of cause (if found). *Finalized by the predictable outcome of management,* e.g. identification of any underlying treatable cause, e.g. tumour or removable haematoma.
Bilateral upper motor neurone lesion (usually in spinal cord)	*Suggested by:* **'scissors'** or **'wading through mud'gait**. Bilateral leg weakness and brisk reflexes. *Confirmed by:* **MRI** of clinically probable site of lesion. *Finalized by the predictable outcome of management,* e.g. identification of any underlying treatable cause, e.g. tumour or removable haematoma.

Pelvic girdle and proximal muscle weakness (e.g. due to hereditary muscular dystrophy)	*Suggested by:* **waddling gait (hip tilts down when leg lifted)**. Hypotonic limb weakness and poor reflexes. *Confirmed by:* EMG. *Finalized by the predictable outcome of management,* e.g. identification of any underlying treatable cause, e.g. tumour or removable haematoma.
Joint, bone, or muscle lesion	*Suggested by:* **hobbling with minimal time spent on affected limb**. Tenderness and limited range of movement. *Confirmed by:* X-rays and response to treatment or resolution of cause. *Finalized by the predictable outcome of management,* e.g. identification of any underlying treatable cause.
Lateral popliteal nerve palsy	*Suggested by:* **unilateral stamping, high-stepping gait with foot drop**. Flaccid weakness around ankle. Loss of sensation of lateral lower leg. *Confirmed by:* **nerve conduction studies.** *Finalized by the predictable outcome of management,* e.g. identification of any underlying treatable cause.
Drug effect	*Suggested by:* wide-based gait, nystagmus, past pointing. History of alcohol intake or other drug. *Confirmed by:* ↑alcohol or other drug level, improvement with withdrawal. *Finalized by the predictable outcome of management,* e.g. stopping drug.

Difficulty in rising from chair or squatting position

Investigations in **bold** below.

Main differential diagnoses and typical outline evidence, etc.	
Polymyositis	*Suggested by:* muscle wasting, weakness, and poor reflexes. *Confirmed by:* **EMG** and **muscle biopsy.** *Finalized by the predictable outcome of management,* e.g. physiotherapy to optimize function.
Carcinomatous neuromyopathy	*Suggested by:* muscle wasting, weakness, and poor reflexes. Evidence of cancer (usually late stage). *Confirmed by:* **EMG** and evidence of carcinomatosis. *Finalized by the predictable outcome of management,* e.g. physiotherapy to optimize function.
Thyrotoxicosis	*Suggested by:* weight loss, tremor, sweating, anxiety, loose bowels. ↑**T3** or **T4** and ↓**TSH.** *Confirmed by:* response to treatment of thyrotoxicosis. *Finalized by the predictable outcome of management,* e.g. non-selective β-blocker, e.g. propranolol followed by carbimazole or propylthiouracil.
Diabetic amyotrophy	*Suggested by:* long history of diabetes mellitus. *Confirmed by:* **nerve conduction studies** and muscle biopsy. *Finalized by the predictable outcome of management,* e.g. physiotherapy to optimize function.
Cushing's syndrome	*Suggested by:* facial and truncal obesity with limb wasting, ↑**midnight cortisol**, ↑**24h urinary free cortisol.** *Confirmed by:* failure of 9 a.m cortisol and failure of 24h urinary cortisol to suppress in **dexamethasone test**. Bilateral adrenal hyperplasia or unilateral adenoma on **CT scan**. *Finalized by the predictable outcome of management,* e.g. stopping or reducing glucocorticoid therapy or surgical removal of cortisol secreting adrenal adenoma or ACTH secreting pituitary adenoma. Metyrapone preoperatively to reduce cortisol.
Osteomalacia	*Suggested by:* ↓**serum calcium** and ↑**alkaline phosphatase.** *Confirmed by:* response to treatment with calcium and vitamin D. *Finalized by the predictable outcome of management,* e.g. treatment with calcium and vitamin D.
Hereditary dystrophy	*Suggested by:* evidence of 1°muscle disease and family history. *Confirmed by:* **muscle biopsy.** *Finalized by the predictable outcome of management,* e.g. physiotherapy to optimize function.

Laboratory test results

Microscopic haematuria 544
Asymptomatic proteinuria 546
Glycosuria 547
Raised urine or serum bilirubin 548
Hepatocellular jaundice 550
Obstructive jaundice 552
Hypernatraemia 554
Hyponatraemia 555
Hyperkalaemia 556
Hypokalaemia 557
Hypercalcaemia 558
Hypocalcaemia 560
Raised alkaline phosphatase 562
Raised serum urea and creatinine 564
Low haemoglobin 566
Microcytic anaemia 567
Macrocytic anaemia 568
Normocytic anaemia 570
Very high ESR, CRP, or plasma viscosity 571

Microscopic haematuria

This is detected on routine urine dipstick testing. Initial investigations (other tests in **bold** below): MSU, FBC.

Main differential diagnoses and typical outline evidence, etc.	
Menstruation	*Suggested by:* history of current, recent or imminent periods, and no urinary symptoms. *Confirmed by:* **dipstick** –ve on repeating in mid-cycle. *Finalized by the predictable outcome of management,* e.g. reassurance.
Urinary tract infection	*Suggested by:* fever, frequency, or dysuria; ↑ nitrites, ↑ leucocytes on **dipstick**. *Confirmed by:* **MSU microscopy and culture**, response to antibiotics. **US scan** for possible anatomical abnormality. *Finalized by the predictable outcome of management,* e.g. increased fluid intake, cranberry juice, and regular bladder emptying. Provisional 1st line antibiotic pending MSU result, e.g. trimethoprim, cefalexin for 3d; 2nd line, e.g. ciprofloxacin bd for 5d.
Recent urethral trauma	*Suggested by:* recent urethral catheterization. *Confirmed by:* history, no infection in **MSU**. *Finalized by the predictable outcome of management,* e.g. explanation, reassurance.
Bleeding diathesis	*Suggested by:* bruising, anticoagulant therapy. *Confirmed by:* abnormal **platelet and clotting screen**. *Finalized by the predictable outcome of management,* e.g. treatment of underlying cause, replacement treatment e.g. vitamin K, platelet transfusion.
Kidney calculus	*Suggested by:* excruciating pain that fluctuates in the back below ribs, cloudy dark urine with a foul smell, recurrent dysuria, gout, persistent x3 microscopic haematuria. *Confirmed by:* **renal ultrasound, intravenous urography (IVU), cystoscopy** by urologist. *Finalized by the predictable outcome of management,* e.g. immediate analgesia, e.g. diclofenac IM or suppository, or pethidine IM with metoclopramide IM, and antibiotics. Emergency surgery if renal tract obstruction was confirmed on imaging.
Glomerulonephritis 1° or 2° to SLE, SBE, etc.	*Suggested by:* persistent x3 microscopic haematuria, associated proteinuria, hypertension. *Confirmed by:* **urine microscopy, renal ultrasound, immunoglobulins, complement, ANA, ANCA** positive **blood cultures**/response to antibiotics. *Finalized by the predictable outcome of management,* e.g. corticosteroids and/or immunosuppression with cyclophosphamide. Plasmapharesis to remove auto-antibodies in rapidly progressive glomerulonephritis.

Nephritis 2° to **NSAIDs, etc.**	*Suggested by:* persistent ×3 microscopic haematuria, taking NSAIDs or other suspicious drug. *Confirmed by:* **urine microscopy, renal ultrasound**, improvement on stopping suspected drug, IVU, etc. *Finalized by the predictable outcome of management,* e.g. eliminate possible causes; treat infection with antibiotics, treat renal failure.
Tumour of kidney	*Suggested by:* flank pain and abdominal mass, dark urine, weight loss, varicocoele (forms blockage of testicular vein), persistent ×3 microscopic haematuria. *Confirmed by:* **renal ultrasound, IVU, then cystoscopy** by urologist. *Finalized by the predictable outcome of management,* e.g. treat infection. Stenting, surgical resection, radio- or chemotherapy as single or combined treatments.

Asymptomatic proteinuria

Total protein excretion is usually <50mg/24h, of which albumin alone is normally <30mg/24h. Abnormal proteinuria is regarded as >150mg/24h. Initial investigations (other tests in **bold** below): urine dipstick ± MSU, FBC, U&E.

Main differential diagnoses and typical outline evidence, etc.	
Postural or orthostatic proteinuria	*Suggested by:* specimen from ambulant person <40y. *Confirmed by:* protein testing –ve on early morning urine specimen. *Finalized by the predictable outcome of management,* e.g. explanation to patient and reassurance.
Non-specific febrile illness	*Suggested by:* known febrile illness. *Confirmed by:* normal when illness resolved. *Finalized by the predictable outcome of management,* e.g. no change when temperature is back to normal.
Urinary tract infection	*Suggested by:* strong urge to pass urine, dysuria, increased frequency and fever; ↑nitrites, ↑leucocytes on dipstick. *Confirmed by:* **MSU microscopy and culture,** response to antibiotics. **US scan** for possible anatomical abnormality. *Finalized by the predictable outcome of management,* e.g. increased fluid intake, cranberry juice, and regular bladder emptying. Provisional 1st line antibiotic pending MSU result, e.g. trimethoprim, cefalexin for 3d. 2nd line, e.g. ciprofloxacin bd for 5d.
Glomerulonephritis 1° or 2° to SLE, etc.	*Suggested by:* proteinuria >1g/24h, persistent x3 microscopic haematuria, hypertension. *Confirmed by:* **urine microscopy, renal ultrasound, immunoglobulins, complement, ANA, ANCA, etc.** *Finalized by the predictable outcome of management,* e.g. corticosteroids and/or immunosuppression with cyclophosphamide. Plasmapheresis to remove auto-antibodies in rapidly progressive glomerulonephritis.
Nephritis 2° to NSAIDs, etc.	*Suggested by:* proteinuria >1g/24h, taking NSAIDs or other suspicious drug. *Confirmed by:* **urine microscopy, renal ultrasound,** improvement on stopping suspected drug, IVU, etc. *Finalized by the predictable outcome of management,* e.g. elimination of causes; treatment of renal failure.
Nephrotic syndrome due to minimal change glomerulonephritis, diabetes mellitus, etc.	*Suggested by:* frothy urine, oedema of legs, and swelling around the eyes, reduced quantity of urine, high blood pressure, and blood in urine. *Confirmed by:* **proteinuria** >3g/24h. **Serum albumin** low (<30g/L), and elevated total cholesterol and ↑triglycerides. *Finalized by the predictable outcome of management,* e.g. treat specific disease. Monitor U&E, BP, fluid balance, and weight. Lifestyle advice: no smoking, exercise, and low-fat diet. Restricted salt and normal protein intake, consider diuretics and ACE inhibitors.

Glycosuria

Almost always indicates diabetes and blood sugar has to be tested, but consider other possibilities. Initial investigations (other tests in **bold** below): urine dipstick ±MSU, FBC, fasting glucose, U&E.

Main differential diagnoses and typical outline evidence, etc.	
Diabetes mellitus	*Suggested by:* fatigue or other unexplained symptoms, thirst, polydipsia, polyuria. *Confirmed by:* **fasting blood glucose** ≥7.0mmol/L OR random or **2h glucose tolerance test (GTT)** glucose ≥11.1mmol/L once only with symptoms or on two occasions if no symptoms OR HbA1c ≥6.5% (48mmol/mol). *Finalized by the predictable outcome of management,* e.g. lifestyle advice—stop smoking, exercise, and weight reduction. Dietary advice, ↓saturated fat, ↓glucose, and ↑carbohydrate. When dietary measures are not enough in type 2 diabetes, oral treatment, e.g. metformin or sulphonylurea. Insulin for all type 1 diabetics, and if ↑HbA1c despite oral treatment in type 2 diabetics.
Renal glycosuria	*Suggested by:* patient well or renal disease or pregnant. *Confirmed by:* glycosuria when blood sugar shown to be normal on **glucose tolerance test**. *Finalized by the predictable outcome of management,* e.g. explanation and reassurance.

Raised urine or serum bilirubin

Initial investigations (other tests in **bold** below): US scan of liver.

Main differential diagnoses and typical outline evidence, etc.	
Hepatocellular jaundice (due to hepatitis or very severe liver failure) (see ➔ Hepatocellular jaundice, p.550)	*Suggested by:* jaundice with dark stools and dark urine. Also ↑urine urobilinogen (you can check this immediately). *Confirmed by:* **↑serum bilirubin** and **↑urine urobilinogen**. Highly abnormal **LFT**. Normal bile ducts but abnormal liver parenchyma on **US scan**. *Finalized by the predictable outcome of management,* e.g. treatment of the cause.
Obstructive jaundice due to intrahepatic causes (drugs, hepatitis, etc.) or extrahepatic (stones, tumours, etc.) (see ➔ Obstructive jaundice, p.552)	*Suggested by:* jaundice with pale stools and dark urine. Also NO ↑ urine urobilinogen. *Confirmed by:* ↑plasma bilirubin but ↑↑alkaline phosphatase, otherwise slightly abnormal LFT. Dilated bile ducts on US scan. *Finalized by the predictable outcome of management,* e.g. treatment of the cause.

Hepatocellular jaundice

Suggested by: jaundice with dark or normal stools and dark urine.
Confirmed by: ↑serum bilirubin and ↑ urine urobilinogen. Highly abnormal LFT. Normal bile ducts on US scan.

Main differential diagnoses and typical outline evidence, etc.

Acute (viral) hepatitis A	*Suggested by:* flu-like illness, pruritus, loss of appetite, jaundice, and tender hepatomegaly. *Confirmed by:* presence of **hepatitis A IgM antibody** suggests acute infection. *Finalized by the predictable outcome of management,* e.g. supportive care, rest, nutritious diet, and no alcohol. General hygiene. Liver transplantation for fulminant hepatic failure. Immunize contacts with hepatitis A vaccine.
Acute hepatitis B	*Suggested by:* history of IV drug use, transfusion, needle punctures, tattoos, tender hepatomegaly. *Confirmed by:* presence of **HBsAg** in serum. *Finalized by the predictable outcome of management,* e.g. conservative advice—no alcohol. Chronic despite antiviral treatment: pegylated interferon alfa, entecavir, or tenofovir disoproxil fumarate. Immunize sexual contacts.
Acute hepatitis C	*Suggested by:* history of transfusion or other blood products. Tender hepatomegaly. *Confirmed by:* presence of **anti-HCV antibody and antigen.** *Finalized by the predictable outcome of management,* e.g. combination of ribavirin + pegylated interferon alfa for moderate and severe chronic hepatitis (response depends on ethnic group, age, viral load, and HCV genotype).
Alcoholic hepatitis	*Suggested by:* history of drinking, presence of spider naevi, and other signs of chronic liver disease. *Confirmed by:* **raised GGT, raised ALT, liver biopsy**. *Finalized by the predictable outcome of management,* e.g. stop alcohol, treatment of alcohol withdrawal, high dose vitamin B, steroids in severe disease if no infection.
Drug-induced hepatitis, e.g. paracetamol (dose-dependent), halothane (dose-independent)	*Suggested by:* drug history, recent surgery. *Confirmed by:* improvement after stopping the offending drug. *Finalized by the predictable outcome of management,* e.g. stop causative agent, conservative treatment.

1° **hepatoma**	*Suggested by:* weight loss, abdominal pain, heaviness feeling in right upper abdomen, excessive alcohol intake, right upper quadrant (RUQ) mass.
	Confirmed by: **US scan/CT liver, liver biopsy, ↑alpha-fetoprotein**.
	Finalized by the predictable outcome of management, e.g. resection for solitary tumour <3cm diameter. Liver transplantation, chemotherapy, percutaneous ablation, tumour embolizations.
Right heart failure (due to pulmonary hypertension, COPD, tricuspid incompetence, worsened by anaemia, infection	*Suggested by:* shortness of breath, fatigue, tachycardia, rapid weight gain, ↑JVP, hepatomegaly, ankle oedema.
	Confirmed by: **CXR, ECG, echocardiogram, radionuclide ventriculography.**
	Finalized by the predictable outcome of management, e.g. diuretics, β-blockers, and digoxin. Treatment of cause. Lifestyle advice on weight reduction, diet, and smoking cessation.

Obstructive jaundice

Suggested by: jaundice with pale stools and dark urine.
Confirmed by: ↑**urine and serum bilirubin** but NO ↑**urobilinogen in urine.** ↑↑**alkaline phosphatase**, otherwise slightly abnormal **LFT.** Dilated bile ducts on **US liver scan.**

Main differential diagnoses and typical outline evidence, etc.

Common bile duct stones	*Suggested by:* pain in RUQ ± Murphy's sign. *Confirmed by:* **US scan liver/biliary ducts.** *Finalized by the predictable outcome of management,* e.g. analgesics, anti-emetics, and antibiotics. Emergency or elective cholecystectomy.
Cancer of head of pancreas	*Suggested by:* progressive painless jaundice, itching, ↓appetite and weight loss, development of diabetes mellitus, palpable gallbladder (Courvoisier's law). *Confirmed by:* **CT pancreas, ERCP or MRCP.** *Finalized by the predictable outcome of management,* e.g. relief of symptoms caused by jaundice with an endoscopic or percutaneous stent insertion. Pain control with opiates. Surgery if patient fit with no metastases and tumour is <3cm.
Sclerosing cholangitis	*Suggested by:* progressive fatigue, pruritus, dark urine, right upper abdominal pain, and jaundice. *Confirmed by:* ↑**serum alkaline phosphatase**, no gallstones on **US scan**, normal **anti-mitochondrial antibodies, ERCP** (beading of the intra- and extra-hepatic biliary ducts). *Finalized by the predictable outcome of management,* e.g. colestyramine for pruritus. Ursodeoxycholic acid to improve LFT and jaundice. Antibiotics for infection, endoscopic stenting for strictures, yearly follow-up, and liver transplantation for end-stage disease.
1° biliary cirrhosis	*Suggested by:* scratch marks, non-tender hepatomegaly ± splenomegaly, xanthelasmata, and xanthomas, arthralgia. *Confirmed by:* +ve **anti-mitochondrial antibody**, ↑↑**serum IgM, liver biopsy.** *Finalized by the predictable outcome of management,* e.g. colestyramine for pruritus. Codeine for diarrhoea. Vitamins D and K if clotting abnormal. Ursodeoxycholic acid to improve LFT, jaundice, and spironolactone if ascites.
Drug-induced e.g. oral contraceptive pill, phenothiazines, anabolic steroids, erythromycin	*Suggested by:* drug history. *Confirmed by:* symptoms recede when offending drug is discontinued. *Finalized by the predictable outcome of management,* e.g. improvement after the discontinuation of the causative agent.

Pregnancy (last trimester)	*Suggested by:* jaundice during pregnancy and severe itching.
	Confirmed by: resolution following delivery.
	Finalized by the predictable outcome of management, e.g. explanation and reassurance.
Alcoholic hepatitis/cirrhosis	*Suggested by:* history of drinking, presence of spider naevi, and other signs of chronic liver disease.
	Confirmed by: **liver biopsy**.
	Finalized by the predictable outcome of management, e.g. stop alcohol. Treat withdrawal symptoms. High dose vitamin B, thiamine, and steroid in severe disease if no infection.
Dubin–Johnson syndrome (decreased excretion of conjugated bilirubin)	*Suggested by:* intermittent jaundice and associated pain in the right hypochondrium. No hepatomegaly.
	Confirmed by: normal **alkaline phosphatase**, normal **LFT**. ↑**urinary bilirubin**. Pigment granules on **liver biopsy**.

Hypernatraemia

Initial investigations (other tests in **bold** below): repeat U&E, blood glucose, urine and simultaneous serum osmolality.

Main differential diagnoses and typical outline evidence, etc.	
Hypertonic plasma with hypervolaemia (e.g. excess IV saline) or hypovolaemia (e.g. diabetic polyuria or diabetes insipidus)	*Suggested by:* little hypotonic fluid orally or intravenously and thirsty, high volume of urine with low sodium content (e.g. in diabetic polyuria). *Confirmed by:* **iplasma osmolality** and **urine osmolality** higher (unless diabetes insipidus). *Finalized by the predictable outcome of management,* e.g. replace fluids. Avoid rapid changes. Give water orally or IV in the form of 5% glucose. Monitor serum electrolytes regularly.
Diabetes inspidus with hypovolaemia	*Suggested by:* drinking excessively and passing large volumes of urine (polydipsia and polyuria). Thirsty. *Confirmed by:* ↑plasma osmolality and ↓urine osmolality. *Finalized by the predictable outcome of management,* e.g. replace fluids. Avoid rapid changes. The aim is to reduce sodium at a rate of <10mmol/L per day. Normal saline may be used initially if serum sodium was >170mmol/L. Desmopressin 100–200 micrograms tds orally IM might be used.
Primary aldosteronism due to adrenal hyperplasia or Conn's sydrome with adrenal tumour	*Suggested by:* normal fluid intake, ↑BP. ↓serum potassium, metabolic alkalosis. *Confirmed by:* ↓**plasma renin** activity and ↑**aldosterone** levels. **CT** or **MRI scan** appearance. *Finalized by the predictable outcome of management,* e.g. spironolactone, amiloride, or eplerenone for cases of bilateral adrenal hyperplasia. Adrenalectomy for aldosterone-producing adenoma.

Hyponatraemia

Also usually indicates hypotonicity—low plasma osmolality. Initial investigations (other tests in **bold** below): U&E, blood glucose, urine and simultaneous serum osmolality.

Main differential diagnoses and typical outline evidence, etc.	
Hypotonic with hypovolaemia due to excess renal or non-renal loss (excessive diuretic therapy, history of renal tubular disease, diarrhoea, vomit, fistula, burns, small bowel obstruction, blood loss)	*Suggested by:* ↓**serum sodium** and ↓**osmolality**. Loss of skin turgor, tachycardia, ↓BP. History of possible cause. *Confirmed by:* response to removal or treating of cause. *Finalized by the predictable outcome of management,* e.g. treat the cause. If symptomatic, saline water. In chronic conditions, fluid restriction. Avoid rapid changes, e.g. maximum change of sodium of 12–15mmol/L/d.
Hypotonic with normovolaemia, including pseudohyponatraemia (severe hypothyroidism or glucocorticoid deficiency). Symptoms of severe diabetes mellitus	*Suggested by:* ↓**serum sodium** and ↓**osmolality**. Normal skin turgor, normal pulse and BP. *Confirmed by:* response to treating cause, balancing fluid intake. **Blood glucose** of >20mmol/L in pseudohyponatraemia. *Finalized by the predictable outcome of management,* e.g. treatment of the cause, e.g. hypothyroidism, Addison's disease, or diabetes mellitus.
Hypotonic with hypervolaemia (water overload, cardiac failure, cirrhosis, renal failure, nephrotic syndrome, inappropriate antidiuretic hormone (ADH) secretion)	*Suggested by:* ↓**serum sodium** and ↓**osmolality**. Oedema, basal lung crackles. *Confirmed by:* response to treating cause, reducing fluid intake. *Finalized by the predictable outcome of management,* e.g. treatment of the underlying condition.
Syndrome of inappropriate ADH secretion (malignancy, CNS disorders, chest infections, metabolic problems, drugs)	*Suggested by:* **serum sodium** usually <120mmol/L. Confusion, progressing to coma, mild oedema. *Confirmed by:* **urine osmolality > serum osmolality** despite ↓serum osmolality (<270mmol/L). **Urine sodium** >20mmol/L. *Finalized by the predictable outcome of management,* e.g. fluid restriction. Treat the underlying cause. If not possible, demeclocycline for long-term control.

Hyperkalaemia

Initial investigations (other tests in **bold** below): U&E, blood glucose.

Main differential diagnoses and typical outline evidence, etc.	
Drug effect: potassium administration or other drug effect	*Suggested by:* potassium supplements, blood transfusion, ACE inhibitor, spironolactone, amiloride, triamterene, etc. *Confirmed by:* normal potassium when drug reduced or stopped. *Finalized by the predictable outcome of management*, e.g. stop suspect drug.
Metabolic acidosis, renal failure, diabetic ketoacidosis	*Suggested by:* usually obvious illness and severe metabolic disturbance, $\downarrow$**pH** and $\downarrow$**plasma HCO$_3$**. *Confirmed by:* response to treatment of metabolic disturbance. *Finalized by the predictable outcome of management*, e.g. if K$^+$ >6.5 and not falling, calcium gluconate IV, glucose + insulin, Calcium Resonium®. Treatment of cause.
Addison's disease	*Suggested by:* fatigue, $\downarrow$BP, pigmented buccal mucosa, and palmar creases, $\downarrow$Na$^+$, $\uparrow$K$^+$. *Confirmed by:* $\downarrow$random and **9a.m cortisol**, $\uparrow$**ACTH**, and poor response to **Synacthen® stimulation**. Response to hydrocortisone IV and normal saline. *Finalized by the predictable outcome of management*, e.g. hydrocortisone, e.g. 10–20mg mane and 5–10mg evening. Fludrocortisone, e.g. 50–100 micrograms daily.
Recent blood transfusion	*Suggested by:* history. *Confirmed by:* fall of potassium after few hours. *Finalized by the predictable outcome of management*, e.g. monitor potassium. If K$^+$ >6.5 and not falling, calcium gluconate IV, glucose + insulin, Calcium Resonium®.
Spurious result due to haemolysis in specimen bottle	*Suggested by:* laboratory reporting haemolysis in specimen bottle. *Confirmed by:* normal potassium when repeated with no delay in delivery to lab. *Finalized by the predictable outcome of management*, e.g. repeat potassium.

Hypokalaemia

Initial investigations (other tests in **bold** below): U&E, plasma glucose.

Main differential diagnoses and typical outline evidence, etc.	
Diuretic therapy	*Suggested by:* taking thiazide or loop diuretic (fondness of liquorice or Pernod drink). *Confirmed by:* normal potassium after stopping diuretic. *Finalized by the predictable outcome of management,* e.g. stop suspected cause ± oral potassium supplements.
β-agonist treatment	*Suggested by:* taking high doses of β-agonist, usually in nebulizer for acute asthmatic attack in hospital. *Confirmed by:* normal potassium after stopping drug. *Finalized by the predictable outcome of management,* e.g. stop β-agonist.
Vomiting e.g. pyloric stenosis	*Suggested by:* history of severe vomiting with poor fluid intake. *Confirmed by:* normal potassium without subsequent need for replacement when cause of vomiting treated. *Finalized by the predictable outcome of management,* e.g. depending on severity, replacement of fluids and electrolytes, correction of acid–base imbalance, and dealing with specific underlying causes.
Chronic diarrhoea, purgative abuse, intestinal fistula, villous adenoma of rectum	*Suggested by:* history of severe diarrhoea or mucous loss. *Confirmed by:* normal potassium without need for further replacement when cause treated subsequently. *Finalized by the predictable outcome of management,* e.g. oral potassium supplements if not dehydrated, potassium IV with IV fluid replacement, treatment of cause.
1° hyperaldosteronism due to adrenal hyperplasia or Conn's syndrome with adrenal tumour	*Suggested by:* normal fluid intake, ↑BP, ↓serum potassium. *Confirmed by:* **↓plasma renin activity** and **↑aldosterone. CT or MRI scan** appearance. *Finalized by the predictable outcome of management,* e.g. spironolactone, amiloride, or eplerenone for bilateral adrenal hyperplasia. Adrenalectomy for 'Conn's syndrome' (aldosterone-producing adenoma).
Renal tubular defect (in recovery phase from renal failure, pyelonephritis, associated myeloma, heavy metal poisoning, congenital renal tubular defects)	*Suggested by:* hypokalaemia and history of possible cause. *Confirmed by:* **test for renal concentrating ability**. *Finalized by the predictable outcome of management,* e.g. treatment of underlying cause. If serum K+ <3mmol/L, potassium PO or IV not exceeding 20mmol/L/h. Serum U&E and ECG monitoring during treatment.

Hypercalcaemia

Present when specimen taken without a venous cuff, and calcium result was corrected for albumin concentration. Initial investigations (other tests in **bold** below): U&E, calcium, alkaline phosphatase.

Main differential diagnoses and typical outline evidence, etc.	
Severe hypercalcaemia	*Confirmed by:* calcium >3.5 mmol/L. *Finalized by the predictable outcome of management,* e.g. saline infusion + furosemide to maintain fluid balance and prevent overload. Correct hypokalaemia and hypomagnesaemia. If calcium remains high, pamidronate disodium over 2–3d.
Thiazide diuretics	*Suggested by:* mild hypercalcaemia, drug history, normal phosphate and alkaline phosphatase. *Confirmed by:* normal calcium when drug stopped. *Finalized by the predictable outcome of management,* e.g. stop thiazide.
Bone metastases from breast, bronchus, kidney, thyroid, ovary, colon	*Suggested by:* normal phosphate and ↑alkaline phosphatase. *Confirmed by:* 2°s on **bone scan**. *Finalized by the predictable outcome of management,* e.g. pamidronate to lower calcium over 2–3d. Appropriate treatment of neoplastic process.
Thyrotoxicosis	*Suggested by:* weight loss with good appetite, tremor, palpitation and agitation, goitre, mild ↑calcium. *Confirmed by:* ↑**T4** or ↑**T3** and ↓↓**TSH**. Normal phosphate and alkaline phosphatase. Response to treatment of thyrotoxicosis. *Finalized by the predictable outcome of management,* e.g. propranolol 40–80mg 8mg hourly to control symptoms (avoid in asthmatics). Carbimazole, e.g. 40mg reduced to 10 ± 5mg for 18mo according to test results. Written warning about agranulocytosis.
1° (or tertiary) hyperparathyroidism	*Suggested by:* fatigue, constipation, depression, impaired memory, renal colic and kidney stones, stomach ulcer, ↑BP, pancreatitis, low phosphate, and ↑alkaline phosphatase. *Confirmed by:* ↑**plasma parathyroid levels** with ↑calcium. *Finalized by the predictable outcome of management,* e.g. correct very high calcium. Surgical removal of parathyroid adenoma.

Myeloma	*Suggested by:* low back pain, polyuria and polydypsia, spinal fracture, normal serum phosphate and alkaline phosphatase. *Confirmed by:* paraprotein with immunoparesis on **electrophoresis**, hypercalcaemia, ↓**Hb**, **Bence–Jones protein in urine**, spinal X-ray showing fracture with an osteolytic lesion. *Finalized by the predictable outcome of management,* e.g. correct very high calcium. Analgesics for bone pain. Oral bisphosphonate to keep calcium down. Local radiotherapy in progressive disease. Prompt treatment of infections. Transfusions for anaemia. Chemotherapy using melphalan or cyclophosphamide in conjunction with steroids. More aggressive treatment for fitter patients.
Sarcoidosis	*Suggested by:* cough, weight loss, night sweats, shortness of breath, erythema nodosum, ↑phosphate and alkaline phosphatase. Bilateral hilar shadows on CXR. *Confirmed by:* **lung function tests, Kveim test, biopsy** from a granuloma, ↑vitamin D levels and ↑ACE levels. *Finalized by the predictable outcome of management,* e.g. correct very high calcium. Long-term prednisolone to control calcium. If severe cases, methylprednisolone IV or immunosuppression, e.g. methotrexate and cyclophosphamide.
Vitamin D excess	*Suggested by:* drug history and ↑phosphate. *Confirmed by:* normal calcium when drug stopped. *Finalized by the predictable outcome of management,* e.g. stop suspected drug.
Ectopic parathyroid hormone due to lung cancer usually	*Suggested by:* ↓phosphate and ↑alkaline phosphatase. *Confirmed by:* ↑plasma parathyroid levels with high calcium presence of underlying neoplasm. *Finalized by the predictable outcome of management,* e.g. correct very high calcium. Surgical resection of cancer in appropriate cases.

Hypocalcaemia

Present when specimen taken without a venous cuff and corrected for albumin concentration. Investigations in **bold** below:

Main differential diagnoses and typical outline evidence, etc.	
Vitamin D deficiency— due to dietary deficiency or 1,25 (OH)₂D abnormality	*Suggested by:* diet history, ↓phosphate, and ↑alkaline phosphatase. *Confirmed by:* **↓1, 25(OH)2 vitamin D**, normal calcium after adequate treatment with vitamin D. *Finalized by the predictable outcome of management,* e.g. calcium + vitamin D, 1–2 tablets daily.
Hypoparathyroidism (transient or permanent after thyroid surgery, autoimmune disease, radiations)	*Suggested by:* neck surgery, ↑phosphate. *Confirmed by:* **↓parathyroid hormone** or normal in presence of ↓calcium. *Finalized by the predictable outcome of management,* e.g. alfacalcidol with careful monitoring of calcium levels.
Chronic renal failure	*Suggested by:* **↑phosphate**, **↑creatinine**, **↑alkaline phosphatase**, **↓Hb**. *Confirmed by:* improvement with control of renal failure and phosphate levels. *Finalized by the predictable outcome of management,* e.g. stop nephrotoxic drugs, relieve obstruction; prompt treatment of infections, treat ↑BP with ACE inhibitors or angiotensin receptor blockers (ARBs); hyperlipidaemia with statins. Restriction of fluids and furosemide for oedema. Erythropoietin for severe anaemia. Alfacalcidol for renal bone disease. Dialysis.
Pseudohypo-parathyroidism	*Suggested by:* short stature, obesity, round face, short metacarpals, ↑phosphate. *Confirmed by:* **↑plasma parathyroid levels** with ↓or normal calcium. *Finalized by the predictable outcome of management,* e.g. alfacalcidol with careful monitoring of calcium levels.
Pancreatitis	*Suggested by:* abdominal pain and tenderness, ↓phosphate, normal alkaline phosphatase. *Confirmed by:* **↑↑serum amylase** and **US scan** of abdomen. *Finalized by the predictable outcome of management,* e.g. nil by mouth, nasogastric (NG) tube, saline infusion to correct dehydration, strong analgesics (e.g. pethidine IM), regular monitoring.

Fluid overload	*Suggested by:* history and ↓phosphate and normal alkaline phosphatase.
	Confirmed by: normalization with correction of fluid balance.
	Finalized by the predictable outcome of management, e.g. reduced fluid intake to allow correction use of diuretics.
Rhabdomyolysis	*Suggested by:* severe muscle pains, weakness, dark or cola-coloured urine, racing heart, history of extreme muscle activity, ↑phosphate.
	Confirmed by: ↑↑**CPK, ↑creatinine**, ↑urinary myoglobin, **CT and MRI scans** of the muscles and **muscle biopsy**.
	Finalized by the predictable outcome of management, e.g. correct electrolyte disturbances, e.g. hyperkalaemia. Rehydration to maintain a urine output of 300mL/h until myoglobinuria disappears. Sodium bicarbonate IV ± dialysis.

Raised alkaline phosphatase

Investigations in **bold** below.

Main differential diagnoses and typical outline evidence, etc.	
Paget's disease	*Suggested by:* deformity of skull or tibia typically, ↑alkaline phosphatase.
	Confirmed by: bone deformity, especially on **skull and tibia X-ray** and ↑**urinary hydroxyproline**.
	Finalized by the predictable outcome of management, e.g. analgesics for bone pain. If not enough, try alendronic acid.
Vitamin D deficiency due to dietary deficiency	*Suggested by:* diet history, ↓phosphate and ↑alkaline phosphatase.
	Confirmed by: ↓**1,25 (OH)2 vitamin D level**, and normal calcium after oral vitamin D and calcium supplement.
	Finalized by the predictable outcome of management, e.g. dietary treatment and calcium supplement with vitamin D.
Bone metastases from breast, bronchus, kidney, thyroid, ovary, colon	*Suggested by:* normal phosphate, ↑calcium and ↑alkaline phosphatase.
	Confirmed by: 2°s on **bone scan.**
	Finalized by the predictable outcome of management, e.g. appropriate management of malignancy.
1° or tertiary hyperparathyroidism	*Suggested by:* ↓phosphate and ↑alkaline phosphatase after years of 2° hyperparathyroidism.
	Confirmed by: ↑**plasma parathyroid** levels with ↑calcium.
	Finalized by the predictable outcome of management, e.g. correct very high calcium. Surgical removal of parathyroid adenoma.
Cholestasis	*Suggested by:* jaundice with pale stools and dark urine. Bilirubin (i.e. conjugated and thus soluble) in urine.
	Confirmed by: ↑**urine and serum bilirubin** but NO ↑**urobilinogen** in urine. ↑↑alkaline phosphatase, otherwise slightly **abnormal LFT**.
	Finalized by the predictable outcome of management, e.g. colestyramine for pruritus. Treat infections. Relieve obstruction by stenting or surgery.

Raised serum urea and creatinine

Investigations in **bold** below.

Main differential diagnoses and typical outline evidence, etc.	
High protein load due to gastrointestinal (GI) bleed, catabolism, sepsis, etc.	*Suggested by:* ↑**blood urea** and normal creatinine or urea/creatinine ratio strongly in favour of urea. *Confirmed by:* recovery when catabolism or GI bleeding stops. *Finalized by the predictable outcome of management,* e.g. IV line—IV fluids and then blood transfusion, regular monitoring. Reduce acidity, e.g. with PPI.
Pre-renal failure due to hypovolaemia (due to low fluid intake, or high fluid loss of any cause)	*Suggested by:* ↑blood urea and ↑creatinine. History of fluid imbalance with fluid loss exceeding intake. Urea/creatinine ratio in favour of urea. *Confirmed by:* improvement (↓**creatinine**) with restoration of fluid volume. *Finalized by the predictable outcome of management,* e.g. correction of fluid and electrolyte imbalance. Antibiotics for infection. Stop nephrotoxic drugs. Rehydration orally, via NG tube or IV infusion. Monitor urine output ± central venous pressure (CVP) monitoring.
Chronic renal failure due to pyelonephritis, glomerulonephritis, interstitial nephritis, diabetes mellitus, renovascular disease, analgesic nephropathy, hypertension, etc.	*Suggested by:* ↑**blood urea** and ↑creatinine and not rising rapidly over days. ↓calcium, ↑phosphate, ↓Hb, small renal size on **US scan**. *Confirmed by:* **renal biopsy** appearance. *Finalized by the predictable outcome of management,* e.g. treat infections, stop nephrotoxic drugs, relieve obstruction: treat ↑BP with ACE inhibitors or ARBs, and hyperlipidaemia with statins. Restriction of fluids and furosemide for oedema. Calcium carbonate for hyperphosphatemia. Erythropoietin for severe anaemia. Alfacalcidol for renal bone disease. Dialysis.
Acute tubular necrosis, severe hypotension, nephrotoxins (NSAIDs, aminoglycosides, amphotericin B, etc.)	*Suggested by:* ↑blood urea and ↑creatinine and rising rapidly over days. Hb normal. Recent acute illness with hypotension and oliguria (fall in urine output <1mL/kg/h). **US scan**: normal kidney size and no obstructive uropathy. *Confirmed by:* no improvement when normovolaemic and **renal biopsy**. *Finalized by the predictable outcome of management,* e.g. eliminate any causes. Maintain fluid balance with careful monitoring of output and input + insensible loss (± CVP). Temporary dialysis.

Obstructive renal failure	*Suggested by:* ↑blood urea and ↑creatinine and rising. Hb normal. ↓urine output. *Confirmed by:* **US scan** showing dilatation of renal calyces or ureters. *Finalized by the predictable outcome of management,* e.g. catheterization for acute retention of urine. Ureteric stenting or nephrostomy.

Low haemoglobin

Investigations in **bold** below.

Main differential diagnoses and typical outline evidence, etc.	
Microcytic anaemia (see ⊃ Microcytic anaemia, p.567)	*Suggested by:* history of blood loss or familial microcytic anaemias (especially in Mediterranean origin). *Confirmed by:* ↓Hb and ↓MCV.
Macrocytic anaemia (see ⊃ Macrocytic anaemia, p.568)	*Suggested by:* sore tongue, diarrhoea. Family history of pernicious anaemia (PA), medication or alcohol. *Confirmed by:* ↓Hb and ↑MCV.
Normocytic anaemia (see ⊃ Normocytic anaemia, p.570)	*Suggested by:* history of chronic intercurrent illness, e.g. pancytopaenia, chronic renal failure. *Confirmed by:* ↓Hb and MCV normal.

Microcytic anaemia

Usually accompanied by low mean corpuscular Hb concentration. Investigations in **bold** below.

Main differential diagnoses and typical outline evidence, etc.	
Iron deficiency anaemia	*Suggested by:* history of blood loss (e.g. history of heavy periods, passing blood rectally), or poor diet. *Confirmed by:* ↓**serum iron**, ↓**ferritin**, and ↑**total iron binding capacity**. *Finalized by the predictable outcome of management,* e.g. treat the cause. Iron replacement therapy.
Thalassaemia: α, β, **intermedia, and variants**	*Suggested by:* persistent mild anaemia, failure to thrive, family history, Mediterranean origin. Hepatosplenomegaly, ↓↓MCV for degree of anaemia. *Confirmed by:* **blood film**: target and nucleated cells. **Hb electrophoresis** shows ↑HbF or ↑HbA2, ↑serum iron and iron binding capacity. *Finalized by the predictable outcome of management,* e.g. regular blood transfusions to keep Hb above 9g/dL. Iron-chelating agents, e.g. desferrioxamine infusion 8–10h per day. Splenectomy when increased frequency of transfusions; treat complications such as 2° diabetes mellitus. Bone marrow transplantation.
Sideroblastic anaemia rarely congenital or acquired due to alcohol lead poisoning, etc.	*Suggested by:* history of chronic intercurrent illness, e.g. chronic renal failure. *Confirmed by:* ↑**serum iron**, ↑**ferritin**, and **total iron binding capacity** normal. *Finalized by the predictable outcome of management,* e.g. elimination of the cause. Pyridoxine. Blood transfusion in severe anaemia.

Macrocytic anaemia

Investigations in **bold** below.

Main differential diagnoses and typical outline evidence, etc.	
B$_{12}$ deficiency: pernicious anaemia, intestinal malabsorption	*Suggested by:* associated autoimmune disease, e.g. primary hypothyroidism, vitiligo, etc. ↓Hb, ↓WCC, and ↓platelets.
	Confirmed by: **↓serum B$_{12}$** (± **↓folate** too due to anorexia) + pernicious anaemia diagnosed in absence of general malabsorption.
	Finalized by the predictable outcome of management, e.g. treat any malabsorption. In pernicious anaemia, hydroxocobalamin 1mg IM every 3–4mo after loading doses (e.g. 6x 1mg IM over 2wk).
Folate deficiency	*Suggested by:* poor diet, pregnancy, lactation, general malabsorption.
	Confirmed by: **↓folate** but serum B$_{12}$ normal.
	Finalized by the predictable outcome of management, e.g. eliminate cause + folic acid, e.g. 5mg daily for 4mo. Correct any B$_{12}$ deficiency before starting folic acid.
Antifolate drugs	*Suggested by:* phenytoin typically, barbiturates and similar, methotrexate and similar.
	Confirmed by: response to high dose folic acid treatment or stopping drug (**serum folate** may be normal).
	Finalized by the predictable outcome of management, e.g. stopping antifolate drug.
Alcohol abuse	*Suggested by:* history of abuse and poor diet.
	Confirmed by: response to abstinence (**serum folate** may be normal).
	Finalized by the predictable outcome of management, e.g. stop alcohol; treat withdrawal symptoms—high dose vitamin B.
Hepatitis and liver disease	*Suggested by:* abnormal liver enzymes.
	Confirmed by: normal (or ↑) **serum B$_{12}$** and poor response to folic acid.
	Finalized by the predictable outcome of management, e.g. conservative treatment. Advise no alcohol. If chronic, trial of interferon alfa or antiviral treatment.
Hypothyroidism	*Suggested by:* **↓FT4** and **↑TSH**.
	Confirmed by: **normal B$_{12}$** and response to treatment with thyroxine.
	Finalized by the predictable outcome of management, e.g. levothyroxine replacement, e.g. 25–50 micrograms per day and adjust, based on TSH.

Haemolysis	*Suggested by:* **urobilinogen in urine**.
	Confirmed by: ↑reticulocytes on **blood film**, ↓haptoglobin.
	Finalized by the predictable outcome of management, e.g. avoid precipitating factors. Blood transfusion if anaemia is severe. Treatment depends on cause, e.g. steroid and immunosuppressants in autoimmune haemolytic anaemia.
Myelodysplasia	*Suggested by:* hepato- or splenomegaly.
	Confirmed by: **bone marrow examination**, normal B_{12} and folate, pancytopenia in later stages.
	Finalized by the predictable outcome of management, e.g. intensive combination or single-agent chemotherapy. Frequent transfusion of RBC and platelets. Stem cell transfusions if young patient.

Normocytic anaemia

Investigations in **bold** below.

Main differential diagnoses and typical outline evidence, etc.	
Anaemia of chronic disease (e.g. rheumatoid arthritis, hypogonadism, etc.)	*Suggested by:* associated chronic disease. *Confirmed by:* **iron**, **B$_{12}$** normal. ↓**folate** or normal. Normal or ↑ferritin from inflammation. *Finalized by the predictable outcome of management*, e.g. treatment of underlying cause.
Chronic renal failure	*Suggested by:* high **creatinine** and **urea**. *Confirmed by:* response to erythropoietin treatment only. *Finalized by the predictable outcome of management*, e.g. erythropoietin.
'Anaemia of pregnancy'	*Suggested by:* pregnant state. *Confirmed by:* persistence despite folic acid and iron supplements, resolution after birth. *Finalized by the predictable outcome of management*, e.g. explanation, reassurance.
Hypothyroidism	*Suggested by:* ↓**FT4** and ↑**TSH**. *Confirmed by:* **normal B$_{12}$** and response to treatment with thyroxine. *Finalized by the predictable outcome of management*, e.g. thyroxine replacement, e.g. 25–50 micrograms levothyroxine per day and adjust based on TSH.
Haemolysis (e.g. due to reticulosis)	*Suggested by:* urobilinogen in urine. *Confirmed by:* ↑reticulocytes on **blood film**. *Finalized by the predictable outcome of management*, e.g. avoid precipitating factors. Blood transfusion if severe haemolysis. Treat infection depending on the cause, e.g. steroids, immunosuppressants, splenectomy, anticoagulation, and stem cell transplantation.
Bone marrow failure	*Suggested by:* pancytopaenia. *Confirmed by:* **bone marrow examination**. *Finalized by the predictable outcome of management*, e.g. blood cell transfusion to support blood count. Immunosuppression (e.g. ciclosporin) may be effective but not curative. Allogeneic marrow transplantation for younger patients who are severely affected.

Very high ESR, CRP, or plasma viscosity

An ESR or CRP or plasma viscosity which is just above normal is non-specific as it is associated with any cause of inflammation, including infection—but an ESR near 100 or above is a good lead. Initial investigations (other tests in **bold** below): FBC.

Main differential diagnoses and typical outline evidence, etc.

Severe bacterial infection, e.g. osteomyelitis empyema, peritonitis	*Suggested by:* high fever, ↑leucocytes. *Confirmed by:* positive **bacterial culture** from blood and/or site of infection and response to antibiotics and/or **surgical drainage**. *Finalized by the predictable outcome of management,* e.g. antibiotics according to culture and sensitivity. Clearance of pus.
Giant cell arteritis	*Suggested by:* localized headache, especially over temple, late loss of vision ± muscle pain and stiffness in shoulder area. *Confirmed by:* vessel wall inflammation on **biopsy**. *Finalized by the predictable outcome of management,* e.g. prednisolone 40–60mg per day and reduce the dose gradually after a week. Bisphosphonates as a prophylaxis for osteoporosis.
Bacterial endocarditis	*Suggested by:* fever, changing heart murmurs, nail splinter haemorrhages. *Confirmed by:* bacterial growth from several **blood cultures**, **echocardiogram** may show vegetations. *Finalized by the predictable outcome of management,* e.g. aggressive antibiotic treatment, e.g. benzylpenicillin 1.2g/4h IV + gentamicin 1mg/kg/8h IV for 4wk. Addition of flucloxacillin 2g qds IV in acute causes. Surgical treatment, e.g. if unstable infected prosthetic valve.
Myeloma	*Suggested by:* bone pain or fractures. **Bence–Jones protein** in urine and monoclonal protein band on **electrophoresis**. *Confirmed by:* myeloma cells on **bone marrow examination**. *Finalized by the predictable outcome of management,* e.g. treat severe hypercalcaemia (see ➔ Hypercalcaemia, p.558). Analgesics for bone pain. Bisphosphonates to reduce fracture rates. Local radiotherapy in rapidly progressive disease. Prompt treatment of infection. Transfusions for anaemia, chemotherapy using melphalan or cyclophosphamide in conjunction with steroids. More aggressive treatment for fitter patients.
Prostatic carcinoma	*Suggested by:* bone pain, few urinary symptoms. *Confirmed by:* sclerotic changes in **pelvic bones X-ray** and ↑**prostatic-specific antigen (PSA)** and prostatic biopsy. *Finalized by the predictable outcome of management,* e.g. for localized disease, radical prostatectomy or radiotherapy with hormonal therapy. For metastatic disease, hormonal therapy.

Chest X-rays

The general approach 574
Area of uniform lung opacification (whiteness) with a
   well-defined border 576
Round opacity (or opacities) >5mm in diameter 582
Multiple 'nodular' shadows and 'miliary mottling' 586
Diffuse poorly defined hazy opacification 590
Increased linear markings 594
Symmetrically dark lungs 596
Single area of dark lung 598
Enlarged hilar shadowing 600
Abnormal hilar shadowing—streaky 604
Upper mediastinal widening 606
Abnormal cardiac silhouette 610

The general approach

- Use good viewing conditions. Nearly all systems are now electronic, but monitors (especially on wards) can be of variable quality, so don't look at screens with any electronic interference!
- Check the patient's name, gender, and age to ensure correct identity, and correct date of the scan.
- Check if the film is marked P–A (X-rays passing from posterior to anterior in a standard way) or A–P (X-rays passing from anterior to posterior). A–P views are done when the patient is ill, using a portable X-ray tube—these will often be semi-erect films with suboptimal exposure factors. This projection magnifies the mediastinum so A–P films should not be used to assess cardiac size or hilar configuration.
- Check which sides are marked left and right, and whether the cardiac apex is on the left (if not, the patient may have dextrocardia).
- Check the patient's positioning. Are the sternoclavicular joints equidistant from the spinous processes of the vertebral column? If not, then the patient was rotated. Rotation causes asymmetry of shoulder girdle muscles projected over the lung fields. The side that has the less space between the end of the clavicle and spinous process has more muscle projected over the lung fields and should be whiter than the other side. Be cautious in the interpretation of a rotated chest radiograph.
- Can you see the vertebral column through the heart shadow? If not, then it is 'under-penetrated' (the X-ray beam was too weak). This means that normal lung tissue will look abnormally opaque (white).
- If the lungs appear dark, the vertebral column can be seen very clearly and the heart shadow is vague, it was over-penetrated and abnormalities may be missed.
- Is the diaphragm between the 5th/6th anterior rib ends? If it is higher, then the patient did/could not take a deep breath, and interpretation of the appearance of the lungs and mediastinum will be suboptimal. If the diaphragm is flattened, then emphysematous changes are likely.
- Having considered the technical issues, is there anything that strikes you immediately? Check for foreign bodies, e.g. endotracheal tubes, chest drains, monitoring wires, oxygen tubes, masks, pacemakers, central lines, etc. A striking radio-opaque (white) or lucent (dark) area is likely to be a good lead.
- After noting the obvious finding or if there is nothing dramatic, assess the X-ray systematically as there could well be more subtle abnormalities.
- Compare the lung fields in the lower zones, mid-zones, and upper zones, and check 'behind' the heart.
- Look at the superior mediastinum, the hilum, the heart, the cardiophrenic angles, the diaphragms, and the costophrenic angles.
- Lastly, look at the ribs, the shoulders, the overlying soft tissue from the neck down to the upper abdomen. Note artefacts from skin folds, electrodes, hair and clothing, especially braids, piercings, and buttons.

- Initially, try to look at the film without considering the clinical setting (otherwise, there is a tendency to miss obvious things, which do not fit in with your differential diagnosis), then look again with the clinical setting in mind.
- Remember to compare any chest film with an abnormality with any previous X-rays. Progression, or more importantly stability, over time will often hold the key to the correct diagnosis.
- This brief account only includes some common X-ray features of some common diagnoses. Get the X-rays formally reported by a radiologist urgently if you do not recognize a sign and the patient is unwell. Remember that all radiation exposures have to be justified by clinical benefit to comply with IR(ME)R (Ionizing Radiation (Medical Exposure) Regulations).

Abnormal chest X-ray (CXR) appearances

Many CXR appearances may be recognizable immediately as indicating a specific diagnosis but if not, classify an appearance into one of the leads on the following pages, and then approach the lead systematically.

X-rays cannot be used to decide management alone. Their appearances can be used as diagnostic leads—the symptoms, signs, and other test results being differentiators between the diagnoses. The X-ray appearance can also be used to differentiate between differential diagnoses provided by symptoms and signs. Some patients with highly abnormal CXR may be relatively well and have self-limiting conditions, and monitoring only is needed. In immunocompromised patients, the findings are altered so that diagnostic leads may have wider (or longer) differential diagnoses that include many other infections (think also of mycobacterial disease such as TB-MAI (mycobacterium avium Intracellulare), fungal, lymphoma, and Kaposi's sarcoma, etc). Do not treat X-rays but patients!

Area of uniform lung opacification (whiteness) with a well-defined border

This typically occurs when there is abnormal substance (liquid, cells, pus, blood) in the alveolar spaces next to an anatomical border (e.g. a fissure), causing a sharp border definition. The silhouette sign consists of loss of normal demarcation between white tissue and darker lung due to latter's abnormal opacification. The position of this sign can help localize an affected lobe as follows: loss of a diaphragm silhouette ⇒ (implies) lower lobe consolidation same side; loss of right (R) heart border silhouette ⇒ (R) middle lobe consolidation; loss of left heart border silhouette ⇒ lingular segment consolidation; loss of upper (R) mediastinal border silhouette ⇒ (R) upper lobe consolidation. A veil-like shadow over the whole left hemithorax ⇒ left upper lobe opacification. Investigations in **bold** below.

Main differential diagnoses and typical outline evidence, etc.	
Consolidation (usually due to lobar pneumonia), Fig. 12.1a and Fig. 12.1b	*Suggested by:* well-demarcated uniform whiteness, with a straight border (due to containment by fissural pleura) **with no volume loss** ± air bronchograms. History of productive cough, chest pain, breathlessness, bronchial breathing, fever, ↑neutrophils.
	Confirmed by: clinical resolution on antibiotics and clearing of opacification; repeat **CXR after 8wks** in smokers.
	Finalized by the predictable outcome of management, e.g. analgesia and provisional antibiotic, e.g. amoxicillin/ clarithromycin PO for 5d. If >2 features of **C**onfusion, **R**esp rate >30/min, **B**P <90/60, age >**65**y, then antibiotic IV, e.g. amoxicillin/co-amoxiclav or cefuroxime + controlled O_2 and fluids. If suspected aspiration, then anaerobic antibiotic, e.g. cefuroxime/metronidazole IV. If hospital/nursing home acquired, cefuroxime or piperacillin with tazobactam IV.
Collapsed lobe due to bronchial obstruction from carcinoma, mucus plugs, foreign body, misplacement of endobronchial tube, Fig. 12.2	*Suggested by:* dense, well-demarcated whiteness with straight borders (due to containment by fissures **with volume loss**). Background clinical picture suggestive of cause (e.g. cachexia, monophonic wheeze, and central soft tissue opacity in carcinoma or inhalation of foreign body, recent endotracheal intubation, etc).
	Confirmed by: **CT thorax** and/or **bronchoscopy** or CXR resolution following appropriate treatment for intraluminal blockage, e.g. clearing of foreign body, mucus impaction.
	Finalized by the predictable outcome of management, e.g. if suspected aspiration, then anaerobic antibiotic, e.g. cefuroxime/metronidazole IV.

Pulmonary infarction/ embolus	*Suggested by:* wedge-shaped regions of opacification peripherally ± atelectasis and pleural effusion. History of pleuritic chest pain, breathlessness, haemoptysis. May have hypoxia, tachycardia, signs of deep vein thrombosis (DVT). *Confirmed by:* **CT pulmonary angiogram** (**V/Q** is only helpful when CXR is completely normal). *Finalized by the predictable outcome of management,* e.g. LMW heparin, then warfarin for 3mo. Thrombolysis if ↓BP, large bilateral clots, or acutely dilated right ventricle on echocardiogram.
Dense pulmonary fibrosis, Fig. 12.3	*Suggested by:* bilateral parenchymal opacification (i.e. reticulonodular shadowing), usually with volume loss, often shrunken against apical pleura. Often idiopathic, but may have history of previous TB exposure, radiation, extrinsic allergic alveolitis, chronic sarcoid, ankylosing spondylitis, pneumoconiosis, etc. *Confirmed by:* **high resolution CT thorax**. *Finalized by the predictable outcome of management,* e.g. address cause, immunosuppression. Controlled O_2 therapy if hypoxic.
Pleural effusion: transudate due to heart failure or exudate due to tumour/ pneumonia, etc., Fig. 12.4	*Suggested by:* homogeneous dense area of opacification, obscuring the hemidiaphragm in erect position, less dense superiorly with concave meniscus. No air bronchogram. Shift with change of position ± interfissural or subpulmonary loculation. Stony dullness to percussion. *Confirmed by:* aspiration of fluid in diagnostic tap ± **US scan** to differentiate from consolidation. *Finalized by the predictable outcome of management,* e.g. controlled O_2 therapy if breathless/hypoxic. If heart failure: diuretics, β-blockers, and ACE inhibitors; if pneumonia/ TB: antibiotics; if cancer, pleural drainage and pleurodesis; if autoimmune disease, immunosuppression.
Empyema	*Suggested by:* large, lentiform pleural opacification. Recent chest infection, spiking temperature. *Confirmed by:* **pleural tap** (pus cells, ↓pH, bacteria present). *Finalized by the predictable outcome of management,* e.g. drainage with intercostal (IC) drain. High dose antibiotics IV according to cultures/sensitivity. If slow/poor drainage and loculated effusion, intrapleural thrombolytics or surgical decortication.
Pneumonec- tomy, Fig. 12.5	*Suggested by:* dense white area over entire lung with ipsilateral displacement of mediastinal structures and trachea towards side of surgery. *Confirmed by:* history of pneumonectomy.
Complete lung collapse	*Suggested by:* dense white area over entire lung, trachea and heart (mediastinum) shifted towards affected side, dullness to percussion, ↓ or absent tactile vocal fremitus, absent breath sounds. *Confirmed by:* **CT thorax** and complete obstruction of main bronchus at **bronchoscopy**. *Finalized by the predictable outcome of management,* e.g. controlled O_2 therapy, analgesia. Management of underlying cause, e.g. carcinoma.
Drugs	Amiodarone, nitrofurantoin, etc.

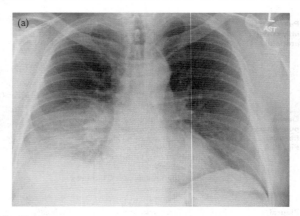

Fig. 12.1a Right lower lobe pneumonia, silhouetting the right hemidiaphragm (frontal image). Reproduced from Lipschik, G., Feldt, J., *et al.*, *Oxford American Handbook of Clinical Diagnosis* (2009), with permission from Oxford University Press.

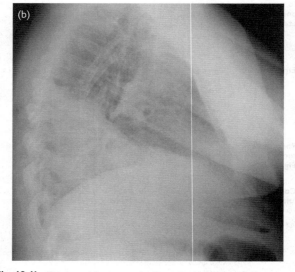

Fig. 12.1b Right lower lobe pneumonia, silhouetting the right hemidiaphragm (lateral image). Reproduced from Lipschik, G., Feldt, J., et al., *Oxford American Handbook of Clinical Diagnosis* (2009), with permission from Oxford University Press.

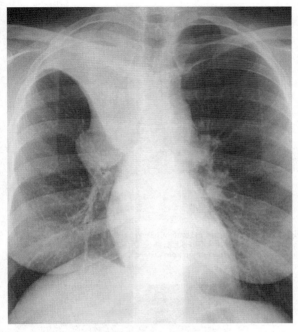

Fig. 12.2 Right upper lobe atelectasis resulting from a large right hilar cancer forming the classic 'Golden's S sign'. Reproduced from Lipschik, G., Feldt, J., *et al.*, *Oxford American Handbook of Clinical Diagnosis* (2009), with permission from Oxford University Press.

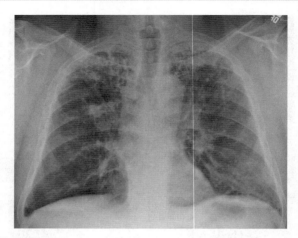

Fig. 12.3 Apical fibrosis and bilateral hilar retraction due to stage 4 sarcoidosis. Reproduced from Lipschik, G., Feldt, J., et al., *Oxford American Handbook of Clinical Diagnosis* (2009), with permission from Oxford University Press.

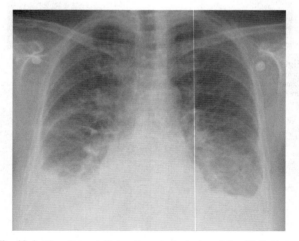

Fig. 12.4 Bilateral pleural effusions due to congestive heart failure (CHF). Note that there is a pulmonary linear septal pattern with Kerley B lines. Reproduced from Lipschik, G., Feldt, J., et al., *Oxford American Handbook of Clinical Diagnosis* (2009), with permission from Oxford University Press.

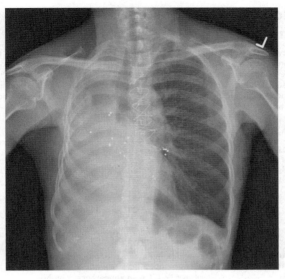

Fig. 12.5 Pneumonectomy resulting in mediastinal shift to the right. Note multiple BB pellets in the chest and median strenotomy wires. Reproduced from Lipschik, G., Feldt, J., et al., *Oxford American Handbook of Clinical Diagnosis* (2009), with permission from Oxford University Press.

Round opacity (or opacities) >5mm in diameter

Beware skin/rib lesions or artefact from hair, braids, or clothing, which can mimic intrathoracic pathology. Positron Emission Tomography (PET) scans are being increasingly used in assessing solitary pulmonary nodules to help distinguish between malignant (increased metabolic uptake in, for example, lung cancer) and benign (low/no metabolic activity) causes. Investigations in **bold** below.

Main differential diagnoses and typical outline evidence, etc.	
Carcinoma of bronchus, Fig. 12.2, Fig. 12.6	*Suggested by:* solitary opacity with irregular or lobulated or spiculated border ± other features of metastases (hilar enlargement, destructive bone changes in ribs, etc.). Often smoker, symptoms of cough, chest pain, haemoptysis, weight loss. *Confirmed by:* tissue diagnosis via **sputum cytology, bronchoscopy** or **CT guided biopsy**. *Finalized by the predictable outcome of management,* e.g. controlled O₂ therapy if breathless/hypoxic. Analgesia. Staging and other therapies.
Pulmonary metastasis	*Suggested by:* multiple rounded opacities ± background history of neoplasia or lymphoma. *Confirmed by:* **CT scan appearance ± biopsy**. *Finalized by the predictable outcome of management,* e.g. controlled O₂ therapy if breathless/hypoxic. Analgesia. Staging and other therapies.
'Rounded pneumonia' or lung abscess	*Suggested by:* round opacity in child, cavitating thick-rimmed lesion in adult. Background of raised inflammatory markers, neutrophilia and cough, pyrexia, spiking (in abscess). *Confirmed by:* **sputum microscopy**, culture and sensitivity resolution following appropriate antibiotic therapy. *Finalized by the predictable outcome of management,* e.g. antibiotics IV according to cultures/sensitivity. Analgesia.
TB granuloma, Fig. 12.7	*Suggested by:* coin lesion ± cavitation in upper lobe. History of TB exposure, weight loss, lymphadenopathy (if calcified, suggests old/healed TB scar). *Confirmed by:* **CT scan** appearance. Acid-fast bacilli (AFB) on Ziehl–Neelsen (ZN) **smear** or **culture**. *Finalized by the predictable outcome of management,* e.g. nursing in isolation if hospitalized until smear status is known. Rifampicin, pyrazinamide, isoniazid, ethambutol PO ± pyridoxine if malnourished.
Rheumatoid nodule	*Suggested by:* peripherally positioned, multiple soft tissue nodules ± cavitation. History/signs of rheumatoid arthritis. *Confirmed by:* **CT scan** appearance and +ve **rheumatoid serology**. **PET scan** if evidence equivocal.

Histoplasmosis	*Suggested by:* coin lesion ± cavitation, mainly in upper lobe. Patient from USA, Africa, or HIV +ve.
	Confirmed by: **CT scan** appearance. Yeast-like organisms in sputum; +ve complement fixation test.
	Finalized by the predictable outcome of management, e.g. itraconazole/ketoconazole PO. Amphotericin B if very ill/ immunosuppressed.
Wegener's granuloma, Fig. 12.8	*Suggested by:* multiple rounded opacities ± cavitation with background of proteinuria, nasal/skin lesions, etc.
	Confirmed by: **biopsy of lung lesion or kidney**.
	Finalized by the predictable outcome of management, e.g. immunosuppression with cyclophosphamide, steroids, azathioprine.
Klebsiella pneumonia	*Suggested by:* multiple cavitating opacities, especially in the upper lobes in an elderly person. History of aspiration/ hospitalization/institutionalization.
	Confirmed by: growth of *Klebsiella* on **blood culture** and response to antibiotics.
	Finalized by the predictable outcome of management, e.g. cefuroxime IV ± metronidazole.
Hydatid cyst (echinococcus)	*Suggested by:* opacity in a lower lobe with dark cavity ± daughter cysts within large cyst. Water lily sign may be seen. Patient from endemic area in contact with working sheep dogs.
	Confirmed by: **CT scan** appearance; +ve **complement fixation test** or **ELISA.**
	Finalized by the predictable outcome of management, e.g. albendazole ± surgery if symptomatic or enlarging.
Pulmonary A–V malformation	*Suggested by:* other symptoms or signs ± occasional haemoptysis.
	Confirmed by: **CT thorax** showing feeding blood vessel on contrast-enhanced scan.
	Finalized by the predictable outcome of management, e.g. embolization.
Benign tumours	*Suggested by:* no other symptoms and no change over 6mo.
	Confirmed by: **excision and histology**.
	Finalized by the predictable outcome of management, e.g. excision if symptomatic.
Also	Thymoma, Kaposi's sarcoma, carcinoid, drugs (including amiodarone).

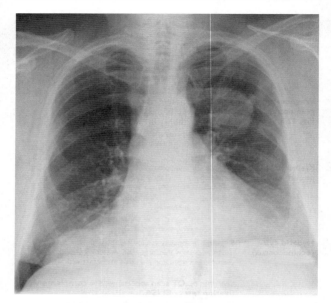

Fig. 12.6 Upper lobe primary bronchogenic carcinoma on frontal image of the chest. Reproduced from Lipschik, G., Feldt, J., et al., *Oxford American Handbook of Clinical Diagnosis* (2009), with permission from Oxford University Press.

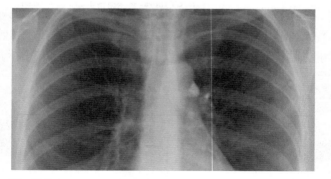

Fig. 12.7 Small, calcified nodule in the left upper lobe laterally with a calcified mediastinal lymph node, a result of granulomatous disease. This particular radiologic appearance is known as a 'Ghon' or 'Ranke Complex'. Reproduced from Lipschik, G., Feldt, J., et al., *Oxford American Handbook of Clinical Diagnosis* (2009), with permission from Oxford University Press.

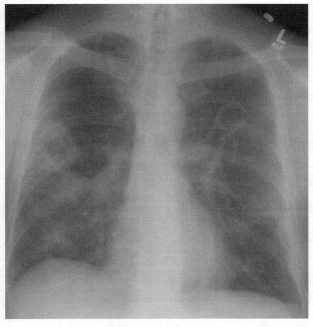

Fig. 12.8 Wegener's granulomatosis with large bilateral cavitary masses.
Reproduced from Lipschik, G., Feldt, J., et al., *Oxford American Handbook of Clinical Diagnosis* (2009), with permission from Oxford University Press.

Multiple 'nodular' shadows and 'miliary mottling'

These are round lesions 2–5mm in diameter of variable density, from small and soft in miliary (<2mm) mottling to larger and calcified in old chickenpox. Investigations in **bold** below.

Main differential diagnoses and typical outline evidence, etc.	
Metastases, Fig. 12.9	*Suggested by:* low-density nodules more profuse in the lower lung zones ± mediastinal widening and other manifestations of malignancy, e.g. lytic lesions in ribs. History of malignancy, e.g. thyroid or renal cell carcinoma. Anorexia and weight loss. *Confirmed by:* **histological** diagnosis. *Finalized by the predictable outcome of management,* e.g. controlled O_2 therapy if breathless/hypoxic, analgesia ± chemotherapy.
Miliary TB, Fig. 12.10	*Suggested by:* innumerable, grain-like, low density, discrete nodules with background history of TB contact. Weight loss. *Confirmed by:* AFB in **sputum, culture of bone marrow or biopsy** specimens from pleura, lung, liver, or lymph nodes. *Finalized by the predictable outcome of management,* e.g. nursing in isolation if in hospital until sputum smear results known ± quadruple therapy (rifampicin, pyrazinamide, isoniazid, and ethambutol), notification, and contact tracing.
Sarcoidosis, Fig. 12.11	*Suggested by:* low-density nodules more profuse in the perihilar and mid-lung zones. Bilateral hilar ± paratracheal lymph node enlargement. Background of rash, uveitis, etc. *Confirmed by:* **histology** showing non-caseating granuloma with no AFB, ↑serum angiotensin-converting enzyme (ACE). *Finalized by the predictable outcome of management,* e.g. long-term steroids if evidence of end-organ damage, e.g. low transfer factor.
Past chickenpox	*Suggested by:* very dense opacities suggesting calcification. No current symptoms. Past history of chickenpox. *Confirmed by:* no change over months on **serial X-rays**. *Finalized by the predictable outcome of management,* e.g. self-limiting illness after explanation and reassurance.

Pulmonary haemosiderosis from mitral stenosis with pulmonary hypertension, Fig. 12.12	*Suggested by:* dense opacities due to calcification. Background of tapping left ventricular impulse (palpable 1st heart sound), ECG findings—M-shaped P wave. *Confirmed by:* **echocardiogram** and **cardiac catheterization**. *Finalized by the predictable outcome of management*, e.g. aspirin, diuretics ± ACE inhibitors. Anticoagulation if atrial fibrillation ± valvotomy/replacement.
Pneumoconiosis	*Suggested by:* discrete (worsening) opacities mainly in upper lobe. Employment history of >10y (coal mining, metal mining, quarrying). *Confirmed by:* comparison with previous CXR. High resolution CT scan. *Finalized by the predictable outcome of management*, e.g. controlled home O_2 therapy if breathless/hypoxic ± industrial compensation.

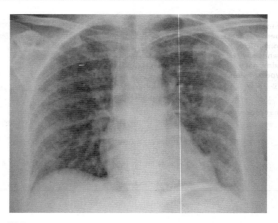

Fig. 12.9 Multiple micronodular lung cancer metastasis with left PICC (peripherally inserted central catheter) line. Reproduced from Lipschik, G., Feldt, J., et al., *Oxford American Handbook of Clinical Diagnosis* (2009), with permission from Oxford University Press.

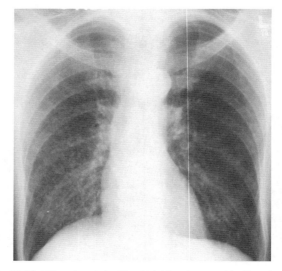

Fig. 12.10 Miliary tuberculosis with multiple bilateral micronodules. Reproduced from Lipschik, G., Feldt, J., et al., *Oxford American Handbook of Clinical Diagnosis* (2009), with permission from Oxford University Press.

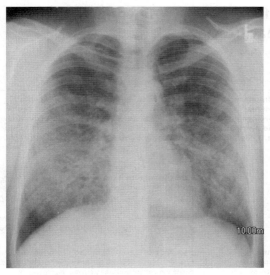

Fig. 12.11 Sarcoidosis with airspace disease showing the typical pattern of midlung involvement; in this particular case there is no adenopathy (stage 3). Reproduced from Lipschik, G., Feldt, J., et al., Oxford American Handbook of Clinical Diagnosis (2009), with permission from Oxford University Press.

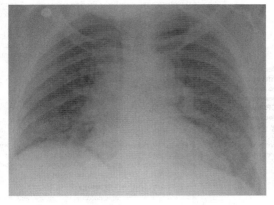

Fig. 12.12 Pulmonary haemosiderosis at lung bases as a result of mitral valve stenosis. Reproduced from Lipschik, G., Feldt, J., et al., Oxford American Handbook of Clinical Diagnosis (2009), with permission from Oxford University Press.

Diffuse poorly defined hazy opacification

Investigations in **bold** below.

Main differential diagnoses and typical outline evidence, etc.

Pulmonary oedema: (cardiogenic or fluid overload or both), Fig. 12.13	*Suggested by:* symmetrical haziness more florid in a perihilar distribution, fluffy alveolar opacities ± confluence, (if fluid is in air spaces), Kerley B lines or peri-bronchial cuffing (if in interstitium), or effusion (if in pleural space). Cardiomegaly if cardiogenic. Background history of fluid overload ± heart disease ± abnormal ECG, S3, fine bibasal crackles in lungs.
	Confirmed by: ventricular dysfunction on **echocardiogram** if cardiogenic, and response to diuretics or vasodilators.
	Finalized by the predictable outcome of management, e.g. stopping any IV fluids. Controlled O_2 therapy if breathless/hypoxic, diuretics IV, nitrates IV. Long-term diuretics, ACE-inhibitors, β-blockers according to BP and renal function.
Acute respiratory distress syndrome (ARDS), Fig. 12.14	*Suggested by:* symmetrical, diffuse, poorly defined opacities, which become confluent. Normal heart size. Acutely ill patient with severe hypoxia. History of precipitating cause (e.g. smoke inhalation, aspiration, drug exposure, fat/amniotic fluid emboli, viral infection, disseminated intravascular coagulation (DIC)), no clinical signs of left ventricular failure.
	Confirmed by: (1) acute onset, (2) bilateral infiltrates, (3) **pulmonary capillary wedge pressure** <19mmHg or no congestive cardiac failure, (4) P_aO_2:FiO_2<200 in the presence of good left ventricular function.
	Finalized by the predictable outcome of management, e.g. intubation; ventilation with small volumes and consider prone ventilation/steroids. Treatment of underlying cause.
Infective infiltration due to viral pneumonia, PCP, bacterial pneumonia, Fig. 12.15	*Suggested by:* region of patchy pulmonary infiltrate ± air bronchogram ± pleural effusion. History of cough, increased sputum; fever, ↑inflammatory markers, neutropaenia (viral) or neutrophilia (bacterial).
	Confirmed by: +ve **cultures**.
	Finalized by the predictable outcome of management, e.g. or resolution following appropriate antibiotics or antivirals.
Alveolar cell carcinoma	*Suggested by:* region of poorly defined opacification, which may contain air bronchogram. Background of progressive breathlessness, copious watery productive cough, weight loss. No resolution with antibiotic therapy.
	Confirmed by: **sputum cytology, lung biopsy**.
	Finalized by the predictable outcome of management, e.g. analgesia. Surgery ± radiotherapy ± chemotherapy.

Lung haemorrhage, Fig. 12.16	*Suggested by:* region of poorly defined opacification ± air bronchogram. Background history of trauma/contusion, clotting abnormality, necrotizing pneumonia or rarer causes such as Hamman–Rich/Goodpasture's syndrome.
	Confirmed by: haemoptysis or profuse bleeding through endotracheal tube. Resolution if trauma/clotting corrected. CT appearances + renal/lung biopsy (for Goodpasture's syndrome, Hamman–Rich).
	Finalized by the predictable outcome of management, e.g. correction of reversible causes and clotting disorders; steroids and management in HDU/ITU.

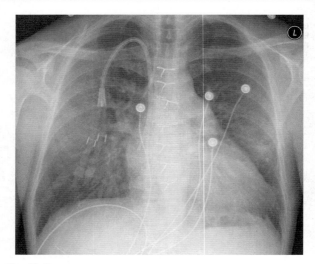

Fig. 12.13 Pulmonary oedema and Kerley B lines in a patient on hemodialysis.
Reproduced from Lipschik, G., Feldt, J., et al., *Oxford American Handbook of Clinical Diagnosis* (2009), with permission from Oxford University Press.

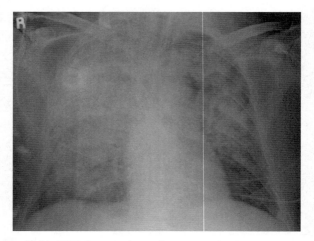

Fig. 12.14 ARDS, showing patchy opacificaton in an intubated patient.
Reproduced from Lipschik, G., Feldt, J., et al., *Oxford American Handbook of Clinical Diagnosis* (2009), with permission from Oxford University Press.

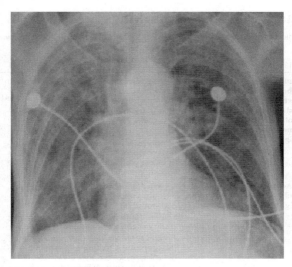

Fig. 12.15 Herpes simplex virus (HSV) pneumonia with diffuse infiltrates.
Reproduced from Lipschik, G., Feldt, J., et al., *Oxford American Handbook of Clinical Diagnosis* (2009), with permission from Oxford University Press.

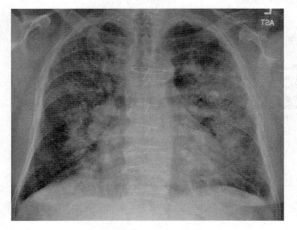

Fig. 12.16 Diffuse pulmonary haemorrhage of uncertain etiology. Reproduced from Lipschik, G., Feldt, J., et al., *Oxford American Handbook of Clinical Diagnosis* (2009), with permission from Oxford University Press.

Increased linear markings

Indicates thickening of the interstitial tissues. Investigations in **bold** below.

Main differential diagnoses and typical outline evidence, etc.	
Pulmonary fibrosis: idiopathic or 2° to, extrinsic allergic alveolitis, asbestosis, sarcoidosis, collagen vascular disease, pneumoconiosis, etc., Fig. 12.17	*Suggested by:* increased interstitial markings with relevant exposure history and clinical/X-ray features of above conditions. *Confirmed by:* typical appearances on **high resolution CT scan**. **Lung biopsy**. *Finalized by the predictable outcome of management,* e.g. removing birds, immunosuppression if autoimmune disease, etc. Controlled home O_2 therapy if breathless/hypoxic, palliation.
Interstitial fluid = pulmonary oedema, Fig. 12.4, Fig. 12.13	*Suggested by:* smooth thickening of the interlobular septa (Kerley B lines) with background lung crackles. *Confirmed by:* rapid resolution following diuretic therapy or correct fluid balance or dialysis. *Finalized by the predictable outcome of management,* e.g. controlled O_2 therapy if breathless/hypoxic, diuretics IV, nitrates IV. Long-term diuretics, ACE-inhibitors, β-blockers according to BP and renal function.
Metastatic cells = lymphangitis carcinomatosis	*Suggested by:* irregular thickening of the interlobular septa (Kerley B lines) with background of other features of malignancy. Usually no crackles. *Confirmed by:* **high resolution CT**, **lung biopsy**, or progressive malignant disease. *Finalized by the predictable outcome of management,* e.g. steroids and palliation.
Bronchiectasis, Fig. 12.18 (congenital, e.g. cystic fibrosis; post-infective, e.g. post-whooping cough; obstruction, other, e.g. hypogammaglobulinaemia)	*Suggested by:* tram lines and rings with background of cough with high volume of sputum ± foul and purulent (if super-added infection). *Confirmed by:* High resolution CT (bronchiole bigger than its accompanying artery). *Finalized by the predictable outcome of management,* e.g. sputum cultures and often prolonged, high dose antibiotics according to results when symptomatic. Chest physiotherapy. Bronchodilator and mucolytics if wheeze/airways obstruction.

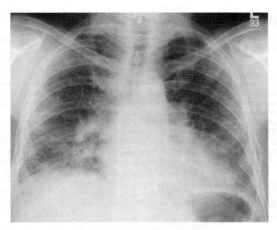

Fig. 12.17 Idiopathic pulmonary fibrosis with a peripheral and basilar predominance. Reproduced from Lipschik, G., Feldt, J., et al., *Oxford American Handbook of Clinical Diagnosis* (2009), with permission from Oxford University Press.

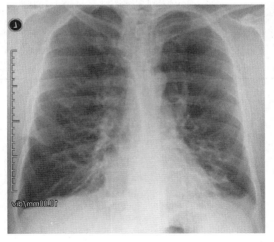

Fig. 12.18 Extensive bronchiectasis with cylindrical and cystic features in this 34-year-old male with cystic fibrosis (note that markings on film are reversed). Reproduced from Lipschik, G., Feldt, J., et al., *Oxford American Handbook of Clinical Diagnosis* (2009), with permission from Oxford University Press.

Symmetrically dark lungs

CXR film exposure is correct. Another clue to presence of pathology is abnormal lung size. Investigations in **bold** below.

Main differential diagnoses and typical outline evidence, etc.	
Chronic obstructive pulmonary disease (COPD), Fig. 12.19a, Fig. 12.19b	*Suggested by:* long, narrow heart and chest, flat diaphragms, ribs horizontal, 7th rib visible anteriorly and 11th rib visible posteriorly. Prominent pulmonary arteries with paucity of interstitial markings, peripheral pruning (in pulmonary hypertension). Large, thin-rimmed, dark areas with no lung markings are bullae. History of smoking at least 10 pack years. *Confirmed by:* **High resolution CT** and lung function tests showing fixed obstructive deficit **FEV$_1$<80%, FEV$_1$/FVC <70%.** *Finalized by the predictable outcome of management,* e.g. no smoking, bronchodilators (short-acting prn, then regular long-acting bronchodilators), inhaled steroids if FEV$_1$ <50–60% predicted and recurrent exacerbations.
Asthma	*Suggested by:* hyper-expanded lungs. No loss of lung markings. Background history of variable wheeze, cough, and breathlessness. *Confirmed by:* peak flow/FEV$_1$ improvement following appropriate treatment. *Finalized by the predictable outcome of management,* e.g. removing allergen if possible (e.g. occupation, stopping NSAIDs, stopping smoking, etc). In acute attacks: controlled O$_2$ if breathless/hypoxic, nebulized/high dose repeated inhaled bronchodilators, systemic steroids. Treating infection, dehydration, and monitoring clinical response, ABG, and K+. Long term: stepwise increase in treatment starting with inhaled bronchodilators prn, then regular inhaled steroids, then combination inhaler: long-acting B-agonist and inhaled steroids.

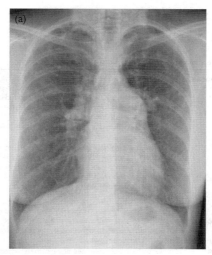

Fig. 12.19a COPD with pulmonary hypertension as evidenced by enlarged central pulmonary arteries and peripheral arterial pruning (frontal image). Reproduced from Lipschik, G., Feldt, J., *et al.*, *Oxford American Handbook of Clinical Diagnosis* (2009), with permission from Oxford University Press.

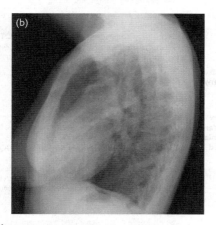

Fig. 12.19b COPD with pulmonary hypertension (lateral image) as evidenced by enlarged pulmonary arteries and flattening of the diaphragms. Reproduced from Lipschik, G., Feldt, J., *et al.*, *Oxford American Handbook of Clinical Diagnosis* (2009), with permission from Oxford University Press.

Single area of dark lung

Investigations in **bold** below.

Main differential diagnoses and typical outline evidence, etc.	
Pneumothorax, Fig. 12.20	*Suggested by:* visible lung edge with absence of lung markings peripheral to this. Central mediastinum. Beware skin folds, which may mimic a lung edge. History of sudden onset of breathlessness and/or pleuritic chest pain. Hyper-resonance and reduced breath sounds. *Confirmed by:* convincing appearances on CXR. Hint—best seen in an expiration film. *Finalized by the predictable outcome of management,* e.g. controlled O_2 therapy if breathless/hypoxic, analgesia. Aspiration if symptomatic, >15% collapse or co-existing lung disease. If aspiration fails, insertion of intercostal (IC) drain through the 'triangle of safety'. If <15%, monitor for 12–24h and repeat CXR.
Tension pneumothorax (medical emergency: this should have been diagnosed clinically before doing the CXR)	*Suggested by:* visible lung edge with absence of lung markings peripheral to this, mediastinal shift away from the black lung. Background of acute progressive dyspnoea, tachycardia, ↓BP. Shifted mediastinum away from collapsed lung. *Confirmed by:* relief when needle or catheter inserted and re-expansion of lung when chest tube inserted later. *Finalized by the predictable outcome of management,* e.g. inserting large Venflon into 2nd IC space, mid-clavicular line (on side with absent breath sounds), then inserting IC chest drain before requesting CXR.
Bulla, Fig. 12.21	*Suggested by:* loss of lung markings inside lucent, thin-rimmed, circular region ± background history of COPD. *Confirmed by:* comparison with previous CXR, **CT thorax.** *Finalized by the predictable outcome of management,* e.g. endobronchial valve or bullectomy if very large or symptomatic (e.g. recurrent pneumothorax).
Mastectomy	*Suggested by:* no breast shadow. *Confirmed by:* history of mastectomy.
Large pulmonary embolus (area of oligaemia on affected side)	*Suggested by:* wedge-shaped regions of opacification peripherally ± atelectasis and pleural effusion. History of pleuritic chest pain, breathlessness, haemoptysis. May have hypoxia, tachycardia, signs of DVT. *Confirmed by:* **CT pulmonary angiogram (V/Q** is only helpful when the CXR is completely normal). *Finalized by the predictable outcome of management,* e.g. LMW heparin, then warfarin for >3mo. Thrombolysis if ↓BP, large bilateral clots, or acutely dilated right ventricle on echocardiogram.
Lobar collapse	*Suggested by:* usually not whole lung looks dark. Signs of volume loss, e.g. 'sail' sign, raised diaphragm, etc. *Confirmed by:* CXR appearance. **CT chest** and/or **bronchoscopy** to establish cause. *Finalized by the predictable outcome of management,* e.g. treatment of underlying cause.

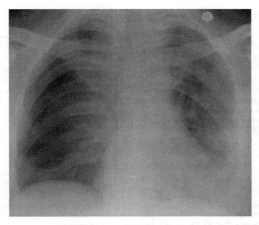

Fig. 12.20 Right lateral pneumothorax with loss of lung markings and visible lung edge. Reproduced from Lipschik, G., Feldt, J., et al., *Oxford American Handbook of Clinical Diagnosis* (2009), with permission from Oxford University Press.

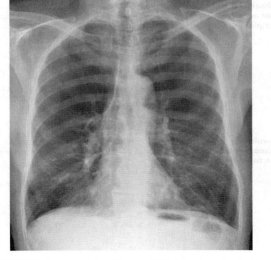

Fig. 12.21 Emphysema with large bilateral apical bullae and vascular distortion. Reproduced from Lipschik, G., Feldt, J., et al., *Oxford American Handbook of Clinical Diagnosis* (2009), with permission from Oxford University Press.

Enlarged hilar shadowing

Check that the film is not rotated—this can give a false-positive diagnosis. Compare with old films, if possible, for duration of abnormality. Investigations in **bold** below.

Main differential diagnoses and typical outline evidence, etc.	
Metastatic lymphadenopathy, bronchial carcinoma, Fig. 12.22	*Suggested by:* unilateral hilar opacity ± lung opacity or bilateral hilar opacity ± evidence of metastatic deposits, e.g. lytic rib lesions. Background history of neoplasia.
	Confirmed by: **bronchoscopy ± CT staging**. **Sputum cytology/biopsy** showing cancer cells.
	Finalized by the predictable outcome of management, e.g. controlled O_2 therapy if breathless/hypoxic, analgesia ± surgery, radiotherapy ± chemotherapy.
Hodgkin's or non-Hodgkin's lymphoma, Fig. 12.23	*Suggested by:* bilateral hilar shadows ± parenchymal opacification. Anaemia, lymph node enlargement elsewhere, hepatosplenomegaly.
	Confirmed by: **histology** (Reed–Sternberg cells in Hodgkin's or without in non-Hodgkin's).
	Finalized by the predictable outcome of management, e.g. chemotherapy ± radiotherapy.
Primary TB with hilar node (primary complex)	*Suggested by:* unilateral hilar mass (lymphadenopathy) and poorly defined opacification in peripheral lung field, often with paratracheal nodal enlargement. Clinical features of TB.
	Confirmed by: **CT scan** showing no tumour. AFB on Ziehl–Neelsen **(ZN) stain** and **culture growth from sputum**. Resolution on specific anti-TB therapy.
	Finalized by the predictable outcome of management, e.g. nursing isolation if in hospital until sputum smear results known ± quadruple therapy (rifampicin, pyrazinamide, isoniazid, and ethambutol), notification, and contact tracing.
Prominent pulmonary artery due to embolus	*Suggested by:* smooth, non-lobular appearance tapering off peripherally with dark peripheral lung fields.
	Confirmed by: **CT pulmonary angiogram**.
	Finalized by the predictable outcome of management, e.g. LMW heparin, then warfarin for 3mo. Thrombolysis, e.g. if ↓BP, large bilateral clots, or acutely dilated right ventricle on echocardiogram.

Prominent pulmonary arteries due to pulmonary hypertension	*Suggested by:* bulky, bilateral hila with outline suggestive of prominent pulmonary arteries, tapering off peripherally with dark peripheral lung fields ± widening of upper mediastinum (superior vena cava) ± bulging right heart border. *Confirmed by:* **echocardiogram** and **CT pulmonary angiogram**. *Finalized by the predictable outcome of management*, e.g. treating cause; controlled O_2 therapy if breathless/hypoxic. Referral to specialist centre.
Sarcoidosis, Fig. 12.24	*Suggested by:* bilateral, hilar, convex shadows, possibly with other lung changes of sarcoid. Erythema nodosum, arthralgia, uveitis, etc. *Confirmed by:* histology showing non-caseating granuloma with no AFB. *Finalized by the predictable outcome of management*, e.g. long-term steroids if end-organ damage, e.g. low transfer factor.

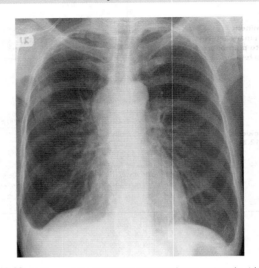

Fig. 12.22 Right upper lobe primary lung cancer with metastasis to the right side of the mediastinum and right hilum (note right hilar fullness and small right pleural effusion). Reproduced from Lipschik, G., Feldt, J., *et al.*, *Oxford American Handbook of Clinical Diagnosis* (2009), with permission from Oxford University Press.

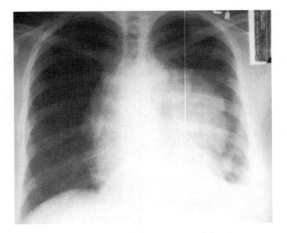

Fig. 12.23 Left hilar mass in a patient with non-Hodgkin's lymphoma. Reproduced from Lipschik, G., Feldt, J., *et al.*, *Oxford American Handbook of Clinical Diagnosis* (2009), with permission from Oxford University Press.

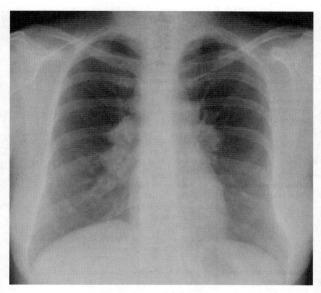

Fig. 12.24 Bilateral hilar and right paratracheal lymphadenopathy in patient with sarcoidosis (stage 2). This pattern is known as the '1,2,3 sign'. Reproduced from Lipschik, G., Feldt, J., et al., *Oxford American Handbook of Clinical Diagnosis* (2009), with permission from Oxford University Press.

Abnormal hilar shadowing—streaky

Investigations in **bold** below.

Main differential diagnoses and typical outline evidence, etc.	
Left ventricular failure (due to myocardial infarction, arrhythmia, fluid overload)	*Suggested by:* smooth thickening of the interlobular septa (Kerley B lines), cardiomegaly, bilateral fine lung crackles. *Confirmed by:* rapid resolution following diuretic therapy or correct fluid balance or dialysis. *Finalized by the predictable outcome of management,* e.g. controlled O_2 therapy if breathless/hypoxic, diuretics IV, nitrates IV, treating cause, long-term diuretics, ACE inhibitors, β-blockers according to BP and renal function.
Bronchopneumonia (bilateral)	*Suggested by:* breathlessness, chest pain, productive cough. *Confirmed by:* +ve **sputum/blood cultures**, atypical serology. *Finalized by the predictable outcome of management,* e.g. controlled O_2 therapy if breathless/hypoxic, antibiotics to cover *Streptococcus pneumoniae* (penicillins) and other organisms (e.g. clarithromycin).
Pneumocystis carinii pneumonia	*Suggested by:* breathlessness, chest pain, dry cough, known immunosuppression (or risk factors), and lymphopaenia. *Confirmed by:* +ve **sputum/bronchial washings**, cultures, immunostaining. *Finalized by the predictable outcome of management,* e.g. controlled O_2 therapy if breathless/hypoxic, co-trimoxazole.
Also	Histioplasmosis, pulmonary alveolar proteinosis.

Upper mediastinal widening

Investigations in **bold** below.

Main differential diagnoses and typical outline evidence, etc.

Retrosternal goitre, Fig. 12.25	*Suggested by:* superior mediastinal mass shadow extending from the neck.
	Confirmed by: clinical examination, **US or radioisotope scan**.
	Finalized by the predictable outcome of management, e.g. surgery if local symptoms of compression. Correction of thyroid function if hypothyroid (↑TSH, ↓FT4) or thyrotoxic (↓TSH, ↑FT4, or ↑FT3).
Hodgkin's or non-Hodgkin's lymphoma or metastatic lymphadenopathy	*Suggested by:* dense, often multinodular masses, causing mediastinal widening. CT scan appearances.
	Confirmed by: **mediastinoscopy** or surgical removal showing **histology**.
	Finalized by the predictable outcome of management, e.g. chemotherapy ± radiotherapy.
Thymoma, Fig. 12.26a, Fig. 12.26b (30% complicated by myasthenia gravis)	*Suggested by:* clearly outlined opacity (calcification in 20%). Background features of myasthenia gravis (in 30%).
	Confirmed by: **CT scan** appearance and **histology** from **mediastinoscopy** or surgical removal.
	Finalized by the predictable outcome of management, e.g. surgical removal ± chemo-radiotherapy according to histological subtype and staging. Treatment of any myasthenia gravis.
Teratoma: benign or malignant	*Suggested by:* anterior mediastinal opacification, rarely with calcification, e.g. in teeth.
	Confirmed by: **CT scan** appearance ± fat, hair, teeth, and histology from **mediastinoscopy** or surgical removal.
	Finalized by the predictable outcome of management, e.g. surgical removal, ± chemo-radiotherapy according to histological subtype and staging.
Aortic aneurysm, Fig. 12.27	*Suggested by:* opacification continuous with descending aorta shadow. Risk factors for aneurysms (↑BP, smoker, trauma, syphilis, collagen disease, etc). Signs of aortic valve regurgitation.
	Confirmed by: CT scan appearance.
	Finalized by the predictable outcome of management, e.g. vascular surgery if aneurysmal and reducing risk factors.

| Mediastinal lymphadenopathy from primary bronchogenic carcinoma, Fig. 12.22 | *Suggested by:* pulmonary nodule or mass that may appear after symptoms, e.g. dry cough, fatigue, weight loss, hyponatraemia of SIADH.

Confirmed by: CT scan appearance, mediastinoscopy or surgical biopsy or removal.

Finalized by the predictable outcome of management, e.g. surgery, radiotherapy or chemotherapy with prognosis depending on cell type. |

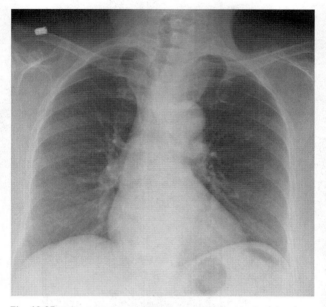

Fig. 12.25 Substernal goitre with tracheal deviation to the right. Reproduced from Lipschik, G., Feldt, J., et al., *Oxford American Handbook of Clinical Diagnosis* (2009), with permission from Oxford University Press.

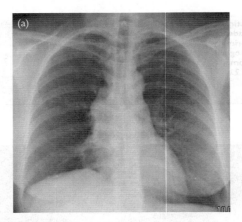

Fig. 12.26a Anterior mediastinal mass; differential includes thymoma, teratoma, lymphoma, and thyroid gland. (This case was a partially calcified thymoma; frontal image.) Reproduced from Lipschik, G., Feldt, J., et al., *Oxford American Handbook of Clinical Diagnosis* (2009), with permission from Oxford University Press.

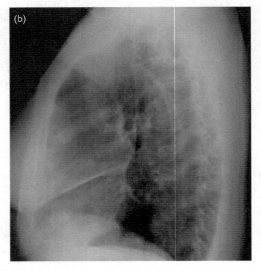

Fig. 12.26b Anterior mediastinal mass (partially calcified thymoma; lateral image). Reproduced from Lipschik, G., Feldt, J., et al., *Oxford American Handbook of Clinical Diagnosis* (2009), with permission from Oxford University Press.

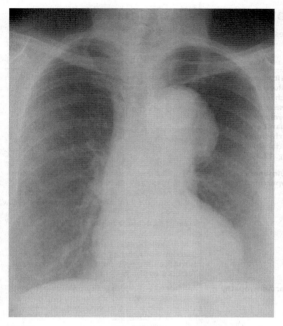

Fig. 12.27 Aortic aneurysm involving the arch and proximal descending thoracic aorta. Reproduced from Lipschik, G., Feldt, J., *et al.*, *Oxford American Handbook of Clinical Diagnosis* (2009), with permission from Oxford University Press.

Abnormal cardiac silhouette

Investigations in **bold** below.

Main differential diagnoses and typical outline evidence, etc.

Left ventricular failure due to ischaemic heart disease, recent myocardial infarction, arrhythmia (e.g. atrial fibrillation), Fig. 12.28	*Suggested by:* large heart, mainly to left of midline (with central trachea), linear upper lobe opacities, and fluffy lung opacities—centrally more than peripherally. *Confirmed by:* **echocardiogram** showing poor contraction of left ventricle. *Finalized by the predictable outcome of management,* e.g. controlled O_2 therapy if breathless/hypoxic, diuretics IV, nitrates IV. Long-term diuretics, ACE inhibitors, β-blockers according to BP and renal function. Treating cause.
Pulmonary hypertension	*Suggested by:* prominent right heart border (of right ventricle), upwardly rounded apex and bilateral prominence of hila. Loud S2 (pulmonary valve closure), ↑JVP ± history of pulmonary embolus, tall R waves in V1 to V3 and right axis deviation on ECG. *Confirmed by:* **echocardiogram** (estimated pulmonary pressure >25 mmHg at rest). *Finalized by the predictable outcome of management,* e.g. controlled O_2 therapy if breathless/hypoxic, treat reversible causes, e.g. pulmonary emboli, vasculitis. Diuretics if swollen legs.
Cardiomyopathy	*Suggested by:* generally large heart with clear borders (indicating poor contraction). Predisposing condition, e.g. ischaemia, chronic alcohol abuse, amyloid, leukaemia, rheumatoid arthritis, etc. *Confirmed by:* **echocardiogram** showing poor contraction of left ventricle. *Finalized by the predictable outcome of management,* e.g. controlled O_2 therapy if breathless/hypoxic, diuretics IV, nitrates IV. Long-term diuretics, ACE inhibitors, β-blockers according to BP and renal function.
Pericardial effusion	*Suggested by:* large globular cardiac outline and clear borders (indicating little or no contraction). Quiet heart sounds, impalpable apex. Low-voltage **ECG** complexes. *Confirmed by:* echocardiogram. *Finalized by the predictable outcome of management,* e.g. if distressed, emergency pericardiocentesis. If stable, echocardiogram-guided drainage and pericardial window.
Atrial septal defect	*Suggested by:* unusually convex right heart border, upwardly rounded cardiac apex, and bilateral prominence of hila. *Confirmed by:* **echocardiogram**. *Finalized by the predictable outcome of management,* e.g. surgical correction.

Mitral stenosis	*Suggested by:* large heart, enlarged left atrium (rounded opacity behind the heart, which 'splays' the carinal angle) ± calcification in position of mitral valve and dense nodules due to haemosiderosis. History of rheumatic heart disease.
	Confirmed by: **echocardiogram** and **cardiac catheterization**.
	Finalized by the predictable outcome of management, e.g. aspirin, diuretics, and ACE inhibitors. Warfarin if AF ± valvotomy/valve replacement.
Left ventricular aneurysm, Fig. 12.29a, Fig. 12.29b	*Suggested by:* bulge in left ventricular border ± calcification. Background history of ischaemic heart disease ± myocardial infarction. Persistent ST elevation on ECG.
	Confirmed by: **echocardiogram**.
	Finalized by the predictable outcome of management, e.g. surgical repair. Warfarin if associated thrombus.
Mediastinal emphysema	*Suggested by:* gas around the mediastinal contour ± surgical emphysema. Background history of acute asthma, OGD, oesophageal rupture, etc., signs of surgical emphysema.
	Confirmed by: **CT thorax**.
	Finalized by the predictable outcome of management, e.g. nil by mouth, prophylactic cefuroxime IV and metronidazole if oesophageal rupture. Surgical repair if no spontaneous healing after 2–3d.
Hiatus hernia	*Suggested by:* circular shadow behind the heart ± air/fluid level, absent gastric bubble. Intermittent appearance on previous CXR.
	Confirmed by: **barium swallow**, **endoscopy**.
	Finalized by the predictable outcome of management, e.g. lifestyle modification. Antacids, e.g. PPI if symptoms continue.
Also	Diaphragmatic hernia, atrial myxoma, radiation pneumonitis.

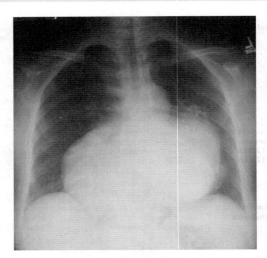

Fig. 12.28 Cardiomegaly involving all four cardiac chambers due to tricuspid and mitral regurgitation. Reproduced from Lipschik, G., Feldt, J., *et al., Oxford American Handbook of Clinical Diagnosis* (2009), with permission from Oxford University Press.

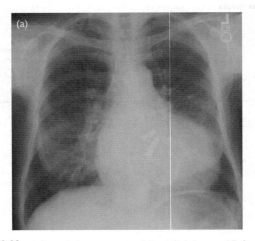

Fig. 12.29a Left ventricular aneurysm, partially calcified, due to an MI after cardiac valve replacement (frontal image). Reproduced from Lipschik, G., Feldt, J., *et al., Oxford American Handbook of Clinical Diagnosis* (2009), with permission from Oxford University Press.

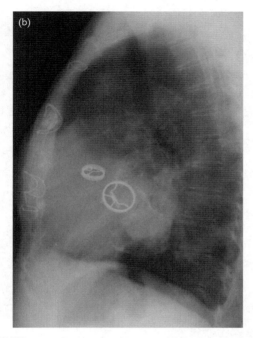

Fig. 12.29b Left ventricular aneurysm, partially calcified, due to an MI after cardiac valve replacement. Note in situ valve rings (lateral image). Reproduced from Lipschik, G., Feldt, J., et al., *Oxford American Handbook of Clinical Diagnosis* (2009), with permission from Oxford University Press.

Making the diagnostic process evidence-based

Evidence-based diagnosis and decisions 616

Grappling with probabilities 617

Picturing probabilities 618

Bayes' and other rules 620

Reasoning by elimination 622

A worked example 623

Using very low frequencies or probability densities 624

Evidence for a finding's role in reasoning by elimination 625

Differential likelihood ratios make use of 'complementing'
    differentiation 626

Things that affect 'differential' and 'overall' likelihood ratios 627

Findings that lead to a 'common cause' 628

Statistical independence versus statistical dependence 629

Reasoning with numerical test results 630

Reasoning by elimination to arrive at 'stratified' diagnostic
    criteria 632

Analysing clinical trials to 'stratify' diagnostic and treatment
    criteria 633

How to improve treatments by better selection or 'stratification'
    of patients 634

Studies to establish treatment indication and diagnostic cut-off
    points 635

Estimating the probability of replication with reasoning by
    elimination 636

Reasoning with hypotheses 637

Proof for the reasoning by probable elimination theorem 638

Evidence-based diagnosis and decisions

The purpose of this chapter is to explain how the diagnostic and treatment selection process can be made 'evidence-based'.

The first chapter explained how a diagnostic lead can be used to provide a differential diagnosis; examples of such diagnostic leads and their differential diagnoses are shown throughout this book.

Each page shows how other findings can be used to 'suggest' a diagnosis by probably differentiating between diagnoses in a list so that one becomes more probable and others less probable.

A diagnosis can be 'confirmed' by the presence of findings that occur by definition only in patients with that diagnosis and not in others. Such a definition is a matter of convention and the term used is also the title to what is imagined or predicted after suitable follow-up with and without treatment or advice.

A diagnosis is the title to a group of predictions about a number of phenomena in the past, present, and future, with or without interventions of various kinds. The purpose of most diagnostic predictions is to help the patient but the predictions arising from a diagnosis may also be of relevance to other parties such as social services, insurance companies, disability pension services, the police, and the courts. Post-mortem diagnoses also provide groups of predictions, none of which benefit the patient of course.

A diagnosis, e.g. 'Type 2 diabetes mellitus', means that its recognized treatments, advice or other actions should be considered but these should only be suggested to the patient if other findings also indicate a significant chance of benefit (e.g. by being treated with insulin). The combination of findings that suggest that an action may benefit (called an indication) are sometimes also regarded as criteria for a sub-diagnosis, e.g. 'Type 2 diabetes mellitus with severe insulin deficiency'.

If a diagnosis is to be of some practical value to the patient then patients with its 'sufficient' diagnostic criteria should have a significant chance of benefit from at least one of the treatments, advice, or other actions suggested by that diagnosis. If some patients are labelled with a diagnosis but do not stand to benefit in any practical way (and may even be exposed to unnecessary harm from the labelling), then this would be an example of 'over-diagnosis'. Over-diagnosis and under-diagnosis represent the two sides of 'mis-diagnosis'.

Conversely if a diagnosis is excluded by the absence of its 'necessary' criteria then no patients should lose out by not being offered any of its treatments, advice, or other actions. Therefore such 'necessary' criteria should not exclude patients with some prospect of benefit. If such patients are excluded, this would represent 'under-diagnosis'.

In order to make each of the above ·steps 'evidence-based' we have to show some track record for each prediction based on the combination of findings (symptoms, signs, or test results) used to make each prediction. Ideally this track record would be the proportion of times each such prediction was correct.

In other words, we must match the feeling of certainty about each prediction with an observed proportion of times that prediction was correct. This means that we must have a clear understanding of the arithmetic of proportions and probabilities.

Grappling with probabilities

Probabilities are abstract representations of mental processes. Thinking about thinking may strike some as being excessively introspective and doing so with mathematics would be too much to bear.

It is simpler than it sounds, however, because the mathematics of probability obeys the same rules as the arithmetic of proportions. For example, a probability of 0.33 that a patient has appendicitis is the degree of certainty that one would experience if there were 300 people admitted to an emergency ward in a month, 100 had appendicitis and all one knew about a person was that he or she was one of the people admitted to that ward.

The correspondence between observed proportions and probability means that we can reason with proportions instead of abstract degrees of belief. For example assume that 60 patients admitted to an emergency ward had the findings of localized right-lower quadrant pain and guarding, and of these 57 had appendicitis. If we came across a patient from this group and were only told that he or she had these findings then the probability of appendicitis would be 57/60 = 0.95.

The mental feeling of certainty of 0.95 would be based upon the external physical 'evidence' of an observed population of 57/60 = 95%. Thus, a belief of 0.95 would have 'given substance' or 'substantiated' by the real tangible population of 57/60. If there were 100 patients with appendicitis in the ward and 57 of these had the three findings, then the converse probability (known as the 'likelihood') of one of these patients having the three findings would be 57/100 = 0.57.

If a new patient was admitted to the ward with the three findings then the number would increase from 60 to 61. If the patient had appendicitis then the new proportion would become 58/61 = 0.951 = P_H and if not it would be 57/61 = 0.934 = P_L so that the 'future probability' would be either 0.934 or 0.951, the pair of values reflecting the uncertainty. If the highest of the two probabilities is called P_H and the lowest is P_L, then this pair of values allows one to calculate the original proportion on which that 'future probability' pair of values is based. The original numerator could be calculated as $(1/(P_H/P_L))-1 = 57$, the denominator being $(1/(P_H-P_L))-1 = 60$. This information in turn would allow confidence intervals and other statistics to be calculated for the 'future probability'.

In the remainder of this chapter we will do all arithmetic with proportions instead of probabilities. When we apply the result of such reasoning to an individual patient, we will convert the proportion, e.g. 57/60 = 95% to a probability, e.g. 0.95. Sometimes we will use guesswork based on careful assumptions. By doing this we aim to maintain good judgement in that if we check the different predictions that we make with a probability of 0.95, then in the long run, we should be correct about 95% of the time. We could do this as part of audit. If we found that for all 0.95 probabilities we were only correct 75% of the time for example, then this would be poor judgement and we could investigate where we are getting it wrong and why.

Picturing probabilities

Proportions and their associated probabilities can be represented pictorially by a Venn diagram, as shown in Fig. 13.1.

The big box is the set of 300 patients studied. The 11 numbers inside each of the 11 sectors sector add to 300. The total number with 'guarding' is 34+3+3+57+23 = 120. The total number with localized right-lower quadrant (LRLQ) pain is 120+3+57+18+2 = 200. The total number with non-specific abdominal pain is 120+3+3+24 = 150 and the total number with appendicitis is 18+57+23+2 = 100.

It can be seen from the Venn diagram in Fig. 13.1 (and by reading the top arrow from left to right in the 'P' map in Fig. 13.2) that of patients with LRLQ pain, a proportion of 75/200 have appendicitis. Reading the P map from right to left, of the patients with appendicitis a proportion of 75/100 had LRLQ pain, and (reading down from right to left) a proportion of 80/100 had guarding. Of the patients with guarding (reading up from left to right), 80/120 had appendicitis. Finally, of patients with LRLQ pain, 60/200 had guarding and of the patients with guarding, 60/120 had LRLQ pain.

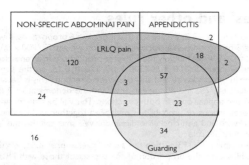

Fig. 13.1 A Venn diagram.

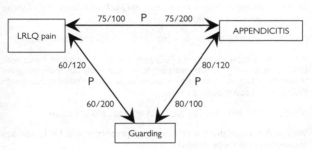

Fig. 13.2 A 'P map'.

Bayes' and other rules

If we examine Fig. 13.2, we will see that it displays 6 proportions. If we multiply the 3 proportions in a clockwise direction we get $75/200 \times 80/100 \times 60/120 = 0.15$. If we multiply the 3 inverse proportions in an anti-clockwise direction we get $75/100 \times 60/200 \times 80/120 = 0.15$, so the product is the same in the clockwise and anti-clockwise direction. This is because the numerators 60, 75, and 80 appear once and the denominators 100, 120, and 200 also appear once in both directions. This will be true for any number of proportions or probabilities multiplied together in the same circuit in a clockwise and anti-clockwise direction. We shall call this the 'inverse probability circuit rule'.

If we examine Fig. 13.3, then the same 'inverse probability circuit rule' applies. However, the proportion of the sub-set of those with LRLQ pain who are in the study set is 200/200 and the proportion of the sub-set of those with appendicitis who are in the study set is 100/100. By rearranging this special case and cancelling out, we get Bayes' rule that the proportion of those with appendicitis in those with LRLQ pain (the 'converse' of those with LRLQ pain in appendicitis) is:

$$75/200 = (100/300 \times 75/100 \times 200/200) / (100/100 \times 200/300).$$

If those with appendicitis and LRLQ pain are also a subset of those with LRLQ pain, as in Fig. 13.4, by rearranging and cancelling out again, this gives 'Aristotle's syllogism', that the proportion of all those studied in those with RLQ pain and appendicitis is:

$$75/75 = (75/300 \times 75/75 \times 200/200) / (200/300 \times 75/200).$$

We can also reason that the 'converse' (the proportion with LRLQ pain and appendicitis in all those studied) is:

$$75/300 = 200/300 \times 75/200 \times 75/75 / (75/75 \times 200/200).$$

This 'proportion syllogism' (or 'probability syllogism') is also used widely in probability calculations, especially 'decision analysis'.

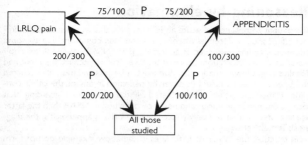

Fig. 13.3 A P map of Bayes' rule.

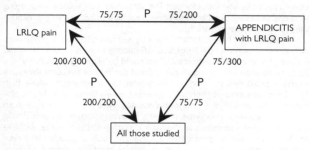

Fig. 13.4 A P map of Aristotle's syllogism.

Reasoning by elimination

If a patient complained of acute abdominal pain, this would suggest a number of possible differential diagnoses: a spurious complaint due to some misunderstanding, non-specific abdominal pain (NSAP), appendicitis, cholecystitis, peptic ulceration, pancreatitis, diverticulitis, etc. If the patient had localized right-lower quadrant abdominal tenderness and this only occurred in appendicitis and NSAP but never by definition in any of the other conditions, then the latter are 'eliminated'. If the patient had 'guarding' that occurs often in appendicitis and never by definition in NSAP, then the latter is eliminated so that the only remaining possibility is appendicitis; the diagnosis is then certain.

In practice, the 'eliminating' findings in the above example do not form part of the definitions of diseases, so the reasoning has to be qualified by saying that each of the diagnoses is 'probably' eliminated and that the diagnosis is 'probably' appendicitis. This also applies when the reasoning process is applied by Sherlock Holmes! The same reasoning is used when trying to predict a patient's response to some treatment or when trying to explain the results of a scientific study.

If a patient with Type 2 diabetes mellitus was found to have a 24h urinary albumin excretion rate (AER) of over 20 micrograms/min, then this could be due to a spurious chance result (that could be eliminated 'probably' if a repeat measurement was also high). It could also be due to recent excessive exercise, prolonged standing, a urinary infection, fever, heart failure, high blood pressure, chronic nephritis, any recent severe illness, or a chronic glomerular albumin leak due to diabetes mellitus (who would benefit from an angiotensin converting enzyme inhibiting or an angiotensin receptor blocking drug). In order to show that the latter is as probable as possible, we have to show that the other possibilities are as improbable as possible by a process of 'probable elimination'. This process of identifying patients responsive to treatments is now called 'stratified' or 'personalized' medicine.

If we read in a paper describing a scientific study on patients with type 2 diabetes mellitus and treated hypertension that only 1 out of 77 patients had an AER between 20 and 40 micrograms/min, then this could mean that if we went on to study 77 patients in our own clinic, then we might be able to replicate the result by observing 3/77 or less again (or fail to do so by getting a result greater than 3/77). This might occur due to chance or because our patients are very different to those in the paper, or because the methods section of the paper was inaccurate so that we could not repeat the study properly, or because there were other studies with results of greater than 3/77 that we had not taken into account. In order that the probability of replication is high, we have to show that the probability of non-replication for all other reasons (including chance) is low.

Reasoning by probable elimination uses the idea that if a *single* finding occurs infrequently in those with a diagnosis (or some other phenomenon) then a *combination* of findings that includes that *single* finding will occur *even less frequently*. If a finding never occurs in a diagnosis, then a combination of findings that includes that finding will never occur in the diagnosis either.

It is important therefore to understand clearly the reasoning process of probable elimination. It is easier to illustrate it with an example from differential diagnosis, e.g. of RLQ abdominal pain.

A worked example

If a patient has LRLQ pain then this is a good short lead, the differential diagnosis being probably appendicitis or non-specific abdominal pain (NSAP). If there is guarding, then as this is likely to occur in appendicitis but less likely in NSAP, the diagnosis is probably appendicitis.

This can be stated in terms of proportions too. Most patients with LRLQ pain have appendicitis or NSAP. Guarding occurs commonly in appendicitis but less commonly in NSAP, so in those with LRLQ pain and guarding the diagnosis is usually appendicitis. We have thus 'stratified' patients with LRLQ pain to improve a prediction. There is intense research interest in such 'stratified' or 'personalized' medicine at present in order to improve response to treatments.

We can also repeat this reasoning process in more detail using the data from Fig. 13.1. Most patients arriving in a surgical admission unit with LRLQ abdominal pain would have appendicitis (e.g. 75/200) or NSAP (e.g. 123/200) with a few (e.g. 2/200) having something else. If the proportion with LRLQ pain in the studied population was 200/300, then the proportion with 'something else' in those with LRLQ pain and guarding can be *no more than* 2/200 x 200/300 = 2/300.

If the patient had 'guarding' and this only occurred in 6/150 patients with NSAP, then the combination of 'guarding' with LRLQ pain can occur *in no more more* than 6/150 of those with NSAP. If the proportion with NSAP in the surgical admission unit was 150/300, then the proportion with NSAP and guarding and LRLQ pain and anything else could be *no more* than 6/150 x 150/300 = 6/300 (the lowest frequency).

If 'guarding' occurred in 80/100 of those with appendicitis and LRLQ pain occurred in 75/100, then both must occur together in at least 80/100 + 75/100 − 100/100 = 55/100 even if they occur together as infrequently as possible. If the proportion with appendicitis in the study population was 100/300, then the proportion with appendicitis, guarding, and LRLQ pain would be at least 100/300×55/100 = 55/300.

If the proportion with LRLQ pain and guarding and appendicitis in the study population was exactly 55/300, the proportion with LRLQ pain and guarding and NSAP was exactly 6/300, and the proportion with LRLQ pain and guarding and 'something else' was exactly 2/300, the proportion of patients with LRLQ pain and guarding who had appendicitis would be: 55/300 / (55/300 + 6/300 + 2/300) = 55/63 = 0.87. But as 55/300 was a minimum value and as 6/300 and 2/300 were maximum values, then at least 87.3% must have appendicitis. (The actual proportion in this example data set is 57/60 = 0.95 = 95% as shown in Fig. 13.1). This reasoning, *using the lowest available 'eliminating' frequencies always*, will produce a proportion of *at least*:

$$1 / \left\{ 1 + \frac{[150/300 \times 6/150] + [200/300 \times 2/200]}{100/300 \times [75/100 + 80/100 - 100/100]} \right\} = 55/63 = 0.873 \quad \text{(A)}.$$

The corresponding probability would be *at least*:

$$1 / \left\{ 1 + \frac{[0.5 \times 0.04] + [0.67 \times 0.01]}{0.33 \times [0.75 + 0.80 - 1]} \right\} = 0.873 \quad \text{(B)}.$$

The formal proof is given in ➲ Proof for the reasoning by probable elimination theorem, p.638.

Using very low frequencies or probability densities

It is not always possible to count all proportions. For example, we can count the proportion of men and women who are taller than 1.5m but it would be difficult to count the proportions that are exactly 1.50000m as such people would be very rare or might not even exist. However, we can estimate the proportion by plotting the continuous distribution of heights in men and women and using this distribution to estimate the proportion at 1.50000m. The proportion would be very low of course and if we used them in the calculations for reasoning by elimination (➔ A worked example, p.623) then we would only get a result of ≥ 0. However, we would have known this already.

We can use an estimate during reasoning by elimination by assuming that a ratio of 4% (e.g. the proportion with guarding in NSAP) to 80% (e.g. the proportion with guarding in appendicitis) has the same effect on the probability of a diagnosis as if the ratio was 0.0004% to 0.008% or if it was a ratio of $(0.04/0.8 = 0.05)$ to 1. In the same way, a ratio of 0.01 to 0.75 could be assumed to have the same effect on the probability of a diagnosis as a ratio of $(0.01/0.75 = 0.013)$ to 1. If we make these assumptions about 'a ratio to 1', then the expression:

$$1/\left\{1+\frac{[0.5\times0.04]+[0.67\times0.01]}{0.33\times[0.75+0.80-1]}\right\} = 0.873 \quad (B)$$

can be replaced by the expression:

$$1/\left\{1 + \left([0.5\text{x}0.04\,/\,0.8] + [0.67\text{x}0.01\,/\,0.75]\right)/\left(0.33\text{x}[1+1-1]\right)\right\} \quad (C).$$

By rearranging (C) we get (see ➔ Proof for the reasoning by probable elimination theorem, p.638, for the formal proof):

$$1/\left\{1+\frac{0.5\times0.04}{0.33\times0.8}+\frac{0.01}{0.375}\right\} = 0.908 \quad (D).$$

Expression (D) gives an estimate of 0.908, which is a closer to the actual value of 0.95 shown in Fig. 13.1.

From Bayes' rule in Fig. 13.3:

$$150\,/\,300\text{x}6\,/\,150 = 200\,/\,300\text{x}6\,/\,200 \text{ is the same as } 0.5\text{x}0.04 = 0.4\text{x}0.05$$

and

$$100\,/\,300\text{x}80\,/\,100 = 120\,/\,300\text{x}80\,/\,120 \text{ is the same as } 0.33\text{x}0.8 = 0.4\text{x}0.67.$$

Thus by replacing [0.5x0.04] by [0.4x0.05] and replacing [0.33x0.8] by [0.4x0.67] in expression (D) we get:

$$1/\{1 + (0.4\text{x}0.05)\,/\,(0.4\text{x}0.67) + (0.01\,/\,0.375)\}.$$

The 0.4s cancel each other out to an expression with no 'likelihoods':

$$1/\left\{1+\frac{0.05}{0.67}+\frac{0.01}{0.375}\right\} = 0.908 \quad (E).$$

Evidence for a finding's role in reasoning by elimination

The conventional wisdom is that it is the 'likelihood ratio' that is the best 'evidence' of the performance of a finding in diagnosis or other predictions. However, there are two types of 'likelihood ratio'.

Type 1. The first is the 'overall' likelihood ratio, which is the frequency of a finding in those with a diagnosis divided by the frequency of the same finding in those without the diagnosis (also called the 'sensitivity' of a test divided by its 'false positive rate' (i.e. 1 minus the specificity).

Type 2. The second type is the 'differential' likelihood ratio, which is the frequency of the finding in those with a diagnosis divided by the frequency of the same finding in those without a rival differential diagnostic possibility. This involves one 'sensitivity' being divided by another 'sensitivity'.

It is the second type—the differential likelihood ratio that allows a finding to be assessed for use in diagnosis by probable elimination. This ratio needs to be as high as possible; if it is infinity, then it shows that the rival diagnosis is impossible. When a likelihood ratio is used in calculations, it is the rival diagnosis's sensitivity that is put on top, so that the likelihood ratio of infinity becomes a likelihood ratio of zero.

This means that the evidence for a finding's role in reasoning by probable elimination is the magnitude of its differential likelihood ratio—the lower the better. The finding with the lowest ratio available should be used in the eliminating process—a ratio of zero, if available. The differential likelihood ratio will only be zero, however, if it forms a part of the definition of a diagnosis, e.g. if it has been deemed a 'necessary' condition of that diagnosis. For example, when considering the differential diagnosis of proteinuria, if there is blood in the urine, then that patient cannot have diabetic microalbuminuria as its defintion specifies that all such patients must not have blood in the urine. Provided that the diagnosis being considered (e.g. glomerulonephritis) sometimes has blood in the urine, the likelihood ratio will be zero.

A finding (F1) that provides the lowest differential likelihood ratio for a pair of diagnoses (D1 and D2) will also provide the best differential probability ratio (or differential odds) for that pair of diagnoses because according to Bayes' rule:

$$\frac{p(D1) \times p(F1 / D1)}{p(D2) \times p(F1 / D2)} = \frac{\cancel{p(F1)} \times p(D1 / F1)}{\cancel{p(F1)} \times p(D2 / F1)}$$

differential likelihood ratio   *differential probability ratio or odds.*

Before a differential likelihood ratio can be used, there must be a finding that suggests a list of differential diagnoses so that the probability of each diagnosis adds to as near to 1 as possible (i.e. so that the probability of something not in the list is very low). This is the second type of evidence of a finding's performance in reasoning by probable elimination—its ability to act as a good 'lead'.

If a finding is a good lead then the probability of each differential diagnosis in its list will be higher than the probability of the diagnoses not in the list. These ratios are the differential probability ratios (or the differential odds). A finding that acts as a good lead will, therefore, be a finding that has a low likelihood ratio between each diagnosis in the list and all other diagnoses not in that list.

Differential likelihood ratios make use of 'complementing' differentiation

Assume that localized LRLQ *tenderness* (as opposed to LRLQ *pain*) occurs in 50/100 patients with appendicitis, in 100/150 patients with 'non-specific abdominal pain' (NSAP), and in 0/50 patients (i.e. never) with 'all other diagnoses'.

Assume also that a raised neutrophil count (RNC) occurs in 25/100 patients with appendicitis, in 0/150 patients (i.e. never) with NSAP, and in 50/50 patients with 'all other diagnoses'.

This means that LRLQ tenderness AND a RNC can only occur together in appendicitis, which makes the diagnosis of appendicitis certain. Note that the list of 2 diagnoses linked to LRLQ tenderness is different to the list of 2 diagnoses linked to RNC, so their lists are 'independent'. This is analogous to solvable simultaneous equations being 'independent'. So, each list 'complements' the other by eliminating different diagnoses.

However, the overall likelihood ratio of LRLQ tenderness regarding appendicitis is 50/100 divided by 100/200 = 1 suggesting that it is a useless test! Furthermore, the overall likelihood ratio of a RNC regarding appendicitis is 25/100 divided by 50/200 = 1, also suggesting that it is a useless test!

If we assume statistical independence between the occurrence of both these findings in those with and without appendicitis, then their combined likelihood ratio is 1 × 1 =1 and by Bayes' rule the probability of appendicitis, given both findings, will be the same as its frequency in the study population of 100/300 = 0.33. But this is wrong as we know the diagnosis is certain. This means that using the overall likelihood ratio with Bayes' rule gives us a false result because it fails to model 'complementing' differentiation.

The differential likelihood ratio for LRLQ tenderness between NSAP and appendicitis is 100/150 divided by 50/100 = 1.33 and between appendicitis and 'all other diagnoses' it is 0/50 divided by 50/100 = 0. If LRLQ tenderness is used as a lead, then the probability of appendicitis is 50/150 = 0.33, the probabililty of NSAP is 100/150 = 0.67, and the probability of 'all other diagnoses' is 0/150 = 0.

The differential likelihood ratio for a RNC between NSAP and appendicitis and NSAP is 0/150 divided by 25/100 = 0 and between appendicitis and 'All other diagnoses' it is 50/50 divided by 50/100 = 2.

When the lowest differential likelihood ratios or odds are used in the expression (D) to calculate the probability of a diagnosis by elimination and thus using 'complementing' differentiation, the probability of appendicitis is:

$$1/\left\{1+\frac{P(\text{NSAP/Study}) \times P(\text{RNC/NSAP})}{P(\text{Appx/Study}) \times P(\text{RNC/Appx})} + \frac{P(\text{'All other } \Delta s'/\text{LRLQ tend})}{P(\text{Appx/LRLQ tend})}\right\}$$

which by inserting the numbers is:

$$1/\left\{1+\frac{150/300 \times 0/150}{100/300 \times 25/100} + \frac{0/150}{50/100}\right\} = 1.$$

The use of differential likelihood ratios with the reasoning by probable elimination theorem to model diagnostic thinking (instead of Bayes' rule) gives the correct result. This is because unlike Bayes' rule with 'overall likelihood ratios', it makes use of 'complementing' differentiation.

Things that affect 'differential' and 'overall' likelihood ratios

The 'overall likelihood ratio' is the frequency of a finding occurring in a diagnosis (e.g. 'guarding' in appendicitis) divided by the frequency of that finding *in all those without* the diagnosis (e.g. 'guarding' in those without appendicitis).

In 300 patients admitted to a surgical department over a month (see Fig. 13.1), 120 had 'guarding' and 100 patients turned out to have appendicitis. Eighty patients had both appendicitis and 'guarding'. This meant that of those 100 patients with appendicitis, 80/100 = 80% had 'guarding'. Also, of the 120 patients with 'guarding', 80/120 = 66.67% also had appendicitis.

The frequency of 'guarding in those *without appendicitis* was 40/200 = 20%, corresponding to a probability of 0.20 (because many patients had other conditions that can cause guarding). Therefore, the 'overall' likelihood ratio would be 0.80/0.20 = 4.

If the 300 patients had been admitted to the surgical ward in a month and 100 of these had appendicitis, then the incidence per month would be 100/300 = 0.33. If 120 of these 300 patients had 'guarding', then its incidence would be 120/300 = 0.40%. However, if *all patients with appendicitis and all patients with 'guarding'* during the same month had been sent to hospital from a catchment area of 300,000, then the incidence of appendicitis in the catchment population would be 100/300,000 = 0.00033 and the incidence of guarding would be 0.00040 per month.

In the catchment area, the proportion of those with appendicitis who had guarding would also be 80/100 = 80%. The proportion of those *without* appendicitis who had 'guarding' would be 40/299,900 = 0.00013. Therefore, the likelihood ratio would be 0.8/0.00013 = 5998 (five thousand nine hundred and ninety eight!)—compared to a ratio of 4 inside the surgical department. Despite this, the probability of any patient in the catchment area having appendicitis who is known to have guarding would still be 80/120 = 66.67%, which is exactly the same as for patients in the hospital. If the frequency of guarding in those with NSAP is also 4% in the community, the differential likelihood ratio, differential odds and probability of the diagnosis will also the same.

So, the overall likelihood ratio will be greater if the population contains larger numbers of patients *without the diagnosis or the finding* (e.g. healthy people). It is best used as evidence for the ability of a test to screen such populations for asymptomatic diseases and should only be applied in the population from which it was derived.

The above example assumed that all patients with guarding and appendicitis seen in the community were sent into hospital. However, if the primary care physicians had been able to send all patients with appendicitis but only those with severe forms of NSAP and other diagnoses into hospital, then this may create a difference in the differential likelihood ratios between the community and the hospital. It is important, therefore, to check whether all likelihood ratios—overall and differential, are the same in other populations.

Findings that lead to a 'common cause'

Diagnoses are often pursued actively by looking for findings that are 'likely' to occur in patients with the diagnosis that one is trying to confirm, and 'unlikely' to occur in those with diagnoses that one is trying to 'eliminate'. However, another approach is to think of each of the patient's findings in turn (e.g. LRLQ pain, guarding, etc.), and to consider if there is only one diagnosis that is common to some lists of differential diagnoses. This approach only depends on 'differential probability ratios' (see equation (E) in ➲ Using very low frequencies or probability densities, p.624).

If only a single diagnosis (e.g. appendicitis) occurs commonly in a number of leads (e.g. LRLQ pain and guarding), it follows that that single diagnosis will become probable, i.e. it will occur very frequently in a group of patients with those lead findings (e.g. appendicitis will occur frequently in those with a combination of LRLQ pain and guarding). The frequency with which the diagnosis will be found can be estimated by using equation (E).

In order to estimate the frequency given a combination of findings by using observed frequencies given single lead findings, choose the best lead (i.e. the finding with shortest list of differential diagnoses). Thus the shortest list of differential diagnoses is that of LRLQ pain—the list is appendicitis (in 37.5%) or NSAP (in 61.5%). These account for 99% of patients with LRLQ pain, the other 1% not being in the list. For each other diagnosis in the list (i.e. NSAP alone in this case), choose another finding that provides the best (i.e. the lowest) 'differential probability ratios'. For example, guarding is associated with NSAP in only $6/120 = 5\%$ of cases and appendicitis occurs in $80/120 = 66.67\%$ of patients with guarding, so the differential probability ratio is $0.05/0.67 = 0.075$.

It is this lowest differential probability ratio that is required in order to probably eliminate each rival diagnoses (e.g. NSAP) and thus to estimate the probability of the diagnosis to be confirmed (e.g. appendicitis). This is done by first adding up the lowest differential probability ratio for each differential diagnosis as follows:

$$1/[1 + \text{sum of all the lowest differential probability ratios}].$$

If the sum of all the lowest differential probability ratios is zero, then the probability of the diagnosis will be one, of course—certainty.

The lowest differential probability ratio for NSAP is 0.075 (provided by guarding) and the lowest differential probability ratio for the 'unlisted' diagnoses is provided by LRLQ pain is $1/37.5 = 0.027$. Therefore, the estimated probability of appendicitis give LRLQ pain and guarding is $1/(1 + 0.075 + 0.027) = 0.908$ (see equation (E) in ➲ Using very low frequencies or probability densities, p.624). Note that this calculation does not use incidence or prevalence and only a small number of frequencies, minimizing the task of data collection when seeking evidence for the usefulness of tests.

Data are therefore needed to find the frequency with which patients with each differential diagnosis occur in those with a lead finding in different clinical settings (i.e. to calculate the various differential probability ratios). Data are also needed on the frequency of findings in patients with diagnoses to calculate the differential likelihood ratios. These may vary between different communities, hospitals, parts of the country, etc.

Statistical independence versus statistical dependence

Statistical independence plays an important role in the arithmetic of probability. For example, if the probability of throwing an even number on a die is 1/2 and the probability of throwing a 'five' is 1/6, then the probability of throwing an even number followed by a 'five' is $1/2 \times 1/6 = 1/12$. This is because it is assumed that the result of each throw is statistically independent of any other result. The same assumption is sometimes made in diagnosis, so that if the frequency of LRLQ pain in NSAP is 1/2 and the frequency of guarding is 1/6, then the frequency of both is guessed as being $1/2 \times 1/6 = 1/12$.

During reasoning by probable elimination, we do not guess but rely on the fact that the frequency of LRLQ pain and guarding in NSAP can be no more than 1/6. However, if there was statistical dependence, then we could assume that both findings did occur together 1/6 of the time. If we did this we would probably overestimate the true frequency of both. It also has the advantage of only using a small amount of information, i.e. one finding per rival diagnosis to be eliminated.

If we assume statistical independence, then we usually include all the patient's findings and multiply together all their frequencies of occurrence in each possible diagnosis. This is well known to over-estimate probabilities, e.g. so that the probability of appendicitis would be 0.999 and its rivals would be 0.001 or less. Also it is not feasible to find the frequency of all findings that exist in all diagnoses that exist. A compromise would be to use the known best two likelihood ratios for the rival diagnosis, especially if each differential likelihood ratio is weak. For example, if rebound tenderness occurs in 0.1 of those with NSAP and 0.9 of those with appendicitis, the ratio is $0.1/0.9 = 0.111$. If we keep to a dependence assumption then the estimated probability of appendicitis remains (using equations (D) and (E) in ➲ Using very low frequencies or probability densities, p.624):

$$1 / \left\{ 1 + \frac{0.5 \times 0.04}{0.33 \times 0.8} + \frac{0.01}{0.375} \right\} = 1 / \left\{ 1 + \frac{0.05}{0.67} + \frac{0.01}{0.375} \right\} = 0.908.$$

If we assume statistical independence between rebound tenderness and guarding in those with appendicitis and NSAP, then the estimated probability of appendicitis is (using equations (D) and (E)):

$$1 / \left\{ 1 + \frac{0.5 \times 0.04 \times \mathbf{0.1}}{0.33 \times 0.8 \times \mathbf{0.9}} + \frac{0.01}{0.375} \right\} = 1 / \left\{ 1 + \frac{0.05 \times 0.1}{0.67 \times 0.9} + \frac{\mathbf{0.01}}{\mathbf{0.375}} \right\} = 0.966.$$

It should be noted that the estimate is now already slightly higher than the true value of 0.95. Again by using equation (E) in ➲ Using very low frequencies or probability densities, p.624, the incidence or prevalence of a diagnosis is not used in the calculation.

A better approach would be to combine weak diagnostic findings to try to form more useful numerical tests and to test their ability to create differential likelihood or probability ratios.

Reasoning with numerical test results

Fig. 13.5 shows the proportion of patients with acute abdominal pain at different ages that turn out to have each diagnosis. In the range 0–9 years of age, 48.6% of patients will have appendicitis, 49.8% of patients will have 'non-specific abdominal pain' (NSAP), and 1.6% will have small bowel obstruction. Acute abdominal pain under the age of 10 is thus a very good lead with only 3 differential diagnoses. However, over the age of 70 years, the differential diagnosis was appendicitis (4.6%), diverticulitis (7.6%), perforated duodenal ulcer (4.4%), 'non-specific abdominal pain' (32.2%), cholecystitis (35.2%), small bowel obstruction (9.1%), and pancreatitis (6.9%). In the intervening ages, the proportions change as shown in Fig. 13.5.

Fig. 13.5 is a histogram prepared by dividing the ages into ranges and counting the proportions with each diagnosis in each range. However, it is also possible to create smooth curves to display the probabilities. This can be done by plotting the distribution of the ages in a group of patients with each diagnosis; for example, by using kernel spline functions. This can be done by placing a 'Gaussian bell' over each data point and then adding the height of the curve for each 'bell' at each value (each age of the patient in this case). If the summit of each Gaussian kernel 'bell' is set to a value of 1, then the sum of the height of each Gaussian kernel distribution gives the estimated number of the patients whose data contributed to that result. The smoothness of the curve is controlled by varying the standard deviation of each Gaussian curve kernel – the wider the standard deviation, the smoother the curve and the greater will be the estimated number of patients contributing to each point on the curve.

The estimated number of patients at each value for a diagnosis is then divided by the total number of patients with that diagnosis. This gives the 'estimated' likelihood of that value (e.g. of a patient being that age). For the sake of simplicity, only three of these distributions are shown in Fig. 13.6; those for non-specific abdominal pain (NSAP), appendicitis, and cholecystitis. The age distribution of patients with NSAP and appendicitis peak at about 14 years of age, whereas the peak age distribution for cholecystitis is at about 70 years of age.

If the estimated number of patients with a diagnosis, e.g. appendicitis, is divided by the total estimated number of patients at each age, then this gives the proportion with each diagnosis at that age. These values are plotted in Fig. 13.7. It can be seen that at the age of 10, the proportion with appendicitis and NSAP are almost the same but they diverge at older ages.

The likelihoods in Fig. 13.6 and the probabilities in Fig. 13.7 can be used in reasoning by probable elimination, as described in previous pages. The methods used here can be applied to numerical test results, and clinical scores (e.g. the Wells' score). The same approach can also be used on estimated probabilities (plotted on the X axis) to see if they are equal to the proportion of correct predictions (plotted on the Y axis) as part of an audit of the accuracy of probabilities.

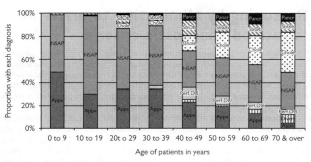

Fig. 13.5 Differential diagnosis of acute abdominal pain at different ages.

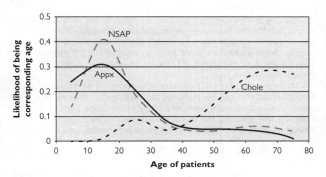

Fig. 13.6 Likelihood distirbution of ages for different diagnoses in acute abdominal pain.

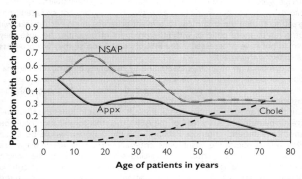

Fig. 13.7 Proportion of patients with each diagnosis at each age in patients with acute abdominal pain.

Reasoning by elimination to arrive at 'stratified' diagnostic criteria

The diagnosis of 'diabetic albuminuria' is based on 'stratifying' patients based on the presence of 'diabetes mellitus' and 'albuminuria', and also on the absence of other causes of 'albuminuria', such as transient rises in urine albumin, recent exercise, prolonged standing, urinary tract infection, other infectious illnesses, other severe illnesses, dehydration, hypertension, heart failure, nephritis, or other chronic renal disease.

'Diabetes mellitus' is assumed to be present if at least two fasting or random blood glucose levels exceed 7mmol/L or 11mmol/L, respectively, so that a transient or self-limiting glucose rise is probably eliminated. 'Microalbuminuria' is assumed to be present if 2 out of 3 albumin excretion rates (AER) exceeds 20 micrograms/min (or an albumin–creatine ratio of >2.5 in females or >3.5 in males), which means that a transient self-limiting rise in albumin excretion is probably eliminated.

Collecting a specimen overnight or on rising means that 'recent prolonged standing' or 'heavy exercise' is probably eliminated. The absence of any symptoms, signs, or test results solely attributed to the other diagnoses (e.g. no breathlessness or ankle swelling, a controlled BP, negative urine tests for blood, or leucocytes, etc.) means that the other diagnoses too are probably eliminated.

This means that there is 'persistent albuminuria' in the presence of diabetes mellitus that can be explained by a leakage of albumin from renal glomeruli due to damage from persistently raised blood glucose. It is also imagined that lowering the blood pressure within each glomerulus with a drug will reduce this leakage and prevent progression until the albumin excretion is over 200 micrograms/min (which would mean by definition they have 'diabetic nephropathy'). These patients are thus identified by 'stratification'.

Some patients may not progress on placebo, some may progress unless they are treated, and some may progress despite being treated (these are 'triage' groups as used in emergency situations). If patients with the 'other causes' of microalbuminuria (e.g. excessive exercise) are not excluded from treatment, then the treatment to prevent progressive glomerular leak will be given to more patients with little prospect of benefiting because they would not have progressed in the first place or because they will progress despite the treatment.

A combination of findings assembled by reasoning by probable elimination that predicts probable benefit from treatment can by common agreement be regarded as a 'sufficient' diagnostic criterion. All those with this criterion would then 'definitely' have the diagnosis.

If there is another combination of findings (e.g. that includes the albumin–creatinine ratio (ACR) instead of the AER), then this combination could be another 'sufficient' criterion. Patients with the diagnosis would be those with at least one of these 'sufficient' criteria. In order to exclude diagnoses we need a 'necessary' criterion that includes virtually all those who benefit so that if that finding is absent, virtually no patients miss out. These criteria depend on careful analysis and 'stratification' of clinical trials based on the principles of 'triage'.

Analysing clinical trials to 'stratify' diagnostic and treatment criteria

Patients with provisional criteria of 'diabetic microalbuminuria' were randomized to have an angiotensin receptor blocker (ARB) or placebo included in their BP control treatment[1]. The proportion developing diabetic nephropathy within 2 years were 'stratified' to those starting with an AER of 20–40, 41–80, 81–120, and 121–200 micrograms/min and were plotted as shown in Fig. 13.8. Only 1/77 developed nephropathy on placebo after starting with an AER between 20 and 40 micrograms/min and 1/127 developed nephropathy on an ARB, so that only 0.5% gained from treatment. However, above 40 micrograms/min, more progressed to nephropathy without treatment and more benefited from treatment. This suggests that the cut-off point should have been 40 micrograms/min and that about 1/3 of the patients already offered an IRB do not benefit much within 2 years. The risk of nephropathy and the proportion benefiting from treatment is more at higher levels of AER; this also shows that AER is a good predictor of outcome. This approach is the aim of 'stratified or 'personalized' medical research.

The response to treatment used here was based on the same biochemical measurement (AER) that was used to establish the diagnosis and treatment indication. The same analysis can be carried out on clinical trials where the outcome was based on symptoms or a well-being score. However, not all patients with a diagnosis are offered all the treatments linked to it. Patients with a diagnosis make up a set that encloses sub-sets of patients who benefit from various actions. In the case of 'diabetic microalbuminuria', each level of severity (each AER) can be regarded as a 'stratified' or 'personalized' diagnostic sub-set with its own probability of benefit from 0.5% to 27%. Few patients with the diagnosis would opt for a treatment with a probability of benefit that was about 0.5%.

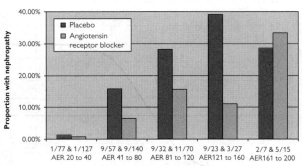

Fig. 13.8 Histogram showing proportions of patients with different degrees of albuminuria getting nephropathy within 2 years.

How to improve treatments by better selection or 'stratification' of patients

The role of a doctor is to recommend treatments to patients by arriving at diagnoses and advising them on the probability of success. This 'stratification' can be improved by predicting more accurately the 'triage' groups of (1) those who will get better without treatment, (2) those who will get better only with treatment, and (3) those who will fail to get better and may have some other progressive illness that might respond to something else, e.g. an unknown renal disease. Its discovery might result in another diagnosis being added to the list of a raised AER. It is also possible that the differential diagnoses might change for different values of AER as in Fig. 13.4, Fig. 13.5, and Fig. 13.6. This would allow more patients who do not respond to treatment with an ARB being excluded from the criterion for 'microalbuminuria'.

The clinical trial results in Fig. 13.8 still showed a high probability of benefit between 120 and 200 micrograms/min but the data were sparse at high levels. If more data had been available, then it might have been possible to create a set of curves as shown in Fig. 13.9. The broken curve of those on treatment shows that the proportion with an adverse outcome is lower than the unbroken curve of those on placebo.

If the treatment had been ineffective, then the broken sigmoid curve would have been superimposed on the continuous curve. However, if the test result did not predict the outcome, then both curves would have been flat. If the treatment was effective, then the flat, broken line would be below the continuous flat line as shown; if not they would be superimposed. A poorer test would result in a shallower curve between the flat and sigmoid curve. A better test with fewer untreatable causes would produce a sigmoid curve with longer horizontal segments at the top and bottom with a steeper rise between. A perfect test would give a vertical rise. A number of such tests could be compared in a RCT, e.g. by doing an AER, albumin–creatinine ratio, etc.

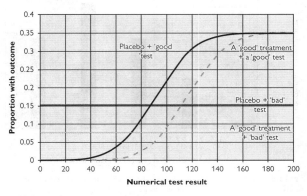

Fig. 13.9 Idealized curves from a randomized controlled trial.

Studies to establish treatment indication and diagnostic cut-off points

The current cut-off for diagnosing and treating patients with diabetic micro-albuminura is 20 micrograms/min. Fig. 13.8 showed that many patients are diagnosed and treated between 20 and 40 micrograms/min when there is no difference between treatment and placebo. In Fig. 13.9 the treatment and placebo curves are also close between '160' and '200' where the condition is therefore too advanced to benefit from treatment.

If a cut-off was placed at 40, then few patients would lose out by not being offered the treatment. However, if the test result was above the cut-off point, then it is important to consider the actual test result, e.g. '100', and to estimate the probability of benefit by subtracting the probability of the outcome on placebo from the probability of the outcome on treatment. At a value of '100' in Fig. 13.9, the probability of the outcome on placebo is about 0.22, whereas on treatment it is 0.09, the difference being 0.22–0.09 = 0.13. This means that the number needed to treat is about 1/0.13 = 7.7 for one to benefit. This would be put to the patient in shared decision-making.

If '100' had been chosen as the cut-off for not considering treatment and the result of a study of the proportion with each outcome plotted as shown in Fig. 13.10, then the marked discontinuity at '100' indicates that the cut-off is too high. This would result in 'under-diagnosis' so that many patients would miss out. If the same study was conducted with a cut-off at '20', then the curve would follow the course of the broken line in Fig. 13.9 with no discontinuity, suggesting 'under-diagnosis' or that the treatment was ineffective in this range at least. A series of studies could be done by moving the cut-off point in stages to assess treatment effectiveness at various cut-off points. This could be used to check that the result of a published RCT was borne out in other centres or to compare tests.

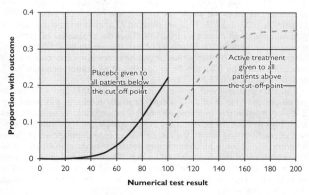

Fig. 13.10 Idealized curves from a 'cut off' study.

Estimating the probability of replication with reasoning by elimination

If a patient presents with acute abdominal pain, then there will be a list of possible explanations. These include appendicitis, a self-limiting condition, and a 'spurious symptom', so that when the patient is asked again, it is met by a denial. In the latter case, the finding has failed to be replicated. A doctor listening to a story or looking at test results should consider their reliability—or their probability of replication. The same happens with scientific studies. There may be many reasons for a low probability of replicating a study result, one important cause being that if the number of observations in the study were few, then chance variation would probably lead to a different repeat result.

Chance variation is often assessed by asking what 'true' AER value in the total population would result in the observed proportion of 1/77, or something more extreme (i.e. 0/77), being seen 2.5% of the time if 77 patients were drawn at random from that total population. The lower 2.5% confidence interval (CI) in this case would be 0.0003. The upper 2.5% CI calculated in the same way would be 0.0702.

Bayesians think that this approach is wrong and maintain that one should first guess 'subjectively' the prior probability of all the possible results in the total population (i.e. of it being 0%, 1%,...15%,...100%) on the basis of the evidence of other studies, personal experience, etc. The likelihood of getting the observed result of 1/77 from each of these possibilities is calculated and then Bayes' rule is used to get an estimate of the probability of each possible outcome (or by adding several outcomes, a range of them, e.g. from 0/77 to 4/77).

There are objections to both these approaches. Another approach would be to regard the observed outcome of 1/77 developing nephropathy as a member of the set of all observations of 1/77 (about asthma, deep vein thrombosis, etc.), the combined set of all these sets containing 1/77 = 0.013% getting the predicted outcome. We can then calculate the proportion of times we would get an outcome reasonably near to 1/77 (e.g. 0/77, 1/77, 2/77, 3/77) if we selected 77 at random from the pooled population with an outcome of 0.013%. Thus the probability of getting a repeat result between 0/77 and 3/77 inclusive would be 0.98 from the binomial theorem. The probability of getting a repeat result between 0/77 and 2/77 would be 0.92 and the probability of replication between 0/77 and 4/77 would be 0.99.

This 0.01 probability of non-replication between 0/77 and 4/77 based on an observed result of 1/77 would 'probably eliminate' this possibility if it were used in the 'probable elimination expressions'. If we could also probably eliminate the other causes of non-replication: inaccurate description of methods and results, the author's patients or population being very different, the absence of contradictory results in other studies, etc, then the probability of replication would be high. The differential probability or differential likelihood ratios for this reasoning would have to be guessed in most cases (unless, for example, some journal editors collected such data from past experience).

Reasoning with hypotheses

Hypotheses are guesses or predictions about currently inaccessible phenomena that are still being investigated. In medical practice, these are 'working' diagnoses. A 'theory' is a prediction that is not currently being investigated (this is 'final' diagnosis in clinical reasoning).

If a patient presents with acute abdominal pain there will be past experience of the diagnoses being considered, so that if all but one are 'probably eliminated', the high probability of the remaining diagnosis can be supported by a track record. With novel scientific hypotheses we may not have thought of all the possibilities, so that even if all but one of those being considered is shown to be improbable, we cannot conclude that the remaining hypothesis is probably correct.

Karl Popper made this point by saying that it was not possible to confirm hypotheses but only to 'refute' or 'falsify' them This implied that such reasoning used definitive criteria. For example, if we postulated that undiagnosed diabetes had caused nephropathy in a group of patients, then this hypothesis could be falsified if a high HbA1c was a 'necessary' criterion for diabetes and the HbA1c was normal in each member of the group. If a high HbA1c was simply frequent in diabetes then the hypothesis would be 'probably eliminated', not falsified.

If a diagnosis or novel hypothesis is still possible (or even 'confirmed' in the case of a diagnosis) there is added uncertainty. This is because diagnoses and hypotheses are titles to many things that we imagine (i.e. predict) about the present, past, and future in terms of phenomena that can or cannot be verified directly by observation.

All probabilities represent a degree of uncertainty about a predicted event. The only highly certain thing about probabilities is that if they are derived appropriately they can predict accurately the frequency of correct predictions of various kinds in the long run. (This is why bookmakers make a profit.) This may well happen if the probabilities are based on past experience. However, probabilities are usually estimates, e.g. the probability of nephropathy based on an AER of 102 micrograms/min when no past patients may have had this actual result.

The only way to assess the accuracy of all probabilities is to check how often all similar probabilities (e.g. of 0.8) are linked to correct predictions in the long run (it should be 80% of the time). This would be a 'probability audit'. If all probabilities have a corresponding predictive success rate, then a plot of probability against correct predictions should be a straight line from 0 to 1 (or a line of identity). If it is not, then the plot can act as a calibration curve to correct the probability.

A 'probability audit' can be done for all predictions made by a person, or those only connected to medicine, or a speciality in medicine, or even a single diagnosis. However, some predictions cannot be verified to see if they are 'correct' (e.g. molecular changes). We then have to assume that our probabilities connected with non-verifiable events are equally accurate to our verifiable probabilities.

People appear to conduct informal 'probability audits' subconsciously during their day to day lives by modulating their sense of certainty to avoid being over-confident or under-confident. If we fail to do this, we would make more misjudgements than necessary.

Proof for the reasoning by probable elimination theorem

The aim of the arguments below is to prove expression (1), which is explained in footnote *. When (a) F_i is any of the 'findings' F_1, F_2,...F_n actually observed (e.g. symptoms), (b) D_j is a hidden phenomenon (i.e. making up a diagnostic criterion), (c) when $\check{D}_x$ = 'not D_x' such that $p(\check{D}_x) = 1-p(D_x)$ and when D_x is a suspected diagnosis chosen from the list D_1, D_2, D_m, (d) when F_L is one of the findings represented by F_i chosen as a 'diagnostic lead' F_L being chosen so that the value of 'm' (the number of diagnostic possibilities linked to it) and $p(D_0/F_L)$ (the proportion of patients without one of these diagnostic possibilities) are both as low as possible and so that $_{j=1}\Sigma^m\ p(D_j/F_L) + p(D_0/F_L) \geq 1$, (e) when $p(F_i/D_j)$ for each D_j other than D_x can use any F_i although the lowest $p(F_i/D_j)$ for each D_j will give the highest lower bound for $p(D_x/(F_1\cap...F_n))$:

(1) $p(D_x\ /\ (F_1\cap...F_n)) \geq$

$$\left\{1+\frac{_{j=1,\ j\neq x}\Sigma^m\ p(D_j).p(F_i\ /\ D_j)_{\text{[i giving lowest likelihood]}}+p(F_L).p(D_0\ /\ F_L)}{p(D_x).\ \text{max of } [_{i=1,\ i\neq L}\Sigma^n\ p(F_i\ /\ D_x)+p(F_L\ /\ D_x)-n+1]\ \text{or } 0}\right\}^{-1}.$$

Proof:

(2) $p(D_x\ /\ (F_1\cap...F_n)) = \left\{1+\dfrac{p(\check{D}_x).p(F_1\cap...F_n\ /\ \check{D}_x)}{p(D_x).p(F_1\cap...F_n\ /\ D_x)}\right\}^{-1}$ (Bayes' rule).

(3) $p(\check{D}_x).p(F_1\cap...F_n\ /\ \check{D}_x) \leq_{j=1,j\neq x}\Sigma^m\ p(D_j).p(F_1\cap...F_n\ /\ D_j) + p(F_1\cap...F_n).p(D_0\ /\ F_1\cap...F_n).$

(4) $_{j=0}\Sigma^m\ p(D_j).p(F_1\cap...F_n\ /\ D_j) \leq_{j=1}\Sigma^m\ p(D_j).p(F_i\ /\ D_j)_{\text{[i giving lowest likelihood]}}+p(D_0).p(F_L\ /\ D_0).$

(5) $p(D_0).p(F_L\ /\ D_0) = p(F_L).p(D_0\ /\ F_L)$ (Bayes' rule).

Substituting (5) in (4) gives:

(6) $_{j=0}\Sigma^m\ p(D_j).p(F_1\cap...F_n\ /\ D_j) \leq_{j=1}\Sigma^m\ p(D_j).p(F_i\ /\ D_j)_{\text{[i giving lowest likelihood]}}+p(F_L).p(D_0\ /\ F_L).$

Substituting (6) in (2) gives:

(7) $p(D_x\ /\ (F_1\cap...F_n)) \geq \left\{1+\dfrac{_{j=1,\ j\neq x}\Sigma^m\ p(D_j).p(F_i\ /\ D_j)_{\text{[i giving lowest likelihood]}}+p(F_L).p(D_0\ /\ F_L)}{p(D_x).p(F_1\cap...F_n\ /\ D_x)}\right\}^{-1}.$

(8) $p(F_1\cap...F_n\ /\ D_x) \geq \text{max of } [_{i=1}\Sigma^n\ p(F_i\ /\ D_x)-n+1]\ \text{or } 0.$

---

* Expressions (1) and (9) are inequality identities based on probability axioms alone and involve no potentially false assumptions but the denominator can be zero or less when the denominator likelihoods are low e.g. when they are probability densities, giving a correct but unhelpful result e.g. $p(D_x/F_1\cap...F_n) \geq$ -2.

Substituting (8) in (7) proves that:

(9) $p(D_x / (F_1 \cap \ldots F_n) \geq$

$$\left\{ 1 + \frac{\sum^m_{j=1,\, j \neq x} p\left(D_j\right).p\left(F_j / D_j\right)_{[j\ giving\ lowest\ likelihood]} + p\left(F_L\right).p\left(D_0 / F_L\right)}{p\left(D_x\right).\ max\ of\ [\sum^n_{i=1,\, i \neq L} p\left(F_i / D_x\right) + p\left(F_L / D_x\right) - n + 1]\ or\ 0} \right\}^{-1}.$$

[see footnote *]

Make a 'likelihood ratio equivalence assumption' that a differential likelihood ratio of x_i / y_i and $(x_i.k_i)/(y_i.k_i)$ result in the same value of $p(D_x / F_1 \cap \ldots F_n)$ and provided that $1 \geq p(F_i / D).k_i \geq 0$; $1 \geq p(F_i / D_x).k_i \geq 0$ and $1 \geq p(F_L / D_0).k_L \geq 0$ and $1 \geq p(F_L / D_x).k_L \geq 0$ then:

(10) $\dfrac{p\left(F_i / D_j\right)}{p\left(F_i / D_x\right)} \equiv \dfrac{p\left(F_i / D_j\right).k_i}{p\left(F_i / D_x\right).k_i}$ and $\dfrac{p\left(F_L / D_0\right)}{p\left(F_L / D_x\right)} \equiv \dfrac{p\left(F_L / D_0\right).k_L}{p\left(F_L / D_x\right).k_L}.$

Substituting (10) in (9):

(11) $p(D_x / (F_1 \cap \ldots F_n) \geq$

$$\left\{ 1 + \frac{\sum^m_{j=1,\, j \neq x} p\left(D_j\right).p\left(F_j / D_j\right).k_{j\,[j\ giving\ lowest\ likelihood]} + p\left(F_L\right).p\left(D_0 / F_L\right).k_L}{p\left(D_x\right).\ max\ of\ [\sum^n_{i=1,\, i \neq L} p\left(F_i / D_x\right).k_i + p\left(F_L / D_x\right).k_L - n + 1]\ or\ 0} \right\}^{-1}.$$

Now let $k_i = 1/p(F_i/D_x)$ and $k_L = 1/p(F_L/D_x)$ so that:

(12) $\dfrac{p\left(F_i / D_j\right).k_i}{p\left(F_i / D_x\right).k_i} = \dfrac{p\left(F_i / D_j\right)\ /\ \cancel{p\left(F_i / D_x\right)}}{p\left(F_i / D_x\right)\ /\ \cancel{p\left(F_i / D_x\right)}} = \dfrac{p\left(F_i / D_j\right)\ /\ p\left(F_i / D_x\right)}{1}$

and

$\dfrac{p\left(F_L / D_0\right).k_L}{p\left(F_L / D_x\right).k_L} = \dfrac{p\left(F_L / D_0\right)\ /\ p\left(F_L / D_x\right)}{1}.$

Substituting (12) in (11) when the term 'likelihood ratio' means the 'differential likelihood ratio', which is the same as a ratio of two 'sensitivities':

(13) $p(D_x / (F_1 \cap \ldots F_n) \geq$

$$\left\{ 1 + \frac{\sum^m_{j=1,\, j \neq x} p\left(D_j\right).p\left(F_j / D_j\right) / p\left(F_j / D_j\right)_{[j\ giving\ lowest\ likelihood\ ratio]} + p\left(F_L\right).p\left(D_0 / F_L\right) / p\left(F_L / D_0\right)}{p\left(D_x\right)[n - n + 1]} \right\}^{-1}.$$

But as:

$$\frac{p\left(F_L\right).p\left(D_0 / F_L\right).\ /\ p\left(F_L / D_0\right)}{p\left(D_x\right)} = \frac{\cancel{p\left(F_L\right)}.p\left(D_0 / F_L\right)}{\cancel{p\left(F_L\right)}.p\left(D_x / F_L\right)}$$

and simplifying (13):

$$(14) \quad p(D_x / (F_1 \cap \ldots F_n)) \geq \left\{ 1 + \frac{\sum^m_{j=1,\, j \neq x} p(D_j).p(F_i / D_j)_{[i\, giving\, lowest\, likelihood\, ratio]}}{p(D_x).p(F_i / D_x)} + \frac{p(D_0 / F_L)}{p(D_x / F_L)} \right\}^{-1}.$$

[see footnote †]

But:

$$(15) \quad \frac{p(D_j).p(F_i / D_j)}{p(D_x).p(F_i / D_x)} = \frac{p(D_j / F_i)}{p(D_x / F_i)}.$$

Substituting (15) in (14):

$$(16) \quad p(D_x / (F_1 \cap \ldots F_n)) \geq \left\{ 1 + \sum^m_{j=1,\, j \neq x} \frac{p(D_j / F_i)_{[i\, giving\, lowest\, probability\, ratio]}}{p(D_x / F_i)} + \frac{p(D_0 / F_L)}{p(D_x / F_L)} \right\}^{-1}.$$

[see footnote †]

It is noteworthy that expression (16) does not use 'likelihoods' at all. Equations (14) and (16) always provide estimates of $p(D_x / F_1 \cap \ldots F_n)$ that are greater than or equal to zero even when the values of the denominator likelihoods are low (e.g. in probability densities). Any F_i can be chosen to 'probably eliminate' a D_j by showing that each $p(D_j / F_1 \cap \ldots F_n)$ is low but in expressions (1) and (7), the closest upper bound for each $p(D_x / F_1 \cap \ldots F_n)$ and the closest lower bound for $p(D_x / F_1 \cap \ldots F_n)$ will be obtained from using the lowest $p(F_i / D_j)$ for each D_j in the numerator. However, in the simpler expressions (14) and (16), the closest estimate for $p(D_x / F_1 \cap \ldots F_n)$ will be obtained from using the lowest ratio of $p(F_i / D_j)$ / $p(F_i / D_x)$ in expression (14) or the lowest probability ratio of $p(D_j / F_i)/p(D_x / F_i)$ in expression (16). When these ratios are actually zero, then $p(D_x / F_1 \cap \ldots F_n) = 1$ providing a perfectly accurate result.

If $p(F_i / D)$ or $p(D / F_i)$ is not known for some values of 'i' then the expressions still hold true for the value of 'i' that provides the lowest *known* likelihood or likelihood ratio. It should be noted that expression (14) provides an estimate of the upper bound of the likelihood ratio of the total evidence (i.e. all the symptoms, signs and test results etc.) and thus expressions (14) and (16) estimate the lower bound of the probability of the diagnosis given the total evidence even though many of these findings will not be used in the calculation.

Expressions (14) and (16) are inequalities but if the lowest known likelihood ratio is assumed (by a '*dependence*' assumption) to be EQUAL to the likelihood ratio for the total evidence, then expression (14) provides an

---

† Expressions (14) and (16) are approximations based on an assumption of 'likelihood equivalence', which is only known to be true when $p(F_i / D_j)$ or $p(D_j / F_i)$ or $p(F_L / D_0)$ or $p(D_0 / F_L)$ are zero. The assumption of 'likelihood equivalence' assumes that a likelihood ratio of $p(F_i / D_j)/p(F_i / D_x) = x/y$ or x.k/y.k give the same probability of $p(D_x / F_1 \cap \ldots F_n)$. This will also be true for example when there is statistical independence between $p(F_i / D_j)$ and the remaining findings in $p(F_1 \cap \ldots F_n)$ and $p(F_i / D_x)$ and the remaining findings in $p(F_1 \cap \ldots F_n)$.

estimate of the probability of the diagnosis given the total evidence. Thus the 'inequality' (14) after a dependence assumption becomes an 'equality':

$$(17) \quad p(D_x / (F_1 \cap \ldots F_n) =$$

$$\left\{ 1 + \frac{\sum^m_{j=1,\ j\neq x} p(D_j) . p(F_i / D_j)_{[i \text{ giving lowest likelihood ratio}]}}{p(D_x) . p(F_i / D_x)} + \frac{p(D_0 / F_L)}{p(D_x / F_L)} \right\}^{-1}$$

and the 'inequality' (17) gives rise to the 'equality' (18):

$$(18) \quad p(D_x / (F_1 \cap \ldots F_n) = \left\{ 1 + \frac{\sum^m_{j=1,\ j\neq x} p(D_j / F_i)_{[i \text{ giving lowest probability ratio}]}}{p(D_x / F_i)} + \frac{p(D_0 / F_L)}{p(D_x / F_L)} \right\}^{-1} .$$

The principle of using the most highly predictive combination of findings (which can be described as the 'central' or 'most relevant' evidence) as an estimate of the probability given the total evidence can be regarded as a 'heuristic' that simplifies the interpretation of the 'total evidence'.

A further assumption of statistical independence can be made between $p(F_i / D_j) / p(F_i / D_x)$ and $p(F_{i+1} / D_j) / p(F_{i+1} / D_x)$ in expression (17) when F_{i+1} provides the next lowest likelihood ratio to that provided by F_i. Expression (17) will then become:

$$(19) \quad p(D_x / (F_1 \cap \ldots F_n) \approx \left\{ 1 + \frac{\sum^m_{j=1,\ j\neq x} p(D_j) . p(F_i / D_j) . p(F_{i+1} / D_j)}{p(D_x) . p(F_i / D_x) . p(F_{i+1} / D_x)} + \frac{p(D_0 / F_L)}{p(D_x / F_L)} \right\}^{-1} .$$

By applying the same assumption to expression (18) we get:

$$(20) \quad p(D_x / (F_1 \cap \ldots F_n) \approx \left\{ 1 + \frac{\sum^m_{j=1,\ j\neq x} p(D_j / F_i) \ p(F_{i+1} / D_j)}{p(D_x / F_i) . p(F_{i+1} / D_x)} + \frac{p(D_0 / F_L)}{p(D_x / F_L)} \right\}^{-1} .$$

An assumption of statistical independence can be made between any number of $p(F_i / D_j)$ and $p(F_i / D_x)$ up to 'n'. When the maximum of 'n–1' such assumptions are made we get the following result from expression (17):

$$(21) \quad p(D_x / (F_1 \cap \ldots F_n) \approx \left\{ 1 + \frac{\sum^m_{j=1,\ j\neq x} p(D_j)_{i=1} \prod^n p(F_i / D_j)}{p(D_x)_{i=1} \prod^n p(F_i / D_x)} + \frac{p(D_0 / F_L)}{p(D_x / F_L)} \right\}^{-1} .$$

The corresponding result from expression (18) is:

$$(22) \quad p(D_x / (F_1 \cap \ldots F_n) \approx \left\{ 1 + \frac{\sum^m_{j=1,\ j\neq x} p(D_j / F_i)_{i+1} \prod^n p(F_{i+1} / D_j)}{p(D_x / F_i)_{i+1} \prod^n p(F_{i+1} / D_x)} + \frac{p(D_0 / F_L)}{p(D_x / F_L)} \right\}^{-1} .$$

The value of $p(D_x/F_1 \cap \ldots F_n)$ can be estimated for each D_j in turn using any of the above approaches and each $p(D_x/F_1 \cap \ldots F_n)$ divided by the sum of all the $p(D_x/F_1 \cap \ldots F_n)$ for different values of x from 1 to m to give a normalised estimate $p_{ne}(D_x/F_1 \cap \ldots F_n)$ where they all sum to 1.

The probability estimates arising from any of the expressions given here can be calibrated against the frequency of correct predictions.

These expressions and their proofs have also been published elswhere.[2,3,4]

References

1. Llewelyn DEH, Garcia-Puig J (2004) How different urinary albumin excretion rates can predict progression to nephropathy and the effect of treatment in hypertensive diabetics. *J Renin Angiotensin Aldosterone Syst* 5, 141–5.
2. Llewelyn, DEH (1979). Mathematical analysis of the diagnostic relevance of clinical findings. *Clin Sci* 57, 477–9.
3. Llewelyn, DEH (1981). Applying the principle of logical elimination to probabilistic diagnosis. *Med Inform* 6, 25–32.
4. Llewelyn, DEH (1988). Assessing the validity of diagnostic tests and clinical decisions. MD thesis. University of London.

Index

A

abdomen 52
see also under
  gastrointestinal
  symptoms and physical
  signs
abdominal:
aortic aneurysm or
  dissection, ruptured
  355, 361, 362
aortic dissection 326
bruising 355
bruit 384
movement, poor 356
pain
  acute, in children 329
  acute central 326
  acute lateral 327
  acute lower central
    (hypogastric) 328
  acute pain in upper
    abdomen 324
  non-specific 300, 623,
    624, 626, 627, 628,
    629, 630
  recurrent, in children 330
  severe upper abdominal
    pain 176
striae 112
veins, distended 354
see also under
  gastrointestinal
  symptoms and physical
  signs
abducent (6th cranial nerve)
  paresis 504
abscess 107
  acute 102, 103
  dental 95
  subcutaneous 95
  tuberculoid ('cold') 102,
    103
acanthosis nigricans 126,
  132, 170
ACE inhibitors 250
achalasia 295, 296
  progressive 322
acne 130, 134
  vulgaris 148
acromegaly 80, 208, 252
acromio-clavicular joint 434
ACTH deficiency 466
actinic prurigo 164
activities of daily living:
  history taking 38

inability to carry out
  the 456
acuity, loss of 497
acute coronary syndrome
  324
acute respiratory distress
  syndrome 590, 592
Addison's disease 114, 170,
  210, 290, 304, 308,
  466, 556
adenosis, sclerosing 107
adhesive capsulitis 434
adrenal:
  adenoma 112, 292
  carcinoma 111, 112
  disease, primary 466
  failure 466
  hyperplasia 557
aerotitis 78
agoraphobia 458
agranulocytosis 92, 320
  clinical opinion 46
  investigations 31
  problem-structuring notes
    30, 37, 39, 41
AIDS 116
albinism 172
albumin states, low 194,
  220, 268
alcohol:
  abuse 568
  intake, high 108
  withdrawal 458, 466,
    480, 515
alcoholism 116, 290
aldosteronism 554
alimentary:
  symptoms 34
  system 52
alkaline phosphatase, raised
  562
allergic contact dermatitis
  154, 156
allergy 411
  conjunctivitis 86
alopecia:
  areata 74
  totalis 74
alveolar cell carcinoma 590
alveolitis, fibrosing 66
Alzheimer's disease 468
amenorrhoea, secondary
  406
amyloidosis 366, 370, 374
anaemia 242, 476
  acquired haemolytic 312

of chronic disease 570
clinical 90
haemolytic 370
hereditary haemolytic 312
hypoplastic or aplastic
  90, 146
iron deficiency 567
macrocytic 90, 484, 566,
  568
microcytic 90, 484, 566,
  567
normocytic 90, 484,
  566, 570
of pregnancy 570
severe 200, 205
sideroblastic 567
anal:
  fissure 342, 348, 351
    acute 390
  swelling 390
anaphylaxis 178, 184, 238,
  240, 274, 282, 286, 308
anarthria 489
aneurysm 215
  anterior communicating
    artery 512
  aortic 376, 384
  dissecting thoracic aortic
    174, 215
  femoral artery 386
  subclavian cavity 104
  ventricular 224
    left 610, 612–13
angina 174
angiodysplasia 396
angioedema, hereditary
  160
angle-closure glaucoma,
  acute 86, 470
anisocoria 503
ankle swelling:
  bilateral 194, 220
  unilateral 218
ankylosing spondylitis 424
anomalies, congenital 76
anorectal pain 351
anorexia nervosa 116, 458
anterior cruciate ligament
  tears 446
antibiotic-induced bacterial
  opportunists 332
antifolate drugs 568
anxiety 154
  acute 458
  disorder, generalized 458
  hyperventilation 476

anxiety (Cont.)
  with semi-voluntary
    resistance 72
  state 515
aorta:
  coarctation 215
  dissecting 384
aortic:
  aneurysm 376, 384, 606,
    609
  arch syndrome 214
  incompetence 205, 228
  sclerosis 230
  stenosis 188, 206, 230
  supravalvular 214
apex:
  impulse, abnormal 224
  and palpating hand, fat,
    fluid, or air between
    224
aphasia 489
aphonia 489
aphthous ulcers, local 92
appendicitis 327, 363
  acute 300, 329
  'common cause' 628
  elimination, reasoning by
    623, 624
  likelihood ratios 626, 627
  numerical test results,
    reasoning with 630
  statistical independence
    versus statistical
    dependence 629
appendix mass 377
Argyll Robinson pupil 503
Aristotle's syllogism 620,
  621
arm 49
  see also under psychiatric
    and neurological
    symptoms and physical
    signs
arterial obstruction 197
arteriosclerosis 205
arthritis:
  acute 446
  acute septic 426
  reactive 426
  septic 434
  tuberculous 442
  see also osteoarthritis;
    rheumatoid: arthritis
ascites 352
asthma 180, 596
  chronic 250
  exacerbation 184, 240,
    286
  precipitated by allergens
    242
  severe 274
athletic heart 202

atrial:
  ectopics 204
  fibrillation 182, 204, 222
    with cerebral embolus 482
  flutter with variable heart
    block 204
  septal defect 230, 610
auditory canal trauma 80
auscultation 51, 52
autoimmune diseases 88, 91

B

B$_{12}$ deficiency 568
Bacillus cereus 332
back pain see under joint,
  limb, and back symptoms
  and signs
bacteraemia 466
bacterial:
  endocarditis 571
  infection:
    conjunctivitis 86
    severe 571
Baker's cyst, ruptured
  192, 218
barotrauma 78
Bartholin's cyst 412
basal cell carcinoma 95, 132,
  134, 162, 168
Bayes' rule 620, 621, 625,
  626, 636
Bazin's disease 144
Beau's lines 64
Becker's melanocytic naevus
  166
Bell's palsy 508
benign:
  essential tremor 515, 516
  positional vertigo 478
  tumours 582
berloque dermatitis 126
β-agonist treatment 557
biceps, rupture of long head
  of 434
bigemini, ventricular or
  supraventricular 202
bile duct stones, common
  316, 552
biochemistry 59
bipolar disorder 464
bites, insect 130, 138
bladder:
  calculus 400
  distension 378, 380
    acute 357
  'neurogenic' 402
  'spastic', due to upper
    motor neurone lesion
    400
  tumour 404
blisters 138

blood:
  gas disturbance,
    appearance suggestive
    of 255
  passage of rectally 348
  pressure see under
    cardiovascular
    symptoms and physical
    signs; hypertension;
    hypotension
  tests 59
  transfusion, recent 556
  volume, low circulating
    210, 212
bone:
  disease, adjacent 524
  marrow failure 570
  metastases 558, 562
botulism 332
bowel:
  chronic infection of 340
  habit, change in 344
  infarction 382
  sounds, high-pitched 383
Bowen's disease 150
brachial plexus lesion 518
bradycardia 202, 205
brain:
  injury 487
  stem dysfunction, severe
    502
  stem ischaemia or
    infarction 478
  tumour 480
branchial cyst 102
breast lump(s) 107
breath sounds, reduced 274
breathing, bronchial 277
breathlessness:
  acute 184
    with wheeze ± cough
      240
  chronic 242
  sudden, onset over
    seconds 178, 238
Briquet's syndrome 458
bronchial carcinoma 66, 108,
  600, 602
bronchiectasis 66, 244, 280,
  594, 596
bronchitis:
  acute bacterial 248
  acute viral 248
  bacterial 184, 240, 244
  chronic 248, 278
  viral 184, 240, 244
  wheezy 286
bronchoconstriction 274
bronchopneumonia, bilateral
  604
bronchus carcinoma 579,
  582, 584

brucella 370
buccal mucosa 114
bulbar palsy 322
bulimia nervosa 458
bullae 598, 599
  large 272, 276
bullous:
  drug eruption 140
  impetigo 140
  myringitis 78
burns:
  chemical 138, 142
  sunburn 142
  thermal 138, 142
bursitis 446
  post-calcaneal 450
  prepatellar 446

C

C5 posterior root lesion 533
C5/6 prolapsed disc 436
C5/6 root lesion 522
  posterior 539
C6 posterior root lesion 533
C6/7 prolapsed disc 436
C7 root lesion 522
  anterior 514
  posterior 534
C7/8 posterior root lesion
  539
C8/T1 root lesion 522
C-reactive protein, very
  high 571
cachectic 116
caecum carcinoma 377
café-au-lait spot 126
calcaneal tendon tear 450
calcaneum disease 450
calf, unilateral swelling 192
calorie intake:
  excessive 292
  low 116
Campbell-de-Morgan spots
  130, 168
Campylobacter enteritis 335
cancer somewhere 68
Candida albicans 411
candidiasis 92, 148, 156, 320
  investigations 31
capsule cerebral lesion,
  internal 490
capsulitis, adhesive 434
carbon dioxide:
  narcosis 256
  retention 255, 516
carcinoid syndrome 338
carcinoma rectum 348
carcinomatosis 381
carcinomatous
  neuromyopathy 542
cardiac:

arrhythmia 180, 238
contractility, poor 206
failure, congestive 220,
  222, 292, 302, 381
output:
  examination 50
  low 197
silhouette, abnormal 606
cardiogenic low output
  210, 212
cardiomyopathy 226, 610
cardiovascular symptoms
  and physical signs:
  acute breathlessness,
    wheeze ± cough 184
  ankle swelling, bilateral 194
  apex impulse, abnormal
    224
  blood pressure:
    high—hypertension 208
    postural fall in 212
    very low 210
  blood pressure/pulse:
    difference between
      arms 214
    difference between arm
      and legs 215
  bradycardia 202
  calf or leg swelling,
    unilateral 192
  chest pain—alarming and
    increasing over minutes
    to hours 174
  cough and pink frothy
    sputum 186
  cyanosis:
    central 198
    peripheral 197
  heart sounds, extra 226
  interpreting cardiovascular
    signs 196
  jugular venous pressure,
    raised 222
  leg and ankle swelling:
    bilateral 220
    unilateral 218
  leg pain:
    on standing—relieved by
      lying down 191
    on walking—intermittent
      claudication 190
  leg veins, prominent, ±
    unilateral leg swelling
    216
  lower chest or upper
    abdominal pain, severe
    176
  murmurs:
    diastolic 228
    mid-systolic 230
    not entirely in systole or
      diastole 233

pansystolic 232
orthopnoea and
  paroxysmal nocturnal
  dyspnoea 180
palpitations 182
pulse:
  high volume 205
  irregular 204
  low volume 206
  rate >120bpm 200
sudden breathlessness,
  onset over seconds
  178
syncope 188
systems enquiry 33
cardiovascular system 50
carious teeth 92
carotenaemia 170, 310
carotid:
  body tumour 102
  sinus hypersensitivity 476
  sinus syncope 188
carotinaemia:
  diagnostic pathway 19
  diagnostic table 18
carpal tunnel syndrome
  430, 518
case 45
case history 29
cataract 492, 498
  diabetic 494
'cauliflower' ear 76
cellulitis 142, 192, 218
  bilateral 194
  orbital 84
central nervous system
  diseases 212
cerebellar:
  disease 516, 539
  lesion 490, 521, 540
  ipsilateral 523
  stroke 474
cerebello-pontine lesion
  508, 512
cerebral:
  artery:
    anterior infarction 530
    posterior infarction 530
  embolus 474
  haemorrhage 474
  infarction 474
  ischaemic attack, transient
    474
  lesion 344
cerebrovascular accident 188
cerumen 76
cervical:
  carcinoma 410, 414, 420
  cord trauma 256
  dystonia 436
  ectropion 414
  erosions 420

cervical: (Cont.)
  intraepithelial neoplasia
    414
  nerve root lesion 532
  polyps 414
  rib 436, 518
  root pain, referred 236
  spondylitis:
    acute 72
    with osteophytes,
      chronic 72
  spondylosis 434, 436
    compressing nerve
      root 518
  ulcers and lumps 414
cervicitis 414, 420
chair, difficulty in rising
  from 542
Charcot–Marie–Tooth
  disease 528
chemodectoma 102
chest:
  expansion:
    bilateral poor 260
    unilateral poor 262
  infections 242
  inspection 51
  pain:
    alarming and increasing
      over minutes to
      hours 174
    severe 176
    sharp and aggravated
      by breathing or
      movement 236
  wall:
    abnormalities 258
    bone structure, absence
      of part of 258
    pain 174, 236
  X-rays see radiology
chickenpox 138
  past 586
chlamydia:
  cervicitis 420
  peritonitis 357
chloasma 126, 166
cholangitis, acute 324
cholecystitis:
  acute 298, 324, 357
  numerical test results,
    reasoning with 630
cholestasis 562
cholesteatoma 80, 508
chondrodermatitis nodularis
  168
  chronica helicis 76
  helicis externa 134
chondromalacia patellae 446
choroiditis 499
choroidoretinitis 492,
  498, 499

Christmas disease 146
chronic fatigue syndrome
  484
chronic obstructive
  pulmonary disease 116,
  180, 242, 250, 596, 597
  exacerbation 184, 240
cirrhosis 366, 372, 381
  alcoholic 316, 552
  hepatic 66, 68, 108, 268,
    292
  primary biliary 161, 170,
    316, 366, 552
  shifting dullness 381
claudication 190
  intermittent 190
claw toes 450
clinical opinions 46
clinical trial:
  ideal 16
  stratifying diagnostic and
    treatment criteria by
    analysis of 633
closed-angle glaucoma, acute
  86, 470
Clostridium difficile 332
Clostridium perfringens 332
clotting disorder 146
clubbing 64, 66
coagulopathy:
  acquired 118
  congenital 118
coccydynia 351
coeliac disease 340
cognitive impairment 468
colic:
  biliary 176
  infantile 329
colitis
  infective 328
  see also ulcerative: colitis
colon/colonic:
  carcinoma 334, 342, 344,
    348, 396
  of descending or sigmoid
    379
  descending, tumour of 350
colorectal carcinoma 334
'common cause' 628
common peroneal nerve
  lesion 526
communicating artery
  aneurysm, anterior 512
condylomata acuminata 412
confirmatory evidence see
  evidence: that confirms a
  diagnosis
confusion:
  acute 466
  chronic 468
congenital:
  anomalies 76

enzyme defect:
  diagnostic table 18
  diagnostic pathway 19
heart disease 66
ptosis 500
vasculopathy 118
congestive cardiac failure
  220, 222, 292, 302, 381
conjunctivitis 86
Conn's syndrome 208,
  554, 557
consciousness, disturbed
  487
consent 21
consolidation 576, 578
  due to bacterial infection
    270, 276, 277, 278
  extensive 262, 267
constipation 330, 342
contact, prolonged 122
context information,
  faulty 22
contralateral:
  cortical lesion 532, 536
  pyramidal tract lesion
    538, 540
cor pulmonale 220, 222
corneal:
  opacity in quiet eye 492
  ulcer 86
coronary syndrome, acute
  174
corrosives, ingestion of
  346, 392
cortical lesion 490
  contralateral 532, 536
cortico-cavernous fistula
  84
coryza 491
cough 184, 186
  breathlessness, acute 240
  persistent dry, with no
    sputum 250
  with sputum 248
  syncope 188
cow's milk protein
  intolerance 340
coxa vara 442
crackles:
  coarse 280
  fine inspiratory 278
cranial:
  arteritis 472, 497
  nerve lesions 512
  nerves 56
C-reactive protein, very
  high 571
creatinine, raised 564
Creutzfeldt–Jakob disease
  468
Crigler–Najjar syndrome
  313

Crohn's disease:
acute central abdominal
pain 326
clubbing 66
passage of blood rectally
348, 396
polyarthritis 428
recurrent diarrhoea 334
Crohn's granuloma 377
croup 282
CSF:
low pressure 470
otorrhoea 80
Curtis–Fitz-Hugh syndrome
357
Cushing's syndrome:
abdominal striae 112
difficulty in rising from
chair or squatting
position 542
hirsutism 111
hyperpigmentation 170
hypertension 208
obesity 113
pigmented creases and
flexures 114
striking facial appearance
80
weight gain 292
cyanosis:
central 198
peripheral 197
cystic fibrosis 340
cystic hygroma 102, 103
cystitis 357, 400, 401,
403, 404
due to bacterial infection
328
cystocoele 413
cysts 107
epidermal 168
sebaceous 134
cytotoxic drugs 75

D

Darier's disease 132
De Quervain's syndrome
430
deafness 489
decision analysis 16
proportion syllogism 620
decision trees 16
deep vein thrombosis 192,
216, 218, 220
dehydration:
clinical opinion 46
problem-structuring
note 43
delusions 464
dementia 402
dental abscess 95

depression 154, 290, 344,
455, 462, 484
agitated 458
major 462
psychotic 464
manic 464
mild to moderate 462
secondary 462
severe 402
dermatitis:
allergic contact 154, 156
atopic 138
berloque 126
contact 138
herpetiformis associated
with gluten enteropathy
140, 148, 156
seborrhoeic 150, 156
dermatofibroma 134, 168
dermatomyositis 162
dermatosis, juvenile plantar
150
developmental history 27
dextrocardia 224
diabetes:
insipidus with
hypovolaemia 554
mellitus 68, 484
clinical opinion 46
confirmatory findings
based on general
evidence 10
diagnostic criteria 632
gastroparesis 298
hyponatraemia 555
laboratory tests 547
problem-structuring
notes 37, 39, 41, 43
undiagnosed or
uncontrolled 290
diabetic:
amyotrophy 542
autonomic neuropathy 338
hard exudates 494
ketoacidosis 304, 556
macular exudates 494
microalbuminuria 632, 633,
634, 635
micro-aneurysm 494
nephropathy 633
new vessel 494
ophthalmoscopy 494
soft exudates 494
diagnosis:
in dermatology 124
dynamic 20
explaining to patients 21
and hypotheses and
theories 15
ruled in 10
ruled out 10
writing the 44

diagnostic classifications 18
diagnostic criteria 616
stratified 632–4
diagnostic cut-off points 635
diagnostic errors:
faulty context information
22
faulty information
gathering and
processing 23
faulty triggering 22
faulty verification 22
minimizing 22
no fault errors 23
diagnostic leads:
changing 7
differentiating between
diagnoses 6
'transparent' reasoning 5
useful 3
diagnostic pathways 18
jaundice 19
diagnostic process:
changing diagnostic leads 7
confirmatory findings
based on general
evidence 10
confirming a diagnosis 8
diagnoses, hypotheses, and
theories 15
diagnostic classifications,
pathways, and tables 18
differentiating between
diagnoses 6
dynamic diagnoses 20
evidence-based diagnosis
and plan 13
see also evidence-based
diagnosis and plan
evidence that 'suggests' a
diagnosis 9
explaining a diagnostic
thought process 12
explaining diagnoses to
patients 21
findings that suggest
diagnoses based on
general evidence 11
imagining an ideal clinical
trial 16
informed consent 21
medical and surgical
sieves 14
minimizing diagnostic
errors 22
purpose of this book 2
reasoning:
'intuitive' 4
'transparent' 5
understanding others'
reasoning 2
using this book 3

diagnostic reasoning:
checking 2
transparent 2
understanding others'
reasoning 2
diagnostic tables 18
jaundice 18
diarrhoea:
chronic 557
in children 340
traveller's 336
see also under
gastrointestinal
symptoms and physical
signs
diastolic murmurs 228
diathesis, bleeding 392, 404,
408, 544
diet, change in 342, 344
differential likelihood ratio
11, 625, 626–7, 628, 636
diffuse oesophageal spasm
(intermittent) 322
diffuse poorly defined hazy
opacification 590
digoxin 108
diplopia 504
disc:
prolapse 436, 529
protrusion 191, 438
dissecting:
abdominal aortic aneurysm
215, 355, 361, 362
aorta 384
thoracic aortic aneurysm
174, 215
disseminated intravascular
coagulation 146
diuretic therapy 557
diverticular abscess 379
diverticular disease 334
diverticulitis 334, 348,
363, 396
numerical test results,
reasoning with 630
dizziness 476
dorsal column loss 536, 540
drug/drug effects:
bullous drug eruption 140
confusion, acute 466
constipation 342
dizziness 476
dysarthria 490
eczema 156
eruptions 142
fatigue 484
gait abnormality 540
headache 473
hepatitis 314
hyperkalaemia 556
hyperkeratosis, scales and
plaques 152

hyperpigmentation 170
hypertension 208
large pupil with no ptosis
502
lymphadenopathy:
axillary 110
generalized 120
photosensitivity 164
phototoxicity 142
purpura 118
purpura and petechiae 146
pustules 148
small pupil with no ptosis
503
thrombocytopenia 146
vomiting 308
weight gain 292
drug/drugs:
abuse 116
bradycardia 202
galactorrhoea 105
history 27, 38
-induced symptoms:
ankle swelling, bilateral
194
blood pressure fall 212
bowel habit 344
diarrhoea 338
jaundice 316
ototoxicity 478
overdose 304
pulse rate 200
radiology 576
reactions and allergies 128
polyarthritis 428
respiratory rate 256
see also drug/drug effects
Dubin–Johnson syndrome
316, 552
duct:
ectasia 106
papilloma 106
ductal cancer 107
ductus arteriosus, patent
233
dullness:
central 380
shifting 381
duodenal ulcer 298, 361
bleeding 346, 392
perforated 630
Dupuytren's contracture 430
dynamic diagnoses 20
dysarthria 489, 490
dysentery:
amoebic 335
bacillary 335
dysphagia:
for fluids and solids 322
for fluids and solids which
do not stick 319
for solids which stick 318

dysphonia 489
dysplasia, developmental
442
dystrophia myotonica 500
dystrophy, hereditary 542
dysuria 400, 403

E

ear:
discharging 80
external abnormalities 76
foreign bodies 76
painful 78
swimmer's 78
echinococcus 582
ectopic:
ACTH secretion 114
parathyroid hormone 558
pregnancy 302, 328,
363, 416
thyroid tissue 98
ectropion:
cervical 414
cervical erosions 420
eczema:
acute 138
asteatotic 156
atopic 150
contact 150
discoid 156
drug-induced 156
herpeticum 156
seborrhoeic 154
varicose 156
elbow:
lumps around 71
pain or limitation of
movement at the 432
electrolyte disturbance
200, 202
severe 480
elimination, reasoning by
622
evidence for a finding's role
in 625
example 623
probability of replication
estimation 636
proof of theorem 638
'stratified' diagnostic
criteria 632
using very low frequencies
or probability densities
624
emphysema 260, 272,
276, 278
mediastinal 610
see also chronic obstructive
pulmonary disease
empyema 66, 268, 576
encephalitis 472

endobronchial:
carcinoma 284
obstruction 274
endocarditis 146
bacterial 66, 69, 370
endocervicitis 420
endocrine findings *see*
general and endocrine
findings
endocrine symptoms 32
endometrial:
carcinoma 408, 410
polyp 420
proliferation 416
tuberculosis 416
endometriosis 408
endometritis 415
Entamoeba histolytica 335
enterocoele 413
environment, change in 342
enzyme defect, congenital:
diagnostic pathway 19
diagnostic table 18
ependymoma in spinal
cord 512
epicondylitis 432
epidermolysis bullosa 140
epididymal cyst 388
epididymitis:
acute 388
chronic 388
epigastrium:
localized tenderness 361
masses in 376
epiglottitis 282
epilepsy 188, 306, 476
due to meningitis 480
due to old brain scar
tissue 480
idiopathic epilepsy—new
presentation 480
known idiopathic 480
temporal lobe 478
epileptic fits 402
episcleritis 86
episodic heart block 182
Erb's palsy 522
erythema 142
ab igne 142
chronicum migrans 144
induratum 144
multiforme 140
due to sarcoidosis 142
nodosum 134, 144
palmar 142
viral toxic 142
erythrocyte sedimentation
rate, very high 571
erythroderma 152
Escherichia coli:
enteroinvasive 335
enterotoxigenic 336

type 0157
(enterohaemorrhagic)
335
essential tremor, benign
515, 516
euthyroid goitre 99
evidence 9
general 9, 10–11
particular 9
that confirms a diagnosis
6, 8, 9
that suggests a diagnosis
6, 9
evidence-based diagnosis
and plan 13
Bayes' and other rules 620
clinical trials analysis to
'stratify' diagnostic and
treatment criteria 633
'common cause', findings
that lead to a 628
decisions 616
'differential' and 'overall'
likelihood ratios, things
that affect 627
differential likelihood
ratios make use of
'complementing'
differentiation 626
elimination, reasoning
by 622
evidence for a finding's
role in 625
example 623
probability of replication
estimation 636
'stratified' diagnostic
criteria 632
using very low
frequencies or
probability densities
624
hypotheses, reasoning
with 637
improving treatments by
better patient selection
or 'stratification' 634
numerical test results,
reasoning with 630
probabilities:
grappling with 617
picturing 618
probability elimination
theorem, proof for
reasoning by 638
statistical independence
versus statistical
dependence 629
treatment indication and
diagnostic cut-off
points, studies to
establish 635

examination:
alimentary and
genitourinary systems
52
blood and urine test
results 59
cardiovascular system 50
chest X-ray appearances,
abnormal 60
general 48–9
investigations, interpreting
the 42
mental state 58
motor function 57
nervous system 54, 56
neurological system 56
physical 40, 48–9
problem-structuring
note 43
respiratory system 51
'routine' physical 48–9
sensation 57
exanthema, viral 128
exercise, strenuous, normal
response to 424
exophthalmos 84
exostosis 76
explaining a diagnostic
thought process 12
extension injuries, neck 436
extradural haemorrhage 474
extrapyramidal dysarthria
490
exudates 268
eye:
exophthalmos 84
general examination 49
iritis (anterior uveitis) 88
opening 488
proptosis 84
red 86
strain 473

F

face 49
see also facial
facial:
appearance, striking 82
canal lesion 512
lump 95
muscle weakness 508
nerve palsy 508
from brain stem
ischaemia 508
from parotid swelling 508
nerve swelling, from
demyelination 508
sensation, loss of 506
faecal impaction 352, 379,
383
with overflow 338, 402

Fallopian tubes 416
falsifying facts 15
family history 36
　plan for writing out the
　　history 27
fat necrosis 107
fatigue—'tired all the time'
　484
faulty:
　context information 22
　information gathering and
　　processing 23
　triggering 22
　verification 22
febrile convulsion 480
febrile illness, non-specific
　546
femoral:
　artery aneurysm 386
　epiphysis, slipped 442
　hernia 386
　nerve see L1/2; L3/4
　nerve lesion 526
fever 91, 200
fibroadenoma 107
fibroids 352, 408, 416
fibromyalgia 424
fibrosis, severe 270
finger:
　melaena 392
　vasculitic nodules 69
fingernail:
　abnormalities 64–9
　clubbing 66
　fold infarcts 64, 69
　pitting 64
　Terry's lines 68
fit 480
　epileptic 402
flail segment following
　trauma 262
flank, resonance in 380
flatus (gas) 352
fluid:
　intake, poor 342
　overload 560
　volume overload 222
foetus 352
folate deficiency 568
folliculitis 148
food poisoning 300, 332
foot:
　movements, bilateral
　　weakness of all 528
　pain or limitation of
　　movement 450
foreign bodies 420
　in ear 76
　inhaled 178, 238, 282,
　　283, 284
frank haemoptysis (sputum
　streaking) 244

freckles 126, 166, 170
　Hutchinson's 126
frontal lobe:
　lesion 466
　tumour 491
frozen shoulder 434
'functional' fit 480
fungal infection 150, 154
furunculosis 78

G

gait:
　abnormality 540
　arms, legs, spine (GALS)
　　system 54
galactorrhoea 105
gallbladder, distended 375
gallstone colic 324
ganglion 430
gastric:
　carcinoma 295, 324, 346,
　　376, 392
　erosion 346, 392
　outlet obstruction 298
　ulcer 298, 361, 392
　　bleeding 346
gastritis 176, 298, 324, 361
gastroenteritis 300, 308, 329
　viral 332
gastrointestinal bleed,
　massive upper 348
gastrointestinal symptoms
　and physical signs:
　abdomen:
　　central, acute pain in 326
　　central, localized
　　　tenderness in 361
　　children, acute pain
　　　in 329
　　children, recurrent pain
　　　in 330
　　distended 352
　　lateral, acute pain in 327
　　lower, acute pain in 328
　　silent, with no bowel
　　　sounds 382
　　upper, acute pain in 324
　abdominal:
　　bruising 355
　　/loin bruit 384
　　movement, poor 356
　　veins, distended 354
　anal swelling 390
　anorectal pain 351
　bilateral mass in upper
　　abdomen 374
　blood, passage of rectally
　　348
　bowel habit, change in 344
　bowel sounds, high-pitched
　　383

constipation 342
diarrhoea:
　acute bloody, ± mucus—
　　'dysentery' 335
　chronic, in children 340
　recurrent, with blood
　　± mucus—bloody
　　flux 334
　recurrent, with no blood
　　in the stools, no
　　fever 338
　sudden, with fever and
　　vomiting 332
　watery 336
dullness:
　central, resonance in
　　flank 380
　shifting 381
dysphagia:
　for fluids and solids 322
　for fluids and solids that
　　do not stick 319
　for solids that stick 318
epigastrium:
　localized tenderness
　　in 361
　mass in (umbilical area)
　　376
groin, lump in the 386
haematemesis ± melaena
　346
hepatomegaly:
　irregular, not tender 368
　smooth and tender 364
　smooth but not tender
　　366
hypogastrium, localized
　tenderness in 357
jaundice 310
　hepatic, due to
　　congenital enzyme
　　defect 313
　hepatocellular 314
　obstructive 316
　pre-hepatic, due to
　　haemolysis 312
left upper quadrant,
　localized tenderness
　in 360
loin, localized tenderness
　in 362
mass:
　in hypogastrium 378
　in lower quadrant 377,
　　379
　in upper quadrant 375
melaena on finger 392
prostate enlargement 391
quadrant, lower, localized
　tenderness in 363
rectal examination, fresh
　blood on finger in 396

right upper quadrant, localized tenderness in 358
scrotal swelling 388
splenomegaly:
  massive 373
  moderate 372
  slight 370
tenesmus 350
throat, sore 320
vomiting 294
  alone 308
  shortly after food 298
  with abdominal pain alone— non-metabolic causes 302
  with abdominal pain alone—metabolic causes 304
  with abdominal pain and fever 300
  with headache 306
  with weight loss 295
  without weight loss 296
weight gain 292
weight loss, unintentional, over weeks or months 290
gastro-oesophageal reflux 176, 250, 346, 392
gastroparesis 298
Gaussian distribution 630
general and endocrine findings:
  abdominal striae 112
  anaemia, clinical 90
  anterior triangle, lump in 102
  body temperature, low 91
  breast lump(s) 107
  clubbing 66
  ear:
    abnormalities, external 76
    discharging 80
    painful 78
  elbow, lumps around the 71
  eye:
    proptosis or exophthalmos 84
    red 86
  facial:
    appearance, striking 82
    lump 95
  fever 91
  fingernail abnormality 64
galactorrhoea 105
general principles 62
groin lymphadenopathy, localized 122

gynaecomastia 108
hair loss:
  diffuse 75
  in specific area 74
hand arthropathy 70
hirsutism in female 111
iritis 88
lymphadenopathy 120
  axillary 110
mouth lesions 92
neck lump:
  anterior 98
  bilateral 100
  moving with swallowing but not with tongue 99
neck stiffness 72
nipple abnormality 106
obesity 113
parotid swelling 94
pharynx and tonsils, red 93
pigmented creases and flexures 114
posterior triangle of neck, lump in 103
pressure sores 122
purpura 118
spider naevi 115
submandibular lump 96
supraclavicular lump(s) 104
Terry's lines 68
thin, wasted, cachectic 116
thyroid nodule, solitary 101
vasculitic nodules on fingers 69
general examination 48–9
  see also general and endocrine findings
genitourinary:
  symptoms 34
  see also urological and gynaecological symptoms and physical signs
  system 52
giant cell arteritis 472, 497, 571
giant papillary conjunctivitis 86
Gilbert's syndrome 313
gingivitis 92
glandular fever 92, 120, 314, 320, 364, 370
  clinical opinion 46
  investigations 31
  problem-structuring notes 30, 37, 39, 41, 43
Glasgow Coma Scale 54, 487
glaucoma 492, 498
  acute 306

  acute closed-angle 86, 470
  diabetic 494
glenohumeral joint, osteoarthritis 434
glioma in spinal cord 529
globus pharyngeus 319
glomerulonephritis 544, 546
glossopharyngeal (9th cranial) nerve lesion 511
glucocorticoid steroid therapy 80, 112
glycosuria 547
goitre 99, 100
  retrosternal 606, 607
gonococcal cervicitis 420
gout 142, 426
gouty tophi 71, 134
Gradenigo's syndrome 512
granulomas 134, 252
Graves' disease 80, 84, 100, 504
groin:
  lump 386
  lymphadenopathy, localized 122
Guillain–Barré syndrome 256, 260, 528
guttate psoriasis 130, 150
gynaecomastia 108

H

haemarthrosis, traumatic 426
haematemesis 346
  false 346, 392
haematocoele 388
haematology 59
haematometra 416
haematuria:
  microscopic 544
  painful 403
  painless 404
haemochromatosis 366
haemoglobin:
  abnormalities 198
  low 566
haemolysis 568, 570
  septicaemic 312
  in specimen bottle, spurious result due to 556
haemolytic uraemic syndrome 300
haemophilia 146
haemorrhage 197, 200
  retroperitoneal 355
haemorrhagic:
  stroke 306
  telangiectasia, hereditary 92

haemorrhoids 342, 351, 396
  bleeding 348
  prolapsed internal 390
hair loss:
  diffuse 75
  in specific area 74
hallux:
  rigidus 450
  valgus 450
halo melanocytic naevus 166
hammer toes 450
hand:
  arthropathy 70
  coarse tremor 516
  diminished sensation 534
  fine tremor 515
  general examination 49
  pain or limitation of
    movement 430
  at rest, odd posture of 514
  tapping 523
  wasting of small muscles
    518
hand, foot, and mouth
  disease 138
Hashimoto's thyroiditis 100
head:
  general examination 49
  injury 256
    with cerebral contusion
      470
  lice 154
headache see migraine; and
  under psychiatric and
  neurological symptoms
  and physical signs
hearing loss 510
  see also deafness
heart:
  athletic 202
  block:
    complete 222
    episodic 182
    variable, with atrial flutter
      204
    Wenkenbach 204
  disease, cyanotic
    congenital 66
  examination 50
  failure 200, 226
    congestive 68
    right 314, 364, 550
  normal young 226
  sounds, extra 226
Heberden's nodes 134
hemidiaphragm, elevated
  270
hemiparesis 530
Henoch–Schönlein purpura
  146
hepatic:
  carcinoma 302

failure 516
  jaundice due to congenital
    enzyme defect:
    diagnostic pathway 19
    diagnostic table 18
hepatitis 568
  A 300, 370
    acute viral 314, 357, 550
    acute alcoholic 357
  alcoholic 314, 316, 364,
    550, 552
  B 300, 357, 370
    acute 314, 550
  C 357, 370
    acute 314, 550
  D 357, 370
  drug-induced 314, 550
  E 357
  infectious 364
hepatoma 368
  primary 368, 550
hepatomegaly see under
  gastrointestinal
  symptoms and physical
  signs
hernia:
  femoral 386
  hiatus 324, 346, 392, 610
    sliding 308
  inguinal 386
    descended into scrotum
      388
  strangulated 386
hernial orifice strangulation
  383
herpes:
  simplex 138, 148, 412
  zoster 138, 148, 154, 478
herpetic whitlow 138
hiatus hernia 324, 346,
  392, 610
  sliding 308
hilar shadowing, abnormal:
  homogeneous 600
  streaky 604
hip:
  congenital dislocation 442
  pain or limitation of
    movement of the 442
  replacement, problems
    442
hirsutism in a female 111
histoplasmosis 582
history of presenting
  complaints 27
history taking skills:
  case history, interpreting
    the 29
  completed history 38
  drug history 38
  past medical history 36
  plan 26, 27

problem-structuring note
  30, 37, 39, 41, 43
sore throat 31
systems enquiry 32
thoughtful 26
HIV infection 142, 338
hoarseness 252
  functional 252
Hodgkin's or non-Hodgkin's
  lymphoma 102, 103, 120,
  161, 366, 372, 386, 600,
  602, 606
Hoffa's fat pad syndrome
  446
Holmes–Adie pupil 502
Horner's syndrome 500
housemaid's knee 446
Huntington's chorea 80, 468
Hutchinson's freckle 126
hydatid cyst 368, 582
hydranitis suppurativa 148
hydrocoele 388
hydronephroses:
  bilateral 374
  unilateral 375
hyperaldosteronism, primary
  208, 557
hypercalcaemia 304, 344,
  558
hyperemesis gravidarum 308
hyperhidrosis 161
hyperkalaemia 556
hyperkeratosis 150
hyperkinetic circulation 205
hypernatraemia 554
hyperparathyroidism 558,
  562
hyperphoto-sensitivity, plant
  chemical 126, 164
hyperpigmentation 170
hyperprolactinaemia 105,
  406
hypertension 208
  essential 208
  portal 354, 372
  of pregnancy 208
  pulmonary 610
  renal 208
  severe 306
  temporary 208
  vascular 208
hypertensive:
  ophthalmoscopy
    appearance 496
  retinopathy 496
hyperthyroidism 344
hypertonic plasma with
  hypervolaemia or
  hypovolaemia 554
hypertrophic
  cardiomyopathy 188,
  224, 230

hypertrophy, prostatic 400, 401, 422
benign 391
hyperventilation 476
hypervolaemia 555
hypoalbuminaemia 64
hypocalcaemia 560
hypocapnia 255
hypogastrium:
localized tenderness 357
mass 378
hypoglossal (12th cranial) nerve lesion 511
hypoglycaemia 188, 466, 480
hypoglycaemic episode 482
hypogonadism 75, 108
hypokalaemia 344, 557
hypomania 464
hyponatraemia 482, 555
hypoparathyroidism 560
hypopigmentation 172
post-inflammatory 129
hypotension:
idiopathic orthostatic 212
severe 564
sudden severe 480
transient 482
hypothermia 91, 202
severe 256
hypotheses 15
reasoning with 637
hypothyroid 202
goitre 99
hypothyroidism 80, 113, 292, 342, 344, 466, 568, 570
primary 105, 161, 408, 424, 484
hypotonic hyponatraemia 555
hypovolaemia 206, 555
hypoxia 200, 255, 466, 476

I

ichthyosis 152
idiopathic thrombocytopenic purpura 146
ileotibial band syndrome 446
illness:
prolonged systemic 518
severe 75
immobility 218, 220, 342, 344
impetigo 148
bullous 140
impingement syndrome 434
inattention 489
incontinence:
of urine alone 401

of urine and faeces 402
incoordination 523
infection 88, 91, 92, 110, 122
infective:
infiltration 590, 593
space-occupying lesion 529
inflammatory bowel disease 330, 340
information gathering and processing, faulty 23
informed consent 21
infraspinatus tendon 434
insect bite 130, 138
inspection:
alimentary and genitourinary systems 52, 53
respiratory system 51
intermenstrual bleeding 410
internal capsule:
bleed, infarct, or tumour 514
cerebral lesion 490
internuclear ophthalmoplegia 504
interstitial:
fluid 580, 592, 594
lung disease 242, 250, 260, 277, 278, 280
intestinal:
fistula 557
malabsorption 338
tumour, small 295, 298
intracerebral space-occupying lesion 482
intracranial:
haemorrhage 470
pressure, raised 256, 306, 472
intrauterine contraceptive device 408
'intuitive' reasoning 4
explaining 12
intussusception 329, 348
in children or elderly 396
inverse probability circuit rule 620
investigations:
interpretation 42
problem-structuring note 43
iridoplegia, traumatic 502
iritis 86, 88
iron deficiency 75, 161
irritable bowel syndrome 338, 383
ischaemic colitis 396
itchy scalp 154
itchy skin:
with lesions but no wheals 156

with no lesions 161
with wheals 160

J

jaundice 310
diagnostic pathway 19
diagnostic table 18
drug-induced 552
hepatic, due to congenital enzyme defect 310, 313
hepatocellular 310, 314, 548, 550
diagnostic pathway 19
diagnostic table 18
obstructive 310, 316, 548, 552
pre-hepatic, due to haemolysis 310, 312
jaw muscle weakness 507
joint lesion 540
joint, limb, and back symptoms and signs:
back, pain or limitation of movement of:
with sudden onset over seconds to hours originally 438
with onset over days to months originally 440
with onset over years 441
elbow, pain of limitation of movement of 432
foot, pain or limitation of movement of 450
hand, pain or limitation of movement in 430
hip, pain or limitation of movement of 442
knee, pain or limitation of movement of 446
monoarthritis 426
muscle stiffness or pain 424
neck, pain or limitation of movement of 436
polyarthritis 428
shoulder, pain or limitation of movement in 434
jugular:
foramen syndrome 512
vein obstruction 222
venous pressure, raised 222
jumper's knee 446
junctional naevus 126
juvenile plantar dermatosis 150

K

kala-azar 373
Kallman's syndrome 491
keloid 168
keratoacanthoma 134, 168
keratoderma 152
keratosis pilaris 132
kidney:
  calculus 544
  transplanted 377
  tumour 544
Klebsiella pneumonia 582
Klinefelter's syndrome 108
Klumpke's paralysis 522
knee, pain or limitation of
  movement of 446
koilonychia 64
kyphosis 258
kyphotic pain 441

L

L1 posterior root lesion 536
L1/2 root lesion 526
L2/3 posterior root lesion
  536
L2/3 root lesion 526
L3/4 posterior root lesion
  539
L3/4 root lesion 526
L4/5 posterior root lesion
  536
L4/5 root lesion 526
L5/S1 root lesion 526
laboratory tests:
  alkaline phosphatase,
    raised 562
  anaemia:
    macrocytic 568
    microcytic 567
    normocytic 570
  C-reactive protein, very
    high 571
  erythrocyte sedimentation
    rate, very high 571
  glycosuria 547
  haemoglobin, low 566
  hypercalcaemia 558
  hyperkalaemia 556
  hypernatraemia 554
  hypocalcaemia 560
  hypokalaemia 557
  hyponatraemia 555
  jaundice:
    hepatocellular 550
    obstructive 552
  microscopic haematuria 544
  plasma viscosity, very
    high 571
  proteinuria, asymptomatic
    546

serum urea and creatinine,
  raised 564
urine or serum bilirubin,
  raised 548
labyrinthitis, acute viral 308
lactose intolerance 340
large bowel obstruction 302,
  328, 352, 356, 383
laryngeal:
  carcinoma, 252
  oedema 282
  papillomas 282
laryngitis, chronic 252
laryngomalacia, rapidly
  progressive 282
lateral:
  collateral ligament tear 446
  medullary syndrome 512
  popliteal nerve palsy 526
lead poisoning 304, 528
leads, diagnostic see
  diagnostic leads
leg:
  arterial disease 190
  examination 49, 57
  oedema 138
  pain:
    on standing—relieved by
      lying down 191
    on walking—intermittent
      claudication 190
  sensation 57
  swelling:
    bilateral 220
    unilateral 192, 216, 218
  veins, prominent 216
leishmaniasis, visceral 373
lentigines 126, 170
leprosy 134
Leriche's syndrome 190
leukaemia 90, 366
  acute lymphoblastic 120
  acute myeloid 120
  chronic 372
  chronic lymphocytic 120
  chronic myeloid 120, 373
leukaemic joint deposits 426
leukoplakia 411
Lewy body dementia 468
lichen:
  planus 130, 150, 156, 170
  sclerosus 156, 411
  simplex chronicus 150,
    154, 158
lifestyle, change in 342
ligament tears 446
likelihood 617
likelihood ratios 11
  differential 11, 625, 626–7,
    628, 636
  elimination, reasoning
    by 625

overall 625, 627
limb:
  lower:
    disturbed sensation 536
    weakness 57, 526
    see also leg
  upper:
    disturbed sensation
      in 532
    examination 57
    sensation 57
    weakness 57
    see also arm
linear IgA disease 160
linear markings, increased
  594
lipoma 134, 168
livedo reticularis 142
liver:
  abscess 357
  congestion, acute 357
  disease 146, 568
    chronic 161
  failure 115
lobar:
  cancer, invasive 107
  pneumonia 576, 578
lobe, collapsed 576, 579,
  598
  with no consolidation 266
locomotor symptoms 32
loin:
  bruit 384
  localized tenderness 362
longitudinal lines 64
loose bodies 446
lumbar:
  disc prolapse 438
  spinal stenosis 440
lung:
  abscess 66, 244, 248, 582
  carcinoma 244, 250, 558
  cavity 277
  collapse, complete 576
  disease, interstitial 242,
    250, 260, 277, 278, 280
  haemorrhage 590, 593
  single area of dark 598
  symmetrically dark 596
lupus:
  erythematosus, systemic
    69, 70, 142, 162, 164,
    268, 428
  scleritis 86
  vulgaris 134
Lyme disease 144
lymph node:
  inflammation 96, 102, 103,
    104, 386
  pre-auricular 95
  malignancy 96
  metastasis in 103

secondary to gastric or
   lung carcinoma 104
systems enquiry 32
lymphadenopathy:
   axillary 110
   generalized 120
   localized groin 122
lymphangitis carcinomatosis
   594
lymphatic:
   drainage 192, 194, 218, 220
   obstruction 218, 220
lymphoblastic leukaemia,
   acute 104
lymphoma 95, 102, 103,
   104, 120, 161, 366, 372,
   386, 600, 602, 606

M

macular degeneration 498
   age-related 492
macule:
   brown 126
   pale 129
   red 128
malabsorption 338
malaria 300, 312, 373
malignancy 116, 161
   advanced 290
mallet toes 450
Mallory–Weiss tear 346, 392
mammary dysplasia, benign
   fibrous 107
mammillary fistula 106
management 44
   sieves 14, 42
mandibular branch of
   trigeminal nerve lesion
   506
mania 464
manic depression 464
March fracture 450
mastectomy 598
maxillary branch of
   trigeminal nerve lesion
   506
measles 128
mechanical pain 438
Meckel's diverticulum 346,
   348, 392, 396
medial:
   collateral ligament tear 446
   shelf syndrome 446
median:
   nerve lesion 534
   nerve palsy 518
mediastinal:
   emphysema 610
   masses, extrinsic
      compression by 283,
      284

medical diagnostic sieves
   14, 42
Mee's lines 64
melaena 346
   on finger 392
melanoma, malignant 132,
   134, 166, 168
Ménière's disease 308, 478
meningism due to viral
   infection 72
meningitis 306
   bacterial 72, 470
   epilepsy due to 480
   viral 72, 470
meniscal:
   cyst 446
   tears 446
menopause 182, 406
menorrhagia 408
menstruation 544
mesenteric:
   adenitis 300, 329, 363
   artery occlusion 302, 326
   infarction 396
mesothelioma 270, 275, 281
metabolic:
   acidosis 556
   disturbances 344
metastases 586, 588
metastatic:
   carcinoma 368
   cells 242
   lymphadenopathy 600,
      602, 606
metatarsalgia 450
micro-aneurysm, diabetic
   494
micturition syncope 188
middle:
   cerebral artery 530
   ear disease 478
mid-systolic murmur 230
migraine 306, 473, 478, 482
   bilateral 470
milia 130, 168
miliary:
   mottling 586
   tuberculosis 586, 588
Milroy's syndrome 192,
   218, 220
miosis, age-related 503
miscarriage 302
mitral:
   incompetence 232
   stenosis 186, 224, 228, 610
      with pliable valve 228
      with pulmonary
         hypertension 586,
         589
moles:
   flat 126

pigmented 166
molluscum contagiosum 130
monoarthritis 426
mononucleosis, infectious
   92, 120, 314, 320, 364
   clinical opinion 46
   investigations 31
   problem-structuring notes
      30, 37, 39, 41, 43
Morton's metatarsalgia 450
motor:
   branch of trigeminal nerve
      507
   dysphasia 489
   function 57
   neurone 521
      bilateral upper or lower
         80, 540
      brainstem 490
      disease 260, 322, 518,
         520
      hypoglossal (12th cranial)
         nerve lesion 511
      lesion 524
      paresis 523
   neuropathy 539
   response, best 488
mouth lesions 92
Muehrcke's lines 64
multi-infarct dementia 468
multiple sclerosis 212, 260,
   478, 482
   affecting spinal cord 529
mumps:
   parotitis 94
   sialitis 96
murmurs:
   diastolic 228
   mid-systolic 230
   not entirely in systole or
      diastole 233
   pansystolic 232
muscle:
   deconditioning 242
   disease 524
      adjacent 524
      primary 424, 520, 521,
         539
   stiffness or pain 424
   wasting 524
muscular:
   atrophy, progressive 520
   dystrophy 260
musculoskeletal:
   causes of unilateral poor
      chest expansion 262
   injury or inflammation 236
myasthenia gravis 322,
   500, 504
mycosis fungoides 150
myelodysplasia 568
myelofibrosis 373

myeloma 558, 571
myocardial infarction 176, 202
  acute inferior 302
myopathy 500
myxoedema 252

N

nabothian cysts 414
naevi:
  Becker's melanocytic 166
  blue 132
    melanocytic 166
  dysplastic 166
  halo melanocytic 166
  junctional 126
  spider 115
  Splitz melanocytic 166
nail:
  fold infarcts 64, 69
  pitting 64
nasal:
  allergy 491
  polyps 244
necessary criteria 10
neck:
  general examination 49
  lump:
    anterior 98
    moving with swallowing but not with tongue 99
  mass, bilateral 100
  pain or limitation of movement at the 436
  posterior triangle, lump in 103
  stiffness 72
neoplasms 91, 268
nephritis 544, 546
nephrotic syndrome 268, 292, 381, 546
nephrotoxins 564
nervous system:
  examination 54, 56
  full neurological assessment 56
  short CNS examination 54
  symptoms 35
neurological symptoms
  see psychiatric and neurological symptoms and physical signs
neuromuscular disease:
  acute 256
  complicated by respiratory failure 242
neuropathy, autonomic 212
nipple abnormality 106
no fault errors 23
'nodular' shadows 586

nodules 134
non-differential likelihood ratio 11
non-Hodgkin's or Hodgkin's lymphoma 102, 103, 120, 161, 366, 372, 386, 600, 602, 606
non-malignant gastrointestinal diseases 290
non-parotid lesion 95
non-specific abdominal pain 300, 363
  'common cause' 628
  elimination, reasoning by 623, 624
  likelihood ratios 626, 627
  numerical test results, reasoning with 630
  statistical independence versus statistical dependence 629
non-ST elevation myocardial infarction 174
normovolaemia 555
Norwalk virus 332, 336
numerical test results, reasoning with 630
nutrition, poor 122

O

obesity 108, 112, 113, 242, 260, 275, 352
  hypoventilation syndrome 260, 275
obsessive–compulsive disorder 458
obstructive:
  jaundice:
    diagnostic pathway 19
    diagnostic table 18
  sleep apnoea 208
obturator nerve lesion 526
occult malignancy, early manifestation of 424
ocular palsy 504
oculomotor (3rd nerve):
  lesion 500
  paresis 504
odynophagia 320
oedema, congenital 192, 218, 220
oesophageal:
  carcinoma 295, 318, 346, 392
  compression, external 318
  spasm 174
  stricture 295, 318
  tumours 283, 284
  varices 346, 392
oesophagitis 174, 296, 324

oestrogens 115
old age 68
onset, speed of 3, 26
onycholysis 64
onychomedesis 64
opacity, round 582
'open mind' approach 47
ophthalmic branch of trigeminal nerve lesion 506
ophthalmoscopy 56
  appearance:
    abnormal 492
    abnormal in the diabetic 494
    abnormal in the hypertensive 496
optic:
  atrophy, primary 492, 498
  chiasm lesion 499
  nerve swelling or atrophy 492, 497
  tract lesion 499
orbital:
  cellulitis 84, 504
  tumours 84
orchitis, acute 388
orf 130
orthopnoea 180
Osler nodes 69
Osler–Weber–Rendu syndrome 118
osteoarthritis 71, 432, 442, 446
  acromio-clavicular joint 434
  glenohumeral joint 434
osteoarthrosis, primary (post-menopausal) 70
osteochondritis dessicans 446
osteomalacia 542
otitis:
  externa 78, 80
  media 80, 308
ototoxic drugs 478
outline findings 30
ovarian:
  carcinoma 111
  cyst 352, 378, 380
  failure, premature 406
  mass 416
  tumour 74
overall likelihood ratio 625, 627
over-diagnosis 616

P

P map 618, 619
  Aristotle's syllogism 621
  Bayes' rule 621

Paget's disease 106, 562
palpation:
  alimentary and
    genitourinary systems
    52, 53
  respiratory system 51
palpitations 182
pancoast tumour 518
pancreas:
  carcinoma 376
  head of, cancer of 316,
    552
pancreatitis 176, 361, 560
  acute 298, 324
  numerical test results,
    reasoning with 630
pancytopenia 118
panic:
  attacks 476
  disorder 458
pansystolic murmur 232
papules 130
paraproteinaemia 146
parasagittal cerebral
  meningioma 529
parasomnias 484
Parkinson's disease/
  Parkinsonism 80, 212,
  516, 521, 540
paronychia 64
parotid:
  duct obstruction 94
  infection, suppurative 94
  sarcoidosis 94
  Sjögren's syndrome 94
  swelling 94
  tumour 94
parotitis, non-suppurative 94
paroxysmal nocturnal
  dyspnoea 180
past medical history 27, 36
patella:
  subluxation, recurrent 446
  tendinopathy 446
patent ductus arteriosus 233
Paterson–Kelly syndrome
  319
pathology tests see
  laboratory tests
pectus:
  carinatum 258
  excavatum 258
pellagra 158, 164, 170
pelvic:
  endometriosis 328
  examination 416
  floor muscles, weakness
    401
  girdle muscle weakness
    540
  inflammatory disease 300,
    328, 350, 357

chronic 408
pemphigoid 140, 170
  gestationis 140
pemphigus 138, 164
peptic ulcer 298
percussion:
  alimentary and
    genitourinary systems
    52
  dull to, but not stony
    dull 270
  hyper-resonant 272
  respiratory system 51
  stony dull 268
perianal:
  abscess 351, 390
  haematoma, spontaneous
    390
pericardial effusion 222, 610
pericarditis 236, 268
  constrictive 222, 226
  with pericardial friction
    rub 233
peripheral:
  neuropathy 532, 536, 540
  retinal damage 492
peritoneal dialysis 268
peritonitis 356, 357, 382
  chlamydia 357
peroneal nerve lesion,
  common 526
Perthes' disease 442
pes:
  cavus 450
  planus 450
petechiae 146
Peutz–Jegher's syndrome 92,
  126, 166
phaeochromocytoma 182,
  208, 304, 458
pharyngeal:
  movement, abnormal 511
  pouch 102, 296, 319
  tumours
pharyngitis:
  investigations 31
  problem-structuring notes
    30, 37, 39, 41
  viral 92, 320
pharynx, red 93
phenylketonuria 172
phobia:
  simple 458
  social 458
photosensitive rash 164
physical examination:
  interpretation 40
  'routine' 48–9
pigmented creases and
  flexures 114
pinna haematoma 76
pituitary tumour 512

pityriasis:
  alba 129
  lichenoides chronica 132
  rosea 150
  versicolor 129, 150
plan 26, 27
plant chemical
  hyperphotosensitivity
  126, 164
plantar fasciitis 450
plaques 150
plasma viscosity, very high
  571
platelet dysfunction 118
pleural:
  effusion 262, 266, 275,
    576, 580
  contralateral 264
  rub 281
  thickening, severe 270,
    275, 281
pleurisy due to pneumonia
  236, 281
Plummer–Vincent syndrome
  319
pneumoconiosis 586
Pneumocystis carinii
  pneumonia 604
pneumonectomy 576, 581
pneumonia 244, 248, 300
  with pleurisy 236, 281
  'rounded' 582
pneumothorax:
  chest pain 174, 236
  contralateral tension 264
  hyper-resonant percussion
    272
  ipsilateral 264
  reduced breath sounds 275
  reduced tactile vocal
    fremitus 266
  single area of dark lung
    598, 599
  sudden breathlessness
    178, 238
  tension 598
  unilateral poor chest
    expansion 262
poliomyelitis 441
polyarteritis nodosa 134
polyarthritis 428
polycystic:
  ovary syndrome 74, 111,
    292, 406
  renal disease 374
polymorphic light eruptions
  158, 164
polymyalgia rheumatica 424
polymyositis 542
polyps, cervical or
  intrauterine 410
pompholyx 138, 158

pontine:
  haemorrhage 503
  stroke 474
popliteal nerve palsy, lateral 540
Popper, Karl 15, 637
porphyria 140, 528
  acute intermittent 304
post-coital bleeding 410
post-cricoid web 319
post-ictal state 466
post-nasal drip 250
post-thrombotic syndrome 218
post-traumatic stress disorder 458
post-viral fatigue 484
posterior:
  carotid artery aneurysm 512
  cruciate ligament tears 446
  fossa tumour 72, 478
  root lesion 533, 534, 536
  triangle of neck, lump in 103
postural hypotension 29, 188, 476
  syncope:
    clinical opinion 46
    problem-structuring notes 30, 37, 39, 41, 43
posture, neck pain due to 436
potassium 556
pre-auricular:
  lymph node inflammation 95
  sinus, infected 76
'pre-hepatic' jaundice due to haemolysis:
  diagnostic table 18
  diagnostic pathway 19
pre-renal failure 564
pregnancy:
  abdominal striae 112
  anaemia of 570
  ectopic 302, 328, 363, 416
  galactorrhoea 105
  hypertension 208
  jaundice 316, 552
  recent 75
  secondary amenorrhoea 406
  spider naevi 115
  tender or bulky mass 416
  vomiting 308
  weight gain 292
pregnant uterus 378, 380
premenstrual fluid retention 292
presenting complaint:

case presentations 45
history 27
history taking, thoughtful 26
plan for writing out the history 27
systems enquiry 32
pressure sores 122
prickly heat 132
probabilities:
  audits 637
  grappling with 617
  picturing 618
  syllogism 620
problem-structuring notes:
  case presentations 45
  history taking 30, 37, 39, 41, 43
  investigations, interpreting the 43
  'open mind' approach 47
  physical examination, interpreting the 42
proctalgia fugax 351
proctitis 350, 351
prolactinoma 105
proportions 617
  syllogism 620
proprioception, loss of 523
proptosis 84
prostate enlargement 391, 422
prostatic:
  carcinoma 391, 422, 571
  hypertrophy 400, 401, 422
    benign 391
prostatitis 391, 422
  referred pain 351
protein load, high 564
proteinuria:
  asymptomatic 546
  orthostatic 546
  postural 546
pseudo-acanthosis nigricans 126
pseudobulbar palsy 322
pseudo-fit 480
pseudogout 426
pseudohyponatraemia 555
pseudohypoparathyroidism 560
pseudomonas infection 148
pseudoxanthoma elasticum 132
psoas sheath, cold abscess 386
psoriasis 150, 154, 156, 426, 428, 430
  generalized pustular 148
  guttate 130, 150
  localized pustular 148
psoriatic arthropathy 70

psychiatric and neurological symptoms and physical signs 455
  activities of daily living, inability to carry out the 456
  anxiety, acute 458
  arm:
    dermatome, diminished sensation in 533
    and hand at rest, odd posture of 514
    hemiparesis 530
    and shoulder, wasting of 520
    tone, abnormalities of 521
    weakness around without pain 522
  chair, difficulty rising from 542
  cognitive impairment 468
  confusion:
    acute 466
    chronic 468
  consciousness, disturbed 487
  cranial nerve lesions, multiple 512
  delusions 464
  depression 462
  diabetic, ophthalmoscopy appearance in 494
  dizziness 476
  dysarthria 490
  eye opening 488
  facial:
    muscle weakness 508
    sensation, loss of 506
  fatigue—'tired all the time' 484
  'fit' 480
  foot movements, bilateral weakness of all 528
  gait abnormality 540
  hand:
    coarse tremor 516
    diminished sensation in 534
    fine tremor 515
    wasting of small muscles 518
  headache:
    acute, new onset 470
    chronic and recurrent 473
    subacute onset 472
  hearing loss 510
  hemiparesis 530
  hypertensive, ophthalmoscopy appearance in 496

incoordination 523
jaw muscle weakness 507
leg hemiparesis 530
limb:
  lower, disturbed
    sensation in 536
  lower, weakness around
    526
  upper, disturbed
    sensation in 532
motor response, best 488
muscle wasting 524
nervous system
  examination 486
neurological deficit,
  transient 482
ophthalmoscopy
  appearance, abnormal
  492
ptosis 500
pupil:
  large (mydriatic), with no
    ptosis 502
  small (miotic), with no
    ptosis 503
reflexes:
  brisk 538
  diminished 539
shoulder, weakness around
  without pain 522
smell, absent sense of
  491
spastic paraparesis 529
speech disturbance 489
squatting position, difficulty
  rising from 542
squint and diplopia: ocular
  palsy 504
stroke 474
tongue, uvula, and
  pharyngeal movement,
  abnormal 511
verbal response, best 487
vertigo 478
visual, central and acuity,
  loss of 497
visual field defect,
  peripheral 499
visual loss, gradual onset
  of 498
psychiatric illness 290
psychiatric symptoms 35
psychogenic field defect
  499
psychological causes,
  transient neurological
  deficit 482
psychosomatic cause,
  recurrent abdominal pain
  in children 330
ptosis 500
  congenital 500

pulmonary
  arterio-venous
    malformation 244, 582
  artery, prominent 600
  embolus 174, 178, 188,
    200, 236, 238, 244,
    268, 281, 576, 580
    large 598
  fibrosis 242, 260, 277, 278,
    280, 594, 595
    dense 576, 580
  haemosiderosis 586, 589
  high flow 230
  hypertension 242
  infarction 174, 178,
    188, 200, 236, 238,
    244, 268, 281, 576,
    580
  metastasis 582
  oedema 180, 270, 278,
    286, 580, 590, 592
    acute 186
    reactive, with acute
      urinary retention
      180
  stenosis 230
pulse see under
  cardiovascular symptoms
  and physical signs
pupil:
  large (mydriatic) with no
    ptosis 502
  small (miotic) with no
    ptosis 503
purgative abuse 557
purpura 118, 146
  senile 146
pustules 148
pyelonephritis 300, 327,
  360, 362
pyloric stenosis 557
pyoderma gangrenosum
  162
pyogenic:
  granuloma 134, 168
  spinal infection 440
pyometra 416
pyramidal tract lesion:
  contralateral 538, 540
  high level 538

Q

quadrant:
  lower:
    localized tenderness
      363
    mass 377, 379
  upper:
    localized tenderness
      360
    masses 375

R

racial skin sensitivity 111
radial nerve lesion 514,
  522, 534
radiology:
  abnormal appearance 575
  cardiac silhouette 606
  hilar shadowing—
    homogeneous 600
  hilar shadowing—streaky
    604
  diffuse poorly defined hazy
    opacification 590
  general approach 574
  linear markings, increased
    594
  lungs:
    opacification, with
      well-defined border
      576
    single area of dark 598
    symmetrically dark 596
  mediastinal widening,
    upper 606
  'nodular' shadows,
    multiple, and 'miliary
    mottling' 586
  opacity, round 582
Ramsay Hunt syndrome
  478, 508
ranula 96
rash, photosensitive 164
Raynaud's phenomenon
  197
rectal:
  area, fresh blood in 348,
    396
  carcinoma 396
  inflammation 350
  prolapse 390
  tumour 342, 350
rectocoele 413
reflexes:
  brisk 538
  diminished 539
  examination 57
Reiter's disease 426, 428
renal:
  artery stenosis 384
  calculi 302, 327, 362, 403
  carcinoma 375
  cyst 375
  failure 146, 556
    chronic 161, 308, 560,
      564, 570
    obstructive 564
  glycosuria 547
  tubular defect 557
  tumour 404
replication, probability
  of 636

respiratory:
effort, poor 274
rate low 256
symptoms and physical
signs:
blood gas disturbance
255
breath sounds, reduced
274
breathing, bronchial 277
breathlessness, acute 240
breathlessness, chronic
242
breathlessness, sudden
238
chest expansion, bilateral
poor 260
chest expansion,
unilateral poor 262
chest pain 236
chest wall abnormalities
258
cough, persistent dry,
with no sputum 250
cough, with sputum 248
crackles, coarse 280
crackles, fine inspiratory
278
frank haemoptysis 244
hoarseness 252
percussion, dull, but not
stony dull 270
percussion,
hyper-resonant 272
percussion, stony dull
268
pleural rub 281
respiratory rate low 256
stridor and inspiratory
wheeze 282
systems enquiry 33
tactile vocal fremitus,
increased 266
tactile vocal fremitus,
reduced 266
trachea displaced 264
wheeze, expiratory
monophonic 284
wheeze, inspiratory
monophonic 283
wheeze, inspiratory ±
stridor 282
wheeze, polyphonic,
high-pitched 286
system 51
examination 254
reticulosis 110
retinal:
artery occlusion 492, 497
bleeding 494
haemorrhage and
detachment 494

vein occlusion 492, 494,
497
retinitis pigmentosa 492, 499
retroperitoneal
haemorrhage 355
rhabdomyolysis 560
rheumatic fever 428
rheumatoid:
arthritis 70, 424, 426, 428,
430, 434
scleritis 86
with vasculitis 162
nodules 71, 134, 582
symptoms 268
ribs, fractured 262
right-to-left cardiac shunt
198
right-to-left pulmonary
shunt 198
root lesion 522
rosacea 142, 148
rotator cuff tears 434
rotavirus 332, 336
'routine' physical
examination 48–9
rubella 128
ruling diagnoses in and
out 10
ruptured abdominal aortic
aneurysm 355, 361, 362

S

S1/2 posterior root lesion
539
S1/2 root lesion 526
salivary:
duct obstruction 96
infection, suppurative 96
sarcoidosis 96
Sjögren's syndrome 96
tumour 96
Salmonella typhimurium 332
salpingitis 327
acute 416
chronic 416
saphena varix 386
sarcoidosis 558
generalized
lymphadenopathy 120
hilar mass 600, 603
hypercalcaemia 558
iritis 88
multiple nodular shadows
and miliary mottling
586, 589
parotid 94
salivary 96
scabies 130, 156
scales 150
scalp, itchy 154
schizophrenia, acute 464

sciatic nerve lesion 526
scleritis 86
scleroderma 322
sclerosing cholangitis 316, 552
scoliosis 258, 264
idiopathic, of thoracic or
lumbar spine 441
scoliotic pain 441
scrotal swelling 388
seasonal affective disorder
462
sebaceous cyst 95
self-confidence 455
seminoma 388
sensation 57
sensitivity 6, 11, 625
sensorineural (8th cranial):
lesion 510
nerve conduction defect
510
sensory:
dysphasia 489
neuropathy 539
septicaemia 197, 466
meningococcal 146
septicaemic haemolysis 312
serum:
bilirubin, raised 548
urea, raised 564
Shigella (bacillary) *dysenteriae*
335
shingles 236
shoulder:
frozen 434
general examination 49
pain or limitation of
movement at the 434
wasting 520
weakness without pain 522
sialitis, non-suppurative 96
Sicca syndrome 292
sieves, medical and surgical
14, 42
sigmoid volvulus 383
singer's nodes 252
sinoatrial disease 202
sinus tachycardia 182
sinusitis 470
Sjögren's syndrome 428
parotid 94
salivary 96
skin:
friction 138
melanoma 95
symptoms and physical
signs:
blisters 138
diagnosis in dermatology
124
erythema 142
hyperkeratosis, scales,
and plaques 150

hyperpigmentation 170
hypopigmentation 172
itchy scalp 154
itchy skin, with no wheals
    but no wheals 156
itchy skin, with no lesions
    161
itchy skin, with wheals
    160
macules, brown 126
macules, pale 129
macules, red 128
moles, pigmented 166
nodules 134
papules 130
petechiae 146
photosensitive rash 164
purpura 146
pustules 148
scalp, itchy 154
tumour on the skin 168
ulceration 162
systems enquiry 32
tags 130
skull fracture 491
sleep:
    apnoea syndrome 484
    poor habit 484
small bowel:
    infarction 361
    obstruction 326, 352,
        356, 383
    numerical test results,
        reasoning with 630
smell, absent sense of 491
smoking 250
social:
    history 27, 38
    phobia 458
soft tissue injury or fracture
    430, 432, 434, 442, 450
solar:
    keratosis 150
    lentigines 126
somatization:
    disorder 458
    'functional cause' 540
space-occupying lesion,
    infective 529
spastic paresis 529
specificity 11, 625
speech 487
    disturbance 489
speed of onset 3, 26
spermatocoele 388
spider naevi 115
spinal:
    claudication 190
    cord injuries/disease 210
    lesion 344
    stenosis, lumbar 440
    tuberculosis 440

tumours 440
spinothalamic tract damage
    532, 536
spironolactone 108
splenic:
    infarct 360
    rupture 352, 355, 360
splenomegaly see under
    gastrointestinal
    symptoms and physical
    signs
splinter haemorrhages 64
Splitz melanocytic naevus
    166
spondylitic bone formation
    compressing spinal
    cord 529
spondylolisthesis 438
sputum:
    cough with 248
    pink frothy 186
    streaking 244
squamous cell carcinoma
    134, 162, 168
squatting position, difficulty
    in rising from 542
squint 504
ST elevated myocardial
    infarction 174
staphylococcal infection 162
Staphylococcus aureus 332
statistical independence
    versus statistical
    dependence 629
stenosing tenosynovitis 430
stenosis after ventilation 283
steroids:
    inhaled 252
    therapy 292
Stevens–Johnson syndrome
    140
Stokes–Adams attack 188
stomach, carcinoma of
    cardia of 318
strangulated hernia 386
stratified medicine 622, 623,
    633, 634
stridor 282
stroke 474
    haemorrhagic 306
subacute cutaneous lupus
    erythematosus 164
subarachnoid haemorrhage
    72, 470
    from berry aneurysm 474
subclavian:
    cavity aneurysm 104
    steal syndrome 214
subconjunctival
    haemorrhage 86
subcutaneous abscess 95
subdural haemorrhage 474

submandibular:
    lump—not moving
        with tongue nor on
        swallowing 96
    lymph node:
        inflammation 96
        malignancy 96
submental dermoid 96
subscapularis tendon 434
subtalar joint, arthritis 450
suggestive evidence see
    evidence: that suggests a
    diagnosis
sunburn 142
supraclavicular lump(s) 104
suprapubic region 378
    localized tenderness 357
    mass 378
supraspinatus:
    inflammation and
        calcification, chronic
        434
    tendon 434
supraventricular:
    bigemini 202
    tachycardia runs 182
surgical diagnostic sieves
    14, 42
swimmer's ear 78
sycosis barbae 148
sympathomimetic drugs 515
syncope 29, 188
syndrome of inappropriate
    ADH section 555
synovitis, transient 442
syphilis 162
    secondary 134, 152
syringomyelia 441, 518, 532
systemic lupus
    erythematosus 69, 70,
        142, 162, 164, 268, 428
    scleritis 86
systems enquiry 32

T

T1 lesion 518
    anterior 514
    posterior 533
T2 posterior root lesion
    533
tactile vocal fremitus 51
    increased 267
    reduced 266
Takayasu's syndrome 214
tardive dyskinesias 511
teeth, carious 92
temporal/giant cell arteritis
    472, 497
temporal lobe epilepsy 478
temporomandibular joint
    dysfunction 78

tenderness, localized:
  in epigastrium or central
    abdomen 361
  in hypogastrium 357
  in left or right loin 362
  in left or right lower
    quadrant 363
  in left upper quadrant 360
  in right upper quadrant
    358
tendonitis 434
tenesmus 350
tennis elbow 432
tenoperiostitis 432
tension:
  headache 470, 473
  pneumothorax 598
teratoma 388, 606
Terry's lines 64, 68
testicular:
  torsion 388
  tumours 108
testis, immature 108
thalassaemia 567
theories 15
thiamine deficiency 466
thiazide diuretics 558
thinness 116
thoracic:
  inlet syndrome 214
  nerve root lesion 532
thoracoplasty, previous 262
throat, sore 31, 320
thrombocytopenia 118, 146
thrombo-emboli, chronic 242
thrombophlebitis 216
thrombosis 214, 215
  bilateral 194
  see also deep vein
    thrombosis
thrombus 91
thrush 411, 420
thymoma 606, 608
thyroglossal cyst 98
thyroid:
  adenoma 101
  carcinoma 101
  cyst 101
  enzyme deficiency 100
  nodule 101
thyrotoxic goitre 99
thyrotoxicosis:
  anxiety 458
  breathlessness, chronic
  brisk reflexes 538
  clinical opinion 46
  confusion, acute 466
  fine tremor of hands 515
  hypercalcaemia 558
  palpitations 182
  problem-structuring notes
    30, 37, 39, 41, 43

pulse rate 200
recurrent diarrhoea 338
rising from chair or
  squatting position,
  difficulty in 542
secondary amenorrhoea
  406
severe weight loss 290
striking facial appearance
  80
thin, wasted, cachectic 116
tibial nerve lesion 526
Tietze's syndrome 174, 236
tissue necrosis 91
Todd's paralysis 482
tongue, abnormal 511
tonsillitis:
  acute follicular 92, 320
  clinical opinion 46
  investigations 31
  problem-structuring notes
    30, 37, 39, 41, 43
  writing the diagnosis and
    management 44
tonsils 93
torticollis:
  infantile 436
  spasmodic 436
toxic:
  epidermal necrolysis 140
  shock syndrome 300
toxins 332
trachea displaced 264
tracheal:
  blunt trauma 283, 284
  tumours 283, 284
transient:
  ischaemic attack 482
  neurological deficit 482
'transparent' reasoning 4, 5
transudates 268
trauma 146, 348, 396, 403
  old 432
  surgical 88
traumatic ulceration 92
treatment indication, studies
  to establish 635
triangle, anterior, lump
  in 102
Trichomonas vaginitis 420
tricuspid:
  incompetence 232
  regurgitation 222, 364
trigeminal nerve 506, 507
trigger finger 430
trigger toe 450
triggering, faulty 22
trochlear (4th cranial nerve)
  paresis 504
trunk 49
trypanosomiasis 192, 218,
  220

tuberculosis 116, 144, 268
  endometrial 416
  granuloma 582, 584
  miliary 586, 588
  primary, with hilar node 600
  pulmonary 244, 250, 290
  spinal 440
tuberous sclerosis 132
tubular necrosis, acute 564
tumour:
  compressing nerve root
    518
  ocular palsy 504
  primary 110
  on skin 168

U

ulceration 296
  skin 162
  traumatic 92
ulcerative:
  colitis:
    acute lower central
      abdominal pain 328
    clubbing 66
    iritis 88
    passage of blood rectally
      348, 396
    polyarthritis 428
    recurrent diarrhoea 334
  keratitis 86
ulnar nerve lesion 514,
  518, 534
umbilical area 376
under-diagnosis 616, 635
unilateral mass in upper
  quadrant 375
unipolar disorder 464
upper gastrointestinal bleed,
  massive 396
upper lobe fibrosis 264
upper mediastinal widening
  606
upper respiratory tract
  infection 244, 466
ureteric:
  calculus 327
  tumour 404
urethral:
  calculi 400
  carbuncle 412
  trauma, recent 544
urethrocoele 413
urinary frequency 400
urinary incontinence:
  alone 401
  with faecal incontinence
    402
urinary tract infection:
  abdominal pain in children
    329

confusion, acute 466
incontinence 401
laboratory tests 544, 546
painful haematuria 403
painless haematuria 404
recurrent 330
urinary frequency 400
vomiting with abdominal
  pain and fever 300
urine:
  acute retention with reactive
    pulmonary oedema 180
  raised 548
  tests 59
urological and gynaecological
  symptoms and physical
  signs:
  amenorrhoea, secondary
    406
  cervix, ulcers and lumps in
    the 414
  haematuria:
    painful 403
    painless 404
  incontinence:
    of urine alone (not
      faeces) 401
    of urine and faeces 402
  intermenstrual or
    post-coital bleeding 410
  menstrual loss, excessive—
    menorrhagia 408
  pelvic exam, tender or
    bulky mass on 416
  prostate, enlargement of
    the 422
  urinary frequency ±
    dysuria 400
  vagina, lumps in the 413
  vaginal discharge 420
  vulval:
    skin abnormalities 411
    ulcers and lumps of
      the 412
urticaria:
  acute 160
  chronic idiopathic 160
  physical 160
  solar 164
uterine:
  fibroid 378
  leiomyomata 416
  neoplasm 378
  prolapse 400, 401, 413
uterus, pregnant 378, 380
uveitis, anterior 86, 88
uvula, abnormal 511

V

vaginal:
  carcinoma 413

discharge 420
lumps 413
secretion, excessive
  normal 420
thrush 420
vaginitis 420
vaginosis, bacterial 420
vagus (10th cranial) nerve
  lesion 511
variant Creutzfeldt–Jakob
  disease 468
varicocoele 388
varicose veins 191, 216
  bilateral 220
  unilateral 218
vascular dementia 468
vascular tone, loss of 210,
  212
vasculitic nodules on
  fingers 69
vasculitis 146
vasculopathy:
  acquired 118
  congenital 118
vasovagal attack 188
vena cava obstruction:
  inferior 194, 354
  superior 268, 354
Venn diagrams 618, 619
venous:
  disease, peripheral 191
  insufficiency 218
    chronic 218
  irregularity 494
  pressure, raised 146
  return:
    examination 50
    in the legs 50
    poor 194
ventricle, left: large 224
ventricular:
  aneurysm 224
    left 610, 612–13
  bigemini 202
  dysfunction 242
  ectopics 182, 204
  failure:
    left 184, 240, 268, 604,
      610, 612
    right 194
  hypertrophy:
    left 224
    right 224
  septal defect 232
verification, faulty 22
vertebra, collapsed 529
vertebral displacement or
  fracture, traumatic 529
vertebrobasilar insufficiency
  478
vertigo 478
vestibular neuronitis 478

Vibrio cholera 336
Vibrio para haemolyticus 332
villous adenoma of rectum
  557
viral infection:
  conjunctivitis 86
  recurrent 330
  with slow recovery 250
viruses 428
vision, central, loss of 497
visual:
  cortex lesion 499
  field defect, peripheral 499
  loss, gradual onset of 498
vitamin:
  A intoxication 304
  B12 deficiency 568
  C deficiency 146
  D:
    deficiency 560, 562
    excess 558
  deficiency 92
  K deficiency 146
vitiligo 129, 172
vitreous haemorrhage
  494, 497
vocal cord:
  paralysis, acute bilateral
    283, 284
  paresis 252
Volkmann's ischaemic
  contracture 430
vomiting 294, 557
  see also under
    gastrointestinal
    symptoms and physical
    signs
Von Willebrand's disease
  118, 146
vulval:
  carcinoma 411
  skin abnormalities 411
  ulcers and lumps 412
  warts 412

W

warts 134
  early seborrhoeic 130
  seborrhoeic 166, 168
  viral 130
wasted body 116
wax 76
Weber's syndrome 512
Wegener's granuloma 162,
  244, 582, 585
weight gain 292
weight loss 290
Wenkenbach heart block
  204
Wernicke's area, lesion
  in 489

Wernicke's encephalopathy
  478
wheeze 184
  breathlessness, acute 240
  expiratory monophonic 284
  inspiratory 282
    monophonic 283
  polyphonic, high-pitched
    286
  viral 286

whiplash 436
whiteness with a
  well-defined border 576
whitlow, herpetic 138
whole patient 20
writing out:
  the diagnosis and
    management 44
  the history 26
    plan 27

X

X-rays see radiology
xanthomata 130, 134
xanthomatosis 71
xerostomia 319

Y

'yellow' nails 64